HEALTH ASSESSMENT IN NURSING

Michele McCarthy

ALLIED HEALTH PRESS

Health Assessment in Nursing

Author: **Michele McCarthy**

Allied Health Press
4164 Lakeshore Road
Burlington ON L7L 1A4
Canada
www.alliedhealthpress.com
Email: orders@arclereducation.com

ISBN: 978-1-77956-822-9

ABOUT THE AUTHOR

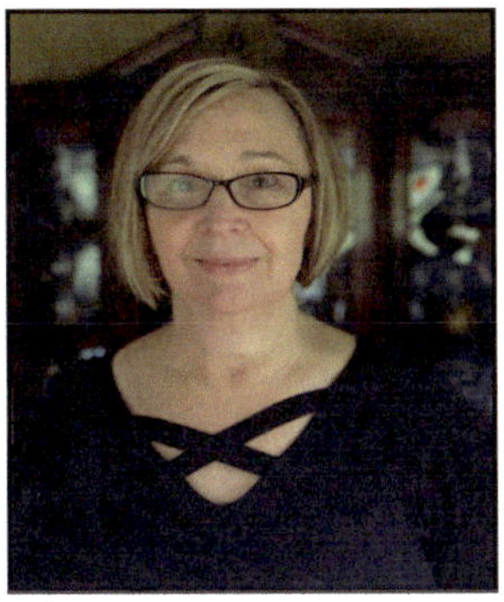

Michele is a registered nurse with over 25 years of clinical experience and a decade of service as a nurse educator. She holds national certifications as a Certified Nurse Educator (CNE) and Certified Healthcare Simulation Educator (CHSE), reflecting her commitment to excellence in teaching and experiential learning. Michele is passionate about advancing nursing education through learner-centered design, curriculum innovation, and the integration of simulation-based strategies.

Brief Table of Contents

1. Foundations of Health Assessment in Nursing	1
2. Interviewing and Communication Techniques in Health Assessment	37
3. Health History Taking	73
4. Techniques of Physical Examination	107
5. General Health Survey and Vital Signs in Nursing	141
6. Skin, Hair, and Nails Assessment in Nursing	175
7. Head, Face, Neck, and Lymphatics Assessment in Nursing	211
8. Eye Assessment in Nursing	245
9. Ear, Nose, Mouth, and Throat (ENT) Assessment in Nursing	279
10. Thorax and Lungs Assessment in Nursing	313
11. Cardiovascular System Assessment in Nursing	347
12. Abdominal Assessment in Nursing	381
13. Musculoskeletal System Assessment in Nursing	415
14. Neurological System Assessment in Nursing	453
15. Breast and Axillae Assessment in Nursing	487
Index	521

Assessment

includes material designed to review and reinforce each content. It includes Critical Thinking
o help test of your understanding of information presented in the chapter and Short answer
o review your understanding of the key concepts presented in the chapter.

Critical Thinking Questions

1. **Who is known as the "Father of Modern Biology"?**
   a. Aristotle
   b. Charles Darwin
   c. Gregor Mendel
   d. Louis Pasteur
2. **What is the basic unit of life?**
   a. Atom
   b. Molecule
   c. Cell
   d. Organism
3. **Which branch of biology studies the interaction of organisms with their environment?**
   a. Genetics
   b. Ecology
   c. Physiology
   d. Botany
4. **Which macromolecule is the main source of energy for living organisms?**
   a. Proteins
   b. Lipids
   c. Carbohydrates
   d. Nucleic acids
5. **DNA is primarily responsible for which function in living organisms?**
   a. Energy production
   b. Protein synthesis
   c. Storing genetic information
   d. Regulating body temperature

Short Answer Questions

1. What is biology, and why is it important to study biology?
2. What are the three main domains of life, and how are they different from one another?
3. Define homeostasis and give an example of how it works in living organisms.
4. What is the cell theory, and why is it fundamental to biology?
5. How do autotrophs and heterotrophs differ in the way they obtain energy?
6. What is the scientific method, and how is it applied in biological research?
7. Discuss how biology helps address global challenges such as climate change, disease, and food security.
8. Explain the levels of biological organization from the smallest unit to the largest. Provide examples at each level.
9. Describe the relationship between structure and function in biology, giving specific examples from cells or organs.
10. How has the discovery of genetics shaped our understanding of inheritance and variation among organisms?

ary Materials

A list of key terms is given for quick reference

KEY TERMS FROM THIS CHAPTER

Annotation enrichment analysis	Biological structure	Cell
Cell theory	Cellular structure	Ecology
Ecosystems	Genetics	Human biology
Microbiology	Natural selection	Organism
Plant biology		

urces: Recommendations for additional readings, websites, and multimedia resources.

References

1. Argelaguet, R., Velten, B., Arnol, D., Dietrich, S., Zenz, T., Marioni, J. C., Buettner, F., et al. (2018). Multi-omics factor analysis—A framework for unsupervised integration of multi-omics data sets. *Molecular Systems Biology, 14*. https://doi.org/10.15252/msb.20178124.
2. Bacher, S., Blackburn, T. M., Essl, F., & Genovesi, P. (2017). *Socio-Economic Impact Classification of Alien Taxa (SEICAT)*. https://core.ac.uk/download/286567949.pdf (accessed on 8th March 2025).
3. Barnett, R., Brace, S., Cucchi, T., & Dobney, K. (2013). *Divergent Evolutionary Processes Associated with Colonization of Offshore Islands*. https://core.ac.uk/download/20664364.pdf (accessed on 8th March 2025).

Getting Started

Chapter Openers

A list of Chapter Outline is presented providing a brief Introduction to what will be covered in the chapter.

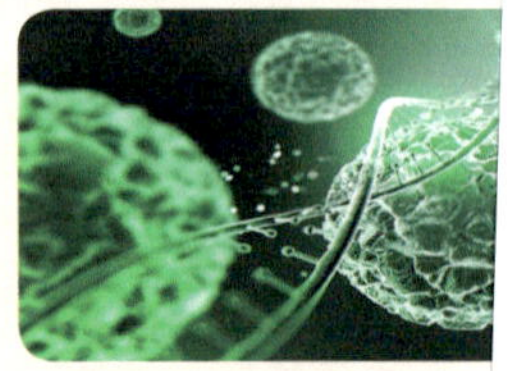

Introduction

Often referred to as the science of life, biolo
of study aimed at comprehending the sev
on Earth, from tiny creatures to sophistic
entities. Comprising several subfields, inc
biology, ecology, and evolutionary biolog
advances our knowledge of living systems,
the mechanisms controlling life events, inclu
reproduction, and interaction with the su
is the central goal of biology. Moreover, b
void between the natural sciences and med
necessary understanding of health, illness, a
between organisms and their environments. I
global issues such as climate change, biodive
diseases depends on an awareness of these
interactions, therefore highlighting the cr
plays in modern civilization. Fundamentall
and tests ideas about the living world u
method. Through methodical observation ar

1.1. The Scientific Method in Biology

Learning Outcome

1. Describe the steps of the scientific method;
2. Focus on hypothesis formation;
3. Learn about experimental design.

Learning Outcomes

The beginning of each section of every chapt
Outcomes that inform students of concepts th
outcomes help students understand what they
have mastered the material in that section.

Test Your Knowledge

Throughout each chapter, Test Your Knowledge cues you to note which topics have been covered and to self-test your understanding of the material presented.

Test Your Knowledge

1. Explain why correlation does not imply causati
2. How does the scientific method help reduce th

Chapter Summary

The Summary Section appear at the end of each chapter and summarize main concepts covered throughout the chapter. These points provide key concepts in an engaging and meaningful way.

Summary

The investigation of biological principles h
reflecting the intricate interactions that o
beyond individual species or systems, as
mold ecosystems and affect biodiversity. F
data using sophisticated technologies lik
mechanisms underlying these interaction
for example, the integration of diverse on
pathways and helps identify important b
and disease (Chong et al., 2018). Additi
component of biological research and a
into unfamiliar habitats has significant
strategies. Examining the origins and e
become a crucial field that highlights the
interactions. As interest in biological i
conventional ecological theories and pra
scientific viewpoints is shown by this
species shape ecosystems and advances
When taken as a whole, these discover
value of multidisciplinary biology resear
technological breakthroughs to improve
crucial as we look to the future of biolo
of the complexities of life, this metho
issues. Future studies can ensure the c
changing by acknowledging the interc
creative solutions that support sustain
thorough comprehension of life that se
investigation and integration of scienti

Knowledg

The chapte
Questions
Questions

Supplemen

Key Terms:

Further Res

Detailed Table of Contents

List of Figures *xvii*
Preface *xxv*

CHAPTER 1

Foundations of Health Assessment in Nursing 1

Introduction **1**
1.1. Historical Context of Health Assessment **5**
1.1.1. Evolution of Nursing Assessments 6
1.1.2. Key Figures in Health Assessment History 7
1.1.3. Impact of Historical Practices on Modern Nursing 8
1.2. Components of Health Assessment **10**
1.2.1. Subjective Data Collection 11
1.2.2. Objective Data Collection 12
1.2.3. Documentation and Reporting 13
1.3. Techniques of Health Assessment **14**
1.3.1. Inspection and Observation 15
1.3.2. Palpation and Percussion 16
1.3.3. Auscultation and Vital Signs 17
1.4. Cultural Considerations in Health Assessment **18**
1.4.1. Understanding Cultural Competence 19
1.4.2. Impact of Culture on Health Beliefs 20
1.4.3. Strategies for Culturally Sensitive Assessments 21
1.5. Technology in Health Assessment **22**
1.5.1. Electronic Health Records (EHR) 23
1.5.2. Telehealth and Remote Assessments 24
1.5.3. Use of Diagnostic Tools and Equipment 25
1.6. Challenges in Health Assessment **26**
1.6.1. Barriers to Effective Assessment 26
1.6.2. Ethical Considerations in Assessment 27
1.6.3. Addressing Biases and Assumptions 28
Summary **29**
References **32**

CHAPTER 2

Interviewing and Communication Techniques in Health Assessment 37

Introduction **37**
2.1. The Role of the Interview in Health Assessment **41**
2.1.1. Establishing Rapport with Patients 42
2.1.2. Gathering Comprehensive Health Histories 43
2.1.3. Identifying Patient Concerns and Symptoms 44
2.2. Types of Interviewing Techniques **45**
2.2.1. Open-Ended Questions 46
2.2.2. Closed-Ended Questions 47
2.2.3. Probing Questions 47
2.3. Nonverbal Communication in Health Assessment **48**
2.3.1. Importance of Body Language 49
2.3.2. Eye Contact and Its Implications 50
2.3.3. Active Listening Skills 51
2.4. Cultural Competence in Health Communication **52**

2.4.1. Understanding Cultural Differences 53
2.4.2. Adapting Communication Styles 54
2.4.3. Overcoming Language Barriers 54
2.5. Ethical Considerations in Health Interviews 56
2.5.1. Informed Consent 57
2.5.2. Confidentiality and Privacy 57
2.5.3. Professional Boundaries 59
2.6. Challenges in Health Assessment Interviews 60
2.6.1. Dealing with Difficult Patients 60
2.6.2. Managing Time Constraints 61
2.6.3. Addressing Sensitive Topics 62
Summary 64
References 67

CHAPTER 3

Health History Taking 73

Introduction 73
3.1. Purpose of Health History Taking 76
3.1.1. Establishing a Patient-Provider Relationship 77
3.1.2. Identifying Health Risks and Concerns 78
3.1.3. Guiding Diagnosis and Treatment Plans 79
3.2. Components of a Comprehensive Health History 80
3.2.1. Demographic Information 81
3.2.2. Medical History and Family History 82
3.2.3. Social History and Lifestyle Factors 82
3.3. Techniques for Effective Health History Taking 84
3.3.1. Active Listening Skills 85
3.3.2. Open-Ended Questioning 86
3.3.3. Building Rapport with Patients 86
3.4. Common Challenges in Health History Taking 88
3.4.1. Patient Reluctance to Share Information 88
3.4.2. Language and Cultural Barriers 89
3.4.3. Time Constraints in Clinical Settings 90
3.5. Role of Technology in Health History Taking 92
3.5.1. Electronic Health Records (EHR) 93
3.5.2. Telehealth and Remote Consultations 93
3.5.3. Mobile Health Applications 94
3.6. Ethical Considerations in Health History Taking 95
3.6.1. Patient Confidentiality and Privacy 96
3.6.2. Informed Consent 97
3.6.3. Cultural Sensitivity and Respect 98
Summary 99
References 102

CHAPTER 4

Techniques of Physical Examination 107

Introduction 107
4.1. Inspection 111
4.1.1. Visual Assessment of the Patient 112
4.1.2. Importance of Body Language and Posture 112
4.1.3. Use of Tools in Inspection (e.g., Otoscope, Ophthalmoscope) 113
4.2. Palpation 115
4.2.1. Techniques for Effective Palpation 116
4.2.2. Areas Commonly Assessed Through Palpation 117
4.2.3. Importance of Patient Comfort During Palpation 118
4.3. Percussion 119
4.3.1. Definition and Purpose of Percussion 120
4.3.2. Techniques for Different Body Areas 120
4.3.3. Interpretation of Percussion Sounds 121
4.4. Auscultation 122
4.4.1. Equipment Used for Auscultation (e.g., Stethoscope) 123
4.4.2. Types of Sounds Assessed (e.g., Heart, Lung) 124
4.4.3. Importance of Quiet Environment During Auscultation 125
4.5. Special Tests 126
4.5.1. Overview of Common Special Tests (e.g., Reflex Tests) 127
4.5.2. Indications for Using Special Tests 128
4.5.3. Interpretation of Results from Special Tests 128
4.6. Documentation 130
4.6.1. Importance of Accurate Documentation 130
4.6.2. Components of a Physical Examination Report 131

4.6.3. Legal and Ethical Considerations in Documentation 132
Summary 134
References 137

CHAPTER 5

General Health Survey and Vital Signs in Nursing 141

Introduction 141
5.1. Purpose of the General Health Survey 144
5.1.1. Assessing Patient Health Status 145
5.1.2. Identifying Risk Factors 146
5.1.3. Establishing Baseline Data 147
5.2. Components of the General Health Survey 148
5.2.1. Patient History and Demographics 149
5.2.2. Review of Systems 150
5.2.3. Physical Examination 150
5.3. Understanding Vital Signs 152
5.3.1. Definition and Importance 153
5.3.2. Key Vital Signs: Temperature, Pulse, Respiration, Blood Pressure 154
5.3.3. Normal Ranges and Variations 154
5.4. Techniques for Measuring Vital Signs 156
5.4.1. Equipment Used in Vital Sign Measurement 157
5.4.2. Proper Techniques for Accurate Readings 157
5.4.3. Common Errors in Measurement 158
5.5. Interpretation of Vital Signs 160
5.5.1. Recognizing Abnormal Findings 161
5.5.2. Correlating Vital Signs with Patient Conditions 161
5.5.3. Clinical Decision-Making Based on Vital Signs 162
5.6. Role of Nursing in Health Surveys and Vital Signs 164
5.6.1. Responsibilities of Nurses in Patient Assessment 165
5.6.2. Documentation and Reporting 166
5.6.3. Patient Education and Communication 166
Summary 168
References 171

CHAPTER 6

Skin, Hair, and Nails Assessment in Nursing 175

Introduction 175
6.1. Anatomy and Physiology of Skin 179
6.1.1. Structure of the Skin Layers 180
6.1.2. Functions of the Skin in the Body 181
6.1.3. Common Skin Conditions and Their Implications 182
6.2. Hair Assessment 183
6.2.1. Types of Hair and Their Characteristics 184
6.2.2. Common Hair Disorders and Their Significance 185
6.2.3. Techniques for Assessing Hair Health 186
6.3. Nail Assessment 188
6.3.1. Anatomy of the Nail Structure 188
6.3.2. Common Nail Abnormalities and Their Meanings 189
6.3.3. Importance of Nail Assessment in Overall Health 190
6.4. Assessment Techniques 191
6.4.1. Visual Inspection Methods 192
6.4.2. Palpation and Its Role in Assessment 193
6.4.3. Use of Diagnostic Tools in Skin, Hair, and Nails Assessment 194
6.5. Cultural Considerations 195
6.5.1. Variations in Skin, Hair, and Nails Across Different Ethnicities 196
6.5.2. Impact of Cultural Practices on Assessment 197
6.5.3. Importance of Cultural Competence in Nursing 198
6.6. Documentation and Communication 200
6.6.1. Best Practices for Documenting Assessments 201
6.6.2. Importance of Clear Communication with Healthcare Team 201
6.6.3. Role of Patient Education in Assessment Findings 202
Summary 204
References 207

CHAPTER 7

Head, Face, Neck, and Lymphatics Assessment in Nursing 211

Introduction 211
7.1. Anatomy of the Head and Neck 214
7.1.1. Key Structures of the Head 215
7.1.2. Anatomy of the Neck 217
7.1.3. Lymphatic System Overview 217
7.2. Assessment Techniques 219
7.2.1. Inspection Methods 220
7.2.2. Palpation Techniques 220
7.2.3. Auscultation in Lymphatic Assessment 221
7.3. Common Conditions and Disorders 223
7.3.1. Headaches and Their Implications 223
7.3.2. Neck Pain and Associated Conditions 225
7.3.3. Lymphadenopathy and Its Significance 226
7.4. Cultural Considerations in Assessment 228
7.4.1. Variations in Anatomy Across Different Populations 229
7.4.2. Cultural Beliefs Affecting Health Assessments 229
7.4.3. Communication Strategies for Diverse Populations 230
7.5. Documentation and Reporting 231
7.5.1. Importance of Accurate Documentation 232
7.5.2. Standardized Assessment Tools 233
7.5.3. Reporting Findings to the Healthcare Team 234
7.6. Nursing Interventions 235
7.6.1. Patient Education on Self-Assessment 236
7.6.2. Referral Processes for Further Evaluation 236
7.6.3. Collaborative Care Approaches 237
Summary 239
References 242

CHAPTER 8

Eye Assessment in Nursing 245

Introduction 245
8.1. Anatomy of the Eye 248
8.1.1. Structure of the Eye 249
8.1.2. Function of Different Eye Components 250
8.1.3. Common Anatomical Variations 251
8.2. Techniques for Eye Assessment 252
8.2.1. Visual Acuity Testing 253
8.2.2. Inspection and Palpation Methods 254
8.2.3. Use of Specialized Equipment 254
8.3. Common Eye Disorders 256
8.3.1. Refractive Errors (e.g., Myopia, Hyperopia) 256
8.3.2. Cataracts and Their Impact on Vision 257
8.3.3. Glaucoma and Its Assessment 258
8.4. Patient History and Eye Assessment 260
8.4.1. Importance of Patient History in Eye Care 261
8.4.2. Key Questions to Ask During Assessment 261
8.4.3. Identifying Risk Factors for Eye Diseases 262
8.5. Documentation and Reporting 264
8.5.1. Importance of Accurate Documentation 265
8.5.2. Standardized Reporting Formats 265
8.5.3. Legal Implications of Documentation Errors 266
8.6. Role of Technology in Eye Assessment 267
8.6.1. Advancements in Diagnostic Tools 268
8.6.2. Telehealth and Remote Eye Assessments 269
8.6.3. Future Trends in Eye Assessment Technology 270
Summary 272
References 275

CHAPTER 9

Ear, Nose, Mouth, and Throat (ENT) Assessment in Nursing 279

Introduction 279
9.1. Anatomy of the Ear, Nose, Mouth, and Throat 282
9.1.1. Structure and Function of the Ear 283
9.1.2. Anatomy of the Nasal Passages 284
9.1.3. Overview of the Oral Cavity and Throat 285
9.2. Common ENT Disorders 286
9.2.1. Ear Disorders: Otitis Media and Hearing Loss 287
9.2.2. Nasal Disorders: Sinusitis and Allergies 288

9.2.3. Throat Disorders: Pharyngitis and Tonsillitis 289
9.3. Assessment Techniques in ENT **290**
9.3.1. Inspection Methods for the Ear, Nose, and Throat 291
9.3.2. Palpation and Percussion Techniques 292
9.3.3. Use of Specialized Tools: Otoscope and Laryngoscope 293
9.4. Patient History and Symptoms **294**
9.4.1. Importance of a Thorough Patient History 295
9.4.2. Common Symptoms to Inquire About 296
9.4.3. Cultural Considerations in Patient Communication 297
9.5. Diagnostic Tests and Procedures **298**
9.5.1. Audiometry and Hearing Tests 298
9.5.2. Nasal Endoscopy and Throat Cultures 299
9.5.3. Imaging Studies: X-Rays and CT Scans 300
9.6. Nursing Interventions and Care Plans **301**
9.6.1. Developing Individualized Care Plans 302
9.6.2. Patient Education on ENT Health 303
9.6.3. Collaboration with Interdisciplinary Teams 304
Summary **305**
References **308**

CHAPTER 10

Thorax and Lungs Assessment in Nursing 313

Introduction **313**
10.1. Anatomy of the Thorax **316**
10.1.1. Structure of the Thoracic Cavity 317
10.1.2. Major Organs Within the Thorax 318
10.1.3. Role of the Thorax in Respiratory Function 319
10.2. Physiology of Breathing **320**
10.2.1. Mechanisms of Ventilation 321
10.2.2. Gas Exchange Process 322
10.2.3. Factors Affecting Respiratory Function 324
10.3. Assessment Techniques **325**
10.3.1. Inspection Methods 325
10.3.2. Palpation and Percussion 326
10.3.3. Auscultation of Lung Sounds 327
10.4. Common Thoracic and Pulmonary Conditions **328**
10.4.1. Asthma and Its Assessment 329
10.4.2. Chronic Obstructive Pulmonary Disease (COPD) 330
10.4.3. Pneumonia and Its Implications 331
10.5. Nursing Interventions **333**
10.5.1. Patient Education on Respiratory Health 333
10.5.2. Techniques for Effective Breathing Exercises 334
10.5.3. Importance of Monitoring and Documentation 335
10.6. Challenges in Thorax and Lung Assessment **337**
10.6.1. Variability in Patient Presentations 338
10.6.2. Limitations of Assessment Tools 338
10.6.3. Cultural Considerations in Assessment 339
Summary **341**
References **344**

CHAPTER 11

Cardiovascular System Assessment in Nursing 347

Introduction **347**
11.1. Anatomy of the Cardiovascular System **350**
11.1.1. Major Components: Heart, Blood Vessels, and Blood 351
11.1.2. Function of the Heart and Its Chambers 352
11.1.3. Role of Arteries, Veins, and Capillaries 353
11.2. Physiology of the Cardiovascular System **355**
11.2.1. Blood Circulation Process 356
11.2.2. Cardiac Cycle and Its Phases 357
11.2.3. Regulation of Heart Rate and Blood Pressure 358
11.3. Importance of Cardiovascular Assessment **359**
Test Your Knowledge **359**
11.3.1. Early Detection of Cardiovascular Diseases 360
11.3.2. Monitoring Patient Health Status 361
11.3.3. Guiding Treatment and Intervention Strategies 362
11.4. Techniques for Cardiovascular Assessment **363**

11.4.1. Patient History and Physical Examination 364
11.4.2. Use of Diagnostic Tools: ECG, Echocardiogram, and Blood Tests 364
11.4.3. Interpretation of Assessment Findings 365
11.5. Common Cardiovascular Conditions 367
11.5.1. Hypertension and Its Implications 368
11.5.2. Heart Failure and Its Management 368
11.5.3. Coronary Artery Disease and Risk Factors 369
11.6. Nursing Interventions in Cardiovascular Care 370
11.6.1. Patient Education and Lifestyle Modifications 371
11.6.2. Medication Management and Adherence 372
11.6.3. Emergency Response and Critical Care 373
Summary 375
References 378

CHAPTER 12

Abdominal Assessment in Nursing 381

Introduction 381
12.1. Anatomy of the Abdomen 384
12.1.1. Major Organs Located in the Abdominal Cavity 385
12.1.2. Anatomical Regions of the Abdomen 386
12.1.3. Relationship Between Anatomy and Assessment Techniques 387
12.2. Techniques of Abdominal Assessment 388
12.2.1. Inspection Methods 389
12.2.2. Palpation Techniques 390
12.2.3. Auscultation Procedures 391
12.3. Common Abdominal Conditions 392
12.3.1. Gastrointestinal Disorders 393
12.3.2. Urinary Tract Issues 394
12.3.3. Reproductive System Concerns 394
12.4. Cultural Considerations in Abdominal Assessment 396
12.4.1. Variations in Abdominal Anatomy 397
12.4.2. Cultural Beliefs Affecting Assessment 397
12.4.3. Communication Barriers in Diverse Populations 398
12.5. Documentation and Reporting 400
12.5.1. Importance of Accurate Documentation 400
12.5.2. Standardized Reporting Formats 401
12.5.3. Legal Implications of Documentation Errors 402
12.6. Challenges in Abdominal Assessment 404
12.6.1. Patient-Related Factors 404
12.6.2. Environmental Influences 405
12.6.3. Limitations of Assessment Techniques 406
Summary 408
References 411

CHAPTER 13

Musculoskeletal System Assessment in Nursing 415

Introduction 415
13.1. Anatomy of the Musculoskeletal System 418
13.1.1. Major Components: Bones, Muscles, and Joints 419
13.1.2. Functions of the Musculoskeletal System 420
13.1.3. Common Anatomical Terms Used in Assessment 421
13.2. Assessment Techniques 422
13.2.1. Inspection and Palpation Methods 423
13.2.2. Range of Motion Evaluations 424
13.2.3. Special Tests for Musculoskeletal Conditions 425
13.3. Common Musculoskeletal Disorders 427
13.3.1. Osteoarthritis and Its Implications 428
13.3.2. Rheumatoid Arthritis and Assessment Challenges 429
13.3.3. Fractures and Their Assessment Protocols 430
13.4. Patient History and Interview 432
13.4.1. Importance of a Thorough Patient History 433
13.4.2. Key Questions to Ask During Assessment 433
13.4.3. Understanding Patient-Reported Symptoms 434
13.5. Documentation and Reporting 436

13.5.1. Importance of Accurate Documentation 436
13.5.2. Standardized Assessment Tools and Forms 437
13.5.3. Communicating Findings to the Healthcare Team 438
13.6. Nursing Interventions 439
13.6.1. Pain Management Strategies 440
13.6.2. Rehabilitation and Physical Therapy Referrals 441
13.6.3. Patient Education on Musculoskeletal Health 442
Summary 444
References 447

CHAPTER 14

Neurological System Assessment in Nursing 453

Introduction 453
14.1. Anatomy of the Neurological System 456
14.1.1. Central Nervous System Components 457
14.1.2. Peripheral Nervous System Components 458
14.1.3. Functional Roles of Different Neurological Structures 460
14.2. Common Neurological Assessment Techniques 461
14.2.1. Patient History and Symptom Evaluation 462
14.2.2. Physical Examination Methods 463
14.2.3. Use of Diagnostic Tools and Technologies 464
14.3. Neurological Assessment in Different Patient Populations 466
14.3.1. Assessing Neurological Function in Pediatric Patients 467
14.3.2. Considerations for Elderly Patients 468
14.3.3. Neurological Assessments in Patients with Chronic Conditions 468
14.4. Interpretation of Neurological Assessment Findings 470
14.4.1. Identifying Normal versus Abnormal Findings 470
14.4.2. Understanding Neurological Signs and Symptoms 471
14.4.3. Correlating Assessment Findings with Potential Diagnoses 472
14.5. Documentation and Communication of Assessment Results 473
14.5.1. Importance of Accurate Documentation 474
14.5.2. Effective Communication with Healthcare Team Members 475
14.5.3. Legal and Ethical Considerations in Documentation 476
14.6. Challenges in Neurological Assessments 477
14.6.1. Variability in Patient Responses 478
14.6.2. Limitations of Assessment Tools 479
14.6.3. Cultural and Language Barriers in Assessment 480
Summary 481
References 484

CHAPTER 15

Breast and Axillae Assessment in Nursing 487

Introduction 487
15.1. Anatomy of the Breast 490
15.1.1. Structure and Function of Breast Tissue 491
15.1.2. Lymphatic Drainage and Its Significance 492
15.1.3. Variations in Breast Anatomy 493
15.2. Importance of Axillary Assessment 494
15.2.1. Role of Axillary Lymph Nodes in Disease Detection 495
15.2.2. Common Conditions Affecting the Axillae 496
15.2.3. Implications of Axillary Assessment in Patient Care 497
15.3. Techniques for Breast Assessment 499
15.3.1. Visual Inspection Methods 499
15.3.2. Palpation Techniques for Breast Examination 500
15.3.3. Use of Imaging Technologies in Assessment 501
15.4. Techniques for Axillary Assessment 502
15.4.1. Inspection of the Axillary Region 503
15.4.2. Palpation of Axillary Lymph Nodes 504
15.4.3. Identifying Abnormalities in the Axillae 505
15.5. Common Findings in Breast and Axillary Assessments 506

15.5.1. Normal Findings and Variations 507
15.5.2. Abnormal Findings and Their Implications 508
15.5.3. Documentation of Assessment Results 509
15.6. Patient Education and Communication 510
15.6.1. Importance of Educating Patients About Self-Exams 511
15.6.2. Communicating Findings to Patients 511
15.6.3. Addressing Patient Concerns and Questions 512
Summary 514
References 517
Index 521

LIST OF FIGURES

Figure 1.1. Health assessment in nursing
Figure 1.2. Importance in nursing practice
Figure 1.3. Historical context of health assessment
Figure 1.4. The evolution of nursing assessment
Figure 1.5. Impact of historical practices on modern nursing
Figure 1.6. Components of health assessment
Figure 1.7. Subjective data collection in the field of nursing
Figure 1.8. Objective data collection in the field of nursing
Figure 1.9. Documentation and reporting in the field of nursing
Figure 1.10. Techniques of health assessment
Figure 1.11. Inspection and observation of health assessment in nursing
Figure 1.12. Palpation and percussion of health assessment in nursing
Figure 1.13. Vital signs
Figure 1.14. Cultural considerations in health assessment in the field of nursing
Figure 1.15. Impact of culture on health beliefs in the field of nursing
Figure 1.16. Technology in health assessment
Figure 1.17. Electronic health records (EHR)
Figure 1.18. Telehealth and remote assessments
Figure 2.1. Interviewing and communication techniques in health assessment
Figure 2.2. Effective communication in health assessments
Figure 2.3. The role of the interview in health assessment
Figure 2.4. Establishing rapport with patients
Figure 2.5. Gathering comprehensive health histories
Figure 2.6. Identifying patient concerns and symptoms
Figure 2.7. Types of interviewing questions
Figure 2.8. Open-ended questions of health assessments in nursing
Figure 2.9. Probing questions
Figure 2.10. Nonverbal communication in health assessment in nursing
Figure 2.11. Eye contact of health assessment in nursing
Figure 2.12. Active listening skills

Figure 2.13. Cultural competence in health communication
Figure 2.14. Adapting communication styles in nursing
Figure 2.15. Ethical considerations in health interviews
Figure 2.16. Informed consent
Figure 2.17. Understanding patient confidentiality and privacy
Figure 2.18. Deal with difficult patients
Figure 3.1. Taking a patient history
Figure 3.2. Clinical practice for health history taking
Figure 3.3. Establish a relationship with your healthcare professional
Figure 3.4. Identifying health risks and concerns in nursing
Figure 3.5. Components of a comprehensive health history
Figure 3.6. Patient demographics
Figure 3.7. Medical history and family history
Figure 3.8. Techniques for effective health history taking
Figure 3.9. Active listening in healthcare
Figure 3.10. Building rapport with patients
Figure 3.11. Patient reluctance to share information
Figure 3.12. Time constraints in clinical settings
Figure 3.13. Role of technology in health history taking
Figure 3.14. Telehealth and remote consultations
Figure 3.15. Patient confidentiality and privacy
Figure 4.1. Techniques of physical examination
Figure 4.2. Clinical practice of physical examination
Figure 4.3. Inspection of physical examination
Figure 4.4. The visual assessment of the patient
Figure 4.5. Tools in inspection
Figure 4.6. Palpation of physical examination
Figure 4.7. Techniques for effective palpation
Figure 4.8. Areas commonly assessed through palpation
Figure 4.9. Percussion method of clinical examination
Figure 4.10. Percussion of techniques for different body areas
Figure 4.11. Auscultation in physical examination
Figure 4.12. Equipment used for auscultation
Figure 4.13. Special tests of physical examination
Figure 4.14. Reflex tests
Figure 4.15. Interpretation of results from special tests

Figure 4.16. Documentation of physical examination
Figure 4.17. Accurate documentation of physical examination
Figure 5.1. General health survey and vital signs in nursing
Figure 5.2. Vital signs in nursing
Figure 5.3. Purpose of the general health survey
Figure 5.4. Assessing patient health status
Figure 5.5. Identifying risk factors within the nursing
Figure 5.6. Components of the general health survey
Figure 5.7. Patient history and demographics
Figure 5.8. The review of systems (ROS)
Figure 5.9. Physical examination
Figure 5.10. Understanding vital signs
Figure 5.11. The assessment of key vital signs
Figure 5.12. Techniques for measuring vital signs
Figure 5.13. Proper techniques for accurate readings vital signs
Figure 5.14. Interpretation of vital signs
Figure 5.15. Correlating vital signs with patient conditions
Figure 5.16. Role of nursing in health surveys and vital signs
Figure 5.17. Responsibilities of nurses in patient assessment
Figure 6.1. Physical assessment – skin, hair, and nails
Figure 6.2. Skin, hair, and nails assessment
Figure 6.3. Anatomy and physiology of skin
Figure 6.4. Structure of the skin layers
Figure 6.5. Functions of the skin in the body
Figure 6.6. Hair assessment
Figure 6.7. Types of hair and their characteristics
Figure 6.8. Common hair disorders
Figure 6.9. Techniques for assessing hair health in nursing
Figure 6.10. Nail assessment in nursing
Figure 6.11. Anatomy of the nail structure
Figure 6.12. Common nail abnormalities
Figure 6.13. Nail assessment techniques
Figure 6.14. Palpation and its role in assessment
Figure 6.15. Variations in skin across different ethnicities
Figure 6.16. Importance of cultural competence in nursing
Figure 6.17. Documentation and communication in nursing

Figure 6.18. Importance of clear communication with healthcare team
Figure 7.1. Head and neck assessment nursing
Figure 7.2. Nursing roles in patient assessment
Figure 7.3. Head and neck anatomy
Figure 7.4. Key structures of the head
Figure 7.5. The anatomy and physiology of the neck
Figure 7.6. Lymphatic system overview
Figure 7.7. Assessment techniques
Figure 7.8. Palpation techniques
Figure 7.9. Inspection and palpation of the lymph nodes
Figure 7.10. Headaches and their implications
Figure 7.11. Neck pain and associated conditions
Figure 7.12. The generalized lymphadenopathies
Figure 7.13. Cultural considerations in assessment in nursing
Figure 7.14. Cultural beliefs affecting health assessments
Figure 7.15. Documentation and reporting
Figure 7.16. Understanding the role of health assessment tools in healthcare
Figure 7.17. Nursing interventions
Figure 8.1. Eye assessment nursing
Figure 8.2. Common eye conditions
Figure 8.3. Anatomy of the eye
Figure 8.4. Structure of the eye
Figure 8.5. Function of different eye components
Figure 8.6. Techniques for eye assessment
Figure 8.7. Visual acuity testing
Figure 8.8. Use of specialized equipment of eye assessment
Figure 8.9. Common eye disorders
Figure 8.10. Refractive errors
Figure 8.11. Cataracts and their impact on vision
Figure 8.12. Glaucoma and its assessment
Figure 8.13. Patient history and eye assessment
Figure 8.14. Key questions to ask during assessment
Figure 8.15. Documentation and reporting
Figure 8.16. Standardized reporting formats in nursing
Figure 8.17. Role of technology in eye assessment
Figure 8.18. Telehealth and remote eye assessments

Figure 9.1. Ear, nose, mouth, and throat (ENT) assessment
Figure 9.2. ENT assessment
Figure 9.3. Structure and function of the ear
Figure 9.4. Anatomy of the nasal passages
Figure 9.5. Overview of the oral cavity and throat
Figure 9.6. Ear disorders: Otitis media and hearing loss
Figure 9.7. Nasal disorders: Sinusitis and allergies
Figure 9.8. Pharyngitis
Figure 9.9. Assessment techniques in ENT
Figure 9.10. Palpation and percussion techniques in ENT
Figure 9.11. Modern laryngoscope with otoscope
Figure 9.12. Importance of a thorough patient history
Figure 9.13. Audiometry hearing test
Figure 9.14. Nasal endoscopy
Figure 9.15. Nursing interventions and care plans
Figure 10.1. Thorax and lungs assessment in nursing
Figure 10.2. Thorax and lungs assessment techniques in nursing
Figure 10.3. Anatomy of the thorax
Figure 10.4. Structure of the thoracic cavity
Figure 10.5. Role of the thorax in respiratory function
Figure 10.6. Physiology of breathing
Figure 10.7. Mechanisms of ventilation of breathing
Figure 10.8. Gas exchange process
Figure 10.9. Assessing the thorax and lungs
Figure 10.10. Inspection methods for the thorax and lungs
Figure 10.11. Auscultation of lung sounds
Figure 10.12. Common thoracic and pulmonary conditions
Figure 10.13. Asthma and its assessment
Figure 10.14. Chronic obstructive pulmonary disease
Figure 10.15. Pneumonia
Figure 10.16. Patient education on respiratory health
Figure 10.17. Techniques for effective breathing exercises
Figure 11.1. Focused cardiovascular physical assessment
Figure 11.2. Cardiovascular assessment in nursing
Figure 11.3. Anatomy of the cardiovascular system
Figure 11.4. Major components: Heart, blood vessels, and blood

Figure 11.5. Function of the heart and its chambers
Figure 11.6. Role of arteries, veins, and capillaries
Figure 11.7. Physiology of the cardiovascular system
Figure 11.8. Blood circulation process
Figure 11.9. Cardiac cycle and its phases
Figure 11.10. Importance of cardiovascular assessment
Figure 11.11. Monitoring patient health status
Figure 11.12. Techniques for cardiovascular assessment
Figure 11.13. Diagnostic tools
Figure 11.14. Common cardiovascular conditions
Figure 11.15. Heart failure and its management
Figure 11.16. Nursing interventions in cardiovascular care
Figure 12.1. Abdominal assessment nursing
Figure 12.2. Abdominal assessment in nursing practice
Figure 12.3. Anatomy of the abdomen
Figure 12.4. Major organs located in the abdominal cavity
Figure 12.5. Anatomical regions of the abdomen
Figure 12.6. Techniques of abdominal assessment
Figure 12.7. Inspection methods of abdominal assessment
Figure 12.8. Palpation techniques of abdominal assessment
Figure 12.9. Auscultation procedures of abdominal assessment
Figure 12.10. Common abdominal conditions
Figure 12.11. Gastrointestinal disorders
Figure 12.12. Urinary tract infection
Figure 12.13. Cultural considerations
Figure 12.14. Concepts of cultural assessment
Figure 12.15. Documentation and reporting during health assessments
Figure 12.16. Legal implications of documentation errors
Figure 12.17. Patient-related factors concerning abdominal assessment
Figure 13.1. Physical assessment – musculoskeletal system
Figure 13.2. Assessment in nursing
Figure 13.3. Anatomy of the musculoskeletal system
Figure 13.4. Bones, muscles, and joints of the musculoskeletal system
Figure 13.5. Functions of the musculoskeletal system
Figure 13.6. Assessment techniques of the musculoskeletal system
Figure 13.7. Inspection and palpation methods

Figure 13.8. Range of motion evaluations of the musculoskeletal system
Figure 13.9. Common musculoskeletal disorders
Figure 13.10. Osteoarthritis
Figure 13.11. Rheumatoid arthritis
Figure 13.12. Fractures and their assessment
Figure 13.13. Patient history and interview
Figure 13.14. Key questions to ask during musculoskeletal system
Figure 13.15. Understanding patient-reported symptoms
Figure 13.16. Accurate documentation is fundamental to nursing practice
Figure 13.17. Communicating findings to the healthcare team
Figure 13.18. Pain management strategies in the nursing assessment
Figure 13.19. Rehabilitation and physical therapy referrals in the nursing assessment
Figure 14.1. Physical assessment – neurological system
Figure 14.2. Neurological exam
Figure 14.3. Anatomy of the neurological system
Figure 14.4. Central nervous system components
Figure 14.5. Peripheral nervous system components
Figure 14.6. Clinical techniques: The neurological assessment
Figure 14.7. Patient history and symptom evaluation of neurological conditions
Figure 14.8. Physical examination methods of neurological conditions
Figure 14.9. Neurological assessment in different patient populations
Figure 14.10. Pediatric neurologic examination
Figure 14.11. Assessing neurological function in elderly patients
Figure 14.12. Understanding neurological signs and symptoms
Figure 14.13. Documentation and communication of assessment results in nursing
Figure 14.14. Effective communication with healthcare team members
Figure 14.15. Challenges in neurological assessments
Figure 15.1. Breast and axillae assessment in nursing
Figure 15.2. Overview of assessment techniques breast and axillae
Figure 15.3. Anatomy of the breast
Figure 15.4. Structure and function of breast tissue
Figure 15.5. Variations in breast anatomy
Figure 15.6. Axillary assessment
Figure 15.7. Role of axillary lymph nodes in disease detection
Figure 15.8. Common conditions affecting the axillae

Figure 15.9. Implications of axillary assessment in patient care
Figure 15.10. Visual inspection methods for breast assessment
Figure 15.11. Palpation techniques for breast examination
Figure 15.12. Inspection of the axillary region
Figure 15.13. Palpation of axillary lymph nodes
Figure 15.14. Normal findings and variations in breast and axillary assessments
Figure 15.15. Patient education and communication in breast and axillae evaluation

PREFACE

The practice of assessing health is a chief responsibility of every nurse that demands both careful observation and reflective judgment. Through rational accumulation of facts—ranging from verbal history to hands-on evaluation—nurses build a clear picture of a person's condition. This process requires critical thinking to decipher signs and symptoms, identify deviations from baseline, and predict potential complications. As the first stage of the majority of care plans, assessment guides all future interventions and ensures that care is individually tailored to suit each individual's specific needs.

Effective health assessment also lies with rapport and trust building. How one poses the questions, the tone, and even the body used all help foster a patient's willingness to disclose personal details. Through verbal and nonverbal practice, nurses create an environment where patients are heard and appreciated. This interpersonal aspect of assessment not only enriches the information collected but creates satisfaction and ownership in patients throughout the care process.

Health Assessment in Nursing presents a formal, systematic analysis of the required skills and knowledge requisite for effective nurse assessment. It combines evidence-based best practice, exemplified with tangible examples and lucid guidelines for both students and practicing nurses. Step-by-step instructions, example cases, and evidence-based explanation are all clearly laid out in this book.

Chapter 1 sets forth the assumptions of assessment, including models of critical thinking, ethical standards, and legal guidelines. It provides a foundation for safe and effective practice through professional performance standards and definition of the clinician-advocate role of the nurse.

Chapter 2 discusses interviewing and communication skills for effective collection of information. Problems discussed include formulation of questions, active listening, cultural sensitivity, and how data collection is done from patients with communication impairments.

Chapter 3 covers health history taking, including methods of eliciting comprehensive details of past illnesses, surgery, medications, family history, and life-style factors. Sorting out and being systematic to prevent omission of any crucial factor is emphasized.

Chapter 4 is devoted to physical examination methods, outlining inspection, palpation, percussion, and auscultation. Examples and tips for attaining utmost precision without detriment to patient comfort are given for each procedure.

Chapter 5 is devoted to the general survey and vital signs, demonstrating how to take temperature, pulse, respiration, blood pressure, height, weight, and pain measurement. Normal parameters and conditions that may influence readings are mentioned.

Chapter 6 deals with skin, hair, and nail examination, including the identification of lesions, rashes, coloration changes, and structural irregularities. Photographic examples and terminology aid in accurate documentation.

Chapter 7 deals with examination of head, face, neck, and lymphatics, such as lymph node palpation, cranial nerve function assessment, and thyroid structure and mobility examination.

Chapter 8 deals with eye examination, defining visualization of visual acuity, extraocular movements, pupil reactions, and fundoscopic examination. It contains standard screening tools as well as interpretation of abnormal findings.

Chapter 9 deals with ENT evaluation, such as approaches to examine tympanic membranes, nasal patency assessment, oral mucosa inspection, and tonsillar and pharyngeal evaluation.

Chapter 10 focuses on examination of thorax and lungs, auscultation of breath sounds, palpation of tactile fremitus, and percussion of lung fields. Precaution is taken to determine normal and adventitious sounds.

Chapter 11 deals with examination of the cardiovascular system, including inspection of the precordium, palpation of pulses and peripheral edema, auscultation of heart sounds, and interpretation of murmurs and rhythm.

Chapter 12 covers abdominal examination, explaining inspection, auscultation, percussion, and palpation to evaluate bowel sounds, organ size, tenderness, and masses. It provides techniques for differentiation of normal variation from pathologic findings.

Chapter 13 covers musculoskeletal assessment, guiding range-of-motion testing, strength evaluation, gait examination, and spine inspection. It recognizes normal joint disease and how to document functional limitation.

Chapter 14 is neurological system assessment, and it discusses mental status examination, cranial nerve examination, motor and sensory function, coordination, and reflexes. It gives screening and comprehensive evaluation strategies.

Chapter 15 is assessment of breast and axillae, and it gives inspection and palpation techniques for identifying lumps, skin changes, and lymph node enlargement. It stresses patient education regarding self-examination procedures.

This book is designed for nursing students, clinical faculty, and practicing nurses who wish to refine their assessment skills. It supplements classroom learning, prepares students for the clinical practicum, and assists in ongoing professional practice.

FOUNDATIONS OF HEALTH ASSESSMENT IN NURSING

1

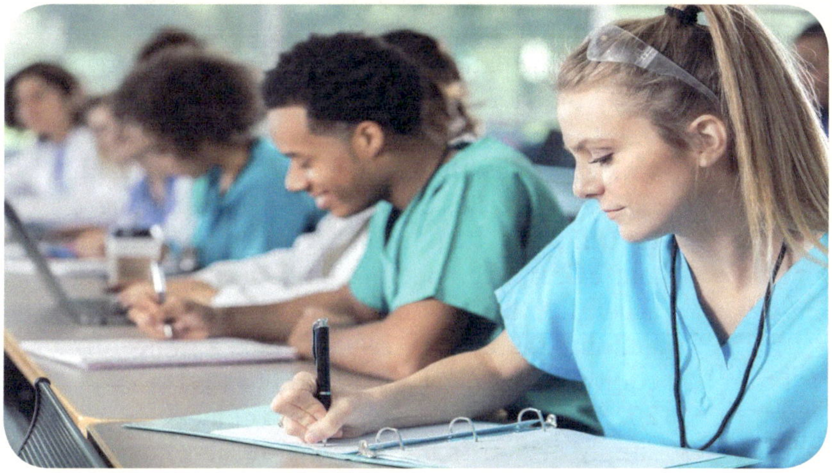

LEARNING OBJECTIVES

After studying this chapter, you will be able to:

1. Give historical context of health assessment;
2. List the components of health assessment;
3. Describe the techniques of health assessment;
4. Discuss about cultural considerations in health assessment;
5. Explore the technology in health assessment;
6. Focus on the challenges in health assessment.

Introduction

The foundation of nursing health assessment is an essential skill set that requires the integration of clinical practice, critical thinking, and interpersonal communications. There are various dimensions involved in a comprehensive assessment of health such as physical examination, patient history, and psychosocial assessment, which allow nurses to identify possible health issues and provide appropriate care. Understanding the finesse of health assessment not only promotes accurate diagnosis but also foster a therapeutic nurse-patient relationship, facilitating patient involvement and compliance. In addition, the orderly process of eliciting and understanding patient data equips nurses with the tools for effective clinical decision-making, which is essential in delivering high-quality care across different environments. In nursing practice, the ability to perform comprehensive health assessments is the very basis of designing individualized care plans. According to nursing regulations evolving at present, it is necessary for these assessments to be evidence-based and to consider various backgrounds and individual needs of patients. Nurses employ a variety of types of assessment, including inspection, palpation, and auscultation, in an effort to gain critical information to guide diagnosis and intervention planning. Such a systematic approach not only allows for the identification of existing health problems, but also for the prevention of resultant complications, thus exemplifying the importance of active assessment in facilitating patient well-being and optimal health outcomes in practice. Alongside this, ongoing practice and education in health assessment techniques are essential to nursing professionals. Combining technological and evidence-based practice improves standard assessment processes through advanced methods. As nursing education evolves, curricula increasingly focus on interprofessional team-based practice, health literacy, and patient-centered care as cornerstones of health assessments. Through the development of these skills, nurses are better equipped to address the challenges of patient care and the polypharmacy demands of complex populations. Emphasizing the qualities of strong health assessment serves ultimately to promote better overall quality of care, referencing back in turn to the broader agendas of health promotion and disease prevention within health care systems (Figure 1.1).

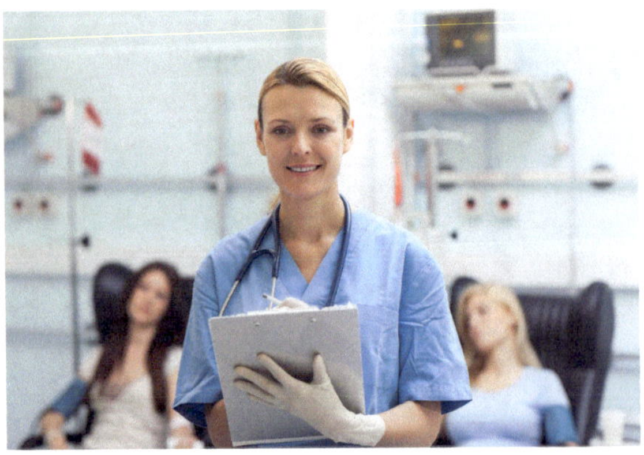

Figure 1.1. Health assessment in nursing.

Source: https://online.utulsa.edu/images/62b725c1-822a-41c4-bf08-f8bae59e9f7e.jpg.

Definition of Health Assessment

Health assessment is the central process in nursing that entails the methodical gathering, organization, and analysis of patient data to assess health status and needs. As a multidimensional process, the use of this allows healthcare professionals to develop individualized care plans responsive to every patient's specific concerns. A general assessment of health is not only comprised of physical examinations but also investigates psychological, social, and environmental factors that may affect the well-being of the patients. By utilizing both subjective and objective approaches to data collection, nurses are able to build a full picture of a patients status. Hence, the achievement of health assessment relies on the ability of practitioners to utilize critical thinking, communication, and cultural competence skills in interpreting accurately health information as required for building therapeutic relationships and healthy equity among diverse populations (Curtis et al., 2019). Additionally, assessment of health is not simply diagnosis but ongoing observation and review to adjust the care plan according to the changing health of the patient. In the current fast-paced, constantly changing healthcare environment, application of health assessment has direct relation to quality measures of care. For instance, correct health assessments not only identify acute health issues but also identify chronic conditions requiring long-term care. As highlighted by the existing literature, the inclusion of cultural competence in health assessment is vital in providing heterogeneous demographic populations (Allen et al., 2016). Culturally competent care provides respectful and responsive care plans to the individual cultural contexts of patients, decreasing health disparities and promoting wellness in various communities. Also, the application of technology within health assessment activities is transforming the way in which nurses receive and analyze patients' information. Electronic health records (EHRs) have transformed the documentation of patients' information in a way that allows for quick access to and transfer of patients' information across healthcare providers. This technology enhances the accuracy and effectiveness of the health assessment process, allowing timely interventions through real-time information. With this transition towards digitalization, there is an increased focus on evidence-based practices which put emphasis on the use of validated instruments highlighting the value of incorporating these in health assessment processes. It is essential to evaluate the validity and reliability of these instruments to ensure that nursing assessment offers valuable insights that inform effective patient care (Allen et al., 2016). In all, the theory and practice of health assessment in nursing reflect a dynamic integration of clinical experience, ongoing assessment, and technological innovation to address patients' diverse health demands.

Importance in Nursing Practice

Nursing practice is founded mostly on the principles of health assessment as it offers crucial skills needed for high-quality patient care. The significance of thorough health assessments can be elucidated using various nursing activities, including the taking of patient histories, physical exams, and analysis of certain health issues. For instance, during the COVID-19 outbreak, healthcare professionals used enhanced assessment strategies to identify and address patients' demands in an effective manner. The implementation of multileveled programs of education that further equip nurses with competence in these assessments demonstrated that the dynamic nature of healthcare necessitates a solid grounding in the competencies of health assessment. Not only does this flexibility make individual nurses more effective in practice, but it also fosters a culture of continuous improvement and professional development within nursing practice (Tiwari et al., 2020). Moreover, the worth of health evaluations is not just in terms of eligibility for medical treatment; it significantly determines the patient's outcomes as well as the quality of care they receive. To illustrate, comprehensive biopsychosocial assessments are important in identifying complex health issues that a patient may have along various dimensions, such as physical, psychological, and social determinants affecting their wellbeing. The application of these tests enables nurses to provide patient-tailored interventions, and therefore improve patient satisfaction as well as health outcomes. The specific knowledge of the chronic disease in the context of a patient can also help with communication and build a collaborative setting between the members of the multidisciplinary team caring for a patient. This combined strategy not only reinforces the nurses role as critical care coordinator but also solidifies the platform for effective nursing practice as discussed in contemporary healthcare paradigms (Allen et al., 2015). Moreover, fostering health assessment competency is vital in sharpening the critical thinking skills that underpin nursing practice. Analyzing and interpreting variable data sets is critical in sound decision-making in patient care. Nurses possessing strong assessment skills are able to quickly identify changes in a patient's condition and take measures proactively to prevent complications. As evident in professional training drills for addressing needs during a crisis like the COVID-19 pandemic, a veteran nursing team showed greater confidence and ability to apply systematic assessment actively. These training programs not only increase individual nurses' skills but also increase the overall effectiveness of healthcare teams in addressing changing situations, ultimately ensuring a safe and effective care environment. This continuous emphasis on evaluation and skill development proves the central role evaluation plays in nursing practice, which guides upcoming trends and modes of healthcare delivery (Tiwari et al., 2020) (Figure 1.2).

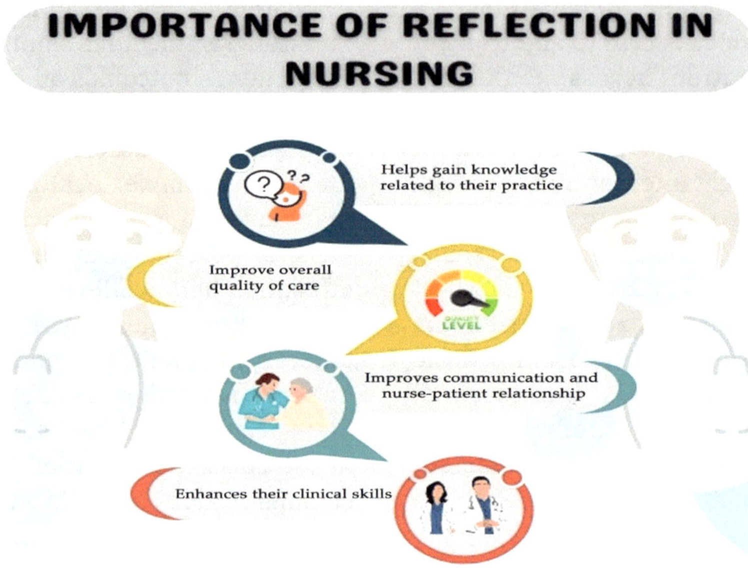
IMPORTANCE OF REFLECTION IN NURSING
Helps gain knowledge related to their practice
Improve overall quality of care
LEVEL
Improves communication and nurse-patient relationship
Enhances their clinical skills

Figure 1.2. Importance in nursing practice.

Source: https://www.tutorsindia.com/blog/wp-content/uploads/2023/09/W11-Inhouse-blog-1.webp.

Overview of Assessment Types

The cornerstones of nursing health assessment are various types of assessments that serve to present an adequate picture of patient health. Among these, the most prominent ones are initial, ongoing, and targeted assessments. Initial assessments provide the foundation for patient care, from which nurses can gather adequate information regarding a patient's clinical history, medications, allergies, and habits. This baseline data is critical, as it determines subsequent care planning and interventions. On-going assessment, on the other hand, consists of regular assessments that track differences or developments in a patient's health over time, care being adjusted in response. As a means of addressing specific health issues or concerns, focused assessments allow clinicians to delve deeper into precise areas, allowing targeted interventions. All these types of assessments combined establish the overall picture of patient health, an essential element of excellent nursing care. Holistic health assessment is particularly vital in nursing practice, highlighting the necessity to take patients into account in a complex context. Such an assessment not only entails physical health but also mental, emotional, social, and environmental factors. Such an approach is commensurate with contemporary health promotion practice, which acknowledges that many interacting factors determine health. For example, in carrying out holistic assessments of patients' health, nurses consider patients' cultural backgrounds, dietary needs, and stages of development so that care becomes tailored to individual circumstances. From nursing education curricula, such a wide understanding optimizes the potential of nurses to communicate effectively with patients using therapeutic communication skills, thereby eliciting relevant subjective information while also collecting objective information. Therefore, holistic health assessment is a sound foundation for delivering quality care that focuses on patients' overall well-being (Krekhovska-Lepiavko et al., 2023). In reality, the integration of varied types of assessment will most certainly lead to improved patient outcomes, particularly for high-risk individuals. For instance, the Northern Territory Diabetes in Pregnancy Partnership explicitly states the need to embrace multiple health assessment models for better coordination of care and quality of care. By employing a systems assessment instrument, practitioners can have a clearer understanding of the effectiveness of existing care models and things that need to be aligned. The outcomes of the collaboration bring out the fact that professional relationships and enhanced communication between caregivers enhance patients' health outcomes, especially in cases of complex health conditions. Also, regular review of care models and stringent integration of information systems has the potential to make healthcare less complex, with regular checks equating to timely and relevant interventions. Hence, it becomes necessary that nursing education programs lay emphasis on such assessment methods as they involve patient care and outcomes (Kirkham et al., 2017).

1.1. Historical Context of Health Assessment

Learning Outcome

1. Evolution of nursing assessments;
2. Key figures in health assessment history;
3. Impact of historical practices on modern nursing.

Health assessment in nursing has evolved significantly over centuries, shaped by numerous historical influences and changes in healthcare practices. In early times, health assessment largely relied on observational routines and patient histories with much integration of rudimentary knowledge of disease. Evolving processes such as pulse-taking and inspection of bodily fluids laid the ground for the next generation of assessments. As the medical sciences were developed in the Renaissance era, the observation process became increasingly systematic in character, courtesy of the anatomical discoveries by early masters like Vesalius. This was the period of transition from mystical descriptions of disease towards a more empirical basis in assessing health, which set the stage for later systematic assessments to take place within nursing. The 19th century also witnessed significant developments in public health and the nursing profession, particularly during the lifetime of Florence Nightingale. She shifted the emphasis from sanitation, organization of patient care, and systematic data collection, which completely transformed the practice of health assessment. Statistical data compiled by Nightingales revealed the impact of environmental factors on health outcomes, highlighting the practice of evidence-based decision making in nursing. The era also saw the creation of formalized nurse training, where health assessment education was incorporated into curricula. With this, the use of scientific principles to guide practice and increased focus on patient-centered care provided an integrative strategy for health assessment that can be used today in nursing. Later technological advancements also reformed practices in health assessment.

The electronic health record and telemedicine innovations have improved data collection and communication between healthcare providers. Additionally, integrating advanced diagnostic equipment has made it easier to assess patient health accurately and on time. Despite this, the above innovations have also created major issues regarding data ethics and the implications of technology in health assessment. As authors like DIgnazio and Klein point out in their explanation of data feminism, consideration must be given to whom these innovations benefit and ensure there is a just approach to health assessment across groups (Catherine et al., 2020). Historical perspective to health assessment prepares nurses with insight into the complexities and challenges inherent within their practice, positioning them to advocate better for continued improvement in the delivery of healthcare (Figure 1.3).

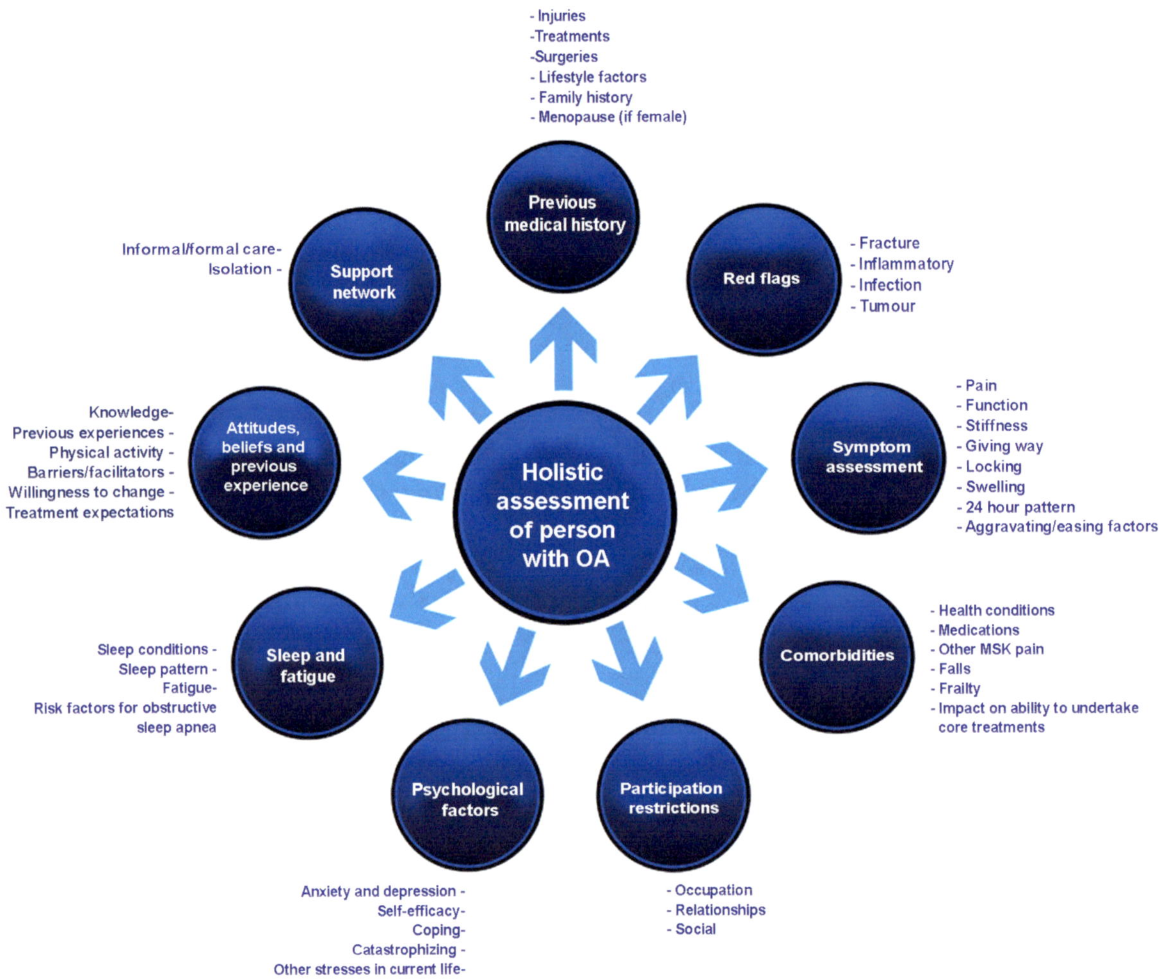

- Injuries
-Treatments
-Surgeries
- Lifestyle factors
- Family history
- Menopause (if female)
Previous medical history
Red flags
- Fracture
- Inflammatory
- Infection
- Tumour
Symptom assessment
- Pain
- Function
- Stiffness
- Giving way
- Locking
- Swelling
- 24 hour pattern
- Aggravating/easing factors
Comorbidities
- Health conditions
- Medications
- Other MSK pain
- Falls
- Frailty
- Impact on ability to undertake core treatments
Participation restrictions
- Occupation
- Relationships
- Social
Psychological factors
Anxiety and depression -
Self-efficacy-
Coping-
Catastrophizing -
Other stresses in current life-
Sleep and fatigue
Sleep conditions -
Sleep pattern -
Fatigue-
Risk factors for obstructive sleep apnea
Attitudes, beliefs and previous experience
Knowledge-
Previous experiences -
Physical activity -
Barriers/facilitators -
Willingness to change -
Treatment expectations
Support network
Informal/formal care-
Isolation -
Holistic assessment of person with OA

Figure 1.3. Historical context of health assessment.

Source: https://ars.els-cdn.com/content/image/3-s2.0-B9780323992695000086-f02-01-9780323992695.jpg.

1.1.1. Evolution of Nursing Assessments

The process of creating nursing assessments is evidence of the paradigm shift in the healthcare system from mere treating of symptoms to being more holistic and considering the patient's general well-being. Previously, nursing assessments were raw, merely touching on the physical presentations of patients. However, as the nursing profession developed, comprehensive assessment became increasingly essential. Nurses are now required to use complex assessment techniques to consider not only the physical but also the psychological, social, and environmental factors that influence patient health. This transformation emphasizes the necessity of preparing nurses who are capable of performing a good health assessment while considering the myriad patient backgrounds and experiences. The procedures employed in assessments of health changed as nursing education developed. The integration of technology and best practice evidence has revolutionized how nurses collect and process patient information. Present education concentrates on clinical decision-making and critical thinking, enabling nurses to consolidate multiple information types. Furthermore, there have been ongoing innovations that have brought competency assessment aimed at responding to racial and ethnic variations in health care. For example, contemporary programs are more focused on ensuring cultural and linguistic competence among nursing professionals to ensure enhanced patient outcomes. Such sensitivity towards the socio-cultural dimensions of healthcare is in congruence with broader campaigns advocating equal access to health. The inclusion of complex care management systems has also influenced the advancements within nursing evaluations, reflecting the need for holistic and personalized patient care. Interventions in managing complex chronic diseases underscore the importance of nurses' findings in developing personalized care plans. Such programs require nurses to assess health holistically against variable interventions with intersections with community support resources and social determinants of health. As mirrored by the growth of programs like the Mount Sinai Visiting Doctors Program and the CARE Partners program, nursing assessment is not merely a diagnostic tool but also a key component in interprofessional health delivery. This revolution brings with it the assumption that health evaluation is not a static process but a dynamic process that reacts in turn to the needs of different populations within a constantly changing healthcare environment (Figure 1.4).

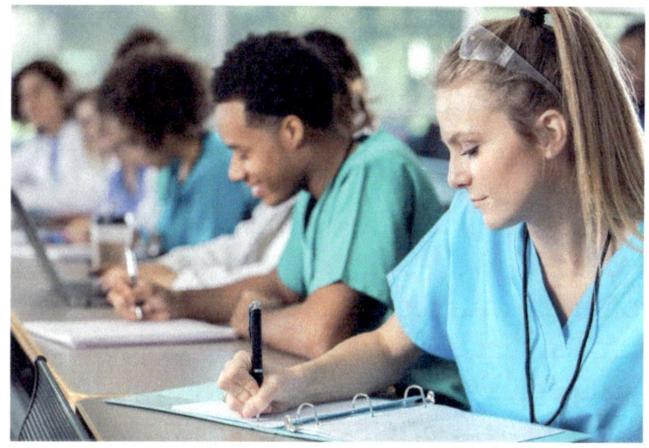

Figure 1.4. The evolution of nursing assessment.

Source: https://nclexnairobi.com/wp-content/uploads/2024/02/nclex.jpg.

1.1.2. Key Figures in Health Assessment History

The history of health assessment within nursing is heavily driven by significant individuals whose works have contributed the discipline with its fundamental grasp. Among the most dominant of these figures is Florence Nightingale, whose attempts to integrate empirical evidence into nursing practice remain unparalleled. Through methodical data collection and examination of mortality rates in military hospitals, Nightingale had developed the paradigmatic relationship between determinants of the environment and the outcomes. Her rigorous approach not only reformed nursing practice but also provided the groundwork for later health assessments, emphasizing the importance of observational information as well as statistical analysis. Such technical exactitude established the precedent in the nursing profession, encouraging nurses to utilize assessment instruments to enhance patient outcomes, emphasizing the important role of data in informing clinical choices. In addition to Nightingale, contemporaries such as Virginia Henderson contributed to the evolution of health assessment. Henderson's definition of nursing as "assisting individuals to achieve health or a peaceful death" highlighted the importance of comprehending the needs of the patient in their totality. She developed the concept of the nursing need theory, which defines 14 basic human needs that formed a basis for comprehensive health assessment. This approach channeled the focus of nursing from the sole amelioration of illness to promotion of overall well-being. Hendersons writing prompted nurses to adopt an evaluation approach that encompasses socio-economic and psychological determinants, thereby promoting a more patient-oriented and multidisciplinary philosophy of care, which remains pertinent in contemporary nursing practices. The efforts of these innovators cannot be downplayed, as they chart a trajectory of growth and improvement in the health assessment approaches in nursing. As health care has evolved through the years, so have the models and mechanisms for assessing patients. The integration of technological advances and evidence-based practice, led by these pioneers, has created efficient evaluation concentrating on patient-centered care. Moreover, the heightened degree of sophistication in health status necessitates a dimensional approach, recalling Nightingale's and Henderson's philosophies. Their legacies continue to pour into present-day nursing education and practice and uphold the crucial relationship between historical information and contemporary health assessment practice. The ongoing development in health assessment still continues to meet the evolving dynamics of health care, allowing the basic principles established by these pioneers to remain current and effective in pursuing effective nursing care.

1.1.3. Impact of Historical Practices on Modern Nursing

The historical development of nursing as a career is closely linked with the past practices that have molded its modern foundations. From the early caregivers, frequently women who cared for the ill in their own homes, to the founding of organized nursing schools during the 19th century, the course of nursing is marked by important societal trends. Ancient nursing practices emphasized holistic care, treating the body, mind, and spirit of patients. This was the basis upon which current health assessments are founded, with continued integration of complete assessments of patient history, lifestyle, and environment. The work of these early nursing practices can still be seen today, where patient-centered care is a key focus, inspiring nurses to form therapeutic relationships and enact the optimal outcomes. Moreover, the legacies of such great people, such as Florence Nightingale, have greatly influenced nursing practice and standards that we witness today. Nightingales' work at the beginning of the Crimean War emphasized the importance of sanitation, diet, and compassionate care. Her meticulous record-keeping and statistical proof laid the groundwork for evidence-based nursing practice. Modern health assessments call to mind her principles, which are highlighted by today's emphasis on critical thought, analysis of data, and the value in comprehending an extensive medical history. Adhering to Nightingales standards of hygiene and diet in assessing patients shows a continued commitment to preventative care and overall patient wellness, illustrating the manner in which practices of days gone by show a lasting impact upon current nursing practices and principles (Valparaiso University, 1990). Along with humane care and hygiene, the historical evolution of nursing has also been marked by increasing recognition of the importance of cultural competence in health assessment. As nursing progressed, it is now imperative that the practitioners be sensitive and respectful to cultural differences influencing patient perception, behavior, and outcomes. Historical atrocities in the healthcare system have served to increase recognition for the need for cultural sensitivity among healthcare providers. Today's nursing education is based on cultural competence, in which nurses are educated to take patient-focused care that considers the social and cultural background of the patients. Hence, the convergence of past practice with contemporary nursing not only reinforces the columns of health assessment but also supports an increased inclusiveness so that nursing remains equally effective at addressing the culturally diverse needs of the populations it serves (Valparaiso University, 2004) (Figure 1.5).

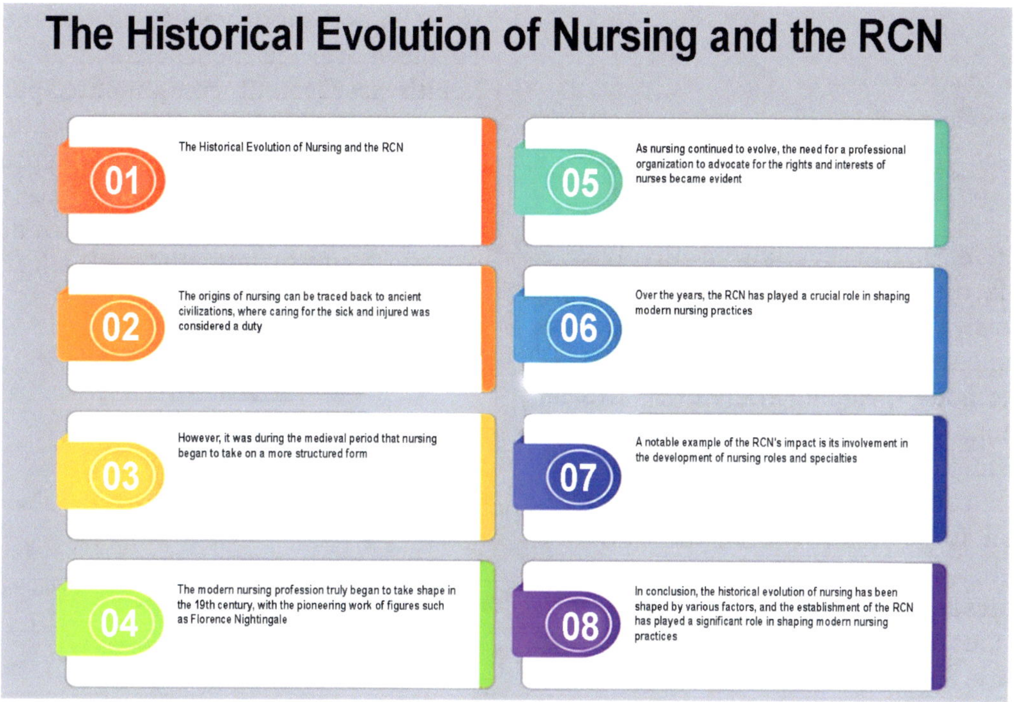

Figure 1.5. Impact of historical practices on modern nursing.

Source: https://fastercapital.co/i/The-Role-of-the-RCN-in-Shaping-Modern-Nursing-Practices--The-Historical-Evolution-of-Nursing-and-the-RCN.webp.

Test Your Knowledge

1. How has the practice of health assessment evolved from traditional methods to modern clinical approaches?
2. What key historical developments have influenced the standards and procedures used in health assessment today?

1.2. Components of Health Assessment

Learning Outcome

1. Subjective data collection;
2. Objective data collection;
3. Documentation and reporting.

An effective health evaluation involves a range of factors that are crucial for obtaining comprehensive patient information. The process most commonly involves data gathering through various methods, including interviews, physical examinations, and laboratory tests. A thorough health history, including the patient's medical history and conditions of lifestyle, provides the foundation for comprehending the patient's health status. This initial step of data gathering allows nurses to evaluate potential health complications and risk factors which can impact patient care. Also, the evaluation must include an evaluation of the psychosocial dimension of the patient because emotional and social issues are an important contribution to general health results. Through the integration of this information, health care providers can create an overall perspective of a patient's requirements, eventually informing effective care plans specific to those requirements. After the initial data gathering, health assessment involves ongoing assessment and monitoring of the patient during the course of his or her care. The ongoing process encompasses not only reevaluation of physical symptoms and signs but also modifying care plans according to changing patient responses. For instance, reassessment can be done through regular check-ups, follow-ups, and implementation of evidence-based practice guidelines that are best practice in nursing. An important aspect of this ongoing process of reassessment is the convergence of community and environmental elements that may affect patient health. This relevance is highlighted in efforts detailed by Potter et al. (2012), which involve nursing course collaboration to ensure student nurses are well equipped to transition into practice, hence enhancing their assessment skills and responsiveness to patients' needs. Furthermore, the incorporation of specialized health assessment components, particularly gerontology care, has also become an area of priority in nursing school. Programs such as the ACE.S initiative demonstrate the value of preparing nursing students to address the distinct health needs of older adults.

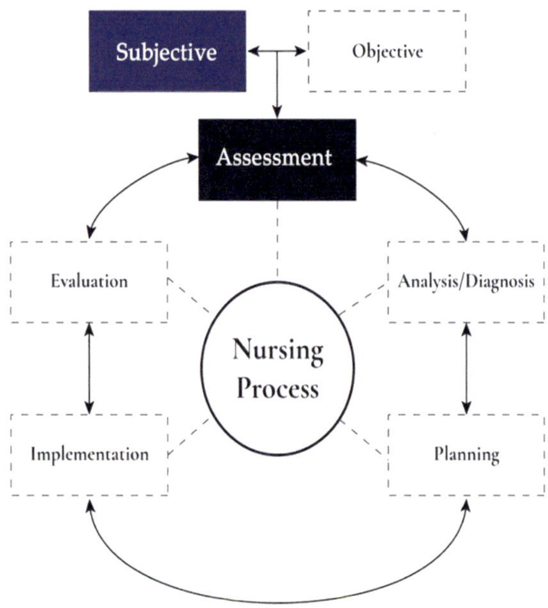

Figure 1.6. Components of health assessment.

Source: https://cod.pressbooks.pub/app/uploads/sites/165/2024/05/TheNursingProcess-1024x788.jpg.

By providing targeted educational materials and teaching tools, such programs enable nursing instructors to integrate geriatric content completely into curriculum, enhancing the competency of emerging practitioners. Concentrating on this population's unique health challenges facilitates a more effective assessment process and supports additional high-quality, patient-focused care. The addition of such specialized training not only addresses the growing demand for elder care but also elevates the overall level of health assessment that is conducted by nursing practitioners, thereby improving patient outcomes across various settings (N/A, 2015) (Figure 1.6).

1.2.1. Subjective Data Collection

Subjective data collection in nursing is a critical component of health assessments, which helps practitioners achieve insight that isn't possible through quantitative data. Personal contact with patients provides room for qualitative data, which introduces nurses to the emotional, psychological, and social environment surrounding patients. Such information can shed light on a patient's feelings about their health situation, such as concerns, fears, and expectations, thereby enabling an integrated perspective of the patient. In addition, the subjective process of data collection depends greatly on good communication skills and establishing trust between the patient and nurse, key in bringing out accurate and broad information. Through attending to physical and non-physical aspects of well-being, nurses are able to create more tailored care plans that are more responsive to the individual needs of the patient, resulting in enhanced health outcomes and patient satisfaction. Secondly, understanding the nuances of subjective data collection is also imperative for nursing practice, particularly with regards to ethical concerns and patient autonomy. Nurses have to be taught how to identify when to explore a patient's subjective states without intruding on their space while remaining respectful in their approach. This is crucial because patients share confidential information that has a significant influence on their care. Through the development of trusting relationships, nurses can encourage patients to respond openly about their symptoms or issues, thereby providing greater insight into their health status. Techniques such as active listening, empathy, and open-ended questioning enhance the authenticity of subjective data collected, illuminating dimensions that can unveil hidden conditions or intricacies not reflected by standard assessments (Khosravi et al., 2022). Therefore, mastering the collection of subjective data is an indispensable nursing expertise. Additionally, the role of subjective data collection is reinforced by the integration into broader healthcare systems and registries that seek to enhance the care of patients. Registries have a tendency to combine both objective and subjective information in order to monitor the health outcomes, thereby obtaining an entire picture that supports evidence-based practice. The Users Guide acknowledges the importance of patient registries and reaffirms the role played by patient registries in understanding complex patient experiences in various contexts (N/A, 2020).

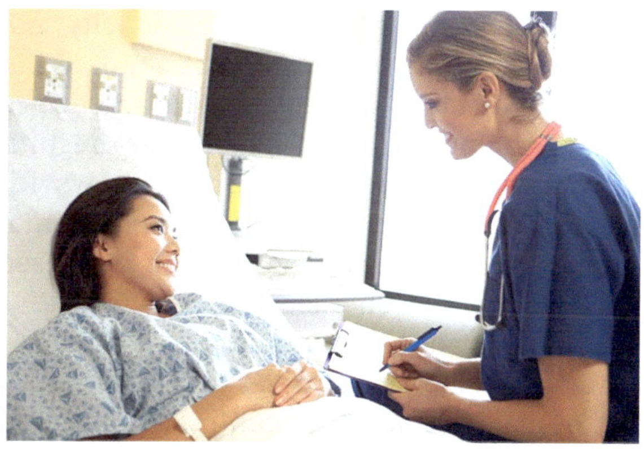

Figure 1.7. Subjective data collection in the field of nursing.

Source: https://www.nursingprocess.org/bimg/subjective-vs-objective-nursing-data.webp.

Subjective data serves an important function in such models of evaluation, offering qualitative information regarding patient experience and attitude that quantitative evidence could never hope to provide. As healthcare continues to advance, the emphasis on patient-centered care demonstrates the significance of subjective assessment in informing clinical decisions, optimizing resource management, and ultimately improving patient satisfaction. The confluence of subjective data collection and broader mechanisms of healthcare shows its essential value in nursing, shaping the way forward in health assessment (Figure 1.7).

1.2.2. Objective Data Collection

The foundation of objective data collection in nursing assessment lies in its ability to provide concrete, quantifiable information which informs clinical decision. Objective data detail the measurable facts which are significant in the development of a whole clinical picture of a patient. Such data is commonly acquired through physical assessment, laboratory results, and imaging studies. By applying empirical measurement, nurses are better able to eliminate subjectivity that is always present in patient-reports. Through its focus on objectivity, not only is the validity of assessment enhanced but also lends itself to evidence-based practice in nursing. Tacking vital signs, laboratory results, and documented medical history allows for an integrated model of patient care such that nursing intervention is being made on fact-based evidence and not on anecdotal or speculative evidence. In health evaluation, systematic gathering of objective facts has to be undertaken methodically to achieve comprehensiveness and reliability. Clinical checklists, standard assessment scales, and computerized medical records are the indispensable tools in gathering precise facts. With the use of these standardized tools, not only is consistency between one assessment and another increased but also trends over time can be identified. Further, as highlighted in the infrastructure produced by contemporary registries, synergy of both existing available data sets as well as newer information accrued is critical to facilitate healthy assessments. Coordination with registry science highlights producing varied methodologies for obtaining objective information in a bid to ensure assessments are practical to modify in response to the dynamic and multifaceted demands of patients. In this sense, application of such methods provides a foundation for building appropriate nursing diagnoses and care plans tailored to the patient's needs. Furthermore, obtaining objective data must be carried out while keeping in mind ethical principles and patient autonomy. Note that although objective observations can bring about unchallengeable facts about a patient's health status, the context in which these data occur is just as significant. Ethical standards in data collection, such as informed consent, privacy, and cultural competence, must inform nursing professionals' practice. As nursing becomes increasingly integrated with cutting-edge data practice, guidelines established in publications such as Data Feminism can inform practitioners how to navigate the ethical subtleties involved. This alignment of objective data with ethical information practice will not only allow nurses to collect and process data in an effective way but also promote the rights and welfare of their patients and develop a culture of trust and respect within healthcare settings (Figure 1.8).

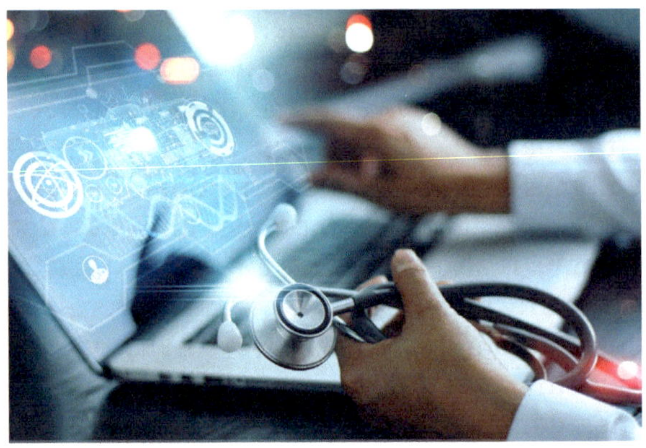

Figure 1.8. Objective data collection in the field of nursing.

Source: https://external-content.duckduckgo.com/iu/?u=https%3A%2F%2Fprognocis.com%2Fwp-content%2Fuploads%2F2022%2F09%2FData-collection-in-healthcare.jpeg&f=1&nofb=1&ipt=678fd39b5b89c1a3196a1fcfc921649e2035cced5713f66255cdc5284ec7d1fd.

1.2.3. Documentation and Reporting

The significance of reporting and documentation in nursing practice cannot be overemphasized, as both are essential components in patient safety and quality of care. Through proper and clear documentation, nurses ensure that critical information about a patient's health status is properly communicated between the multidisciplinary healthcare team. It provides continuity of care, prevents errors, and serves as a valuable resource for future evaluation and intervention. Furthermore, good documentation supports mandatory legal and ethical obligations in that it is a written record to be used in the case of disagreements or audit. Because of increased emphasis on patient safety, organizations have established and prioritized incident reporting systems to identify possible threats and promote improved health outcomes in general. Acquaintance with and use of these reporting processes need to be developed by nursing students in order to practice. Interprofessional teamwork is essential in making documentation and reporting processes better in healthcare settings. Effective information transfer between nursing personnel and other healthcare workers can enhance patient assessment, medication administration, and incident reporting processes. It has been revealed in studies that many pre-registration students are not aware of schemes for reporting, and they may not be given adequate training in documentation practices. Directing learners through methodically designed curricula that integrate patient safety and medication safety education aids in increasing learners' competency in these crucial responsibilities. By applying iterative strategies for obtaining feedback from educators and employers of healthcare, nursing students can be imparted with the significance of thorough documentation and the role played by accurate reporting in preventing adverse outcomes. Hence, making a culture based on accountability and transparency in documentation not only ensures the safety of patients but also promotes a culture of safety among healthcare centers. The assessment and recording of drug harm are a significant area for nursing documentation practice, particularly in hospitals. Knowing a hospitals unique medication-related adverse event profile is crucial in determining good safety strategies. Reports note that, while there are various testing methods, none of them is sufficient to capture the full extent of patient harm. Hence, using systematic methods pilfered from large-scale studies can be extremely useful in obtaining information on the frequency and nature of adverse outcomes in single hospitals. Recording like these illuminates patient safety trends, guiding interventions and facilitating interprofessional collaboration to improve safety standards. Through the integration of these principles into nursing education, future practitioners will be better placed to utilize documentation and reporting not only as a means of communication but as an essential tool in enhancing patient safety and the quality of health care delivery overall (Figure 1.9).

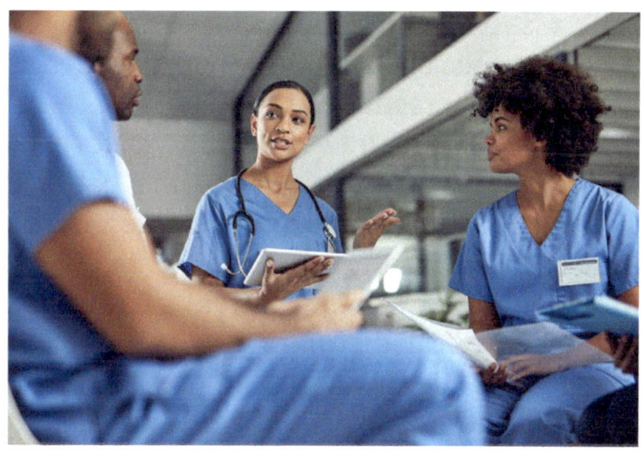

Figure 1.9. Documentation and reporting in the field of nursing.

Source: https://external-content.duckduckgo.com/iu/?u=https%3A%2F%2Fonline.carlow.edu%2Fwp-content%2Fuploads%2F2021%2F10%2Fcar_msn_article_effect-nurse-leader_header.jpg&f=1&nofb=1&ipt=e39f0dd1383612ae89c16d1f517b0ec00a43ba1e0b181a79774758149d94960d.

Test Your Knowledge

1. What are the main components of a comprehensive health assessment, and why is each important?
2. How do subjective and objective data contribute to forming an accurate health assessment?

1.3. Techniques of Health Assessment

Learning Outcome

1. Inspection and observation;
2. Palpation and percussion;
3. Auscultation and vital signs.

For nursing, the health assessment skills are a foundation for delivering excellent patient care. The skills are a sequential method for gathering and interpreting patient data to inform clinical decision. A comprehensive health assessment usually encompasses several approaches like observation, interview, physical exam, and diagnostic tests. Each approach has a unique role but draws together to form an overall picture of the status of the patients. For instance, observation art enables nurses to pick up on non-verbal signals which would inform them about the patient's emotional state or physical discomfort, while effective interviewing skills result in an enhanced comprehension of a patient's medical history and issues. Thus, through incorporation of these techniques, not only is accuracy of assessment enhanced but a therapeutic nurse-patient relationship that is essential for an optimal outcome is also established. A key aspect of health assessment techniques is the emphasis on cultural competence. Cultural competence refers to nurses' ability to communicate with, understand, and provide care for patients of diverse backgrounds. As healthcare environments become increasingly multicultural, culturally sensitive assessments cannot be overemphasized. Techniques like targeted interviews can uncover cultural beliefs influencing a patient's health behaviors and choices. In addition, the use of strategies respectful of differences avoids assessments being disrespectful or irrelevant and facilitates a partnership approach to healthcare. This aspect of the health assessment underpins evidence for context's importance in the implementation of nursing practice, with implications that culturally contextualized assessments may optimize effectiveness and patient satisfaction (Harvey et al., 2015). Integrating technology into methods of health assessment further revolutionizes nursing practice by streamlining data collection and enhancing accuracy.

Electronic health records (EHRs), telemedicine, and mobile health apps significantly enhance efficiency and access to patient records. With these technologies, nurses are able to perform more holistic assessments, maintain accurate records, and share important information easily among healthcare providers. For example, remote monitoring allows continuous monitoring of chronically ill patients, thus allowing for timely interventions and avoiding hospitalization. Further, educational tools that integrate evidence-based practices into regular evaluations allow nurses to remain current and skilled in new procedures (Ozenbaugh et al., 2014). This incorporation of technology not only helps nurses deliver excellence in care but also enhances the overall productivity of health evaluations in all health care environments (Figure 1.10).

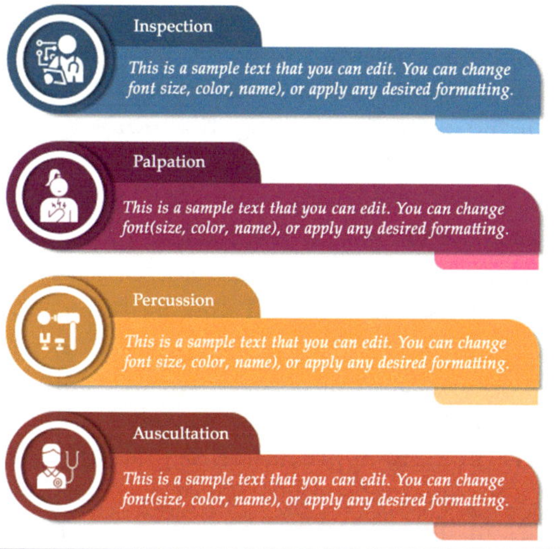

Figure 1.10. Techniques of health assessment.

Source: https://external-content.duckduckgo.com/iu/?u=https%3A%2F%2Fwww.collidu.com%2Fmedia%2Fcatalog%2Fproduct%2Fimg%2F4%2Fc%2F4c8362e5cc2ef29b9f9090b571b85f6096eb1fc285baaae218b38187cac8064b%2Fhealth-assessment-slide3.png&f=1&nofb=1&ipt=a902e952ef7f6dba3f6b8cb6ed68ef7c1bf5dba6a2172bb88560444eceb11244.

1.3.1. Inspection and Observation

The process of observation and inspection forms a foundation for the assessment of health in the nursing profession. Systematic observation enables nurses to gather relevant information concerning a patients physical condition, emotional state, and environment. This first skill is not only about observing but carefully interpreting what is observed, for instance, the change in the color of the skin, the signs of distress, and behavioral responses. To support an all-around understanding of the patient, the nurses must integrate what they observe with clinical experience so that they can identify potential health issues at an early stage. Moreover, this initial evaluation process builds rapport and communicates concern and therefore influences a patient's involvement in their care. As emphasized in recent studies, the usability of such observational skills cannot be overstated since they are also significant determinants of patient health and are bound to have a marked effect on clinical outcomes (Gore et al., 2007). Effective observation and inspection also involve assessment of a patient's environment, which is also crucial in determining what factors can affect health. By noting the patients' environment—e.g., noise levels, lighting, and accessibility—nurses can gain insight into the external threats or support that influence the patients' health. For instance, a very noisy environment within the care environment has been found to lead to excessive levels of stress and compromised recovery, particularly for vulnerable groups like the elderly or dementia patients (Aletta et al., 2017). Accordingly, examining and viewing the physical surroundings plays a twofold function: to enable the identification of concerns immediately and to aid in developing means of promoting patient comfort.

Therefore, the nurses role goes beyond the individual patient and includes working to ensure facility changes to create a more healing environment. In health assessment, observation and inspection are dependent upon each other and should be considered dynamic processes, rather than discrete evaluations. For nurses, proficiency in the skills of observation is something that must be practiced every day and synthesized with clinical practice. Because patient health is dynamic, information gained through inspection may change over time, and repeated measurements should be made to reflect accurately. Also, the ability to perceive fine cues of sickness and health—like patient behaviors within their environment—works to optimize the effectiveness of general nursing practice. As a more complicated health setting, the need for solid observational skill is paramount for obtaining high-quality assessment and interventions tailored to individual patients' requirements (Aletta et al.,

2017; Gore et al., 2007). By regular practice in observation and inspection, the nurses become integral facilitators in the care continuum and ultimately contribute to better health outcomes (Figure 1.11).

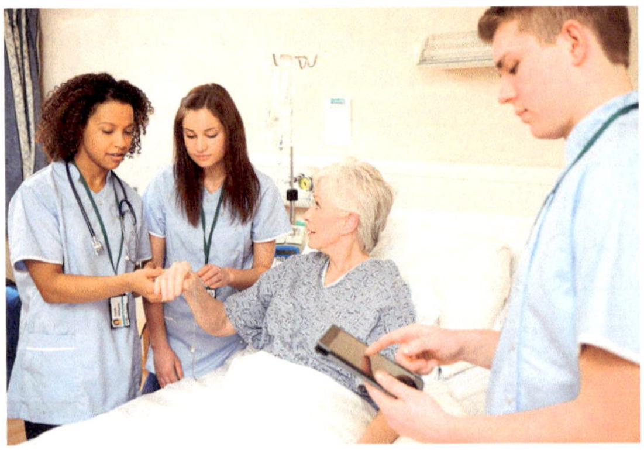

Figure 1.11. Inspection and observation of health assessment in nursing.

Source: https://external-content.duckduckgo.com/iu/?u=https%3A%2F%2Fblogs.biomedcentral.com%2Fon-medicine%2Fwp-content%2Fuploads%2Fsites%2F6%2F2023%2F09%2Fnursing-assessment.jpg&f=1&nofb=1&ipt=536c1b6b490d863674956fdcec2c2d16754211d9553a25357081e036de0fda30.

1.3.2. Palpation and Percussion

Palpation and percussion are simple techniques in the medical examination, providing important information to the diagnosis. Palpation utilizes skilled touch in the exploration of the qualities of body organs and tissues, understanding their shape, size, and consistency. Palpation gives nurses the tools to recognize abnormalities such as swelling, tenderness, or rigidity, indicative of an underlying status. Furthermore, the ability to palpate some anatomical landmarks encourages nurses' familiarity with a patient's anatomy and physiology. These assessments cement the nursing care foundation by encouraging a patient-focused practice where careful observation and tactile evaluations inform clinical decision-making and enhance quality care outcomes. Another core assessment method, percussion, enhances palpation with auditory information on what lies underneath. By percussing or striking the body surface, practitioners can make sounds that reflect texture and consistency of tissue beneath the surface. The technique is particularly valuable in examination for lung and abdominal pathology, where variations in sound may be reflective of fluid accumulation, air, or solid masses. The use of percussion in assessment not only aids localization of abnormality but also promotes a more holistic appreciation of patient status. Through judicious application of percussion and palpation, nurses can build a general impression of the patients' health, ultimately inform their intervention and contribute to enhanced patient outcomes.

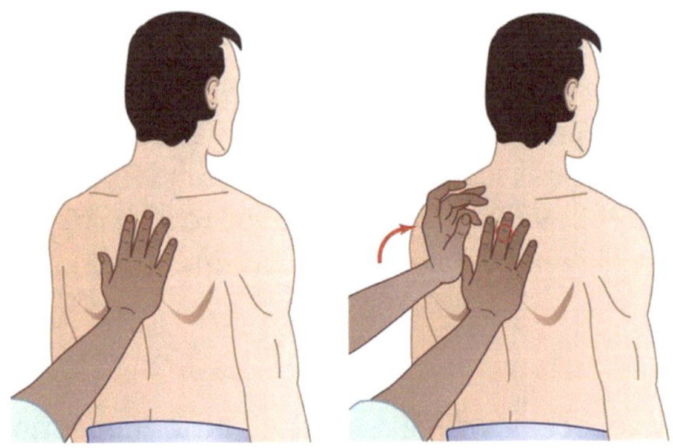

Figure 1.12. Palpation and percussion of health assessment in nursing.

Source: https://external-content.duckduckgo.com/iu/?u=https%3A%2F%2Fnursekey.com%2Fwp-content%2Fuploads%2F2017%2F04%2FB9780323075046000078_f007-003-9780323075046.jpg&f=1&nofb=1&ipt=e41dabd1e4ee98da95e71c991f946f219996c8e19bf5fda306c16662420d36e9.

Palpation and percussion use also mark the broader role of nurses as key agents in the healthcare continuum. Competence in these tools is directly attributable to the quality of nursing practice delivered. As highlighted in nursing process research, compliance with established clinical standards is vital to deliver safe and effective patient care. For instance, if the nurses adhere to the process standards set forth by the regulatory bodies such as the Nurses and Midwives Council of Malawi, then they are going to execute palpation and percussion better, resulting in better patient outcomes from various medical procedures (Lengu et al., 2011; McClave et al., 2015). Thus, ongoing training and education in these skills is a basic requirement for nursing practitioners to offer quality care and to respond effectively to the dynamic demands of their patients (Figure 1.12).

1.3.3. Auscultation and Vital Signs

Auscultation, being an essential part of health assessment in nursing, is a fundamental technique for the assessment of physiological functions via the stethoscope. Not only is this method used for the identification of normal and abnormal sounds from the heart, lungs, and bowels, but it also increases nurses' general knowledge regarding patients' health. Mastering auscultation involves the interplay of theoretical understanding and applied skill so that the nurse can properly interpret different sounds. In addition, proper auscultation can have a great impact on clinical decision making so that early intervention is possible.

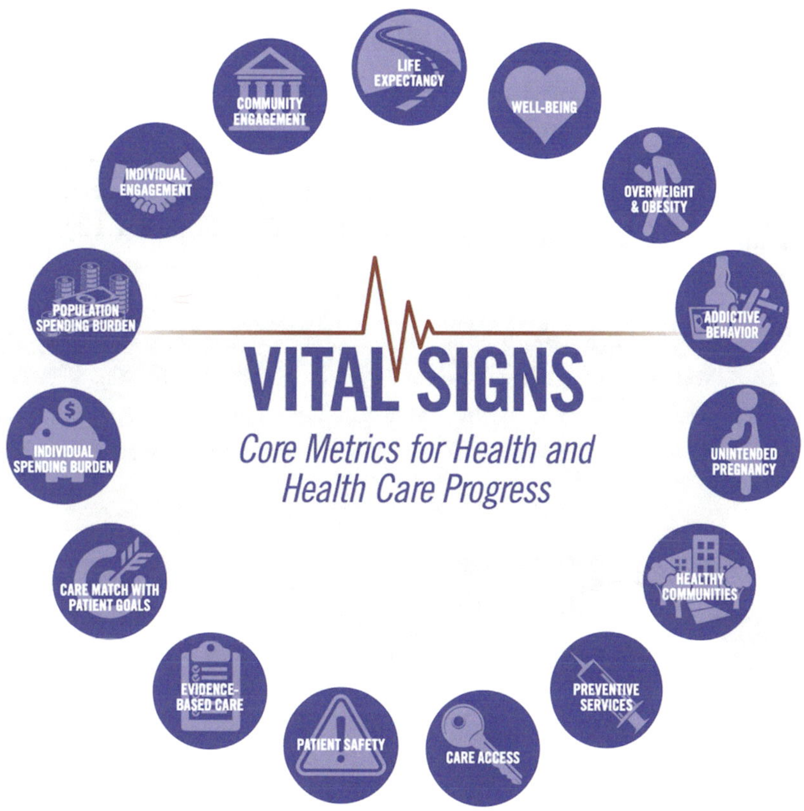
LIFE EXPECTANCY
WELL-BEING
OVERWEIGHT & OBESITY
ADDICTIVE BEHAVIOR
UNINTENDED PREGNANCY
HEALTHY COMMUNITIES
PREVENTIVE SERVICES
CARE ACCESS
PATIENT SAFETY
EVIDENCE-BASED CARE
CARE MATCH WITH PATIENT GOALS
INDIVIDUAL SPENDING BURDEN
POPULATION SPENDING BURDEN
INDIVIDUAL ENGAGEMENT
COMMUNITY ENGAGEMENT
VITAL SIGNS
Core Metrics for Health and Health Care Progress

Figure 1.13. Vital signs.

Source: https://external-content.duckduckgo.com/iu/?u=https%3A%2F%2Fi.pinimg.com%2Foriginals%2F50%2F4e%2F36%2F504e36fb9ca0beb15fce2a77dff8fde8.png&f=1&nofb=1&ipt=5255f31921bb1a03de85b3c5586759bfb9bdedf4b8a97b4efee3bf900c6ba217.

A solid auscultation base is critical in nursing education so that new practitioners can implement this basic assessment tool into the practice environment contextually and with confidence, as outlined in competency profiles articulated in nursing curricula (Bowker et al., 2023). The vital signs of heart rate, respiratory rate, blood pressure, and temperature form another critical element of patient assessment in nursing practice. By monitoring the signs systematically, nurses can quantify patients' physiological state and detect changes from normal ranges that may portend the onset of medical conditions. Not only is the practice useful in the detection of acute illness, but it also plays a crucial role in tracking the effectiveness of treatment regimens.

For instance, alterations in vital signs can be an indication of response to treatment or the development of complications and thus need immediate clinical evaluation. Besides the individual patient evaluation, vital sign aggregate data can also provide a window into general patterns of health and inform nursing care models, making them essential in health assessment (Honeyman, 2021). Also, the inclusion of auscultation and vital sign assessment in nursing care practices shows a holistic patient care approach. Both elements work synergistically to present health care professionals with an enhanced observation of patient health. For example, variations in vital signs may be even better explained by analyzing the results of auscultation to make diagnosis more accurate. Nurses must therefore be technically competent in measuring vital signs and auscultation, but also competent in synthesizing these findings to make effective nursing diagnoses and interventions. Through the acquisition of such critical thinking and integrative abilities, nursing education can prepare practitioners to provide improved patient care and respond effectively to evolving health conditions, making patient safety and health the primary concerns in practice (Bowker et al., 2023) (Figure 1.13).

Test Your Knowledge

1. What are the four primary techniques used in physical health assessment, and how are they applied?
2. How does proper technique in inspection, palpation, percussion, and auscultation improve diagnostic accuracy?

1.4. Cultural Considerations in Health Assessment

Learning Outcome

1. Understanding cultural competence;
2. Impact of culture on health beliefs;
3. Strategies for culturally sensitive assessments.

Cultural influences in health assessment are most vital in guaranteeing the active facilitation of effective practice nursing that responds to diversified patient needs. Failure to appreciate the variations in culture could lead to miscommunication, misinterpretation, and inadequate care, particularly in a contemporary multicultural population. For instance, the variation in belief by various societies concerning health, sickness, and therapy may have significant influences on patients' outlook towards medical prescriptions and intervention. The addition of culturally sensitive practices, such as suggested by Allen et al. (2015), allows nurses to navigate such differences and build trust with patients. Through respecting cultural origins, practitioners of health can modify their assessment methods to better suit values and perspectives of patients, ultimately leading to better health outcomes and patient satisfaction. Moreover, cultural factors recognition transcends being aware and entails becoming involved in the health assessment processes by using empathy and active listening. Culturally competent health assessment requires nurses to use culturally sensitive approaches when assessing or taking patient histories, e.g., by the use of interpreters or cultural liaison persons. It not only legitimizes information gathering but also asserts respect for the patient's culture. Understanding specific cultural practices and cultural health preferences is also crucial in the management of health disparities, as highlighted by Bushy et al. (2000). This way, healthcare providers can make interventions that are culturally appropriate to the patients' cultural identity, thus enhancing compliance with health regimens and offering a more holistic guidance to care. Lastly, the significance of health assessment based on cultural factors is due to their capacity to strengthen the patient-provider relationship, which is crucial in effective healthcare delivery. Culturally responsive assessments form a foundation for free communication and enable patients to express their concerns, resulting in a clearer perception of their health needs. This is a vital link, particularly in rural and underprivileged communities where the differences in culture may be more prominent, as elucidated by Bushy et al. (2000). By prioritizing culturally competent care, nurses not only enhance patient involvement and adherence to treatment plans but also encourage an open healthcare environment that respects and embraces differences. Thus, the inclusion of cultural elements in health assessment becomes the focus of the assumptions of nursing practice so that every patient receives equitable and effective care designed precisely for their unique conditions (Figure 1.14).

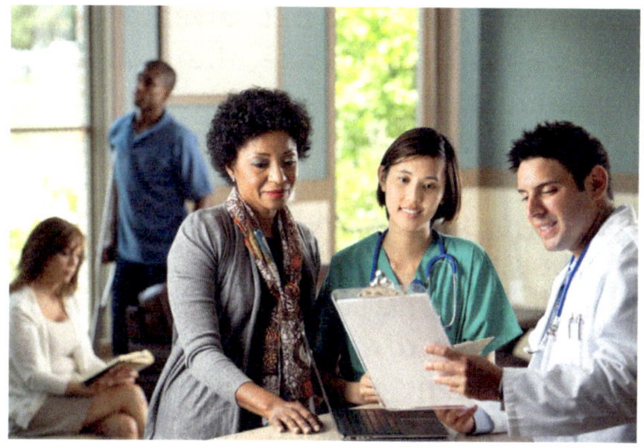

Figure 1.14. Cultural considerations in health assessment in the field of nursing.

Source: https://nevadastate.edu/wp-content/uploads/2024/07/shutterstock_482961049-1-1-scaled.jpg.

1.4.1. Understanding Cultural Competence

Cultural competence is a fundamental aspect of nursing practice, guiding effective health assessment and enabling equitable care for diverse populations. Cultural competence in the healthcare setting is characterized by the capacity to understand and integrate patients' cultural context, beliefs, and values in practice. This information has a tangible impact on the quality of care in the sense that it enables nurses to create an environment in which patients are valued and understood. Lacking cultural competence, miscommunication and misunderstanding may occur, potentially resulting in insufficient assessment and treatment. According to studies, only 30% of acute care nurses are considered culturally competent, creating a huge gap in education and training that needs to be overcome for improving nursing practice and outcomes (Virani et al., 2009). Encouraging awareness of cultural differences not only enhances patient-provider relations but also complies with the ethical responsibilities of nursing in the provision of holistic, patient-focused care. Educational programs aimed at enhancing nurses' cultural competence should tackle diverse cultural practices and emphasize the importance of communication. The provider-patient relationship must be handled with cultural sensitivity since this promotes equitable care across various groups. Public Law 106–129 and Public Law 106–525 underscore the importance of culturally competent communication to bridge barriers to healthcare access among racial and ethnic minorities. By the use of systematic assessment and intervention that is geared towards culturally sensitive practices, healthcare institutions can work to reduce health disparities brought about by cultural misunderstandings (Keys et al., 2012). Successful training interventions should not only include theoretical knowledge but also involve practical experiences in term of training nursing students to work with diverse populations with respect and empathy. Moreover, integrating cultural competence into nursing practice is inevitable in an attempt to tackle health disparities that exist among diverse communities. The evidence indicates that culturally competent behaviors will foster effective intercultural communication, which is a driving factor in improving health outcomes. As nursing educators develop curricula more complex, they must focus on flexibility and cultural humility and encourage future nurses to embrace the complexity of individual patient backgrounds. The findings throughout many studies consistently point toward the necessity of assisting nurses to become culturally competent practitioners because this has long-term patient satisfaction and quality of care consequences (Virani et al., 2009). Lastly, shifting nursing education to further focus on cultural competence will better equip nurses to navigate the nuances of patient interactions, providing the entryway for improved healthcare experiences for all.

1.4.2. Impact of Culture on Health Beliefs

Culture plays a key role in shaping health beliefs, deciding how people perceive illness, treatment methods, and compliance with medical advice. Variations in cultural backgrounds might lead to different explanations of the causation of health issues, influencing how individuals respond to healthcare systems. For instance, a qualitative study among Nigerian immigrants with hypertension in Sacramento demonstrated that participants blamed hypertension on genetics, stress, and eating habits rather than purely lifestyle or individual activities (Iroegbu et al., 2016). These culture-influenced beliefs not only affect the way one understands health but also dictate responses to medical interventions, as the person might engage in traditional treatments as opposed to prescribed medication. This division points to the value placed on healthcare practitioners being aware of the cultural origin for patients' perceptions of health in order to facilitate holistic and patient-tailored evaluations. Cultural beliefs also play an impact on attitudes towards medication compliance, a pivotal factor in effective control of chronic disease. Forgetting and concern about side effects was found to be strong predictors of adherence by patients to antihypertensive medication in the aforementioned study. Respondents showed that while prayer was a cross-cultural practice employed to seek psychological recovery, it did not directly influence adherence to medication schedules (Iroegbu et al., 2016). This highlights the complexity of conceptions of health, whereby religious rituals are coupled with anticipations of medical treatment, normally creating a tension between adherence to instituted interventions and conventional rituals. To ensure proper care, nurses must pick up on these nuances and promote open communication with patients so that means through which cultural beliefs may prove to be obstacles as well as facilitators to effective health management can be discovered. There also cannot be a stronger stress on the role of cultural competence within nursing training because it is directly linked to the potential of nursing professionals in providing culturally suitable care. Research on the effectiveness of Modified Simulation Learning Methods in enhancing cultural awareness of nursing students indicated statistically significant improvement in cultural awareness that supports systematic education can better enlighten health-related cultural variables. Promoting cultural sensitivity through training enables future nurses to deal with variable health beliefs patients can possess. The incorporation of cultural competency in nursing education systems eventually provides support for the delivery of holistic care, enabling practitioners to assess and manage beliefs regarding health and ultimately enhance health outcomes in the varied patient populations. Such alignment with cultural values has the potential to bridge healthcare disparities and build patient trust and compliance with treatment regimens (Figure 1.15).

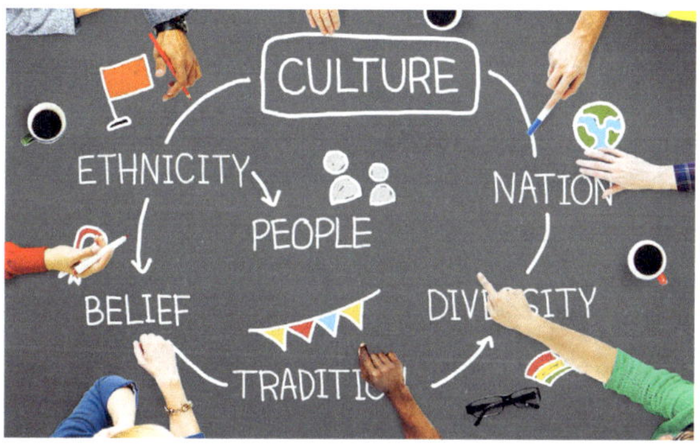

Figure 1.15. Impact of culture on health beliefs in the field of nursing.

Source: https://cdn.statically.io/img/rendia.com/wp-content/uploads/2015/12/patient-education-culture-e1627910739827.jpg?quality=100&f=auto.

1.4.3. Strategies for Culturally Sensitive Assessments

Culturally sensitive nursing diagnoses play a vital role in effective and individualized care for a multicultural population. The first among these is an appreciation of cultural competence, which is the ability of healthcare providers to know and value the values, beliefs, and practices of different cultural groups. One must not only be aware of different cultures but also be self-aware while analyzing one's assumptions and bias. To advance this knowledge, nursing education programs increasingly include cultural training, which allows new nurses to undergo culturally sensitive scenarios. On this foundation, practitioners have a better ability to build trust with patients and provide a platform for open communication and effective assessments to flourish. These efforts can make a significant difference in reducing health disparities and patient outcomes because effective communication is the foundation of good care in nursing environments (N/A, 2020). Another helpful strategy for culturally sensitive assessment is the application of culturally sensitive tools and models. Nurses must adjust their practice of assessment to include measures sensitive to cultural difference and which accommodate variation in manifestation of health problems and symptoms among groups. For instance, employing validated instruments that have been designed for many different cultural contexts not only increases the validity of health assessment but also the reliability of information generated. In addition, collaboration with community leaders can ensure access to culturally tailored resources and information and thereby inform nurses about practice. Involvement of the local organizations ensures that the assessment is tailored to the needs of a population and thus fosters inclusivity and a sense of belongingness in the health care environment (Hossain et al., 2020). Lastly, patient participation in the assessment process becomes unavoidable in creating cultural sensitivity. Through this strategy, nurses are encouraged to employ a participatory approach where patient feedback is integrated in the assessment and planning for care. By querying patients directly about their cultural backgrounds and personal beliefs about health, nurses are able to create individualized care plans that are relevant to the values of the patient. This patient communication not only increases patient satisfaction but also enhances treatment compliance. Furthermore, awareness of the social determinants of health through a patient's culture allows nursing practitioners to address barriers that might hinder access to care. In total, this cooperative strategy promotes nurse-patient relationships and facilitates comprehensive health screenings with sensitivity to cultural variations (N/A, 2020).

Test Your Knowledge

1. How can a nurse ensure that cultural beliefs and practices are respected during a health assessment?
2. What are common cultural barriers that might affect the accuracy of health assessments?

1.5. Technology in Health Assessment

Learning Outcome

1. Electronic health records (EHR);
2. Telehealth and remote assessments;
3. Use of diagnostic tools and equipment.

The application of technology to health screening is essentially transforming the practice of nursing, with the role of electronic health records (EHRs) being quite important in the administration of patient information. Not only are EHRs making it easy to accumulate and store patient data, but they also facilitate improved communication among providers of care. As discussed by Leamon et al. (2016), the increasing application of EHRs mandates adaptation by providers and patients to this model of technology, where the online platform integrates as a part of the healthcare experience. Education programs can help overcome perceived obstacles to effective communication that will enhance both patient and provider satisfaction. This adaptability is needed to improve the quality of care as it encourages even more inclusive and accurate data collection and increases patient satisfaction in general. Technology's function is therefore essential in maximizing nursing workflows and assessments efficiency. The introduction of advanced digital tools and instruments, as well as software, in recent years further increased the role of technology in health assessments in nursing. These technologies permit real-time observation of patient status, providing nurses with the potential to monitor vital signs and other key information around the clock. Using sophisticated analytics, nurses are able to detect patterns and make sound decisions quickly, increasing their capacity for responding to patients' needs. The research conducted by Daily et al. (2019) illustrates how digitization of perioperative processes improves not only the operational effectiveness but also a patient-centric approach to provide optimized results. Such technologically facilitated approaches make it possible to collect comprehensive patient information, thus better evaluation accordingly. The shift towards a digitally facilitated healthcare ecosystem is indicative of commitment towards efficiency as well as enhanced patient care in the course of assessment. Furthermore, developments in telehealth technologies have redefined health assessment by extending the scope of nursing services beyond the walls of health institutions. Telehealth technologies enable nurses to conduct assessments at a distance and provide care to patients in other locations while reducing travel hindrances and access to health facilities. Widening the scope of nursing practice not only provides greater convenience to patients but also facilitates timely interventions based on real-time assessment. The importance of taking advantage of technology in health assessment goes a long way, as evident in the ability to integrate data from telehealth consultations into electronic health record systems and maintain continuity of care and full health histories. Embracing such technological advancements thus presents a critical foundation for future nursing practice, reinforcing the essence of being flexible in an evolving healthcare system (Figure 1.16).

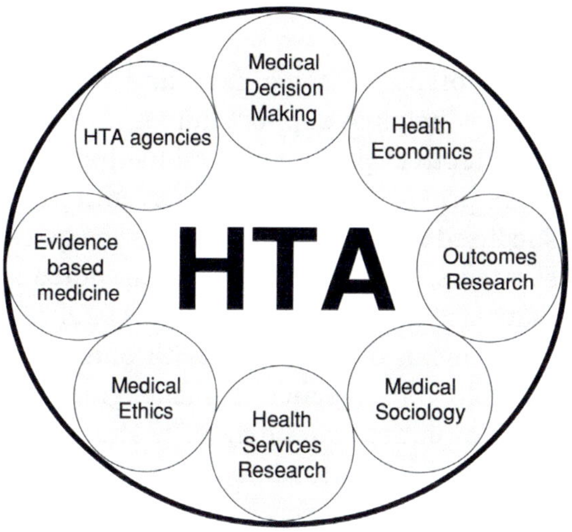

Figure 1.16. Technology in health assessment.

Source: https://about.nested-knowledge.com/wp-content/uploads/2024/03/image1.png.

1.5.1. Electronic Health Records (EHR)

The integration of Electronic Health Records (EHR) into nursing practice significantly enhances health evaluations through the enablement of an expedited documentation process and increased data access. EHRs are digital repositories of patient information that allow for concurrent updates and facilitate informed decision-making by healthcare professionals using up-to-date clinical data. This is particularly relevant to nursing because accurate assessments are vital in the determination of patient need and planning of appropriate interventions. Through the application of EHR systems, nurses can perform more comprehensive assessments and monitor patient outcomes effectively. The interoperability of the systems also enables healthcare professionals working in various facilities to access relevant patient information, ensuring continuity of care and eliminating errors. This way, EHRs fundamentally alter the dynamics of health assessments toward efficiency and accuracy of patient care. One of the primary strengths of EHR systems is the role they play in enhancing better medication management and reducing medication errors. As evidenced by current studies, EHRs incorporating computerized provider order entry (CPOE) have provided a significant reduction in medication errors, besides patient safety. This kind of improvement is significant in nursing, where the administration of medications is a key element in the care of patients. In addition, EHRs facilitate coordination of multi-disciplinary teams by providing access to the shared, up-to-date list of medications. Not only does this minimize redundant testing, but it also encourages communication among providers, resulting in better coordination in addressing patient health assessment. Therefore, the use of EHRs in nursing practice becomes essential not only for quality improvement in assessment but also for creating a safer healthcare environment overall. With all the benefits associated with EHRs are also the persistent challenge in its implementation and ongoing use in nursing settings. Early phases of EHR implementation are usually plagued by user dissatisfaction, as staff usually experiences more documentation time due to the learning process that accompanies new technology. Also, effective utilization of EHRs to facilitate health assessment relies on correct training and acclimatization by nursing staff. To ensure that nurses leverage EHR capabilities to their fullest, organizations must invest in far-reaching training programs for usability and system interoperability. Continuous technical support will also be required to overcome barriers to system use as well as build an adaptive culture within nursing professionals. As EHRs continue to develop, addressing these areas will be pivotal to maximizing their potential for enhancing health assessment in nursing practice (Figure 1.17).

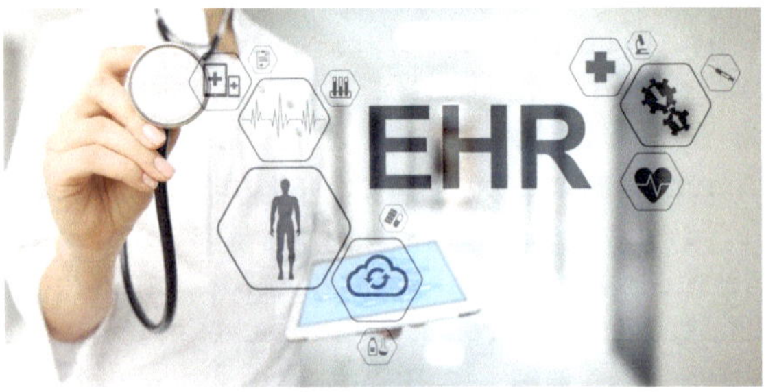

Figure 1.17. Electronic health records (EHR).

Source: https://cdn.prod.website-files.com/650c1bee516c4e723b11b29a/66903433b4ceb00453c8fac2_AdobeStock_286040030.webp.

1.5.2. Telehealth and Remote Assessments

Telehealth has significantly altered the delivery of healthcare, transforming the manner of conducting nursing assessments. Telehealth is a cutting-edge method of utilizing technology to facilitate in-real-time consultations between patients and providers in real-time, providing care conveniently in remote areas. Telehealth has made it possible for nurses to conduct assessments virtually, thereby widening their coverage to underserved populations and facilitating easy access for individuals to seek care. This shift not only enhances the role of patients but also empowers people so that they become active participants in managing their health. With telehealth continuing to develop, it will definitely have an important contribution to make in the shaping of nursing assessment methods so that more patient-centered treatment is embraced and serves the needs of today's diverse population more effectively. Blending telehealth with health screenings is a paradigm shift in the process of obtaining and analyzing healthcare data. With digital platforms, nurses can conduct detailed screenings—collecting vital health information and monitoring chronic conditions—without in-person visits. Telehealth's potential is amplified with the integration of artificial intelligence (AI), which can filter through vast pools of data to assist nurses in making informed clinical decisions. Not only does AI technology make it easier to assess, but it enhances the precision of diagnosis and individualization of care plans as well.

This blend of telehealth and advanced technology helps to support nurses in building more effective patient relationships, since they can provide immediate interventions and personalized health information based on quicker assessments, thus optimizing patient outcomes and satisfaction. While the potential benefits are possible, incorporating telehealth and remote assessment into practice is challenging. Legal and ethical patient confidentiality and security concerns remain foremost, as healthcare systems increasingly rely on digital technology to hold sensitive health information. Nurses must navigate through these complexities while remaining compliant with statutes such as HIPAA. Additionally, there is a critical need to provide massive education and training to health professionals and patients in order to facilitate the effective use of telehealth technologies. In this way, nursing can embrace the potential promises that telehealth holds to offer while patient safety and trust must continue to take precedence in care. With the development of telehealth, its fundamental function in health evaluations will redefine nursing practice, opening avenues for greater health delivery and outcomes in different populations (Bekbolatova et al., 2024; N/A, 2023) (Figure 1.18).

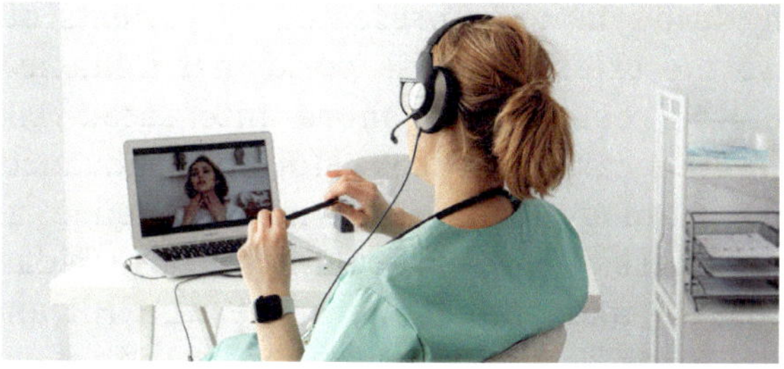

Figure 1.18. Telehealth and remote assessments.

Source: https://solutionchamps.com/blog/wp-content/uploads/2022/03/How-Remote-Patient-Monitoring-1-aspect-ratio-1108-500.jpg.

1.5.3. Use of Diagnostic Tools and Equipment

The use of diagnostic tools and equipment is critical in nursing, as it permits the precise and effective examination of patient health by clinicians. These tools, ranging from the uncomplicated device of a stethoscope to the advanced imaging technology of MRIs and CT scans, all provide critical information that informs clinical practice. With the advent of technology in the health industry, nurses nowadays employ sophisticated diagnostic equipment not only to record vital signs but also to perform sensitive analysis that is advantageous to patient care. Thus, the integration of diagnostic equipment in nursing practice not only facilitates the identification of underlying health conditions but also allows for preventive care of health, eventually resulting in improved patient care and satisfaction. Moreover, diagnostic equipment is not only applicable in-patient care but is also a training and education requirement in nursing education. Simulation teaching, for example, has emerged as a more important component of nursing education, offering the right platform to learn to handle diagnostic equipment in a safe environment without putting patients at risk. As discussed by Heyes et al. (2018), simulations have proven effective in training nursing students with hands-on knowledge for application in real-life situations using the tools as they replicate clinical environments where diagnostic skills are applied. Through the practical sessions, potential nurses acquire skills in the application of various diagnostic tools, hence producing a workforce that is able to deal with patient assessment without any challenges once they join the healthcare sector. The evolving environment of health technology demands from nurses the ability to use diagnostic tools and equipment effectively. There is a need for continuous professional training and development to update nursing professionals on advances in diagnostic technologies. Just as in workforce research, such as that in N/A (2005), demands for nurses with such skills are increasing, thus necessitating the provision of appropriate training. In practice, proficiency in the operation of diagnostic equipment not only enhances clinical judgement but also supports the nurses role as a key member of interprofessional health care teams. As such, ongoing emphasis on the appropriate use of diagnostic devices and apparatus remains a fundamental aspect of nursing, required in providing quality, patient-centered care.

Test Your Knowledge

1. How have modern technologies, such as electronic health records and diagnostic tools, enhanced health assessment?
2. What are the benefits and limitations of using telehealth for conducting health assessments?

1.6. Challenges in Health Assessment

Learning Outcome

1. Barriers to effective assessment;
2. Ethical considerations in assessment;
3. Addressing biases and assumptions.

Nursing health assessment is invariably complex and provides a range of challenges that can distract the precision and effectiveness of care provided. Cultural competency's role in health assessments is one of the highlighted challenges. Cultural origins are varied among health professionals, influencing patient interaction and symptom interpretation. Slightly poor cultural practice and belief knowledge may lead to miscommunication and misdiagnosis, thereby impacting outcomes. As Curtis et al. (2019) puts it, the transition to cultural safety over mere cultural competency is concerned with ensuring healthcare workers critically evaluate power relations and their respective cultures. This shift aims to build a more equitable healthcare culture whereby appraisals are more in line with patients' cultural reality, thereby enhancing the validity of health evaluation. But still another pressing issue in health appraisal is the way to integrate social determinants of health into appraisal. These are social determinants such as socioeconomic status, education, and access to healthcare, which have a strong impact on health outcomes but are normally not considered in appraisal. Integration of these determinants into appraisal is challenging because nurses are not adequately trained to work on the problems of socioeconomic determinants of health. Today, as identified by Allen et al. (2016), there is increased recognition of the interconnected nature of health and the determinants of the social kind, with implications for a biopsychosocial model of evaluation. This transdisciplinary model opens up space for nurses to consider not only physical symptoms presented by patients but also the external social world that influences health, resulting in more integrated and targeted care practices. Moreover, advances in technology bring about new challenges in health assessment, particularly concerning data accuracy and patient privacy. With EHR and telehealth becoming more the reality, using the digital platform brings questions about the management of patient data and potential data entry errors. Inaccurate records can lead to significant discrepancies in health assessments if not effectively managed. Also, technology is the key to more efficient measurements, but it can become a limiting factor in nurse-patient interactions, where focus will be moved away from the patient and towards the display (Gray et al., 2019). The solution to the issue depends on constant training and keeping attention on not letting the human factor in healthcare be passive, so technology becomes an assistive factor and not a reducer of the quality of health assessments (Allen et al., 2016; Curtis et al., 2019).

1.6.1. Barriers to Effective Assessment

Effective health evaluation in nursing is often frustrated by sophisticated obstacles in patient care. Inconsistent assessment practices among medical professionals is one of the foremost obstacles. Variability in assessment techniques can lead to inconsistency among patient results, as nurses will rely on personal subjective experience rather than universally recognized practices. The absence of an ordered framework undermines the authenticity of health evaluations, ultimately leading to potential misdiagnosis or inability to recognize critical health issues. Moreover, without standardizing guidelines, nursing education and training may inadvertently overemphasize generic skills rather than distilling unique assessment skills demanded by different clinical situations, ultimately affecting overall patient safety and patient care quality (N/A, 2020). Cultural dynamics also play an important role in health assessment success in nursing. Cultural competency, as the ability of health professionals to understand, value, and interact with individuals of diverse backgrounds, continues to be unevenly integrated into nursing practice and education. This lack perpetuates miscommunication or misunderstanding of patients' health attitudes and needs. Inadequate training in cultural safety nurses might unconsciously apply stereotypes or biases in assessing, which undermines rapport and trust with patients. Addressing this obstacle involves comprehensive strategies to avoid critical consciousness and ensure that healthcare workers critically reflect upon their own cultural bias. These strategies are crucial for achieving equitable health results (Curtis et al., 2019). Another critical obstacle is suboptimal resource availability, including time, training, and nurse support systems, when conducting assessments. Time is usually scarce in the majority of healthcare environments, especially in those with high patient-to-nurse ratios. Hurrying to meet pressure can lead to rushed encounters, omitting important patient symptoms and lowering the quality of care. In addition, the unavailability of tools and technology to be utilized may make the process of assessment even more difficult. Adequate training for utilizing such means is required to foster a culture of quality in health assessment. It is essential that healthcare organizations invest more in advanced training programs and possess mechanisms to support nurses in their efforts to offer comprehensive assessments and thereby enhance overall patient care and outcomes.

1.6.2. Ethical Considerations in Assessment

The foundation of ethical guidelines in health assessment lies in beneficence, non-maleficence, autonomy, justice, and confidentiality. All of these are necessary in establishing the nursing practices and ensuring that patient assessment is conducted in consideration of people's rights and their welfare. Beneficence refers to the need for the treatment that will bring good to the patient, and non-maleficence refers to the obligation to do no harm. In nursing assessments, these ethical considerations require practitioners to be cautious in their assessment processes, without displaying biases that will lead to discriminatory treatment outcomes. Furthermore, the respect for patient autonomy requires nurses to engage patients in consultations about their care, thus establishing a culture of cooperation that fosters both trust and compliance in health assessments (Alshammari et al., 2024). Conflicts usually arise in interdisciplinary healthcare settings where roles are interchanged, potentially complicating decision-making on ethical matters during assessments. The blending of different professional viewpoints, including pharmacy, laboratory services, and nursing, can lead to role confusion and blurring of responsibilities. These concerns highlight the importance of effective communication among healthcare professionals so that ethical standards are not only recognized but also upheld. For instance, in the assessment of transgender patients, nursing assessments are not only required to acknowledge but also enable gender-affirming care, thus promoting justice and equity in health results. Inadequate understanding or bias can result in significant variability in health among susceptible populations (John et al., 2024). Nursing professionals are thus required to navigate these complexities with a passion-driven commitment to ethical requirements that prioritize patient welfare. Further, technology progress in health evaluation offers challenges and ethical concerns that need to be dealt with cautiously. Telehealth services and electronic health records have transformed the way evaluation is conducted, enhancing efficiency and accessibility. However, the technologies also raise concerns for patient confidentiality and information security. Nurses need to be sensitive to maintaining ethical principles that protect sensitive patient information when working with such emerging technologies. Informed consent issues get complex when technology elements are included, particularly when patients are not fully aware of what happens to their data sharing. As such, while nurses change with emerging equipment and methods of health appraisal, they must stay attentive to ensuring ethical practices at all times and balancing technological benefits against ensuring patient rights and dignity (Alshammari et al., 2024).

1.6.3. Addressing Biases and Assumptions

In nursing practice, assumptions and bias must be dealt with to promote equitable health assessment. Nurses will apply their own individual cultural background, beliefs, and values to patient interactions, leading them to, unconsciously, influence their perceptions and opinions. These biases must be recognized through a conscious examination of one's own values and their impact on patient care. Through the use of models that encourage critical reflection and self-analysis, nursing professionals can start to sort out their own experiences from clinical judgments. When nurses consciously work through this reflective process, they develop a more humane environment that recognizes the diversity of patients' backgrounds, ultimately resulting in better health outcomes. Leadership development, as described in contemporary models of nursing, extends this self-knowledge further by restating the importance of cultural competence in health assessment practice (Miles et al., 2019). Further, the integration of awareness of bias within education is critical to educate the next generation of professionals who will possess profound knowledge of factors that make health assessment complicated. Training workshops on the importance of biases can prepare nursing students to recognize and overcome stereotypes that can be barriers to patient care. For instance, educational curricula can be enriched with case studies highlighting instances in which assumptions have led to discrepancies in treatment or misdiagnosis. In a culture of questioning and challenging assumptions, nursing students can be turned into critical thinkers to deliver patient-centered care. This paradigm change is all about creating a culture of continuous learning and debate among the nursing personnel to ensure competency in preventing biases and providing equal health examinations (Wynsberghe et al., 2012) is enhanced overall. Finally, the ethical impact of omission in areas of bias and assumptions during health examination cannot be overstressed. Such omission not only undermines nursing practice but can actually undermine patient dignity and trust, particularly among marginalized groups. Both care ethics and ethical theories focus on respect, dignity, and empathy in patient care, which necessitates nurses to confront their own intrinsic prejudices. Employing a value-sensitive design approach, healthcare professionals can design systems that prioritize patient-centered care and against which they can defend against prejudicial healthcare behaviors. As technology penetrates more deeply into patient care, ethical examination of these innovations must also consider the potential for design and implementation processes to be biased. Ultimately, by acknowledging and attempting to counteract biases, nurses can fulfill their ethical responsibility to practice compassionate and fair healthcare to all (Wynsberghe et al., 2012).

Test Your Knowledge

1. What are common challenges healthcare providers face in obtaining accurate health assessment data?
2. How can patient-related factors, such as communication difficulties or anxiety, impact the effectiveness of health assessment?

SUMMARY

The controversy over the origins of health assessment in nursing, there is a need to recognize the overall impact that holistic health assessments make on outcomes in patients. Through the application of comprehensive approaches to assessment, nurses can significantly improve the quality of care provided to their patients, particularly in settings dealing with vulnerable populations, i.e., the elderly in long-term care hospitals and nursing homes. Evidence has shown that data-sharing platforms and geriatric assessments contribute to important chronic disease improvement, including diabetes and medication safety. Randomized controlled trials have shown that such interventions contribute to polypharmacy reduction and enhanced cognitive function among elderly individuals, demonstrating the value of a health assessment process in improving patient health and preventing adverse effects (Choi et al., 2024). Furthermore, inclusion of holistic models in health assessment, such as Social Return on Investment (SROI), reflects the paradigm shift of measuring clinical outcomes and other social factors in nursing practice. As the healthcare setting becomes more advanced, incorporating approaches reflecting economic, social, and environmental results is imperative in achieving sustainable public health interventions. This encompasses a balanced analysis that analyzes stakeholder impacts while making sure health measurement is beneficial not just to people's welfare but also community welfare. By entwining SROI analysis and traditional evaluation methods, nurses can more effectively comprehend the intricate value of health interventions as well as align their care with holistic and community-focused goals. Lastly, the conclusion of this essay summarizes the necessity of continued adaptation and refinement of health assessment in nursing. Through the analysis, it is evident that leveraging technological advancements and integrating multidisciplinary models are fundamental steps toward ensuring optimal patient care. Nurses, therefore, are obligated to commit to lifelong learning and embracing innovative assessment methods tailored to new health care needs. By doing so, they will not only advance the profession but also be key to addressing present health problems, providing an integrated patient care approach that ultimately leads to improved health for all populations.

The foundation of nursing health assessment rests on a full understanding of the fundamental principles upon which good practice is based. A key element is the necessity for stringent needs assessments, which situate health assessment activity in the specific needs and priorities of the patient group. Not only will such an approach optimize assessment relevance, but the rate of successful intervention will also be optimized. By identifying local health needs and resources, nurses can tailor their assessment and interventions to community need. Moreover, tailoring these assessments encourages better understanding between healthcare providers and populations being treated, ultimately leading to improved health outcomes and greater public trust in the healthcare system. This emphasis on contextual appropriateness is rooted in the implicit assumption of patient-centered care, a core guiding principle of nursing care. Apart from that, continuous monitoring and evaluation (M&E) of health assessment methods is crucial for the sake of continuing to make nursing practice effective in the long run. M&E allows adjustments and improvement of assessment methods in a bid to catch up with newer trends in health. By adopting regular evaluations, nurses can keep an eye on the effectiveness of their assessment procedures, identify gaps in practice or knowledge, and strive to update their methods accordingly. Furthermore, useful data generated by M&E can attract new partners and investments, thereby supporting the sustainability of health assessment activities. Evidence-based findings enhance the credibility of health programs and can potentially guide further policy enhancement, ultimately amplifying their impacts on public health. This self-reinforcing cycle reflects the usual pursuit of excellence among nurses and is consistent with global goals for improved healthcare systems. Secondly, incorporation of health assessment practice into local health systems can help to optimize resource utilization and sustain it. Incorporation of available resources and infrastructure into planning for health assessment contributes to their efficiency and community responsiveness. According to the Merck Vaccine Networks initiative, interventions must operate with available local resources while simultaneously putting in place enabling supervision systems to facilitate knowledge transfer and utilization among healthcare personnel. Such a strategy not only enhances the capacity of nurses but ensures that interventions achieve long-term impacts over funding cycles. By doing so, health assessment is one activity that translates into part of a comprehensive health initiative, providing a sustained context for providing high-quality care. Embedding such learnings in nursing practice is beneficial to the larger objective of enhancing public health outcomes through strategic and informed health assessment.

KEY TERMS FROM THIS CHAPTER

- Health Assessment
- Subjective Data
- Objective Data
- Nursing Process
- Inspection
- Palpation
- Percussion
- Auscultation
- Vital Signs
- Health History
- Chief Complaint
- Review of Systems
- Physical Examination
- Holistic Assessment
- Cultural Competence
- Clinical Judgment

CRITICAL THINKING QUESTIONS

1. **What is the primary purpose of a comprehensive health assessment in nursing?**
   a. To diagnose the patient's disease
   b. To establish a baseline of health and identify deviations
   c. To prescribe medication
   d. To perform invasive procedures
2. **During a physical assessment, the nurse uses inspection, palpation, percussion, and auscultation. These techniques are collectively known as:**
   a. Laboratory tests
   b. Diagnostic procedures
   c. Physical examination techniques
   d. Health history assessment
3. **Which component of health assessment focuses on the patient's beliefs, values, and cultural practices?**
   a. Physical assessment
   b. Psychosocial assessment
   c. Functional assessment
   d. Vital signs assessment
4. **When collecting subjective data from a patient, the nurse primarily:**
   a. Measures vital signs
   b. Performs a physical examination
   c. Asks about symptoms and health history
   d. Observes laboratory results
5. **Which statement about objective data in health assessment is correct?**
   a. It is based on the patient's feelings and perceptions
   b. It includes measurable and observable findings
   c. It is collected solely through patient interviews
   d. It is less reliable than subjective data

Short Answer Questions

1. What are the primary purposes of performing a comprehensive health assessment in nursing practice?
2. Differentiate between comprehensive, focused, ongoing, and emergency assessments, and give an example of when each would be used.
3. What key components should be included when taking a nursing health history, and why is it important to establish rapport with the patient?
4. What are the four primary techniques of physical assessment (inspection, palpation, percussion, auscultation), and when is each technique used?
5. What are the normal ranges for temperature, pulse, respiration, blood pressure, and oxygen saturation, and how can variations indicate health problems?

Answer to Critical Thinking Questions

1. (b) 2. (v) 3. (b) 4. (c) 5. (b)

REFERENCES

1. Agency for Healthcare Research and Quality. (2020). *Registries for Evaluating Patient Outcomes: A User's Guide.* https://doi.org/10.23970/ahrqepcregistries4 (accessed on 16th July 2025).
2. Aletta, F., Botteldooren, D., De Vriendt, P., Devos, P., et al. (2017). Monitoring sound levels and soundscape quality in the living rooms of nursing homes: A case study in Flanders (Belgium). https://core.ac.uk/download/147044767.pdf (accessed on 16th July 2025).
3. Allen, K., & Spitzer, W. (2016). *Social Work Practice in Healthcare: Advanced Approaches and Emerging Trends.* https://doi.org/10.4135/9781483398532 (accessed on 16th July 2025).
4. Alshammari, K. S. F., Albakr, M. S. B., Almughamis, F. K. S., Albugami, D. M., Alkhabbaz, G. G., Khrami, S. A., Al-Enazi, S. H. S., et al. (2024). Ethical considerations in laboratory, pharmacy, and nursing collaboration: Challenges and solutions. *International Journal of Health Sciences.* https://www.semanticscholar.org/paper/56fe88cb1df11204e5edada16af9da04674cf462 (accessed on 16th July 2025).
5. Al-Shammari, M. A., Jaafar, J. S., & Elfeshawy, R. (2024). The role of electronic health records in improving pediatric nursing care: A systematic review. *Egyptian Pediatric Association Gazette.* https://www.semanticscholar.org/paper/1e9703f65ee7774d3e7739a0ca733faa16efe355 (accessed on 16th July 2025).
6. Ashcroft, D., Howe, A., Pearson, P., Sheikh, A., et al. (2010). Learning about patient safety: Organizational context and culture in the education of health care professionals. https://core.ac.uk/download/2764975.pdf (accessed on 16th July 2025).
7. Atanas, H., Health Wales NHS, Cardiff Trust, Aounallah-Skhiri, H., et al. (2023). Integration of social return on investment with health impact assessment and evaluation frameworks. *The European Journal of Public Health, 33.* https://www.semanticscholar.org/paper/b34d73982c46ef5ab3abd94228c6985ec5377653 (accessed on 16th July 2025).
8. Bekbolatova, M., Mayer, J., Ong, C. W., & Toma, M. (2024). Transformative potential of AI in healthcare: Definitions, applications, and navigating the ethical landscape and public perspectives. *Healthcare, 12,* 125–125. https://doi.org/10.3390/healthcare12020125 (accessed on 16th July 2025).
9. Bowker, D., & Kerkove, K. (2023). Social determinants of health in nursing education: Integrating into curriculum and practice. https://doi.org/10.31274/isudp.2023.147 (accessed on 16th July 2025).
10. Bushy, A., & Baird-Crooks, K. (2000). *Orientation to Nursing in the Rural Community.* https://www.semanticscholar.org/paper/ea4394950d674aef906b3e919f4c9eeaef6480d8 (accessed on 16th July 2025).
11. Choi, J. Y., Kim, H., Chun, S., Jung, Y., Yoo, S., Oh, I. H., Kim, G. S., et al. (2024). Information technology-supported integrated health service for older adults in long-term care settings. *BMC Medicine, 22.* https://www.semanticscholar.org/paper/859556cd0ff482499929e29f7bda9b3ac879b926 (accessed on 16th July 2025).
12. Curtis, E., Jones, R., Tipene-Leach, D., Walker, C., Loring, B., Paine, S. J., & Reid, P. (2019). Why cultural safety rather than cultural competency is required to achieve health equity: A literature review and recommended definition. *International Journal for Equity in Health, 18.* https://doi.org/10.1186/s12939-019-1082-3 (accessed on 16th July 2025).

13. D'Ignazio, C., & Klein, L. (2020). *Data Feminism*. The MIT Press eBooks. https://doi.org/10.7551/mitpress/11805.001.0001 (accessed on 16th July 2025).

14. Daily, S., Doster, B., Lewis, C., Ryan, A., et al. (2019). Business process redesign in the perioperative process: A case perspective for digital transformation. https://core.ac.uk/download/289123784.pdf (accessed on 16th July 2025).

15. Gilmore, J. P., Dainton, M., & McEvoy, N. (2024). Ethical considerations for the nursing care of transgender patients in the intensive care unit. *Nursing in Critical Care, 30*. https://www.semanticscholar.org/paper/febcf036f46a3ff3069bfe845899fddac3ae732c (accessed on 16th July 2025).

16. Gore, J., Komashie, A., & Mousavi, A. (2007). A review of historical developments of quality assessment in industry and healthcare. https://core.ac.uk/download/333784.pdf (accessed on 16th July 2025).

17. Harvey, G., & Kitson, A. (2015). PARIHS revisited: From heuristic to integrated framework for the successful implementation of knowledge into practice. *Implementation Science, 11*. https://doi.org/10.1186/s13012-016-0398-2 (accessed on 16th July 2025).

18. Heyes, M. E., Muckler, V. C., Schnitzen, L., Starr, D., et al. (2018). Recertification and reentry to practice for nurse anesthetists: Determining core competencies and evaluating performance via high-fidelity simulation technology. https://core.ac.uk/download/213088562.pdf (accessed on 16th July 2025).

19. Honeyman, L. (2021). Personal use of handheld fetal Doppler monitors by women in New Zealand. https://doi.org/10.26686/wgtn.14132339.v1 (accessed on 16th July 2025).

20. Hossain, M. S., Muhammad, G., & Guizani, N. (2020). Explainable AI and mass surveillance system-based healthcare framework to combat COVID-19 like pandemics. *IEEE Network, 34*, 126–132. https://doi.org/10.1109/mnet.011.2000458 (accessed on 16th July 2025).

21. Iroegbu, B. (2016). A phenomenological assessment of factors that affect medication adherence among hypertensive Nigerian immigrants. https://core.ac.uk/download/129532354.pdf (accessed on 16th July 2025).

22. Keenan, T. (1992). The promise at hand. https://core.ac.uk/download/71346880.pdf (accessed on 16th July 2025).

23. Keys, T. R. (2012). Behaviors that eliminate health disparities for racial and ethnic minorities: A narrative systematic review. https://core.ac.uk/download/56703666.pdf (accessed on 16th July 2025).

24. Khosravi, H., Shum, S. B., Chen, G., Conati, C., Tsai, Y. S., Kay, J., Knight, S., et al. (2022). Explainable artificial intelligence in education. *Computers and Education Artificial Intelligence, 3*, 100074–100074. https://doi.org/10.1016/j.caeai.2022.100074 (accessed on 16th July 2025).

25. Kirkham, R., Boyle, J., Whitbread, C., Dowden, M., Connors, C., Corpus, S., McCarthy, L., et al. (2017). Health service changes to address diabetes in pregnancy in a complex setting: Perspectives of health professionals. *BMC Health Services Research, 17*. https://www.semanticscholar.org/paper/d5a8ab6d6866c2f34eab846e7c7caee7b768edd0 (accessed on 16th July 2025).

26. Krekhovska-Lepiavko, O., Lokay, B., & Volkov, R. K. (2023). Health assessment and promotion in nursing practice. *Медсестринство.* https://www.semanticscholar.org/paper/626e84a9ffbb556e2248a7f93ba3f6aa7139484b (accessed on 16th July 2025).

27. Leamon, A. E. (2016). The electronic health record scorecard: A measure of utilization and communication skills. https://core.ac.uk/download/79664897.pdf (accessed on 16th July 2025).

28. Lengu, E. S. (2011). The quality of professional practice by registered nurses and midwives in central hospitals in Malawi. https://core.ac.uk/download/654998583.pdf (accessed on 16th July 2025).

29. Mason, M. A. (2007). Equality in health: An annotated bibliography with resources on health disparities and cultural and linguistic competency. https://core.ac.uk/download/71346571.pdf (accessed on 16th July 2025).

30. McClave, L. M. (2015). RN-BSN program: On-demand, online, competency-based modules. https://core.ac.uk/download/217256941.pdf (accessed on 16th July 2025).

31. Miles, J. M., & Scott, E. S. (2019). A new leadership development model for nursing education. https://core.ac.uk/download/286544013.pdf (accessed on 16th July 2025).

32. Mittenthal, R. A. (2002). Effective philanthropy: The importance of focus. https://core.ac.uk/download/75782017.pdf (accessed on 16th July 2025).

33. Miura, T., & Kanoya, Y. (2025). Fall risk assessment and prevention strategies in nursing homes: A narrative review. *Healthcare, 13.* https://www.semanticscholar.org/paper/4c28aa4c6b4c16455c7af01395eb4d0e90f5f84f (accessed on 16th July 2025).

34. Murtiwi, M., Novieastari, E., & Wiarsih, W. (2012). Modified simulation learning method on knowledge and attitude of nursing student's cultural awareness at Universitas Indonesia. https://media.neliti.com/media/publications/149506-EN-modified-simulation-learning-method-on-k.pdf (accessed on 16th July 2025).

35. N/A. (2005). Looking ahead: Workforce supply/demand analysis for New Jersey's pharmaceutical and medical technology industries. https://core.ac.uk/download/71341926.pdf (accessed on 16th July 2025).

36. N/A. (2008). 2008 assessment report. https://core.ac.uk/download/71346066.pdf (accessed on 16th July 2025).

37. N/A. (2013). Complex care management program overview. https://core.ac.uk/download/71362332.pdf (accessed on 16th July 2025).

38. N/A. (2015). Advancing care excellence for seniors: Reflections on a John A. Hartford Foundation-funded nursing education program. https://core.ac.uk/download/80510596.pdf (accessed on 16th July 2025).

39. Organization for Economic Co-operation and Development. (2023). *Health at a Glance 2023. Health at a Glance.* https://doi.org/10.1787/7a7afb35-en (accessed on 16th July 2025).

40. Ozenbaugh, R. L., & Pullen, T. M. (2014). *Developing Practical Nursing Skills.* Routledge eBooks. https://doi.org/10.1201/b16551 (accessed on 16th July 2025).

41. Patty, C. M. (2014). A novel method for assessing medication-related adverse outcomes in a community hospital. https://core.ac.uk/download/70419796.pdf (accessed on 16th July 2025).

42. Potter, H., & Kahlenberg, R. D. (2012). Redesigning nursing education: Lessons learned from the Oregon experience. https://core.ac.uk/download/71358817.pdf (accessed on 16th July 2025).
43. Rinderle, A., Hills, G., & Fiske, L. (2012). Boosting the immunization workforce: Lessons from the Merck Vaccine Network–Africa. https://core.ac.uk/download/71360220.pdf (accessed on 16th July 2025).
44. Tiwari, N., Troth, L., Barclay, A., Chilvers, J., Carpenter, L., & Turner, G. (2020). PP30 Pioneering education in a pandemic–A rapid response unit approach. *BMJ Simulation and Technology Enhanced Learning, 6.* https://www.semanticscholar.org/paper/db1ebbcca4be83803d0fdfb0e1718c5639755163 (accessed on 16th July 2025).
45. Valparaiso University. (1990). *Graduate Catalog, 1990–1991.* https://core.ac.uk/download/144553218.pdf (accessed on 16th July 2025).
46. van Wynsberghe, A. (2012). Designing robots for care: Care centered value-sensitive design. https://core.ac.uk/download/pdf/11487391.pdf (accessed on 16th July 2025).
47. Virani, M. (2009). Assessing culture competence among nurses in an acute care setting. https://core.ac.uk/download/223074332.pdf (accessed on 16th July 2025).

INTERVIEWING AND COMMUNICATION TECHNIQUES IN HEALTH ASSESSMENT

2

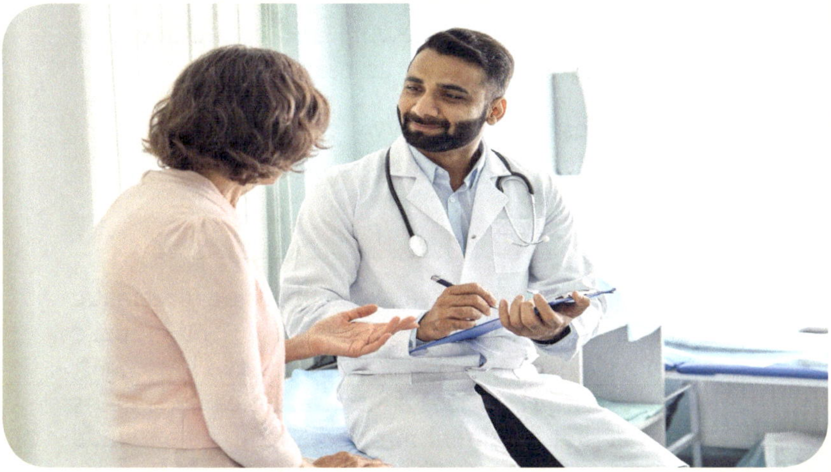

LEARNING OBJECTIVES

After studying this chapter, you will be able to:

1. Define the role of the interview in health assessment;
2. List the types of interviewing techniques;
3. Explain nonverbal communication in health assessment;
4. Describe cultural competence in health communication;
5. Explore ethical considerations in health interviews;
6. Focus on the challenges in health assessment interviews.

Introduction

In the context of health assessment, effective interviewing and communication skills are major elements to constructing healthy clinician-patient relationships. The first step not only sets the platform for gathering important health data but also sets the frame of trust necessary for a therapeutic relationship. Effective communication establishes mutual comprehension among the health professionals and the patients, which is essential in ensuring proper diagnosis and treatment. Given that research has proven communication failures among health teams to be among the most prevalent drivers of medical errors, there is a dire need for brief and compassionate interactions during the process of assessing health (Froehlich et al., 2016). Learning these skills, therefore, is not just a professional necessity but an ethical responsibility in delivering quality care. Active listening is central to effective health interviewing since it significantly enhances the quality of health care encounters. Active listening involves offering undivided attention to the patient, listening to their issues, and validating their experiences. Health professionals can enhance verbal and non-verbal communication skills through methods such as listening partnerships, leading to improved patient satisfaction and health outcomes. These kinds of methodologies create an environment in which patients are listened to and treated with respect, and this can encourage the sharing of information vital to their assessments. A systematic focus on communication skills in health professions programs recognizes a growing recognition of their importance; indeed, structured learning experiences have been shown to enhance students confidence in them (Chambers et al., 2016). Thus, these approaches play a significant role in the perceived and actual effectiveness of communication in health care settings. As health care keeps evolving, it is more important than ever to equip health professionals with quality communication tools.

The sophistication of contemporary healthcare settings, often encompassing interdisciplinary teams and diverse patient populations, necessitates sound communication approaches that transcend simple patient queries. Cultural competence proficiencies can help enable interactions by allowing providers to move through conversations considering the unique backgrounds of their patients. Through ongoing educational courses focusing on communication strategies, health professionals can enhance their capacity to adapt their approaches, ultimately reflecting in improved patient care. Enhanced communication skills can minimize misconceptions that often lead to patient dissatisfaction or disengagement. Thus, inclusion of effective interviewing and communication skills in health screenings not only improves personal interactions but also transcends overall health care delivery systems (Froehlich et al., 2016) (Figure 2.1).

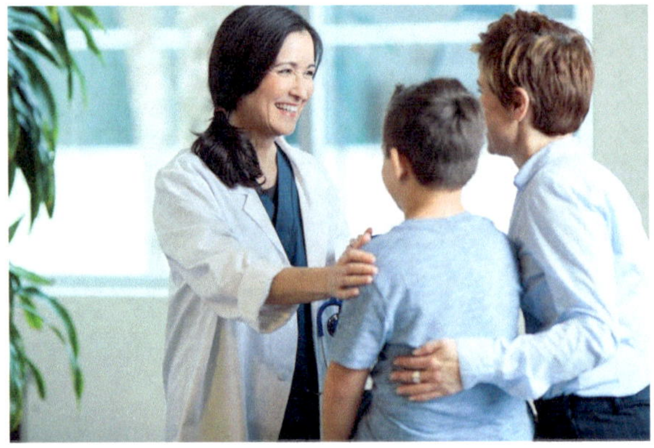

Figure 2.1. Interviewing and communication techniques in health assessment.

Source: https://www.usa.edu/wp-content/uploads/2020/02/Hero-2.jpg.

Definition of Health Assessment

Health assessment can be defined as a systematic and comprehensive review of an individual's physical, psychological, and social well-being. It is a critical part of clinical practice as it helps to gather pertinent information on the patient's health status, thereby helping with making accurate diagnosis and developing effective treatment regimes. Through a combination of interviews, physical examination, and other diagnostic tests, health professionals are in a position to identify health issues early enough so that there can be early intervention. Health testing is also not only concerned with diagnosing disease but also with prevention and promoting health. Through awareness of one's risk factors and health needs, practitioners are in a position to institute interventions that are proactive rather than reactive, eventually enhancing patient outcomes and lifestyle. Health screening success to a large degree relies on interview and communication skills by healthcare providers. A successful interview can establish a rapport between the patient and provider, a mood in which patients are open to sharing sensitive health information. This rapport is essential in gathering accurate information, which is essential in conducting a full health assessment. Effective communication skills such as active listening, open-ended questioning, and empathy can significantly enhance the quality of the health assessment process. Furthermore, such skills are vital in interpreting non-verbal behavior and breaking down possible health literacy barriers that may affect the patient's understanding and engagement in their health care (Brenda, 2020). In conclusion, the relationship between communication skills and the practice of health assessment is vital in providing optimal patient care. In addition to interpersonal skills, health assessments require a strong understanding of valid and reliable assessment tools and methods. Current literature indicates that scale development and validation are important to ensure health assessments are more accurate (Godfred et al., 2018). The use of standardized measures can lead to more consistent evaluations, thereby increasing the entire assessment process's reliability. Furthermore, the use of technology in health assessment, such as electronic health records and telehealth systems, has redefined patient data collection and processing. The new technologies assist in streamlining the assessment process, allowing for better collection and documentation of health information. Ultimately, the solution exists in an integrated method that combines effective communication, proper assessment tools, and technology to optimize the health assessment process and ensure comprehensive patient care.

Importance of Effective Communication in Health Assessments

Effective communication is crucial during health examinations as it has a direct impact on the quality of care offered to patients. When healthcare workers convey information briefly, empathetically to patients, they are able to clearly understand presenting complaints and medical histories. Such an increased understanding could lead to accurate diagnoses and tailored treatment plans. Effective communication also fosters patient-physician trust, which causes patients to question and raise issues freely. Through the application of skills such as active listening and open-ended questioning, healthcare professionals can draw out pertinent information that may otherwise be inadvertently left out. In the absence of strong communication skills, important information can be lost and lead to potential misdiagnosis or ineffective treatment planning across the continuum of care. Effective communication also enables patients to participate actively in health decisions, ultimately enhancing overall patient outcomes. The role of communication becomes even more pertinent when patients with communication impairments are being considered. Research indicates that patients with speech, language, or cognitive disorders report high levels of disability in health care settings, leading to feelings of decreased autonomy in decision-making. Such barriers contribute to increased risk for medical error and decreased overall patient satisfaction. Lack of adequate training among health care professionals on these domains of communication challenge reinforces the demand for curricula on effective communication skills tailored to different patient needs. Consequently, interventions geared towards enhancing medical students' ability to communicate with patients having communication disorders further bridge this gap in care. As evidenced by research assessing a communication curriculum, better student knowledge, self-efficacy, and clinical skills effectively prepare future health professionals to perform these valuable encounters, ultimately serving patient populations. In summary, the need for effective communication in health assessments cannot be stressed enough. It is required to gather accurate patient information, particularly in patients with communication disorders who may require specially adapted methods to facilitate conversation. Teaching health professionals communication skills not only prepares them to serve all patients' needs but also limits the risks of health miscommunication. With attention on effective communication, the healthcare system can move toward a patient-centered, inclusive model of care, further improving the health for all. Overall, the investment in communication training is a central element within the pursuit for enhanced healthcare quality and patient satisfaction, noting that communication is core to the very essence of health assessment (Baylor et al., 2019; François et al., 2019) (Figure 2.2).

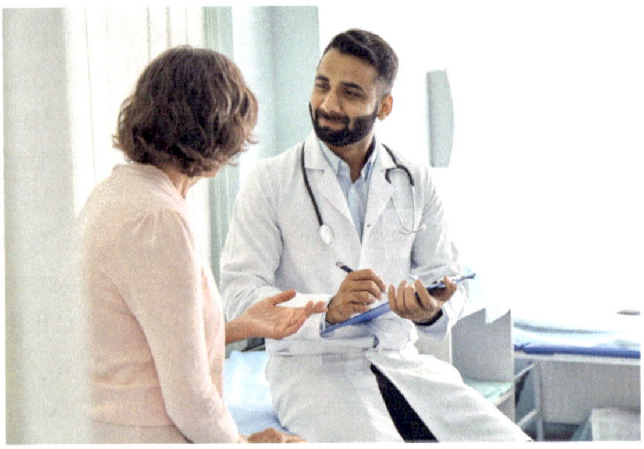

Figure 2.2. Effective communication in health assessments.

Source: https://online-learning-college.com/wp-content/uploads/2024/04/Effective-Communication-Skills-in-Health-and-Social-Care.jpg.

Overview of Interviewing Techniques

Interviewing skills are a part of effective health assessment, and enable clinicians to obtain essential information from patients. The structured interview is one such widely applied method and is a list of predetermined questions used to gain particular information in an effective and efficient way. The method is particularly helpful when time is short, as it allows interviewers to proceed with the essential information without crossing over into areas that are non-relevant. However, the systematic design can limit response quality because it does not leave much space for patient detail regarding experiences. Therefore, while structured interviews provide an advantage in collecting quantitative data, they will not necessarily achieve the rich and qualitative responses patients might provide with a less constrained design. Conversely, semi-structured interviews or unstructured interviews encourage more formal dialogue where patients are at liberty to express themselves. These approaches are particularly effective in health assessment requiring thorough knowledge of a patient's background, emotions, and personal history. Unstructured interviews are more likely to establish rapport between the clinician and the patient, with transparency and trust that could lead to greater insight into the patient's health condition. This kind of understanding is also vital when working with the psychosocial determinants that impact health outcomes and consequently compounding the necessity of the overall approach to patient care. The challenge lies in remaining focused and managing time because such interviews can generate diversionary conversations that might lose track of essential health issues. The use of technology in interview techniques has also transformed the practice of health assessment. For example, e-learning and mentoring have equipped health professionals with innovative strategies for enhancing communication skills, thereby enhancing interviewing as a whole. Digital platforms allow simulations of interactions with patients and practice in different interviewing styles, ultimately getting clinicians ready for adapting to changing patient needs. In addition, embedding mixed-method study approaches, such as assessing the multi-communication online training (MOT) program, can boost contextual fit and method feasibility for increasing competency among health workers (Ogunyemi et al., 2024). Hence, the evolution of interview skills with technological advancement not only promotes better communication but also advances the possibility of extensive and efficient evaluation of health, in line with the ultimate goals of public health promotion (Sinha et al., 2024).

2.1. The Role of the Interview in Health Assessment

Learning Outcome

1. Establishing rapport with patients;
2. Gathering comprehensive health histories;
3. Identifying patient concerns and symptoms.

The interview is the foundation of health assessment, and it provides a standardized yet flexible approach to gathering extensive information about a patient's medical history, symptoms, and psychosocial circumstances. Good interviewing skills allow clinicians to establish rapport, promote open communication, and gather useful information regarding the patient's experiences and perceptions of his or her own health. This first contact not only sets the tone for the helping relationship but also, to a significant degree, the quality of information that is obtained. A well-organized interview enables practitioners to establish relevant health issues, explore lifestyle issues, and define areas that require further investigation, providing the basis for a comprehensive and accurate assessment of health. Through the use of communication techniques such as active listening and empathetic questioning, workers are better able to understand patients unique contexts, a recipe ingredient for the delivery of person-centered care and patient adherence to treatment plans. In health assessment practice, the interview is utilized not only for the collection of factual information; it is a space for exploring patients attitudes, beliefs, and issues regarding their own health status and potential treatments. By adopting a person-centered approach, practitioners can structure their questions to exactly address the individual needs of each patient, resulting in higher levels of participation and trust. It is important to acknowledge the complexity of patient perspectives, particularly when health behavior is influenced by cultural, social, or psychological beliefs. The information that arises from the interview process can determine potential compliance barriers and instigate change, consequently driving the development of effective intervention plans. As has been shown in the context of vaccination communication, identification of underlying drivers of behavior, from lack of knowledge through to emotional response, has a significant impact on the success of healthcare interventions aimed at optimizing patient outcomes (Tuckerman et al., 2022). The effectiveness of interviews in healthcare evaluation can also be further enhanced through the use of motivational interviewing techniques.

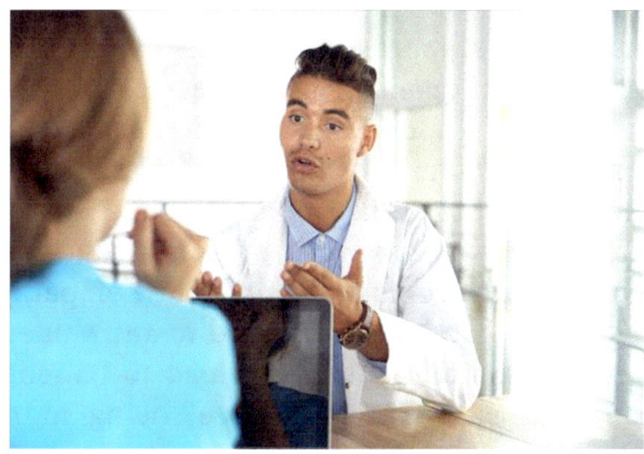

Figure 2.3. The role of the interview in health assessment.

Source: https://p-gpb8fhd4b9fbh6fy.z01.azurefd.net/cms/2a7f87ff-fabd-4664-92c9-b2e6d047e90f/fef6fa82-2d17-43ef-8767-79e502fcc15e-lg.jpg.

This is a technique that motivates clinicians to help patients to explore their motivation for change and resolve ambivalence about healthy behavior. Through the use of open-ended questions and reflective listening, health practitioners can enable patients to express their perceptions and feelings toward their health, leading to further understanding of their motivations and difficulties. This method is aligned with person-centered care, focusing on autonomy and engagement in health management. A study on diabetes education demonstrated how health professionals could enhance their person-centered communicating skills, which directly benefits patients via improved communication and a culture that promotes personal development and change (Stenov et al., 2017). Thus, the role of the interview in health assessment is not only to gather information but to create a partnership relationship that empowers patients and encourages healthier habits (Figure 2.3).

2.1.1. Establishing Rapport with Patients

Establishing rapport with patients is an integral component of quality health assessment, being the basis of good communication. The start of an encounter sets the mood of trust and honesty, vital to gathering good quality health information. Health workers are encouraged to exercise active listening and show empathy, making the patient feel listened to and valued. A positive initial contact can lead to patients feeling at ease and, therefore, being more truthful when asked sensitive questions about their health. The usefulness of the rapport is validated in numerous studies showing that if the patients believe that the doctors are friendly and genuinely care about them, then they are more likely to become participative in the process and supply critical information about their condition. Also, such practices as motivational interviewing have been identified to be crucial in setting up a situation appropriate for establishing rapport. More effectively, practitioners can identify the origin of patients' inherent motivation, and the obstacles to their health behaviors, with the help of this practice. Such practices not only enhance communication but also empower the patients during their healthcare journey. As emphasized in clinical situations, as in case management, gaining the patients trust through mutually respectful and collaborative interpersonal relations diverts attention from the treatment of merely clinical symptoms to an understanding of the patient as a whole. Entire person focus has utility in intervention planning that is suitable to the patient's own lifestyle and needs, eventually leading to sustainability of desired health improvement as referenced in literature on health management. Moreover, the blending of technology, such as clinical video telehealth, creates depths in the establishment of rapport, particularly among special needs populations, such as veterans. As healthcare professionals make the shift toward digital interfaces, the integrity of rapport has to be maintained even in virtual settings. The barriers for the physical assessment and patient assessments under the telehealth context identify preserving effective communication and building relationships through online channels as the problem. Best practices for the establishment of rapport not only remain essential but can also further enhance patient outcomes in distant locations. The recognition of the intricacies of such interactions enables health practitioners to modify their communication methods successfully, being able to address various patient needs, especially among specialized populations confronted with mental and physical complexities of healthcare as described in recent health communication research (Figure 2.4).

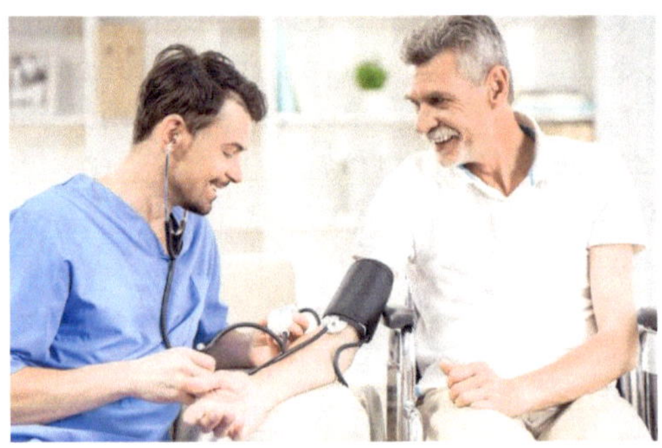

Figure 2.4. Establishing rapport with patients.

Source: https://www.nursebuff.com/wp-content/uploads/2014/03/how-to-build-rapport-with-patients-e1585752674568.jpg.

2.1.2. Gathering Comprehensive Health Histories

The collection of comprehensive health histories is a crucial aspect of successful health assessment since it is used as the foundation for treatment and diagnosis. A comprehensive health history helps the medical practitioners in finding information about the medical history, past diseases, surgeries, and drug history of a patient. All this information is crucial not only to learn about the existing health problems but also to decide upon the likelihood of genetic disorders that can affect the health of the patient. Adequate interviewing skills make it possible to collect such information, with professionals having to create an environment of trust and openness. Through active listening and empathy, health practitioners can encourage patients to talk on sensitive issues that may not have otherwise been expressed. Such comprehensive checks can lead to better health outcomes through the direction of person-centered treatment plans that are suitable to individual patient needs. In addition to history of medicine, collection process entails information regarding the patients psychosocial history, that is, their way of living, social setting, and emotional status. A good health history recognizes that social determinants of health contribute significantly to patient outcomes. Socioeconomic status, education level, housing, and access to resources in a community may influence an individual's access to health care and overall health behavior. Therefore, effective communication skills are necessary when exploring these factors during a health history interview. Having the ability to inquire using open-ended questions and engage patients in dialogue enables greater insight into their health and puts healthcare providers in the position to treat not only medical conditions but also social and emotional ones. This combined model is consistent with today's vision regarding patient-centered care and emphasizes attention to the patients lived experience. Also, the importance of taking in-depth health histories has ramifications that extend beyond caring for individual patients. Accurate documentation of health histories plays a crucial role in disease patterns identification among populations, and information from these histories may be used to inform community health programs as well as policy-making. For instance, understanding the prevalence of disorders such as Fetal Alcohol Spectrum Disorders (FASD) among certain groups can be used to guide preventive interventions in such high-risk groups. Concurrence on problem-solving by healthcare providers and application of diagnostic guidelines can lead to improved diagnosis and care for conditions as per prenatal exposure, as in the developments from (Hoyme et al., 2016).

These recommendations are a consensus from widespread practice and clinical experience, allowing practitioners to deliver informed and equitable care for every patient. The obtaining of comprehensive health histories then is not only a clinical necessity but also a contributing factor to advancing broader health equity efforts (Figure 2.5).

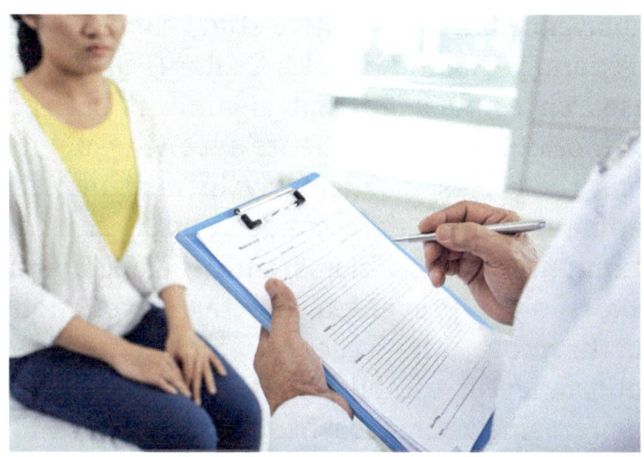

Figure 2.5. Gathering comprehensive health histories.

Source: https://www.unitekcollege.edu/wp-content/uploads/2022/01/shutterstock_454645918-1030x687.jpg.

2.1.3. Identifying Patient Concerns and Symptoms

One of the very key aspects of effectively identifying patient concerns and symptoms is the communication styles of healthcare providers. The quality of interactions between patient and provider significantly affects the quality of information gathered in the health assessment process. For instance, studies have established that physicians utilizing normalization statements and care and concern expressions in assessment are able to enhance the comfort of patients, thereby promoting more detailed discussions regarding sensitive topics such as suicidal ideation among depressed patients. This approach not only fosters a rapport-building environment but also permits a profound probing of concerns that are beneath the surface, permitting healthcare workers to establish concerns that would otherwise remain unspoken (Trena et al., 2023). Lastly, the ability to offer a place where patients feel comfortable sharing weaknesses is critical in ensuring correct diagnosis and care. Identification of patient complaints and symptoms requires a sensitive perception of the diverse population needs, as experienced in a qualitative study conducted at a Federally Qualified Health Center (FQHC). The research established that significant barriers are noticed among patients receiving mental health services, particularly in marginalized populations. Providers' condescending attitude, communication problems, and socioeconomic factors often prevented effective assessment. Furthermore, the research highlighted the importance of establishing rapport and using open, inclusive approaches to communication that have the potential to be enablers of patients' willingness to disclose their mental health problems (So et al., 2022). Through a recognition of these dynamics, healthcare practitioners are in a good position to engage in depth with patients and uncover the rich layers of their illness problems, and thus attain improved outcomes. The combination of sound interviewing skills and awareness of social determinants of health is important in the identification of patient symptoms and concerns. With improved communication skills, healthcare practitioners are also required to be aware of the individual history and situation of their patients. Culturally competent communication and empathic listening play an imperative role in communicating with patients from diverse racial and ethnic backgrounds because such determinants typically travel with the patient's perceived stigma against mental illness. Such appropriateness at inquiry and responsiveness to patient cues can be enhanced by healthcare providers through targeted training, which allows them to identify overt and hidden symptoms. This blended practice facilitates the patients to verbalize their issues, thereby making the health assessment process richer and leading to more individualized and effective interventions for care (So et al., 2022) (Figure 2.6).

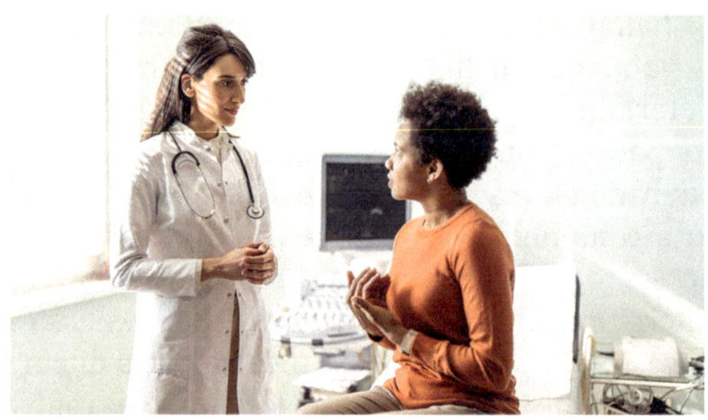

Figure 2.6. Identifying patient concerns and symptoms.

Source: https://www.cdc.gov/me-cfs/media/images/GettyImages-1473559421_1200x675.jpg.

Test Your Knowledge

1. How does a patient interview contribute to identifying the patient's health needs and concerns?
2. In what ways can effective interviewing improve the accuracy of a health assessmen\

2.2. Types of Interviewing Techniques

Learning Outcome

1. Open-ended questions;
2. Closed-ended questions;
3. Probing questions.

Interviewing skills are important components of good health assessment, serving as the cornerstone for establishing rapport, gathering thorough information, and enabling patient-centered practice. Of all the forms, structured interviews are favored since they are systematic in the way that the interviewer employs a set of established questions. Structured interviewing is uniform and simple to compare answers among different patients. By adhering to a specified format, structured interviews prevent variability and minimize bias, and therefore maximize the reliability of data collected. They also enable ease and focus during the interview, thus making patient needs easier to identify in healthcare practice. While structured interviews are useful, they can restrict the quality of patient responses, and therefore flexibility has to be introduced by other interviewing techniques in healthcare practice. Unlike structured interviews, semi-structured interviews offer a mix of focused questioning and conversational flexibility that permits health professionals to collect richer qualitative data. Semi-structured interviews make use of an overarching list of questions but permit interviewers to adapt their questions when gathering answers from patients. The flexibility is particularly beneficial in health assessment since it encourages a more detailed consideration of individual perspectives and experience. Moreover, semi-structured interviews allow the interviewer to react to emergent concerns or themes that arise during the interview, offering a more enhanced understanding of patient health and psychosocial concerns. This approach fosters active listening and responsive dialogue, not only for gathering information but also to facilitate patient engagement, thereby impacting improved health communication tactics required for wider patient care. In certain cases, particularly where sensitive issues are involved, unstructured interviews prove to be very helpful. Using this technique, it is possible to conduct an open-ended discussion where patients freely express their feelings, thoughts, and concerns without being hampered by a pre-set list of questions. In free-flowing conversation of this kind, it is possible to develop a strong therapeutic relationship since patients feel comfortable in offering more personalized and nuanced information about their path of health. Though perhaps time-consuming, unstructured interviews may provide rich information on emotional and social determinants of health lost with more structured interviews. Spontaneous discussion of problems can result in enhanced patient satisfaction and trust with a more holistic approach to assessment of health. For instance, the study highlighted the importance of affect in communication of health, focusing on the power interviewing has in bridging the gap between healthcare providers and patients, thereby meeting their individualized needs and wants in care (Rocha et al., 2024) (Figure 2.7).

Figure 2.7. Types of interviewing questions.

Source: https://pressbooks.library.ryerson.ca/communicationnursing/wp-content/uploads/sites/99/2020/06/Figure-2.4-1024x576.png.

2.2.1. Open-Ended Questions

Open-ended questions serve a fundamental function in the area of health assessments, primarily due to their ability to elicit extensive feedback from patients. The questions encourage individuals to expound on what they are thinking, experiencing, and going through without restrictions of pre-determined answers. When it comes to the area of health communication, the approach allows for a deep understanding of a patients circumstance since it allows space to question beyond symptoms. By having patients speak in detail about their health issues, practitioners can obtain valuable information that won't be found through closed-ended questions. Qualitative information is significant in building a whole picture of the health condition of the patient and can lead to more effective, individualized care plans. Open-ended questions also assist in the establishment of rapport between patients and health professionals. Use of these types of questions demonstrates a clinician's willingness to listen and interact, fostering the therapeutic alliance needed for successful healthcare results. When heard, patients are more likely to offer relevant health information, sustaining the development of trust. The emotional rapport is crucial, especially in delicate health discussions where patients may be hesitant to offer personal information. The merit of powerful interviewing strategies, including open-ended questions, is that effective interaction can significantly affect compliance and satisfaction rates among patients, facilitating good health behaviors and results. In addition to facilitating communication and information gathering, open-ended questions have the potential to empower patients in taking control of health issues. By asking patients to share their concerns and thoughts, health professionals help individuals take charge of their own health narratives. Such facilitation is particularly significant in motivational interviewing, where encouraging self-reflection and change talk are critical to changing behavior. Studies indicate that the incorporation of open-ended questions in health evaluation can enhance patients' knowledge about their health problems so they know the likely remedies and adopt healthier lifestyles (Halbach et al., 2017). Furthermore, the determination of various patient experiences through these questions will enable clinicians to personalize treatment strategies, ultimately producing a more patient-centric care system (Figure 2.8).

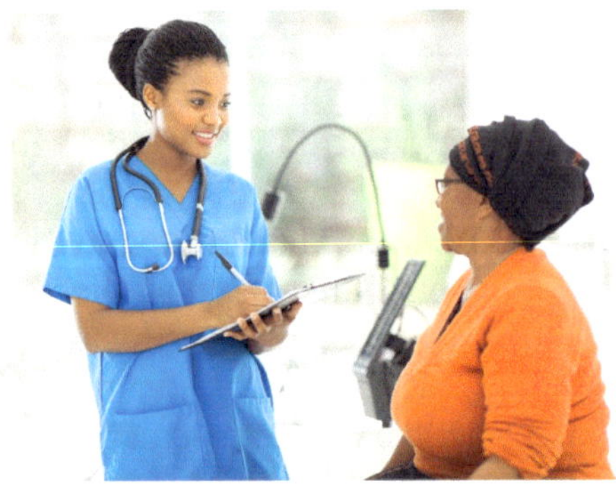

Figure 2.8. Open-ended questions of health assessments in nursing.

Source: https://external-content.duckduckgo.com/iu/?u=https%3A%2F%2Fs3.amazonaws.com%2Futep-uploads%2Fwp-content%2Fuploads%2Fhpu%2F2021%2F07%2F22093327%2Fclinical-nurse-leader-comminicating-patient.jpg&f=1&nofb=1&ipt=6454094001e03efd805c1e9c70d8de50028c86380cb625d5935b483eaeee6895.

2.2.2. Closed-Ended Questions

Closed-ended questions are a key part of health assessments, in that they allow clinicians to quickly get easy, measurable information from patients. Closed-ended questions typically have limited responses available to answer them, e.g., a yes/no or multiple-choice answer. This type of format not only simplifies response for patients, but analysis for medical staff as well. By using closed-ended questions, practitioners can speed up interviews so critical information is obtained in an efficient manner, particularly useful where time is in short supply, such as the emergency care environment. Where conditions of high stress or urgency apply, as in the case of paramedics working during the COVID-19 situation, closed-ended questions will decrease the respondent's mental load and improve the quality of information obtained (Barrett et al., 2024). Moreover, the worth of closed-ended questions is not only in the data gathering but also in personalizing patient communication and establishing rapport. Through effective utilization of such questions, healthcare providers can accurately measure patient experience and feeling. For instance, closed-ended questions can be beneficial in the measurement of lifestyle impacts on health conditions, as applied by research studies on lifestyle evaluation (Barrett et al., 2024). A mix in this case of both open and closed-ended questions can be employed to optimize the assessment process. Closed-ended questions can indicate areas which need further investigation, and therefore cause the clinician to ask more open-ended questions, creating a whole picture of the patient's lifestyle and health. But exclusive use of closed-ended questions can lead to an incomplete picture of the patient experience and feelings. Even though they are extremely proficient at gathering measurable data, they can restrict the patient's freedom to communicate the nuances of their situation or emotions. This limitation may :be so intense when performing health assessments where an understanding of a patient's complexities of their condition is critical. Thus, the inclusion of open-ended questions alongside closed-ended ones improves the assessment process by giving patients an opportunity to elaborate on their responses. By this approach, healthcare professionals can construct a more holistic picture of patients' health, leading to informed treatment and improved communication strategies supported by many studies measuring health outcomes (Kim et al., 2025).

2.2.3. Probing Questions

Among the steps involved in health assessment, the use of probing questions is a crucial approach to gathering adequate information from patients. The probing questions are not meant to evoke only positive or negative answers but comprehensive information that can better guide clinicians regarding patient experiences, symptoms, and issues. By using probing questions, health providers can facilitate open dialogue, through which the patients feel safe articulating themselves and their perceptions. This is consistent with the principles guiding patient-centered care, which involves an understanding of the whole human being as compared to the treatment of individual symptoms in a vacuum. Not only does this kind of interaction promote appropriate diagnosis but also strengthens the clinician-patient therapeutic relationship. The effectiveness of probing questions is also elevated when executed cautiously in addition to appropriate assessment tools and models. For instance, in family nursing cases, interrogation can help disclose family system dynamics so that nurses can assess how family relationships influence individual health outcomes. It has been shown through research that applying systematic techniques of questioning helps nurses gain essential information that supports tailoring of individualized interventions. By establishing an empathic environment where patients feel comfortable expressing themselves, clinicians can effectively deal with immediate physical health challenges as well as with psychosocial determinants that can influence overall well-being. This holistic view emphasizes the significance of competent interviewing competencies in health assessment, particularly in complex family cases (Argent et al., 2017). In addition, the significance of questioning inquiries to clinician training and preparation must not be underestimated. Educational courses that target the training of communication skills, particularly in family assessment, form a significant aspect of the education of future healthcare professionals to perform effective interviews. A case in point is the simulation- and role-playing-based practical training workshops that increase clinicians' confidence and competence in the use of probing questions. Evidence indicates a considerable increase in procedural confidence among practitioners following targeted training in communication skills, and that the integration of probing questions within curricula can lead to more effective and compassionate provision of healthcare (Jeremy et al., 2013). Thus, emphasizing the role of probing questions in health assessments not only enhances clinical practice but also advances a more well-rounded patient care experience (Figure 2.9).

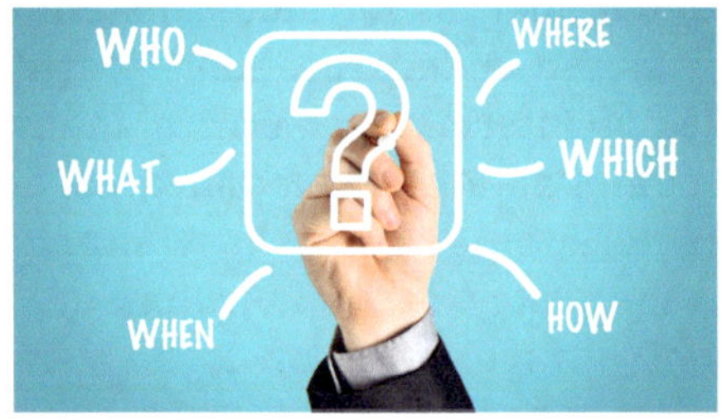

Figure 2.9. Probing questions.

Source: https://themindfool.com/wp-content/uploads/2019/10/400-Probing-Questions-Going-Beyond-Simple-Answers.jpg.

Test Your Knowledge

1. What are the differences between directive and nondirective interviewing techniques, and when is each most appropriate?
2. How can the use of open-ended versus closed-ended questions affect the information obtained during a health assessment interview?

2.3. Nonverbal Communication in Health Assessment

Learning Outcome

1. Importance of body language;
2. Eye contact and its implications;
3. Active listening skills.

Nonverbal communication plays a vital role in the process of health assessment as a very effective complement to verbal communication between medical professionals and patients. Within the professional environment, nonverbal cues such as postures, glances, and facial expressions can significantly enhance the credibility of the assessment process. Nonverbal cues often communicate empathy, concern, and professionalism, which are essential in establishing rapport with patients. When health professionals are sensitive to nonverbal indicators, they can more easily achieve a patient's psychological and emotional state, which is also crucial in getting effective treatment. For instance, anxiety or discomfort by a patient may be communicated by the manner in which they sit or do not make eye contact, providing health professionals with useful information that can be employed in directing the assessment and intervention. Furthermore, adding the nonverbal communication skills to the health assessment process can increase positive patient outcomes. The health care professionals exhibiting effective use of nonverbal communication are more likely to build trust, and these breeds open expression of worries. This openness is vital as it pertains to proper symptom reporting and complete assessments. According to healthcare training studies, emphasis on communication skills, both verbal and nonverbal, with the use of practical assessment modalities enhances the competency of medical professionals to perform optimally in real-life situations. This is particularly observed when one considers the importance of creating a healthy setting where patients are motivated and valued and thus promoted patient satisfaction and adherence to treatment procedures (Monique et al., 2024).

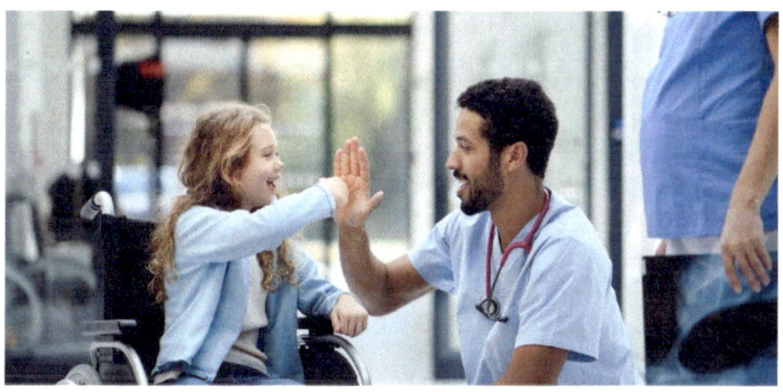

Figure 2.10. Nonverbal communication in health assessment in nursing.

Source: https://cdn.prod.website-files.com/63a1cbc81b0e903002cf9cec/65dd31e09d72b9a23d7c2449_Nursa%20Communicating%20with%20Nonverbal%20Patients.webp.

In health disparity environments, nonverbal communication plays a more critical role. There may be several patients from a variety of different backgrounds, where various nonverbal actions have distinct meanings. Being respectful of these differences then becomes crucial for effective communication. Training programs for healthcare professionals in nonverbal communication can lead to a culturally competent healthcare force. As it has been explored in research examining contextual appropriateness and deliverability of training in resource-poor settings, identification and use of nonverbal cues can bridge communication gaps and achieve health care equity of access (Ogunyemi et al., 2024). Finally, cultivating rich knowledge of nonverbal practices in communication can enhance health assessment so that healthcare is both effective and inclusive (Figure 2.10).

2.3.1. Importance of Body Language

Body language of an individual is one of the main contributors to the process of communication, especially in the case of health assessment. Nonverbal cues often convey feelings and messages that cannot be put into words. Patients' care providers during an interview must observe their own body language and that of patients. For instance, open and loose body position will facilitate a sense of security and trust, allowing patients to voice concerns freely. Closed postures, on the contrary, might induce barriers that will express disinterest or discomfort and negatively influence the interaction. Thus, competency in body language not only creates rapport but also facilitates the provision of correct health information because patients tend to communicate more positively with clinicians who are nonverbally expressive and empathetic. Moreover, the role of body language is also being observed in interpreting patient cues, which is a necessary aspect of health assessment. Patients will also express discomfort, anxiety, or confusion through body stance or positioning, and this generally reflects their psychological and emotional state. Having the capacity to observe these signs allows healthcare workers to intervene appropriately, modifying communication skills in order to serve the patients better. For instance, if a patient is restless or evasive of eye contact, the clinician may question further about such issues that the patient is reluctant to voice in the open. This reading skill of body language makes the clinician more aware and can inform more thoughtful and empathetic care, so that the patient's experience is as comfortable as well as complete. Appreciation of nonverbal communication is thus crucial in health interviewing. Finally, effective health assessment is routinely augmented by application of body language in a deliberate manner. Clinicians can employ gestures, body posture, and facial expressions to reinforce verbal messages, hence making their messages more powerful. For example, a leaning clinician who maintains eye contact can express interest and attention and thus encourage the patient more to give essential information about their health. The relation between verbal and nonverbal communication corroborates prevailing literature that highlights the significance of establishing clear, empathetic channels between healthcare providers and patients. As would have been recognized through the discussion of health science scale development, communication skills validation, including body language, also has the power to dramatically influence clinical practice outcomes, suggesting that effective implementation of these nonverbal methods has far-reaching implications for patient care and assessment (Godfred et al., 2018; Williamson et al., 2017).

2.3.2. Eye Contact and Its Implications

The significance of eye contact in health assessment cannot be overstated because it is a simple nonverbal communication skill. Proper use of eye contact creates a rapport between healthcare providers and patients and supports an environment of trust and honesty. Active and respectful follow-up by the clinician through the application of eye contact encourages patients to reveal more freely. This is particularly crucial when working with older adults with cognitive impairments, who may feel anxious or vulnerable during a clinical evaluation. Research demonstrates how non-verbal communication such as eye contact can significantly impact the participation and satisfaction of patients, improving decision-making within clinical settings (Mishari et al., 2025). In the end, proper eye contact is essential in creating an empathetic atmosphere centered on patient need and affirming the importance of communication in health examinations. Beyond mere attention, the power of eye contact extends to influencing the therapeutic relationship between doctors and patients. In the case of autistic individuals, for instance, even eye contact may be difficult, in that they may have issues with social signals and nonverbal messages (Thahaseen et al., 2025). Such patients must be adjusted to in terms of their eye contact approach by the clinicians in such cases. Intensity and duration modulation of eye contact can help close up communication gaps and decrease anxiety experienced by some clinical patients.

The recognition of these contrasts in preference and response to eye contact enables health practitioners to enhance their communication skills, which will consequently lead to enhanced rapport and patient outcomes. Apart from connecting and being adaptable to individuality, eye contact is crucial in transmitting empathy and empathy during health assessments. A good clinician who utilizes the strength of eye contact not only expresses their interest in hearing a patient's account but also conveys feelings and support by looking at him or her. This nonverbal assurance is also valuable for patients who may be experiencing sensitive health issues, in that it reinforces the notion that their symptoms are being observed and verified. As highlighted within recent literature, the integration of such communication within regular practice can support patient satisfaction, engagement, and general health outcome (Mishari et al., 2025). In general, eye contact is more than an inherent function in communication and is a decisive strategy in creating empathetic relationships in the field of health assessments (Figure 2.11).

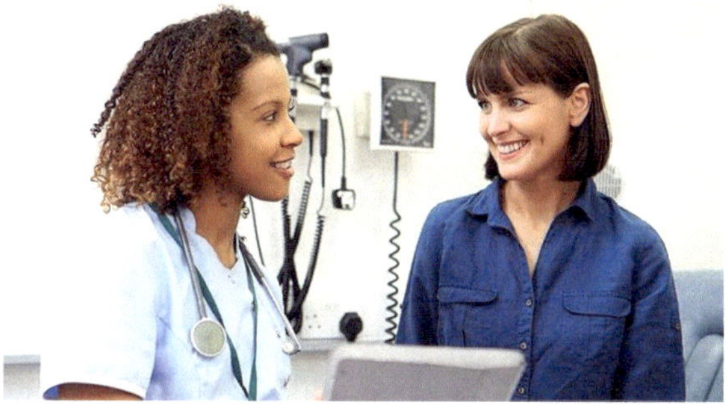

Figure 2.11. Eye contact of health assessment in nursing.

Source: https://media.nurse.org/cache/66/62/6662dd32009cb680737807aeae7f583b.jpg.

2.3.3. Active Listening Skills

Active listening skills are essential aspects of effective health assessment communication, facilitating increased patient participation and comprehension. Active listening in a clinical environment is not merely listening for the patient's words but instead the deliberate focus of the clinician on the speaker, both verbally and non-verbally. By applying skills such as paraphrasing, summarizing, and reflecting emotion, healthcare workers may express empathy and make the patient hear them out, feel valued, and respected. This is important in getting patients to share confidential health details, as it establishes a rapport that deepens the therapeutic bond. Given that the vast majority of healthcare interactions are time-limited, the ability to practice active listening can potentially impact the quality and effectiveness of provided care, patient satisfaction, as well as outcomes of health. Second, incorporating active listening into instructional sessions, even for Physician Assistants (PAs), speaks to its relevance in practice. Research indicates that over 70% of PA programs offer courses that provide training in motivational interviewing (MI) skills, which necessarily rely on active listening. In spite of this fact, there is insufficient comprehensive training in the skill of listening. While lecture remains the prevalent mode of teaching these skills, adding role-play and simulated patient interactions can enhance students' practical skills in active listening. These practice-based learning sessions have been discovered to support the practice of applying MI skills to ensure that subsequent PAs become skilled in communicating with their patients and, therefore, optimize health assessment processes (Halbach et al., 2017). In addition, patient teaching skills theoretical framework demands active listening in various healthcare settings. As outlined in current studies, patient-centered communication, including active listening, is crucial to successful patient care and activation. For patients to receive and comprehend, not merely receive, information, healthcare professionals must possess active listening and quick response skills. Through the utilization of skills borrowed from motivational interviewing, adult learning theory, and the teach-back technique, professionals can tailor communication to meet individual patient needs. This combined strategy not just maximizes patient satisfaction but also ensures ethical health consequences through active and assertive patients assuming control of their well-being (Bobay et al., 2018) (Figure 2.12).

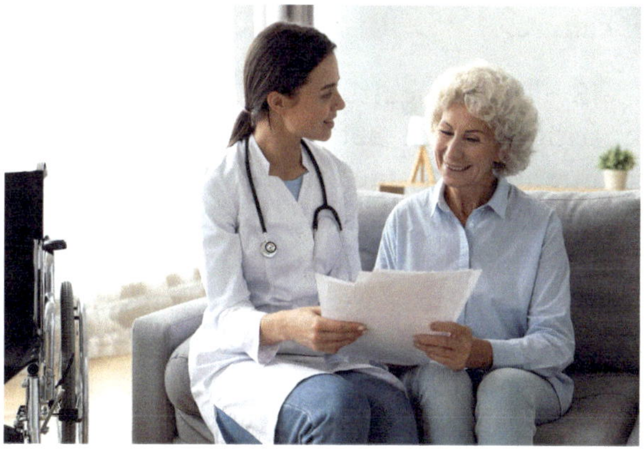

Figure 2.12. Active listening skills.

Source: https://www.oneeducation.org.uk/wp-content/uploads/2021/09/communication-skills-in-healthcare.jpeg.

Test Your Knowledge

1. How can a nurse interpret a patient's body language to gain additional insights into their health status?
2. What nonverbal cues might indicate that a patient is uncomfortable or withholding information during a health assessment?

2.4. Cultural Competence in Health Communication

Learning Outcome

1. Understanding cultural differences;
2. Adapting communication styles;
3. Overcoming language barriers.

Cultural competence is increasingly considered a central element of health communication success, particularly in multicultural health settings. Healthcare providers' ability to understand, communicate with, and engage with individuals from other cultures is part of being culturally competent. This set of skills is essential not only for establishing trust between the provider and patient but also in addressing health disparities that may be induced by miscommunication due to culture.

By being culturally competent, the practitioners can better accommodate their communication modes to the particular requirements of patients, thereby enhancing the overall quality of care. Cultural competence also facilitates patient-centered communication, allowing medical professionals to consider patients' cultural background health belief and practice, ultimately resulting in improved health outcomes (Ayako et al., 2024). Good health communication requires listening, a factor that is extremely crucial while communicating to diverse communities. Listening partnerships, a technique that has been showcased in recent studies, are where participants alternate listening and speaking to improve their communication (Froehlich et al., 2016). This strategy not only helps the provider to listen empathetically to their patient but also encourages a focus on non-verbal communication, which is more culturally dependent. By training medical professionals to employ such strategies, the chances of overcoming communication barriers rise, leading to further participative interaction. Thus, the development of effective listening skills, bolstered by cultural sensitivity, is an integral component of health professional training that ultimately enhances the health assessment process. In addition, the incorporation of cultural competence into health communication planning enables patients to convey their concerns and preferences within a context that is culturally sanctioned. If healthcare providers take the initiative to get familiar with the cultural history of their patients, it establishes an atmosphere of respect and trust. This is crucial, especially when patients are involved in their health experiences, which can be largely controlled by their beliefs and values. Studies indicate that patients have higher satisfaction and treatment compliance with respect to treatment plans when they have good communication because they feel respected and listened to (Ayako et al., 2024). Consequently, health assessment processes ought to prioritize cultural competence and offer practitioners the theoretical and practical competencies needed to effectively communicate in healthcare and eventually achieve equity in healthcare delivery (Figure 2.13).

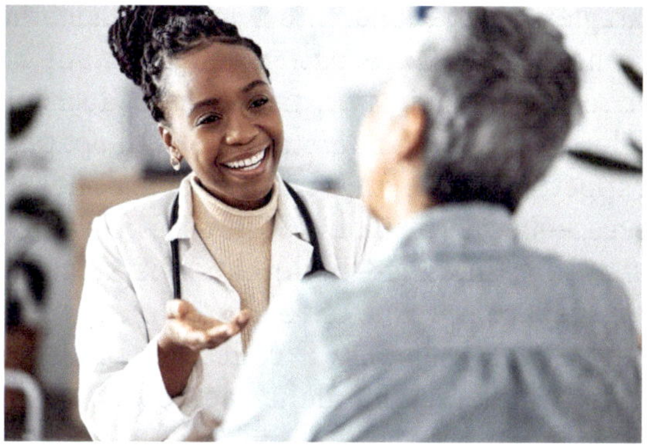

Figure 2.13. Cultural competence in health communication.

Source: https://publichealth.tulane.edu/wp-content/uploads/sites/3/2021/03/How-to-Improve-Cultural-Competence-in-Health-Care.jpg.

2.4.1. Understanding Cultural Differences

Appreciation of cultural differences is a fundamental component in the interviewing and communication competencies applied at the time of health assessment. The health care providers should recognize that patients possess diverse cultural backgrounds, which influence their health attitudes, illness, and health care behaviors. The cultural filter has a bearing on how individuals perceive their symptoms, understand health information, and make decisions regarding their treatment. Culturally sensitive communication optimizes the effectiveness of health assessment to enable the practitioner to build rapport and establish trust with patients. Moreover, it allows a culturally sensitive education and support that honors and respects cultural values. For instance, diabetes education must be tailored to suit the cultural background of families according to language, beliefs, and health customs (Olinder et al., 2022). Through an understanding of these cultural differences, health care providers can make the communication relevant and respectful and, ultimately, produce better health outcomes.

Cultural competence in health assessment is incorporated by ongoing learning and adaptation. Providers cannot have a one-time understanding of a culture; they must engage with patients' unique sociocultural practices throughout the assessment. For instance, adolescents with type 2 diabetes may face varied issues based on their cultural contexts, which may include socioeconomic status and various forms of family structures (Yogesh et al., 2020). To effectively navigate these complexities, health care professionals must apply inclusive communication strategies that are patient-centered to elicit patients' own perspectives and preferences. These talks may provide valuable information regarding the illness management and can be used to guide the development of individualized care plans. By active listening and the integration of this cultural information, practitioners can build a facilitative setting that promotes engaged patient involvement in their own health care and ultimately is improved for the aggregate quality of care. The digital age also poses challenges but presents possibilities for augmenting knowledge of cultural diversity in health assessments. With telemedicine and digital health technologies gaining wider use, providers must be exceedingly sensitive to technology's capacity to span cultural gaps as much as it can also widen them. It is important that effective utilization of digital channels of education and communication, without losing touch with culturally competent resources, is necessary for maintaining patient interest and understanding (Olinder et al., 2022). As seen, online interaction and social media use can foster peer support and exchange of information among patients with common cultural backgrounds. Nevertheless, health care professionals must be vigilant to prevent potential miscommunications arising from differences in language or digital content interpreted in a way other than intended (Yogesh et al., 2020). By engaging these challenges and employing technology in a reflective way, health care professionals can become more culturally competent and improve the health outcomes of diverse populations by respecting each patient's unique context and integrating it into their care.

2.4.2. Adapting Communication Styles

Successful health screenings are built on effective communication, requiring healthcare practitioners to adeptly fit their communication styles to the diverse needs of patients. Variations among patients' cultural backgrounds, reading capabilities, and emotional states prove that formulaic communication is inadequate. Flexible communication styles allow healthcare practitioners not only to facilitate more comprehensible exchanges of information, but also to establish a sense of trust and rapport with patients. This adaptability can incorporate simplification for those with little medical expertise or through the use of visual aids to enhance understanding. Identifying these variations and modifying communication techniques can significantly impact patient understanding and engagement, overall leading to improved health results. Moreover, integration of new communication methods is required in practices of health assessment. For instance, telehealth today is more prevalent, and thus the professionals have to adapt communication to get the best out of digital media. The shift from face-to-face contact to virtual consultation makes health practitioners even more cautious with non-verbal cues, tone, and understanding. Adapting communication in this case involves being brief but providing much detail so that the patients feel taken care of as if they were being seen in person. These procedures not only enhance patient satisfaction but also comply with the evolving technology-laden world of contemporary healthcare, thereby the importance of flexibility in the communication strategies. The problems with these changes are well-documented in literature spanning historical, theoretical, and empirical perspectives (N/A, 2013). Also, some methods, such as motivational interviewing, indicate the significance of individualized communication strategies. Motivational interviewing is a method designed to enhance patient engagement and motivation in their own health care decisions, involving sensitive understanding of the patients perspective. Referring to myths around this process—because it would otherwise be confused with other models—highlights the necessity for transparent, responsive communication. For example, it is not only a collection of generic techniques or a stand-alone method but also a sophisticated process that must be guided by an open and honest cooperative attitude between patient and clinician. This type of clarity in understanding and application of motivational interviewing increases intervention effectiveness and facilitates long-term behavioral changes among patients (William et al., 2009). Thus, by including these techniques in their style of communication, healthcare professionals are able to significantly enhance the health assessment process and general patient interaction (Figure 2.14).

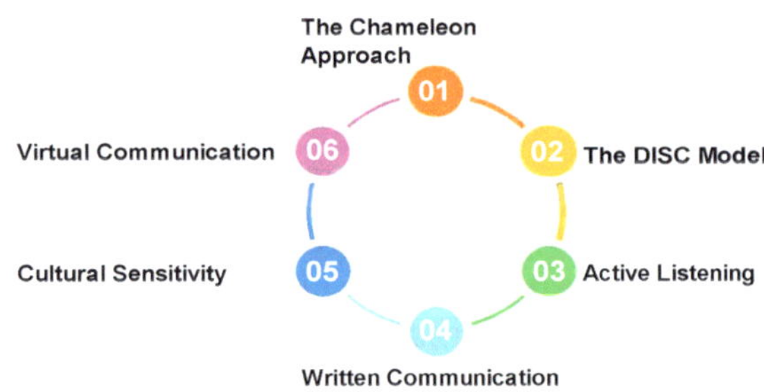
The Chameleon Approach
01
02
The DISC Model
03
Active Listening
04
Written Communication
05
Cultural Sensitivity
06
Virtual Communication

Figure 2.14. Adapting communication styles in nursing.

Source: https://fastercapital.co/i/Sales-communication--How-to-communicate-effectively-with-your-prospects-and-customers-and-build-trust-and-rapport--Adapting-to-Different-Communication-Styles.webp.

2.4.3. Overcoming Language Barriers

Good communication is essential in health assessment, but language barriers present a significant obstacle. The technicality involved in discussions concerning health sometimes requires the application of some specific terminologies and jargon that are not easily understandable to patients. There may be miscommunication when health care providers fail to communicate openly, risking patient safety and the quality of services provided. To meet these demands, practitioners must be patient-focused and emphasize the importance of verbal and non-verbal communication. Good communication, according to the World Dental Federation (FDI), is a process through which patients' needs are understood by using verbal explanations in simple language that fosters rapport and trust, ultimately leading to improved patient compliance with treatment regimens (Ho et al., 2025). Dissecting language barriers in this manner not only maximizes patient understanding but also aids in developing a stronger therapeutic relationship between clinicians and patients. Combining several communication methods can significantly reduce the interruptions caused by language barriers in health interviews. Practitioners can take advantage of translation services, bilingual staff, or technology-based solutions such as language interpretation software to facilitate the transition between clinicians and patients. Further, the application of risk assessment tools in community health interventions, such as the Family Adoption Program (FAP), has been found to enhance the knowledge and clinical skills of the students related to it as well as enhance communication between the health care providers and the community members (Arulmozhi et al., 2025). By engaging the students as well as the patients by culturally adapting conversations, such measures enable effective understanding and trust among the community. Therefore, bridging language gaps not only improves patient outcomes for individual patients but also fosters a more inclusive healthcare culture. Continuous training in communications skills is essential to allow health practitioners to effectively navigate and bridge language gaps. Training courses need to emphasize the development of skills such as motivational interviewing, open-ended questions, and reflective listening, which are important in communicating with diverse patient populations. Training schemes can be designed to combine theory with practice so that healthcare professionals are adequately prepared to confront real communication problems. The complexities of language barriers in dental and community health settings illustrate the necessity of methodical pedagogic interventions to enhance communication skills (Ho et al., 2025). Finally, inculcating a culture of empathy and mutual respect between healthcare professionals is not only capable of helping them manage linguistic barriers more effectively, but also ensures the quality care that all patients are entitled to irrespective of their language background.

Test Your Knowledge

1. How can understanding a patient's cultural background improve the effectiveness of a health assessment interview?
2. What strategies can healthcare providers use to overcome language and cultural barriers during patient interviews?

2.5. Ethical Considerations in Health Interviews

Learning Outcome

1. Informed consent;
2. Confidentiality and privacy;
3. Professional boundaries.

Health interviewing is a central role in health evaluation that demands the utmost level of adherence to ethical standards. Directing ethical health interviewing is the principle of informed consent, which ensures participants' awareness of the reason for the interview, processes involved, and rights to withdraw. Informed consent allows individuals to empower themselves while fostering trust culture in interactions between the health professional and participant in an interview. Such transparency not only enhances the validity of the data gathered but also protects the autonomy of the patient, upholding their right to informed decision-making. This is of special significance in occupational health screening where psychological evaluation can impact work choices, making it crucial to have ethical standards for professionals conducting such evaluations for ensuring best practice (American Psychological Association, 2018). Moreover, cultural problems have to be considered when conducting ethical health interviews, particularly with multi-cultural groups.

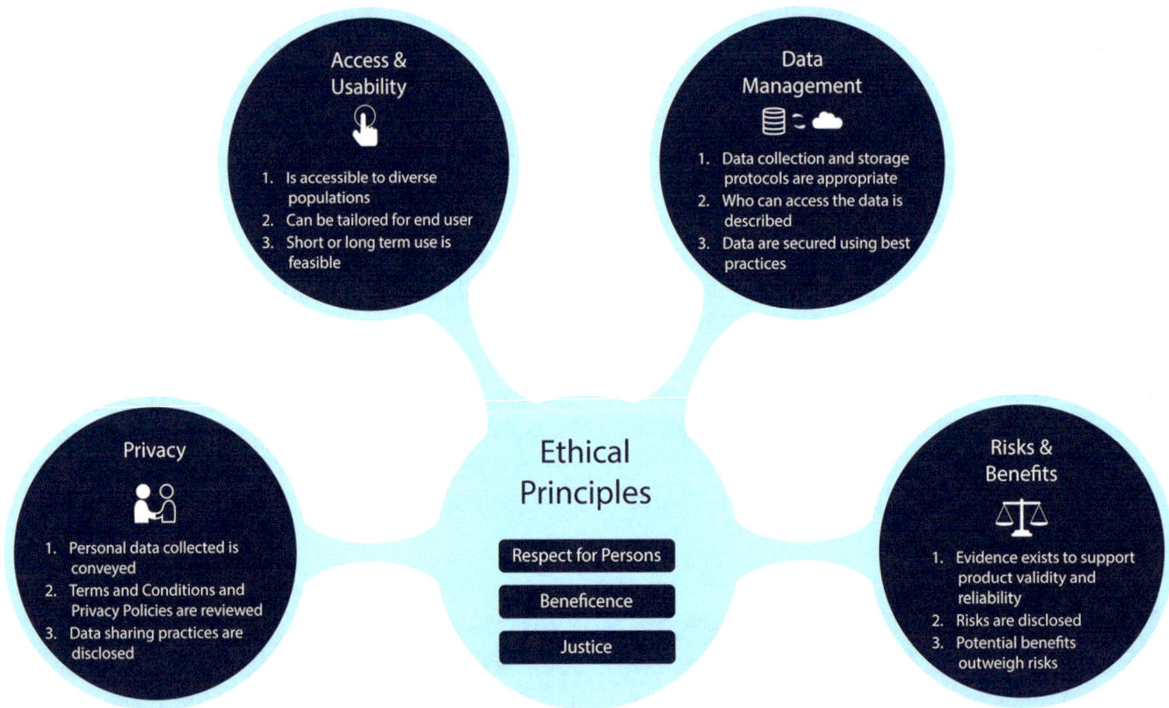

Figure 2.15. Ethical considerations in health interviews.

Source: https://media.licdn.com/dms/image/v2/D4D12AQGZjfAJ0lliCQ/article-cover_image-shrink_720_1280/article-cover_image-shrink_720_1280/0/1697112777430?e=2147483647&v=beta&t=aCm7ctmpYRFKklgwHVvE78Inq1l3rZoRJeRCwLF_Uj0.

2.5.1. Informed Consent

Informed consent is a central concept of health evaluation that underscores respect for the autonomy of patients and the ethical requirements that govern healthcare practice. The process involves ensuring that patients are thoroughly informed about the nature of treatment or evaluation for which they are giving consent to receive. It requires medical practitioners to appropriately explain possible risks, benefits, and alternatives, thereby establishing the feeling of cooperation and trust between the patient and the medical practitioner. With increased focus on patient-centered care within healthcare, informed consent assumes a vital role not just legally but also as an aspect that enhances the therapeutic alliance. In the absence of proper informed consent, there are possible dangers of undermining patient autonomy and compromising the quality of care being offered, which can be linked to undesirable outcomes for both the patient and physician. Proper communication strategies are instrumental in the process of informed consent, particularly in multiculturally diverse clinical settings. Health screenings often encompass patients who have varied backgrounds, individual levels of health literacy, cultural traditions, and ways of communicating. It is crucial that clinicians adopt strategies that harmonize their communication style with the specific needs of their patients. For instance, the development of non-verbal communication styles, as observed in research among children and disabled individuals, has been shown to be instrumental in aiding understanding and cooperation during health assessments (Mitchell et al., 2010). Using visual aids or symbolic communication techniques, providers are able to ensure that all patients, regardless of verbal skills, are involved in the decision-making process, thus improving informed consent on a greater portion of the population. In addition, the incorporation of evidence-based techniques, such as Motivational Interviewing, can also enhance informed consent. This patient-centered approach encourages discussion that respects the patients perspective while actively involving them in their care decisions. Applying Motivational Interviewing in health assessments ensures that not only do patients comprehend the information they require but are also willing to work with their treatment plans (Breckon et al., 2019). By establishing a dialogical environment, health professionals can reduce patient anxieties associated with complex medical information and therefore facilitate informed consent as a participatory and dynamic process. Finally, by prioritizing these communication practices in practice, healthcare practitioners can enhance the process of informed consent, leading to better informed, active, and empowered patients (Figure 2.16).

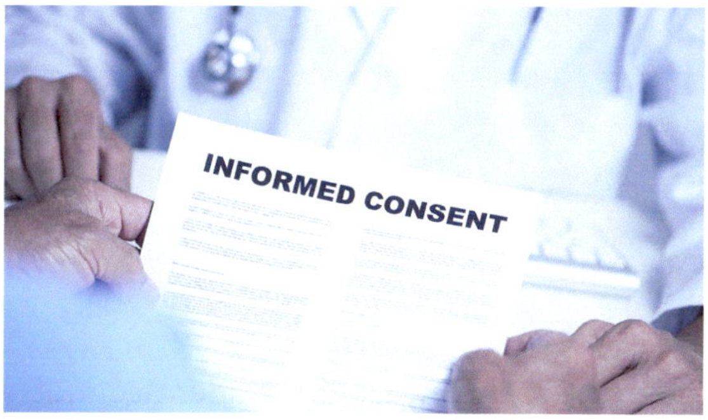

Figure 2.16. Informed consent.

Source: https://www.aamc.org/sites/default/files/d/1/9-informed_consent_redboxxmain.jpg__992x558_q85_crop_subsampling-2_upscale.jpg.

2.5.2. Confidentiality and Privacy

Confidentiality and privacy are the most central pillars of the health assessment profession, particularly while conducting interviews. Healthcare providers must uphold strict codes of ethics that will shield the patient's data and also ensure that personal data is divulged only with express consent from the patient. This practice not only increases trust among health providers and patients but also enhances the quality of the exchange in that it provides patients with a chance to be forthcoming without threats of retaliation. In addition, the expanding role of technology in health assessments, evident in the expanding use of telemedicine and internet-based platforms, necessitates robust privacy controls to protect personal health information from improper observation and theft. The wrong solutions to these problems have profound effects, such as legal ramifications and eroded confidence in healthcare systems. Confidentiality issues are also upheld by the growing ubiquity of the Internet of Things (IoT), which facilitates mass collection and transmission of health data through connected devices. While these innovations offer improved patient monitoring and improved health results, they carry high risks against privacy. They are exposed to high data breach risk since evidence suggests that the majority of IoT devices are susceptible to cyber-attacks, compromising the integrity of private patient records. With growing complexity in managing digital data, health practitioners must become proficient in the nuances of cybersecurity and digital forensics to protect patient confidentiality during tests.

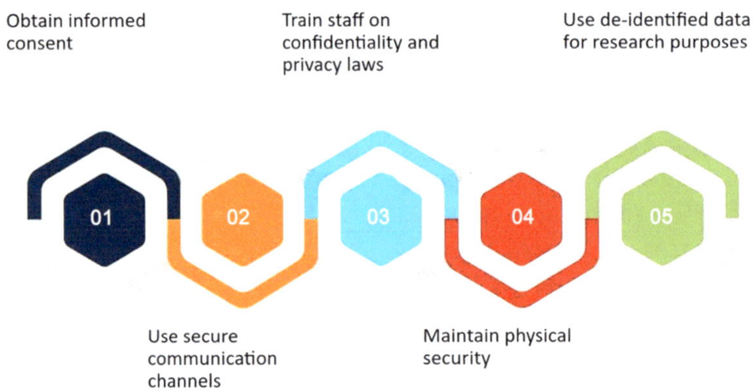

Figure 2.17. Understanding patient confidentiality and privacy.

Source: https://fastercapital.co/i/NDA-in-Medical-Practice--Securing-Patient-Confidentiality-and-Privacy--Understanding-Patient-Confidentiality-and-Privacy.webp.

The nuance of balancing such progress in technology with patient privacy remains a compelling need for comprehensive guidelines and training to stem against the threats posed by IoT devices in healthcare settings (Stoyanova et al., 2020). In the mental health setting, confidentiality is all the more necessary because of the personal and sensitive nature of information typically brought forward in the course of assessment. The newfound emergence of embodied artificial intelligence as a means of therapy serves to complicate matters one step further, as ethical issues related to patient data confidentiality are now concerned. AI technologies can potentially inadvertently disclose patient information or create ambiguity regarding the involvement of non-human agents in the process of healing. Healthcare professionals, while utilizing these sophisticated technologies, must guarantee respect for the autonomy of patients and transparency in the use of algorithms driving AI technologies. Solutions to these ethical problems will not only safeguard patient confidentiality but will also stimulate innovation in the delivery of mental health care (Fiske et al., 2019). Thus, there should be a sound ethical framework in applying technology to psychological assessment to guarantee confidentiality and respect for trust that is essential for patient care (Figure 2.17).

2.5.3. Professional Boundaries

Professional boundaries are important to set and maintain in health evaluation, since this fosters an efficient and safe therapeutic relationship between health practitioners and patients. Professional boundaries demarcate the sphere of accountability and intervention of health providers and also foster respect and understanding of one another. When defining their scope of practice, professionals not only safeguard themselves but also safeguard patients against possible misuse or misinterpretation. Subtlety of working relationships within the healthcare industry demands the establishment of an environment in which emotion boundaries are clearly recognized, and professional codes of practice are maintained. For instance, health literacy education relies heavily on the effective communication of information coupled with emotional support, as cited by Rocha et al. (2024), who emphasize the importance of professional preparedness and the assessment of patient needs as the backbone of the necessary boundaries. Communication channels also illuminate the value of professional boundaries in conducting health assessments, particularly through an interdisciplinary practice perspective. Effective communication among multiple healthcare professionals allows for an integrated approach to considering patient care, improving outcomes. Ineffective communication creates confusion and amplifies poorly coordinated responsibilities, undermining patient-provider trust. The study by Worre et al. (2024) finds that clinical practitioners consider the available channels of communication as inadequate, emphasizing the imperative to problem-free exchange across sector boundaries. By adopting formal systems of communication, healthcare teams are able to ensure that all team members are aware of their individual roles and work toward patient-focused care, strengthening the boundaries that guide professional conduct in collaborative practice. Furthermore, the use of digital communication tools has the potential to facilitate the maintenance of professional boundaries and enhance health assessments. The tools offer health professionals a chance to communicate and collaborate with patients and peers from other settings without compromising the therapeutic relationship. Solutions like eDialogue make timely communication possible that can be designed specifically to suit the individual needs of each patient, addressing both their emotional and health literacy needs (Worre et al., 2024). Although innovative ways of communication are delivered by digital solutions, it is also significant that the deployment must not undermine current professional boundaries among healthcare professionals. Future training programs must work on the incorporation of electronic resources in the context of professional boundaries and ethics to promote a sense of responsibility and respect in patient care.

Test Your Knowledge

1. How does maintaining patient confidentiality influence trust during a health assessment interview?
2. What ethical dilemmas might arise if a patient provides information that could impact their treatment or care?

2.6. Challenges in Health Assessment Interviews

Learning Outcome

1. Dealing with difficult patients;
2. Managing time constraints;
3. Addressing sensitive topics.

During health assessment interviews, health care providers encounter various challenges that can interrupt effective communication and the acquisition of correct information. A key challenge is varying degrees of health literacy among patients. Those with little knowledge of medical terms may not comprehend questions or provide critical information on their health, which creates gaps in knowledge that can slow the assessment process. Also, emotional concerns such as fear of judgment, embarrassment, or anxiety might deter patients from sharing very crucial information about their health history. This level of depth is the explanation for why health care providers need to devise individualized communication plans that are sensitive to the different patient backgrounds and experiences. Unless these obstacles are overcome, health care evaluations might yield partial or incomplete information, eventually affecting the quality of care provided and the management of patient health outcomes. Another significant challenge within health assessment interviews is the potential for cultural differences to impact communication style and interpretation. Patients will have varying perceptions of health, illness, and healthcare systems based on their cultures, which can influence the manner in which they communicate within the interview process. For instance, some individuals may require a more indirect style of communication or may desire emphasis on family involvement in health decision-making. Such approaches may cause misunderstandings when healthcare professionals unknowingly adopt a one-size-fits-all strategy that fails to engage with the patient's culture. It is important to understand such cultural nuances in building a trusting relationship between patient and provider, facilitating open communication, and ultimately better health outcomes. Cultural competence training among healthcare providers may enhance their proficiency in managing these delicate interactions. Lastly, there can also be inherent provider biases and assumptions that may pose significant challenges when performing health assessment interviews. Implicit bias can affect providers' perceptions of patient data as well as possibly the quality of questions asked during assessment. For example, a healthcare provider can unwittingly stereotype a patient's health behaviors according to demographics. This can lead to misinterpretation, with the patients perhaps feeling judged or having their comments misinterpreted, making it even harder for them to be open in offering vital health information. To counter such prejudices, effective self-reflection and constant professional education in the sense of recognizing and dispelling their assumptions is essential for the healthcare providers. Having training sessions on culturally responsive communication and principles of motivational interviewing may facilitate the development of a more inclusive environment by practitioners, resulting in enhanced accuracy and efficacy of health assessments (Stenov et al., 2017; Tuckerman et al., 2022).

2.6.1. Dealing with Difficult Patients

Dealing with complexities of patient interactions is a vital part of health examination, particularly in the presence of difficult patients. They may vary from heightened distress and resentment towards their illness to behavior disorders on the basis of external stress factors. Communication skills prove to be precious in such situations, enabling not only the passing of information but even compassionate understanding of the patient's perspective. Active listening, for instance, can significantly promote the patient-physician relationship so that the latter are heard and appreciated. This realization promotes a more participatory culture, making it easier for patients to communicate freely, which is essential in the acquisition of correct medical histories and the making of appropriate treatment plans. Additionally, the fact that chronic diseases like Alzheimer's disease are so common means that there needs to be a sophisticated way of handling difficult patients. As mentioned, nearly 6.7 million Americans aged 65 and above are presently living with Alzheimer's dementia, a number projected to double by 2060 unless medical advancements are made (N/A, 2023). Patients struggling with such debilitating conditions frequently present behavioral challenges that irritate caregivers as well as healthcare professionals. By utilizing specific interviewing skills, for example, by using open-ended questioning and empathy, employees can alleviate the psychological and emotional burdens of such patients. Trust is essential, which leads to enhanced treatment plan compliance and better understanding of the patients' needs and issues, eventually enhancing their care experience. In addition, incorporation of abilities such as mindfulness in patient interactions has been encouraging to improve results even with challenging patients. Mindfulness interventions can help clinicians remain calm and focused, something that is vital when responding to the typically volatile emotions expressed by challenging patients. Such abilities can de-escalate anxiety on the part of both the patient and provider, which may convert a combative exchange into a useful dialogue. Additionally, mindfulness-based practices have the effect of countering misinformation about a variety of health issues (Nicholas et al., 2017). Lastly, by providing an environment informed by understanding and respect, healthcare providers are able to manage difficult patient encounters more effectively, leading to increased trust, satisfaction, and therapeutic outcomes (Figure 2.18).

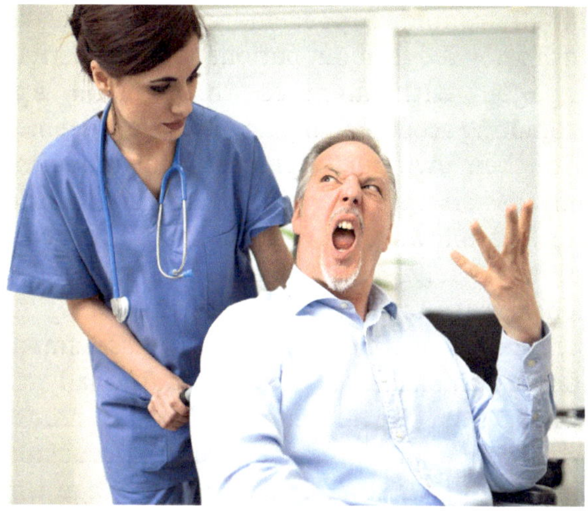

Figure 2.18. Deal with difficult patients.

Source: https://www.goodmanallen.com/wp-content/uploads/2023/08/angry-patient_s.jpg.

2.6.2. Managing Time Constraints

In the health examination sector, dealing with time constraints is essential, particularly while performing patient interviews. Owing to the complexity of full health examinations, experts have a tendency to weigh a range of activities against limited spans of time. Proper management of such constraints not only ensures sturdy data collection but also generates a better patient experience. For instance, interviewing can be made easier by practitioners through the application of structured questioning approaches, which enable guidance with flexibility. Structuring of this sort has been known to enhance the quality of received information while encouraging patient engagement and, as such, minimizing the chances of losing vital health details that have a bearing on patient outcomes. In addition, effective time management within health checks can be significantly improved through the application of technology. Embracing mobile health (mHealth) apps, like that of a study on peer coaching among Parkinson's disease patients, is only one of the ways that digital resources can enhance communication. In such an environment, peer mentors empowered with knowledge about patient needs effectively engaged with mentees through an app, promoting accountability and active engagement with their own health process. This model not only assists in developing a favorable setting but also allows people to be health advocates for themselves, eventually reaping better health results and efficiently managing the constraints of time while making assessments (Colon-Semenza et al., 2018). Additionally, the conservative development of cause models while engaging in focus group discussions can serve as a suitable tactic to manage time limitations. Through systematic identification and elimination of perceived health hazards among stakeholders like caretakers and health workers, practitioners are able to focus efforts on areas most relevant to concerns. This has been proven to resuscitate discussion and ensure that participants remain interested, hence optimizing time spent on evaluations. By examining various health perspectives en masse, practitioners can gather information that is used during individual patient evaluations and helps align healthcare interventions with the needs of the community (de Suremain et al., 2004). In coping with time constraints in a multi-component fashion, eventually enhanced effectiveness of communication practices used during health assessment is attained, prioritizing patient care.

2.6.3. Addressing Sensitive Topics

Managing sensitive issues in the process of health assessment requires a balancing insight in patient psychology and communication tactics. The nature of sensitive issues, i.e., mental illness, drug addiction, or sexual health, tends to elicit fear and vulnerability in the patients. To establish a safe environment, doctors ought to employ active listening and compassionate responses validating the emotional experience of the patient. Building rapport within the early course of the interview is vital; when patients feel they are being heard and respected, they are more willing to share personal details pertinent to their health. It is particularly important when using assessment tools or scales as their validity and reliability to a significant degree depend on patients' cooperativeness in responding and providing honest answers (Godfred et al., 2018). Thus, how experts address sensitive talk has a profound impact on not just immediate treatment but also follow-up adherence to treatments. Moreover, employing a structured method is bound to enhance the efficacy of sensitive issue conversations. Applying models such as the Assess-Ask-Advocate model has the potential to assist health professionals in managing challenging conversations. This strategy requires practitioners to assess the situation in the context, pose open-ended and non-judgmental questions, and voice out on the patient's interest without imposing personal bias. By skillful question design and ordering, clinicians are able to ask patients to reflect on their experience and emotions and hence become more engaged with their health issues. The relevance of selecting the appropriate outcomes within health assessments cannot be overemphasized since the credibility of the conversations lies in their ability to address the wants and needs of both patients and stakeholders in healthcare (Williamson et al., 2017). Thus, this evidence-based communication strategy has an important implication in the improvement of the overall health assessment process and outcomes. In addition to proper use of effective communication skills, healthcare providers should also be culturally competent when handling sensitive information across diverse patient populations. Cultural competency greatly affects how patients interpret and respond to healthcare inquiries regarding personal issues. Healthcare providers need to possess knowledge about cultural values, social norms, and history to ensure that they do not misinterpret and to engage in a respectful discussion. Cultural competence training is able to equip professionals with the skills to manage such complex conversations effectively with empathy and comprehension. Furthermore, familiarity with other people's health practices and beliefs from different cultures can help to create respectful and suitable questions. Integration of cultural considerations into the process of communication facilitates practitioners to enhance patient involvement and foster open and truthful communication of sensitive health matters (Godfred et al., 2018). By so doing, they not only do a better job at evaluating them but also allow patients to become more involved in their health care process.

Test Your Knowledge

1. What are common barriers that prevent patients from sharing complete or accurate health information?
2. How can healthcare professionals manage time constraints while ensuring a thorough health assessment?

SUMMARY

The study of interviewing and communication skills in health assessment, it is apparent that effective communication is the secret to successful patient-provider relationships. The complexity of health assessments demands not only the accurate gathering of information but also the establishment of trust between patients and healthcare providers. Techniques such as motivational interviewing and the use of plain language are directly related to improved patient understanding and comfort, ultimately leading to improved health outcomes. As highlighted in later research, the use of plain language and visual aids has been said to enhance patient understanding, thereby promoting a team culture within healthcare settings (Zhang et al., 2025). This process not only empowers patients but also equips providers with the ability to hold discussions on sensitive topics, thereby enhancing the overall quality of care. Of equal significance is the position patient feedback takes in informing customized communication strategies. Having an understanding of patients' viewpoints and satisfaction levels is key to thorough health assessment strategies. For instance, a survey in ALERT hospital revealed that even though the majority of the patients were satisfied with communication and information, there were still opportunities for enhancement, for instance, waiting times for compounded services (Hirpina et al., 2025). By asking for and using patient feedback, health professionals are able to adjust their skills to fit specific needs and thereby enhance the quality of care. Such a commitment to constant improvement embodies the nature of patient-centered care and enables providers to shape their modes of communication so that they speak with all kinds of patients. As a whole, the marriage of good interviewing and communication skills in health assessment embodies the eminent role played by such skills in the development of good patient outcomes. By focusing on effective communication, patient feedback, and responsiveness in their methods, healthcare providers can render the setting more supportive and interactive. The results of many studies highlight that such interventions, apart from enhancing individual patient satisfaction, also aggregate health outcomes. As health care continues to advance, good communication skills among medical providers need to be a priority so that every patient is enabled with the information and knowledge sufficient to play an effective role in their own health care (Hirpina et al., 2025; Zhang et al., 2025).

Effective interviewing and communication skills are central in health assessment since they enable healthcare providers to gather reliable patient information while fostering empathetic situations. The key here is the structured approach to interviewing, with the insistence that open-ended questions should be used to receive detailed descriptions from patients about their conditions. These techniques not only aid in the discovery of the patients' symptoms but also rapport building, which is essential for quality communication. Active listening is also recognized as an essential skill that aids in understanding and trust building, allowing the healthcare practitioner to interpret non-verbal communication and respond accordingly. Application of these techniques ensures that the process of assessing is prolonged and patient-centered, ultimately resulting in improved health outcomes. Another significant aspect of interviewing in health assessment is the requirement for establishing a good atmosphere. Creating an atmosphere where patients feel at ease to express themselves brings about information flow. This extends not just to verbal communication but also to the non-verbal component of body language and eye contact, which can enhance the interaction quality. The application of reflective statements may also deepen understanding and confirm the patients experience, further optimizing the discussion. The presence of cultural competence is also necessary; awareness and recognition of diversity of backgrounds allow practitioners to modify communication strategies accordingly and counter potential barriers that may affect patient involvement in their care process. Finally, the integration of good interviewing skills with evidenced assessment instruments is critical for accurate health assessments. Scale development and validation ensure that measures are valid and reliable, as per best practice literature for scale development (Godfred et al., 2018). This systematic approach not only strengthens the process of health assessment but also instills evidence-based practice that can be adapted to suit the unique needs of patients. Also, as presented in the taxonomy of behavior change techniques, a more precise framework of classification can complement the implementation of interventions carried out for behavior modification (Michie et al., 2013). Through the integration of these methods, health practitioners are able to improve comprehension and optimize health assessment processes to lead to enhanced health management strategies.

KEY TERMS FROM THIS CHAPTER

- Therapeutic Communication
- Active Listening
- Open-Ended Questions
- Closed-Ended Questions
- Empathy
- Rapport
- Nonverbal Communication
- Verbal Communication
- Clarification
- Reflection
- Summarization
- Silence
- Facilitation
- Therapeutic Relationship
- Cultural Sensitivity
- Paraphrasing

CRITICAL THINKING QUESTIONS

1. **What is the primary purpose of the patient interview in a health assessment?**
   a. To perform physical examinations
   b. To establish a therapeutic relationship and gather health history
   c. To administer medications
   d. To complete laboratory tests
2. **Which interviewing technique is best for encouraging patients to talk freely about their health concerns?**
   a. Closed-ended questions
   b. Leading questions
   c. Open-ended questions
   d. Yes-or-no questions
3. **Nonverbal communication includes all of the following EXCEPT:**
   a. Facial expressions
   b. Body language
   c. Tone of voice
   d. Patient's medical history
4. **Cultural competence in health assessment communication involves:**
   a. Ignoring cultural differences to treat all patients the same
   b. Understanding and respecting patients' cultural beliefs and practices
   c. Using only medical terminology regardless of patient understanding
   d. Avoiding discussion about culture altogether
5. **Which of the following is an ethical consideration during a patient interview?**
   a. Ensuring privacy and confidentiality
   b. Encouraging the patient to answer as quickly as possible
   c. Using medical jargon to assert authority
   d. Conducting the interview in a public area

Short Answer Questions

1. Why is the patient interview considered a critical component of the health assessment process?
2. How does an effective interview contribute to accurate diagnosis and patient-centered care?
3. How can a nurse interpret a patient's nonverbal cues, such as posture or facial expressions, during a health assessment?
4. Give examples of how nonverbal communication can either enhance or hinder effective patient interviews.
5. What strategies can healthcare providers use to ensure culturally sensitive communication with patients from diverse backgrounds?

Answer to Critical Thinking Questions

1. (b) 2. (c) 3. (d) 4. (b) 5. (a)

REFERENCES

1. Adamu, A., Sabo, A., Saad, H., & Shehu, Y. (2024). Assessment of relationship between emotional intelligence and conflict resolution among nurse managers at tertiary health institutions of North Eastern States of Nigeria. *Dutse Journal of Pure and Applied Sciences*. https://www.semanticscholar.org/paper/842e9da00afc1d18d758ebc3e2eaf0594bcfc0de (accessed on 16th July 2025).
2. Alzheimer's Association. (2023). 2023 Alzheimer's disease facts and figures. *Alzheimer's & Dementia, 19*, 1598–1695. https://doi.org/10.1002/alz.13016 (accessed on 16th July 2025).
3. American Psychological Association, & Melchert, T. P. (2018). Professional practice guidelines for occupationally mandated psychological evaluations. https://core.ac.uk/download/231843503.pdf (accessed on 16th July 2025).
4. Argent, K., & Cronin, M. (2017). Working with families. https://www.semanticscholar.org/paper/65ffab8a04232efb84b4134453b2eb122322b6f6 (accessed on 16th July 2025).
5. Arulmozhi, M., Raveendran, A., Ganapathy, K., & Kandasamy, P. (2025). Implementing and evaluating risk assessment as a new learning tool in family adoption program: A qualitative study. *Indian Journal of Community Medicine*. https://www.semanticscholar.org/paper/7528911e625336c853e18b1cd811c780c0f14e85 (accessed on 16th July 2025).
6. Ayako, L. I., Ngari, S., & Asatsa, S. (2024). Parental perceptions on the introduction of competence-based curriculum in public day primary schools in Nairobi County, Kenya. *International Journal of Research and Innovation in Social Science*. https://www.semanticscholar.org/paper/b2812cb98ea477e2a49522cbb5f22c8c09fab9c2 (accessed on 16th July 2025).
7. Barrett, J., Eastley, K. B., Herbland, A., Owen, P., Naeem, S., Mortimer, C., King, J., et al. (2024). The COVID-19 ambulance response assessment (CARA) study: A national survey of ambulance service healthcare professionals' preparedness and response to the COVID-19 pandemic. *British Paramedic Journal, 8*, 10–20. https://www.semanticscholar.org/paper/63cd717df19a8c736c2750a8db2af92908b1d817 (accessed on 16th July 2025).
8. Baylor, C., Burns, M., McDonough, K., Mach, H., & Yorkston, K. M. (2019). Teaching medical students' skills for effective communication with patients who have communication disorders. *American Journal of Speech-Language Pathology, 28*, 155–164. https://doi.org/10.1044/2018_ajslp-18-0130 (accessed on 16th July 2025).
9. Boateng, G. O., Neilands, T. B., Frongillo, E. A., Melgar-Quiñonez, H., & Young, S. L. (2018). Best practices for developing and validating scales for health, social, and behavioral research: A primer. *Frontiers in Public Health, 6*. https://doi.org/10.3389/fpubh.2018.00149 (accessed on 16th July 2025).
10. Bobay, K. L., Candela, L., Piacentine, L. B., Weiss, M., et al. (2018). Teaching students to teach patients: A theory-guided approach. https://core.ac.uk/download/286544047.pdf (accessed on 16th July 2025).
11. Breckon, J., Davidson, M., Holden, J., Monfries, M., et al. (2019). Embedded motivational interviewing combined with a smartphone app to increase physical activity in people with sub-acute low back pain: Study protocol of a cluster randomized control trial. https://core.ac.uk/download/286714043.pdf (accessed on 16th July 2025).

12. César, F. C. R., Oliveira, L., Galvão, M. C., & Lacerda, A. L. A. (2024). How do healthcare professionals develop the communication process to promote patients' health literacy? *International Journal of Environmental Research and Public Health, 21*. https://www.semanticscholar.org/paper/f52efe89a6dd849bf28e2925ff8621a296b96a80 (accessed on 16th July 2025).
13. Chambers, D., Simpson, L., Hill-Briggs, F., Neta, G., Vinson, C., Beidas, R., Marcus, S. C., et al. (2016). Proceedings of the 8th Annual Conference on the Science of Dissemination and Implementation. *Implementation Science, 11*. https://www.semanticscholar.org/paper/87a4a6f590382705c6eeba6305bb861c0379246b (accessed on 16th July 2025).
14. Colon-Semenza, C., Ellis, T. D., Latham, N. K., Quintiliani, L., et al. (2018). Peer coaching through mHealth targeting physical activity in people with Parkinson disease: Feasibility study. https://core.ac.uk/download/215937141.pdf (accessed on 16th July 2025).
15. D'Ignazio, C., & Klein, L. (2020). *Data Feminism*. The MIT Press eBooks. https://doi.org/10.7551/mitpress/11805.001.0001 (accessed on 16th July 2025).
16. de Oliveira e Silva, M., Gomes da Silva Júnior, A., & Koifman, L. (2024). Competencies for the production of comprehensive health care: Analysis of the assessment processes in Medicine Internship at Fluminense Federal University. *Interface–Comunicação, Saúde, Educação*. https://www.semanticscholar.org/paper/0dbb852b9631726487a6e1035f2b67509001915a (accessed on 16th July 2025).
17. de Suremain, C. E., Lefèvre, P., Rubín de Celis, E., Sejas, R., et al. (2004). Combining causal model and focus group discussions: Experiences learned from socio-anthropological research on the differing perceptions of caretakers and health professionals on children's health (Bolivia/Peru). https://core.ac.uk/download/29634988.pdf (accessed on 16th July 2025).
18. Dwivedi, Y. K., Ismagilova, E., Hughes, D. L., Carlson, J., Filieri, R., Jacobson, J., Jain, V., et al. (2020). Setting the future of digital and social media marketing research: Perspectives and research propositions. *International Journal of Information Management, 59*, 102168–102168. https://doi.org/10.1016/j.ijinfomgt.2020.102168 (accessed on 16th July 2025).
19. Fiske, A., Henningsen, P., & Buyx, A. (2019). Your robot therapist will see you now: Ethical implications of embodied artificial intelligence in psychiatry, psychology, and psychotherapy. *Journal of Medical Internet Research, 21*, e13216–e13216. https://doi.org/10.2196/13216 (accessed on 16th July 2025).
20. Froehlich, J., Pardue, K. T., & Dunbar, D. M. (2016). Evaluation of a communication survey and interprofessional education curriculum for undergraduate health professional students. *Journal of Interprofessional Education & Practice, 2*, 4. https://www.semanticscholar.org/paper/b5243d9d705a56d8bdc23097659c4eb88a39f5a9 (accessed on 16th July 2025).
21. Green, A., Green, M., Jerzmanowska, N., Lobb, E., et al. (2018). "Death is difficult in any language": A qualitative study of palliative care professionals' experiences when providing end-of-life care to patients from culturally and linguistically diverse backgrounds. https://core.ac.uk/download/213607752.pdf (accessed on 16th July 2025).
22. Halbach, P., & Keller, A. O. (2017). Evaluating motivational interviewing in the physician assistant curriculum. https://core.ac.uk/download/213073350.pdf (accessed on 16th July 2025).

23. Hirpina, B., Selam, M. N., Fentie, A. M., Wale, M., Tegegne, A. M., & Abera, S. (2025). Assessment of patients' perception and satisfaction with extemporaneous compounding service in ALERT hospital, Ethiopia. *BMC Health Services Research, 25*. https://www.semanticscholar.org/paper/020c71c21cc8cd54c0491261525633c006981920 (accessed on 16th July 2025).

24. Ho, J. C. Y., Chai, H. H., Luo, B. W., Lo, E. C. M., Huang, M. Z., & Chu, C. (2025). An overview of dentist–patient communication in quality dental care. *Dentistry Journal, 13*. https://www.semanticscholar.org/paper/bbee421d7cb88e2f79d730ce04efc3e8f3f5ec39 (accessed on 16th July 2025).

25. Hoyme, H. E., Kalberg, W. O., Elliott, A., Blankenship, J., Buckley, D., Marais, A. S., Manning, M. A., et al. (2016). Updated clinical guidelines for diagnosing fetal alcohol spectrum disorders. *Pediatrics, 138*. https://doi.org/10.1542/peds.2015-4256 (accessed on 16th July 2025).

26. Jensen, L. W. H., Rahbek, O., Lauritsen, R., Kold, S., & Dinesen, B. (2024). Health care professionals' perspectives before and after use of eDialogue for team-based digital communication across settings: Qualitative study. *JMIR Human Factors, 11*. https://www.semanticscholar.org/paper/f40dba8a6ae43b47821e63c32bfc4428e5b8ec1c (accessed on 16th July 2025).

27. Jonassen, D., & Driscoll, M. (2013). *Handbook of Research on Educational Communications and Technology*. Routledge eBooks. https://doi.org/10.4324/9781410609519 (accessed on 16th July 2025).

28. Kim, A. R., Lim, Y. M., & Park, J. H. (2025). Development of lifestyle assessment: A Delphi survey of multi-faceted health experts. *PLOS ONE, 20*. https://www.semanticscholar.org/paper/4836b04a561e18bdf343b5ae09ee1c6a13c098a2 (accessed on 16th July 2025).

29. Mach, F., Baigent, C., Catapano, A. L., Koskinas, K. C., Casula, M., Badimón, L., Chapman, M. J., et al. (2019). 2019 ESC/EAS guidelines for the management of dyslipidemias: Lipid modification to reduce cardiovascular risk. *European Heart Journal, 41*, 111–188. https://doi.org/10.1093/eurheartj/ehz455 (accessed on 16th July 2025).

30. Martínez, R. N., Hogan, T. P., Lones, K., Balbale, S., Scholten, J., Bidelspach, D. E., Musson, N., et al. (2016). Evaluation and treatment of mild traumatic brain injury through the implementation of clinical video telehealth: Provider perspectives from the Veterans Health Administration. *PM&R, 9*, 231–240. https://doi.org/10.1016/j.pmrj.2016.07.002 (accessed on 16th July 2025).

31. Michie, S., Richardson, M., Johnston, M., Abraham, C., Francis, J., Hardeman, W., Eccles, M., et al. (2013). The behavior changes technique taxonomy (v1) of 93 hierarchically clustered techniques: Building an international consensus for the reporting of behavior change interventions. *Annals of Behavioral Medicine, 46*, 81–95. https://doi.org/10.1007/s12160-013-9486-6 (accessed on 16th July 2025).

32. Miller, W. R., & Rollnick, S. (2009). Ten things that motivational interviewing is not. *Behavioral and Cognitive Psychotherapy, 37*, 129–140. https://doi.org/10.1017/s1352465809005128 (accessed on 16th July 2025).

33. Mishari, A. K., & Ali, M. A. K. (2025). Enhancing communication with older adults with cognitive impairment in healthcare settings. *Iraqi Journal of Community Medicine*. https://www.semanticscholar.org/paper/abc4dc7a77b0708017901fa807fdd46e87fba603 (accessed on 16th July 2025).

34. Mitchell, W. (2010). "I know how I feel": Listening to young people with life-limiting conditions who have learning and communication impairments. https://core.ac.uk/download/12461.pdf (accessed on 16th July 2025).

35. Ogunyemi, K., Lokossou, V. K., Sogbossi, L. S., Ohuabunwo, C., Antara, S., Kebede, S., Haley, C., et al. (2024). A pragmatic assessment of contextual fit and feasibility for e-learning implementation among public health workers in 16 West African countries: A mixed-methods study. *Journal of Global Health Economics and Policy*. https://www.semanticscholar.org/paper/7f880a454ffed018f8d19b6632a5595ee071ae63 (accessed on 16th July 2025).

36. Olinder, A. L., DeAbreu, M., Greene, S., Haugstvedt, A., Lange, K., Majaliwa, E., Pais, V., et al. (2022). ISPAD clinical practice consensus guidelines 2022: Diabetes education in children and adolescents. *Pediatric Diabetes, 23*, 1229–1242. https://doi.org/10.1111/pedi.13418 (accessed on 16th July 2025).

37. Pamplin, J. C., Anders, S., Brown, J., Crandall, B., Grome, A., Chung, K., Mann-Salinas, E., et al. (2013). 5: Discovering complexities in critical care and their challenges to health IT design in a burn ICU. *Critical Care Medicine, 41*. https://www.semanticscholar.org/paper/e3161e580bc6f52610922002877280c663884c86 (accessed on 16th July 2025).

38. Paulus, T. M., Al-Khateeb, H., Lester, J., Hess, R., & Williams, A. (2023). A discourse analysis of suicide ideation assessment among first year health professional students enrolled in a communications course. *Qualitative Health Communication*. https://www.semanticscholar.org/paper/12eaa23b660c23bbb52e8995182b878e70c576ef (accessed on 16th July 2025).

39. Sinha, A., & Kumar, Y. D. (2024). Intelligent health assessment based on communication and AI technologies for public health. *South Eastern European Journal of Public Health*. https://www.semanticscholar.org/paper/545cd1f0c783ac74c1d7348fdaa60b64e8a6aeb5 (accessed on 16th July 2025).

40. So, M., & Carlson, K. (2022). "We want to be heard": Perspectives on mental health care among patients at a federally qualified health center. *Annals of Family Medicine, 20*(Suppl 1). https://www.semanticscholar.org/paper/d967c15df808bae7b2569341d66afda7f9a91431 (accessed on 16th July 2025).

41. Stenov, V., Wind, G., Skinner, T., Reventlow, S., & Hempler, N. F. (2017). The potential of a self-assessment tool to identify healthcare professionals' strengths and areas in need of professional development to aid effective facilitation of group-based, person-centered diabetes education. *BMC Medical Education, 17*. https://doi.org/10.1186/s12909-017-1003-3 (accessed on 16th July 2025).

42. Stoyanova, M., Nikoloudakis, Y., Panagiotakis, S., Pallis, E., & Markakis, E. (2020). A survey on the Internet of Things (IoT) forensics: Challenges, approaches, and open issues. *IEEE Communications Surveys & Tutorials, 22*, 1191–1221. https://doi.org/10.1109/comst.2019.2962586 (accessed on 16th July 2025).

43. Tahan, H. A., & Sminkey, P. V. (2012). Motivational interviewing. *Professional Case Management, 17*, 164–172. https://doi.org/10.1097/ncm.0b013e318253f029 (accessed on 16th July 2025).

44. Thahaseen, A. A., Karpagavalli, S. M., Fathima, M. R., Sangeetha, S., & Lidiya, M. (2025). Detecting autism spectrum disorder (ASD) using CNN and its methods in deep learning techniques. *International Research Journal on Advanced Engineering and Management (IRJAEM)*. https://

www.semanticscholar.org/paper/da363fa7bd50e4aa1d07502a45d4c1fe955c3172 (accessed on 16th July 2025).

45. Tuckerman, J., Kaufman, J., & Danchin, M. (2022). Effective approaches to combat vaccine hesitancy. *The Pediatric Infectious Disease Journal, 41*, e243–e245. https://doi.org/10.1097/inf.0000000000003499 (accessed on 16th July 2025).

46. Van Dam, N. T., van Vugt, M. K., Vago, D. R., Schmalzl, L., Saron, C. D., Olendzki, A., Meissner, T., et al. (2017). Mind the hype: A critical evaluation and prescriptive agenda for research on mindfulness and meditation. *Perspectives on Psychological Science, 13*, 36–61. https://doi.org/10.1177/1745691617709589 (accessed on 16th July 2025).

47. Walker, N. E. (2002). Forensic interviews of children: The components of scientific validity and legal admissibility. https://core.ac.uk/download/62568566.pdf (accessed on 16th July 2025).

48. Wiederhold, B. K. (2020). Connecting through technology during the Coronavirus Disease 2019 pandemic: Avoiding "Zoom fatigue." *Cyberpsychology Behavior and Social Networking, 23*, 437–438. https://doi.org/10.1089/cyber.2020.29188.bkw (accessed on 16th July 2025).

49. Williamson, P., Altman, D. G., Bagley, H., Barnes, K. L., Blazeby, J., Brookes, S., Clarke, M., et al. (2017). The COMET Handbook: Version 1.0. *Trials, 18*. https://doi.org/10.1186/s13063-017-1978-4 (accessed on 16th July 2025).

50. Zhang, F., Xie, J. J., Chutinan, S., & Riedy, C. A. (2025). Preferred communication techniques by student-providers and patients during caries management in a teaching practice: A quality improvement study. *BMC Medical Education, 25*. https://www.semanticscholar.org/paper/6af6327914f719fa7a3888ad11915e3fd134dd19 (accessed on 16th July 2025).

HEALTH HISTORY TAKING

3

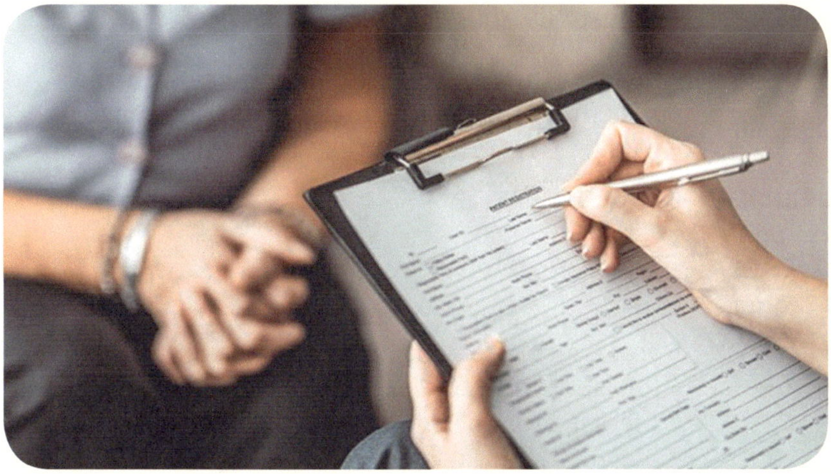

Introduction

The process of taking a health history is the central aspect of medical practice that educates healthcare providers to provide tailored care. The significance of taking a complete health history cannot be overstated, as it provides valuable information on a patient's past medical conditions, family medical history, behaviors, and present state of health. This initial interaction fosters a collaborative environment in which patients are respected and enabled to share information that is pertinent. Knowledge of the patients' experience with health, contextualized, is as important to diagnosis and treatment as it is to a healing relationship. Effective taking of health history by clinicians provides a basis for fully informed clinical decision-making and enhanced patient outcomes, validating the importance of this foundational skill in medical education and practice. Taking health history is not merely a process; it is an ethical practice that must be fulfilled by medical practitioners in order to honor informed consent. Patients have the right to have

LEARNING OBJECTIVES

After studying this chapter, you will be able to:

1. Give purpose of health history taking;
2. Identify the components of a comprehensive health history;
3. Explain the techniques for effective health history taking;
4. Focus on the common challenges in health history taking;
5. Define the role of technology in health history taking;
6. Describe ethical considerations in health history taking.

their health information collected and applied in a manner that honors their autonomy and privacy. Communication throughout the process has a significant influence on trust and rapport, which are key to effective healthcare delivery. By medical ethics studies, the incorporation of culturally sensitive practice in taking health history is capable of reducing miscommunication and enhancing an open healthcare system. By making it topmost, healthcare professionals indicate their commitment to patient-centered care, offering diversified patients equal and respectful treatment. With ethical practice as the focus, the quality of health history taking as an evaluation tool improves. Further, integrating technology into taking health history offers a futuristic model that enhances traditional methods, making patient experience more enriched. Electronic health records (EHRs) minimize information acquisition and storage into efficient processes and facilitate instant access to healthcare professionals.

\This technology facilitates easy documentation of patient histories with accuracy and enhancement of continuity of care. Further, EHRs can be tailored to prompt healthcare professionals with relevant questions that guide the process effectively. But it is critical that technology be balanced with the humanity of care so that patients are not reduced to being mere data points. Through the confluence of technology and compassionate communication, health history taking is an engaged process of not only collecting data but of actively engaging patients in their own care process. Therefore, recognizing this overlap of technology and relationship is vital to modern medical practice, as in most research regarding the success of this paired technique (Corigliano et al., 2017; Szymanski et al., 2002) (Figure 3.1).

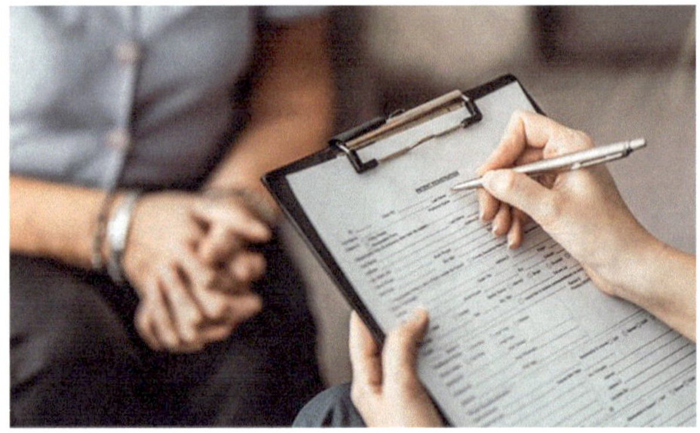

Figure 3.1. Taking a patient history.

Source: https://dm1zcrsul8wju.cloudfront.net/sites/rcn_nspace/files/styles/tile_image/public/Article-images/181691/27508.jpeg?itok=fRXb5WPc.

Definition of Health History Taking

Effective health history taking is a critical patient assessment element that offers the foundation for devising individualized care plans. It is the act of gathering rich information about a patient's medical history, including past disease, surgeries, allergies, medications, and lifestyle concerns. The value of health history cannot be overstated since it assists in making a diagnosis for current conditions and unearthing possible risk elements for future illness. But as earlier research findings inform, there exists a gap between clinical practice guidelines and daily practice within real-world settings, largely on delicate matters of sexual health and taking history (Chastain et al., 2019). The existence of such a gap indicates that health care professionals may find it hard to manage the complexities of taking thorough histories without interrupting the flow of medical interactions, thereby necessitating effective communication measures to optimize patient spontaneity. Apart from physical health measures, taking health history also possesses a wider dimension wherein psychological, social, and environmental factors are considered. The process typically entails questions on mental illnesses, social health determinants, and medical family history of the patient, thereby positioning the patient's overall health status. Awareness of such multifaceted aspects may improve care delivery since it allows practitioners to modify advice based on unique patient situations. Literature shows that patient-provider communication is instrumental to successful taking of the health history; both must be engaged actively to increase information exchange (Mallia et al., 2015). Successful execution of such a conversation fosters trust, allowing patients to make more complete revelations, which ends up in getting an accurate health summary and clinically informed decisions. Overcoming the health history taking challenges must involve recognition of the barriers that have been faced by the patients and providers. Patients may feel apprehensive or stigmatized discussing personal issues, particularly in sensitive areas such as sexual health, and this may discourage collection of essential information. From the providers' viewpoint, time constraints and variation in comfort levels in responding could affect their behavior. Synthesis of evidence from various studies indicates that creating a positive setting and employing empathetic communication skills can enhance the quality of health history taking (Chastain et al., 2019). Furthermore, ongoing education and training in effective history taking can equip providers to better engage with patients, in accordance with clinical guidelines, and ultimately enhance health outcomes through the virtuous effect of an informed appreciation of special patient needs.

Importance in Clinical Practice

Best practice in health history taking is a key foundation for practice that has direct effects on patient outcomes and the overall efficacy of healthcare delivery. Through the accurate gathering of comprehensive health information, healthcare providers are able to identify risk factors, understand patient status, and thus modify interventions. Sexual history taking, specifically, within the field of sexual health, has been found to be plagued by deficiencies in training that lead to significant deficits in patient care. For instance, medical residents have complained about their training in the field, bemoaning discomfort and poor skills as the biggest obstacles to being in a position to start these essential conversations. The discomfort is not just on the part of the clinician to converse with patients but also deters patients from divulging important information about their health, thereby compromising the quality of care received during clinical encounters (Bogaert et al., 2025). In chronic diseases, such as cancer, the importance of complete health history taking is even more well-promoted. Detailed health history taking can enable early detection and correct management through the utilization of appropriate screening and intervention. For instance, in China, inability to understand the natural history of cancers has prompted the shift towards preventive interventions, which stress the requirement of complete health investigations. Once healthcare professionals are invested with proper historical data, they can implement individualized interventions that take into consideration specific patient needs. A well-executed health history, therefore, not only enhances the validity of diagnosis but also becomes part of greater public health goals, like in other types of cancer prevention protocols that summarize patient histories for better screening results (He et al., 2023). Moreover, cultural competency in health history taking shouldn't be exaggerated. With increasing healthcare being delivered to more and more diverse populations, providers must contend with an extensive range of beliefs and practices influencing health behaviors and attitudes that have varied across cultures. The cultural background of a patient is enormously important in creating an improved clinician-patient relationship, where sensitive topics can be openly discussed. Such insensitivity to differences, however, can potentiate existing barriers to provide poor care and also patient dissatisfaction. Training programs for increasing cultural competence in health history taking are therefore of utmost significance in helping clinicians as well as communicate more effectively with patients. Through a concentration on cultural matters, health care providers may render health histories not only complete but also universal, and eventually arrive at better health results for populations with diverse demographics (Figure 3.2).

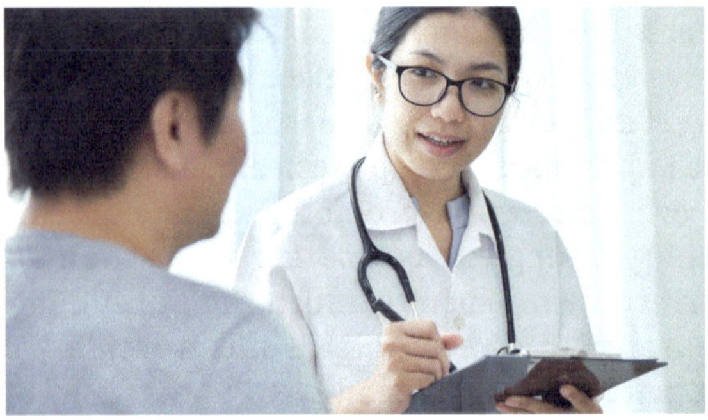

Figure 3.2. Clinical practice for health history taking.

Source: https://www.reading.ac.uk/pharmacy/-/media/project/uor-main/schools-departments/pharmacy/short-courses/taking-patient-notes.jpg?h=675&la=en&w=1200&hash=6DE01C6DE996128D078E3FCA2F8D8A48.

3.1. Purpose of Health History Taking

Learning Outcome

1. Establishing a patient-provider relationship;
2. Identifying health risks and concerns;
3. Guiding diagnosis and treatment plans.

The importance of taking health history lies basically in the establishment of an effective doctor-patient relationship. Through a thorough health history, clinicians gain useful information regarding a patients history, including his or her medical, family, and social history, that collectively affect the health outcome of individuals. It not only allows for diagnosis of the present condition but also for the identification of potential health risks, enabling healthcare providers to tailor preventive measures and interventions. For instance, the familial risk of an individual to suffer from certain diseases allows clinicians to offer customized lifestyle modifications and screening to suit their needs, thus promoting proactivity as opposed to reactivity in the management of healthcare. This abundant information is important to create a trusting setting where patients feel comfortable sharing sensitive details, enhancing the effectiveness of healthcare engagement in general. In addition, health history taking can be an important means of reducing health disparities across various populations.

More particularly, culturally competent communication is essential in being able to effectively communicate with diverse demographic groups, as in the case of the customized means required for Aboriginal and Torres Strait Islander peoples. Creation of communication models that emphasize the relational processes between the patients and the healthcare professionals is essential in ensuring that the delivery of care is appropriate as well as respectful. By using strategies that are sensitive to differences in cultural worldviews about illness and health, such as those highlighted in research among immigrant populations, health care providers are able to create trust as well as adherence from the patients, which ultimately leads to improved health outcomes. This contextual understanding not only enhances better clinical encounters, but also addresses the institutional disparities that often hinder quality access to healthcare. In addition, insights derived from the process of taking health histories become larger than patient encounter boundaries, exerting policy impact on public health programs.

Aggregation of health history information and analysis enables important feed-forward to healthcare systems regarding most frequent issues encountered by populations. It can guide strategic resource allocation, particular health promotion activities, and subsequent research activities, thereby fostering more equitable public health. As in research on medication adherence in ethnically diverse populations, an understanding of culture-specific practices and beliefs has helped illuminate barriers to effective management of health. These findings underscore the importance of utilizing health histories not only as a clinical instrument but as a means to facilitate systemic changes that promote healthier outcomes on all socio-economic and cultural tiers, ultimately pursuing an overall healthier society.

3.1.1. Establishing a Patient-Provider Relationship

The building of a firm patient-provider relationship is the core in health history practice, whose influence directly falls on patient satisfaction and health outcome. The relationship is of trustfulness, compassion, and good communication that provides an open atmosphere where patients are confident to disclose confidential details. The quality of interaction in taking health history can enhance the patients willingness to disclose significant information about their medical history, lifestyle, and problems, thereby making more accurate diagnoses along with customized treatment plans possible. Furthermore, research has indicated that patients who believe their care providers hear and understand them are more likely to comply with medical instructions and aftercare, emphasizing the need for health professionals to gain these interpersonal skills as part of their practice. This encounter lays the groundwork for a continued collaboration aimed at optimizing health and wellness through shared decision-making. Good communication is a key component of the patient-provider interaction, particularly in taking the patient's history. Providers must employ active listening, being genuinely interested in patients' narratives, which allows for the thorough exploration of the patient's issues and history. Employing non-verbal signals such as maintaining eye contact at the level of the other individual and open body posture allows rapport establishment and trust. In addition, professionals also have an obligation to adjust their patterns of communication to address the needs of diverse patient populations. They need to present information in clear, respectful, and culturally competent ways.

By establishing a culture of inclusion where patients feel respected and heard, healthcare providers can maximize the validity and richness of information gained through health history taking, leading to higher-quality patient outcomes and satisfaction. The patient-provider relationship assumptions are not exclusive in the acute situation of history taking but have long-term impacts on patient participation and adherence to treatment plans. Establishing the relationship empowers patients to participate actively in their healthcare. When patients feel they are being partnered with by their providers, they ask questions, clarify, and adhere to treatment plans prescribed. Therefore, this interaction can effectively improve self-management skills and health literacy, which are critical components in the prevention and management of chronic diseases. Talking through with patients their history and preferences not only increases the providers understanding of the patients unique circumstances but allows for a sense of collective responsibility in health outcomes, thereby confirming the importance of establishing and developing a strong patient-provider relationship as foundational to effective health history taking (Visseren et al., 2021; Zhou et al., 2020) (Figure 3.3).

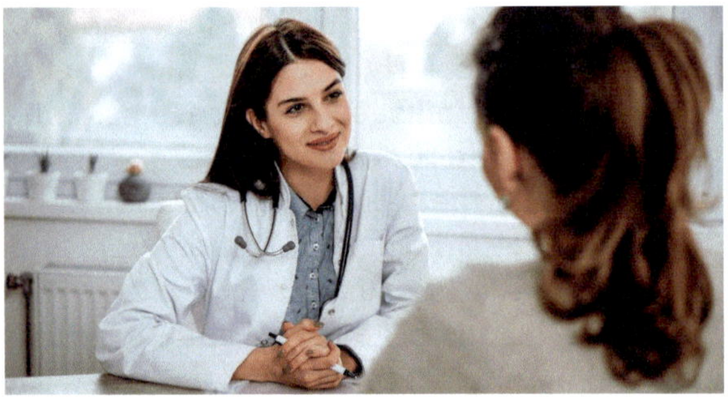

Figure 3.3. Establish a relationship with your healthcare professional.

Source: https://americanmigrainefoundation.org/wp-content/uploads/2018/12/doctor-patient.jpg.

3.1.2. Identifying Health Risks and Concerns

In health history taking, assessing health risks and concerns is paramount to guiding effective patient care. In thorough interviews, health professionals can gain essential information regarding patients' medical histories, lifestyle habits, and family health histories, all of which play pivotal roles in assessing personal risk factors. With these factors, clinicians can initiate targeted screening and prevention programs. For example, differences in healthcare outcomes between persons are often explainable by aspects such as socioeconomic status, age, and underlying conditions. Accordingly, this process serves as a foundation for the formulation of customized care plans addressing the unique health hazards of every patient, thereby maximizing clinical results and improving the potency of healthcare interventions. Moreover, the application of new technologies, particularly AI, to health history taking is promising to be a significant innovation for identifying health dangers. The study on AI in medical anamnesis revealed that physicians increasingly view such technology as being helpful, anticipating higher care quality and efficiency, yet exhibiting initial hesitation regarding the nuances of unique patients' needs and doctor-patient dynamics. Specifically, the expectation is that AI will be able to screen for risk factors better than has been achieved before, thereby leaving health professionals to interact more intensely with patients. However, the successful fulfillment of the potential of AI to do this depends on a careful scrutiny of ethical issues, data privacy, and their effects on patient trust (Felix et al., 2025). At the same time, reducing specific health risks in target populations, such as the elderly, further supports the importance of proper identification of health problems. Specifically, falls are a prevalent issue and can have adverse health effects on this population. The use of tools like the ARMOR intervention highlights the necessity of deprescribing fall risk–augmenting medications (FRIDs) in elderly patients, as a way to decrease such risks. This course not only assists in the prevention of fall events but also serves as a guide for the assessment of general health and medication effectiveness in older patients. Prioritizing risk identification due to polypharmacy enables healthcare professionals to maximize patient safety and improve the quality of life of the older population, which complements broader health care goals in geriatric management and fall prevention strategies (Priyadarshini et al., 2024) (Figure 3.4).

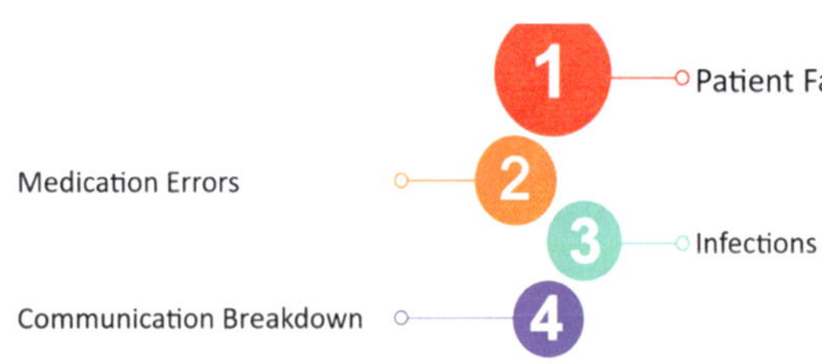

Figure 3.4. Identifying health risks and concerns in nursing.

Source: https://fastercapital.co/i/Risk-Assessment-in-Healthcare--A-Vital-Analysis-for-Patient-Safety--Identifying-Potential-Risks-in-Healthcare-Settings.webp.

3.1.3. Guiding Diagnosis and Treatment Plans

In taking health history, it is important in guiding treatment and diagnosis decisions in the development of a whole picture regarding a patient's status. Good health history is the foundation upon which differential diagnoses may be constructed not merely on the basis of presented symptoms but also on the patient's background, risk factors, and psychosocial setting. Through the acquisition of both contextual and clinical data, practitioners can identify patterns to inform interventions that are suitable to particular needs. For instance, learning about a patients psychosocial context can reveal factors that contribute to their condition and hence lead the clinician to a treatment that moves beyond symptom relief to the identification of causal factors. This preparatory stage is critical in ensuring that the subsequent clinical choices are well-informed and suited to the patient's individual story of health. Effective taking of health histories also supports the partnership relationship between clinician and patient, fostering an attitude of shared decision-making. Patients who demonstrate their health-care professionals take them seriously are likely to optimize participation and concordance with treatment plans. Involving the patient in the process allows them to voice their concerns and preferences, which are focal in the decision-making model of directing diagnosis and treatment. In addition, an interactive style can allow patients to engage actively in the care of their own health, leading to improved outcomes. As is evident in health professions, such as mental health nursing, the relationship between patient narratives and clinical practice is the foundation of effective prescribing practices and signifies the need to integrate theoretical underpinnings with empirical practices to guide treatment interventions (Evans et al., 2009). In addition, the incorporation of incorporating the accommodation of health histories with new medical insights and technologies guides diagnosis and treatment. With new screening tools and treatment options on the horizon, it is more crucial than ever to learn about the social and political context of such innovations. The concept of entrenchment shows how health innovations, such as screening for cystic fibrosis, can be entrenched as routine practices informed by stakeholder relationships and ongoing articulation of demand (Koch et al., 1994). This dynamic relationship highlights the value in staying current with current developments with relevance to patient care. By continuous updating of the knowledge base and integration of new paradigms into health history taking, practitioners are able to sharpen their diagnostic precision and hence maximize the utility and effectiveness of treatment interventions in accordance with their patients' continually evolving requirements.

Test Your Knowledge

1. Why is health history taking considered a critical first step in the patient assessment process?
2. How does obtaining a detailed health history contribute to accurate diagnosis and treatment planning?

3.2. Components of a Comprehensive Health History

Learning Outcome

1. Demographic information;
2. Medical history and family history;
3. Social history and lifestyle factors.

A comprehensive health history is the foundation of establishing a solid foundation for the patient's care and consists of several significant elements. The initial element is the chief complaint, where one mentions the primary reason for the patients visit. Subsequently follows an extended history of present illness (HPI), which is crucial as it delves into the description of the symptoms and incorporates the onset, duration, and other associated factors. Lastly, the taking of a comprehensive past medical history is crucial, documenting significant illnesses, hospital stays, and operations that have bearing on the patient's present health status. Obtaining knowledge of a patient's family history via a family medical history can also be useful in identifying genetic diseases that may affect diagnosis and treatment. Finally, these components work synergistically to provide an entire composite of the patient's health, facilitating clinical decision-making and the possibility of successful treatment result. In the setting of medication documentation, accuracy and completeness are top considerations in achieving optimal patient safety and efficacious treatment. A study on dental students' behavior discovered that even though the majority of students understood the requirement for thorough medication history, they failed to document important factors like possible oral effects and reasons for drugs (Burcham et al., 2019). The significance of these cannot be overstated since they influence not just pharmacological insight but the clinicians' capacity to provide integrative care. Furthermore, barriers such as patients' ignorance about their medication render it harder to cope with, and hence there is an even greater need for a good methodology in history taking. Health practitioners can greatly improve their practice and patient outcomes by filling lacunae and enhancing training around documentation of medication. Furthermore, mental health intake assessment reflects another component of the omnibus history-taking process in which biopsychosocial integration is a critical factor. Results from a study on therapists assessment processes revealed that while some elements of clients biological, psychological, and sociocultural functioning were regularly documented, thoroughness as well as integration of the same were weak (Melchert et al., 2011).

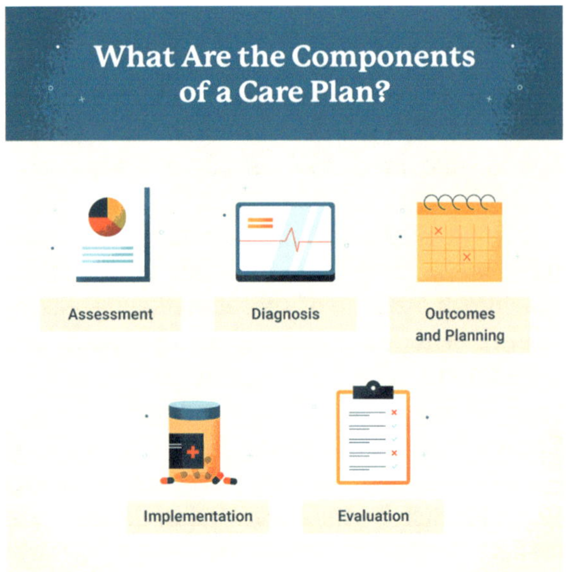

Figure 3.5. Components of a comprehensive health history.

Source: https://i0.wp.com/www.usa.edu/wp-content/uploads/2021/07/1-how-to-write-a-care-plan-1.png?resize=738%2C745&ssl=1.

Such weaknesses are likely to become significant barriers to case conceptualization as well as treatment outcome. This emphasizes the importance of training in collecting and synthesizing total information, which is essential to the capacity to create interventions informed by clients' unique needs. Through the development of a total picture of patients by means of total health histories, clinicians are in better position to address the complex interplay of factors involved in health and well-being, ultimately achieving better therapeutic outcomes (Figure 3.5).

3.2.1. Demographic Information

Understanding demographic information is of the utmost importance in taking health histories since it provides significant context for medical care. Demographics encompass measures such as age, gender, ethnic background, and socioeconomic status, all of which can have drastic impacts on a person's health status and healthcare needs. For instance, the prevalence of Alzheimer's disease demonstrates how important age as a demographic factor is; with approximately 6.7 million Americans aged more than 65 years old presently living with the condition, the demographic composition of seniors such that specialized health care services are required to treat this endemic disease (N/A, 2023). When health professionals obtain demographic data, they can establish risk factors and organize interventions that respond to the needs of specific population groups, demonstrating how demographics coincide with quality delivery of healthcare. Moreover, cultural background and ethnicity also form a pivotal component in the taking of health history. Cultural background and ethnicity not only affect an individual's health belief and practice but also their access to health care resources. For instance, some ethnic populations have higher rates of some chronic illnesses so screening and prevention must be targeted. Health disparities among marginalized groups highlight the necessity for getting inclusive demographics to establish and correct inequities. These disparities appear quite clearly in studies among cancer patients during the COVID-19 pandemic era, with comorbid patients, e.g., cancer, at higher risks of severe illness (Dai et al., 2020). Through incorporation of demographic information, health care professionals can encourage culturally appropriate care, guiding patients appropriately with assistance and counseling according to their backgrounds. Last but not least, socioeconomic status, as a demographic variable, plays a critical role in understanding a patient's health history along with potential barriers towards care. Patients from lower socioeconomic backgrounds have greater challenges with accessing health care, which actually exacerbates existing sickness. Economic factors influence not only the ability to gain access to treatment but also the ability to adhere to medical recommendations, such as for instance paying for meds or attending follow-up appointments. The calculation of the value of unpaid care for dementia at $339.5 billion in 2022 only goes to further establish the economic impact that diseases like Alzheimer's disease can have, particularly on households (N/A, 2023). Thus, the study of demographic information enables health care providers to design interventions that consider the socioeconomic constraints a patient may have, offering equal access to care and increased health benefits (Figure 3.6).

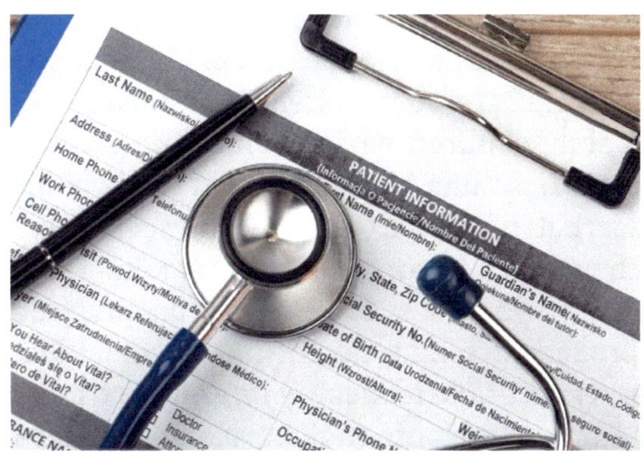

Figure 3.6. Patient demographics.

Source: https://www.eclaimstatus.com/blog/wp-content/uploads/2021/09/patient-demographics.jpg.

3.2.2. Medical History and Family History

Taking of a patient's history of medical and family history is a critical component of taking a health history that immediately translates into effective clinical practice. Medical history includes past and current ailments, surgeries, and treatments, while family history investigates genetic tendencies and disease patterns within the family. Accessing such information is utilized to identify risk factors for various conditions, facilitating timely intervention and control measures. For instance, an accurate understanding of a patient's family patterns can uncover genetic diseases that would otherwise go undetected, enhancing the precision of diagnoses and the efficacy of care interventions. This is especially true in children's health, as certain congenital and genetic disorders become evident early in life, necessitating proactive health interventions based on family history (Il'ya et al., 2022). More importantly, the social determinants context within medical history cannot be overemphasized. While assessing the health of a patient, it is equally essential to determine the part played by socioeconomic factors in individual and family health outcomes. For example, environment, education level, and income levels contribute significantly to a patient's access to healthcare facilities, nutrition, and social support systems. As observed in research, children with chronic illness such as bronchial asthma typically exhibit comorbidities exacerbated by environmental and social factors such as housing conditions and smoking in the family (Il'ya et al., 2022). With an integrated approach in taking health history, healthcare workers are able to identify improved strategies in addressing potential barriers and create interventions that are appropriate for the unique complexities that patients and their families are undergoing. The Inuit Child Health Clinic is an example that integrates medical and family histories with culturally sensitive frameworks, which demonstrate the overlap of health and social complexities. A closer review of both medical and social histories among Inuit families has proven significant gaps in care and service coordination, for which a multidisciplinary treatment modality is required. By addressing these disparities, healthcare professionals can develop targeted screening tools that consider some of these social determinants of health outcomes. The emphasis on comprehensive health history taking, including complete family histories, is central in developing a more just healthcare environment, particularly in addressing those populations that face systemwide health disparities. Practicing diversity on these integrated models of care not only improves clinical effectiveness but also advances the overall objectives of public health—delivering all people with equitable, accessible care regardless of their history (Figure 3.7).

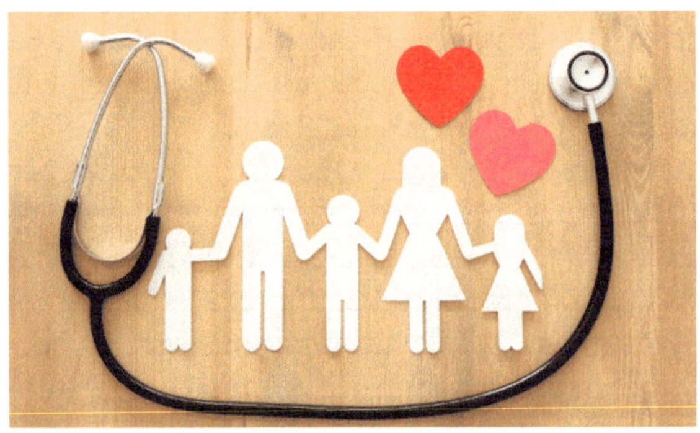

Figure 3.7. Medical history and family history.

Source: https://familytreemagazine.com/wp-content/uploads/2020/09/exploring-family-health-history.png.

3.2.3. Social History and Lifestyle Factors

Social history and lifestyle determinants are significant in the taking of a health history, as they significantly influence patient health outcomes. Social determinants of socio-economic status, education, and ethnicity significantly influence people's health behavior and access to healthcare resources. For instance, individuals with lower socio-economic status can have constraints on healthcare services, which influence their ability to manage chronic health conditions. The integration of social history into a comprehensive health history allows health workers to conceptualize interventions and make recommendations more precisely to the patient context, thus improving the quality of care. Further, identification of lifestyle elements, such as diet, physical activity, and drug abuse, also helps in the assessment of risk factors specific to diseases like cardiovascular disease (CVD) and can better guide prevention efforts as have outlined in literature for effective health history practice (Auerbach et al., 2017). Additionally, intricacies of patients lifestyles, particularly regarding their emotional well-being, are key to keeping them healthy. Evidence indicates that emotional disorders have a dramatic effect on the quality of life in patients with chronic illness, such as stable angina, and are made worse by social isolation or lack of support systems (Ferrari et al., 2020). It is not only important to inquire about physical symptoms during health history taking but also about patients' emotional experiences and support systems. This holistic approach enables health professionals to identify patients who need additional psychological attention, thereby adding to their overall management plan. Through enabling open communication of emotional health and lifestyle concerns, professionals can better respond to the compounded needs of their patients, minimizing health issues and maximizing preventive care. Moreover, integrating social history and lifestyle factors into the taking of health histories can come with improved communication between patients and healthcare providers. When healthcare providers actually take time to discover the lifestyle histories where patients live, it builds a trust culture. More-valued stakeholders in their health care, patients are more likely to share sensitive information related to their health. For instance, diet or exercise discussions can bring intervention opportunities that were not otherwise apparent into view (Auerbach et al., 2017). Second, a clearer image of a patient's social structure can help identify effective stressors that are contributing to decreased health. Thus, through the identification of social history and lifestyle, not only is data collection enhanced but empowered patients to develop more effective and coordinated health management strategies.

Test Your Knowledge

1. What are the key elements included in a comprehensive health history, and how does each element assist in patient care?
2. How does a family history and social history influence the understanding of a patient's current health status?

3.3. Techniques for Effective Health History Taking

Learning Outcome

1. Active listening skills;
2. Open-ended questioning;
3. Building rapport with patients.

Successful taking of a health history is a fundamental competency that medical practitioners must attain to effectively evaluate patients and image for potential health issues. Among the primary techniques is employing open-ended questions when communicating with patients. The process enables patients to present their symptoms, complaints, and histories using their own words without experiencing inhibitions from the limitations of a closed question. By listening and allowing patients to share their health stories, practitioners can extract vital information otherwise lost through limiting yes or no questioning. The qualitative information derived from this exchange is necessary, particularly when confronted with complex medical histories for which a complete understanding must be obtained in order to direct treatment. Thus, blending good communication skills with interview skills would enhance health history taking and lead to more individualized care. Technology application in health history taking, i.e., computer-assisted history-taking systems (CAHTS), provides a new dimension to information quality improvement collected. Research has established that CAHTS can enhance history-taking by making it easier to take more complete patient data. Specifically, evidence indicates that its application has led to better prevention and management outcomes in cardiovascular disease (CVD) patients, such that patients who utilized CAHTS recorded higher rates of engagement in health conversations with health professionals (Auerbach et al., 2017). The technology is able to classify information in an orderly fashion and allow for reduction in the time spent in discussion but intensify the probing into patient concerns rather than expand discussion time. Thus, embracing technological advances in medical practice not only expedites the process of history-taking but also enhances better decision-making and significantly improves patient participation in their own health schemes. Additionally, there is a need to explore the role of empathetic interaction within the process of health history-taking. Building rapport with patients forms the basis of trustful relationship and enables them to share sensitive details about their health. Healthcare professionals are supposed to be sympathetic, compassionate, and interested in-patient histories in order to create a warm atmosphere that encourages open communication. Emotional rapport may relieve the intimidation of the patient during medical interviews.

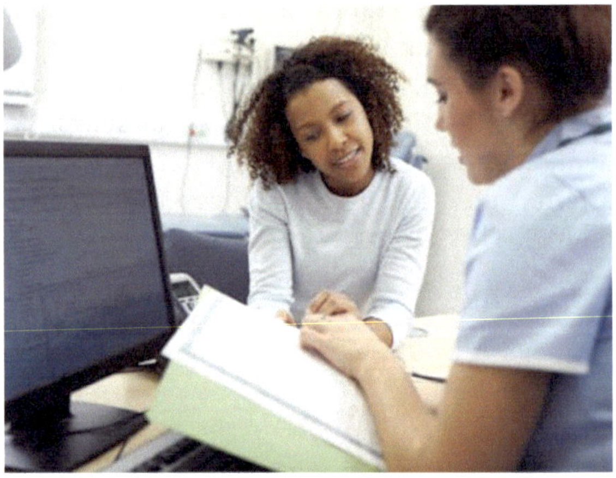

Figure 3.8. Techniques for effective health history taking.

Source: https://emis.imgix.net/emis-health/production/uploads/Primary-care/Patient-grey-jumper-talks-to-nurse.jpg?ar=4%3A3&auto=compress%2Cformat&crop=focalpoint&fit=crop&fp-x=0.5&fp-y=0.5&w=400&s=ee428ee9ae368661a95b8af15771d0cc.

It has been suggested through evidence that patients who are understood and supported are likely to provide honest and truthful feedback regarding their health, and hence the efficacy of the health history taking is enhanced (Escota et al., 2020). All these approaches—open-ended dialogue, technology utilization, and empathetic rapport—form a robust framework to ensure effective health history taking, and subsequently, it further aids in ensuring improved patient outcomes as well as patient satisfaction (Figure 3.8).

3.3.1. Active Listening Skills

Active listening abilities are an essential component of effective health history taking, and they constitute the foundation of patient-provider communication. By active listening, healthcare providers not only obtain required information from the patient but also establish a trusting bond that encourages open communication. It is not just a question of hearing what is being said by the patient, but even perceiving their underlying emotions and issues. While actively listening, clinicians communicate empathy and acknowledge patients experience, which can also be used to greatly enhance the quality of information given. This process of relationship is particularly relevant in cases such as chronic illness care, where comprehending nuances of patient experience are key to successful care. The capacity to reflect upon and interpret what has been communicated allows health professionals to tailor their questioning and interventions better, therefore leading to more accurate diagnoses and treatment strategies. Active listening is particularly worthwhile where there are individuals with unique requirements, e.g., chronic fatigue syndrome or learning disability. Individualized conversation was considered crucial in studies of chronic fatigue syndrome. The treatment process involved describing patients symptoms in plain language and together developing a rehabilitative plan, emphasizing that the effectiveness of any form of communication is required even in clinical trials (Deale et al., 2006). This emphasizes that the process of active listening and supportive communication can achieve greater patient participation and compliance with treatment regimens. Additionally, utilizing these skills to meet the individual perspectives and understanding levels of different patient populations ensures that every opinion is paid attention to and respected in the process of taking the health history. Active listening skills are also utilized in enhancing informed consent procedures, particularly for vulnerable populations. In the case of people with learning disabilities, understanding the concept of research participation and ethical concerns requires an environment where active listening takes precedence. By engaging patients as partners in the conversation, healthcare providers can access their knowledge levels and provide a greater understanding of health information (Cook et al., 2008). Not only does such engagement guarantee ethical research conduct, but it also empowers patients and makes them more informed about their own decisions about their health. This approach is consistent with broader goals of patient-centered care, in which attention is placed on listening to patient stories that inform clinical practice and ultimately improve health outcomes as well as patient satisfaction in the system (Figure 3.9).

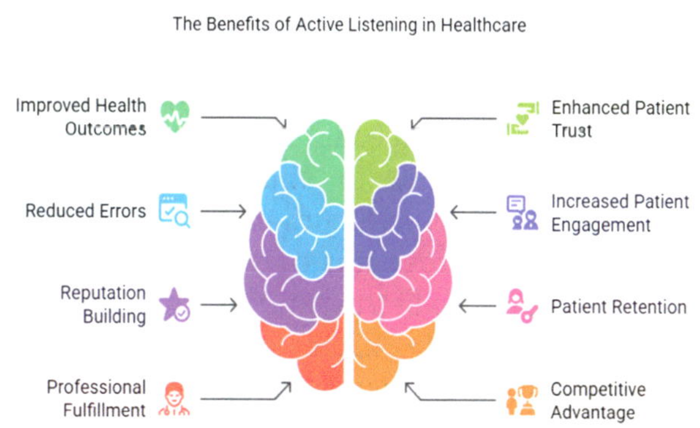

Figure 3.9. Active listening in healthcare.

Source: https://images.squarespace-cdn.com/content/v1/60f38d658275884057b90982/db585f27-1c6d-4892-b625-632604369ea1/active-listening-patient-satisfaction.png.

3.3.2. Open-Ended Questioning

Open-ended questioning is a fundamental technique in the collection of health histories that fosters comprehensive comprehension of patients medical histories. Unlike closed-ended questions that invite brief, sometimes dichotomous responses, open-ended questions enable patients to tell their feelings and thoughts and thereby create an understanding of their health problems. For instance, a clinician can ask, "Tell me about the symptoms you have been experiencing." " Such an approach not only provides the patient the opportunity to give their account but also uncovers information that could prove critical to diagnosis and treatment. The value of open-ended questioning is long established: it promotes communication between health professional and patient, empowers patients, and generates a more compassionate clinical environment, leading ultimately to improved outcomes in healthcare and greater patient satisfaction." Furthermore, open-ended questioning is particularly vital when working with sensitive health topics or complex medical backgrounds. Patients may become uneasy or resistant to sharing information vital to their treatment under these circumstances. Sound approaches such as building rapport and employing open-ended probes will make a significant impact in getting elaborated information from patients, according to researchers who have examined interviewing techniques (Cameron et al., 2015). For example, requesting patients to share their health experience, while inviting them to express any fear or anxiety, does not only collect data; it establishes a sense of trust and alliance between the patient and the health care practitioner. This trust is important in collecting honest and full information, thus enabling a more precise and comprehensive appraisal of the patients' health requirements. Aside from facilitating data collection, open-ended questioning can bring out underlying tendencies or complications that would otherwise remain unheard in a health context. For example, by asking patients to share their perception of their health conditions or treatment protocols, health workers can identify knowledge gaps or misconceptions that may discourage compliance or healing (Lyon et al., 2002). This approach is also consistent with current healthcare practice that aims for patient-centered care, with the patient's perspective being a valuable component of the therapeutic process. With the recent progress in healthcare, the retention of open-ended questioning in health history taking is still an essential practice, enhancing not only the quality of health information that is gathered but also the patient's overall health experience.

3.3.3. Building Rapport with Patients

Establishing rapport with patients is also one of the most important components of effective health history taking since it establishes a relationship built on trust between the health provider and the patient. It begins by establishing an open atmosphere that encourages discussions. When comfortable, patients are relaxed and more likely to divulge personal health-related information. Empathy and active listening are the rudimentary skills with which clinicians should operate to develop such rapport. With sincere expression of concern regarding a patient's welfare, healthcare providers can minimize anxiety, enabling patients to more effectively relate their health histories, contributing significantly to the quality of care with which they are treated. The subtleties of building rapport might be most pronounced in cases with high sensitivity, such as when working with patients who have been exposed to adverse childhood experiences (ACEs) or those faced with social determinants of health (SDOH) challenges. Research affirms that addressing these issues systematically within healthcare organizations is fundamental to providing integral care that considers the patient's life in its entire context. By being attuned to the meaning of ACEs and SDOH, health clinicians will be able to work more effectively with patients. Not only does it help to validate patients' histories but also to guide individualized care plans that address their unique needs, thereby cementing the therapeutic bond critical to effective health history taking. The affective processes between practitioners and patients can also not be overstressed in enabling rapport development. Empathy and feeling are especially critical in managing this relationship, especially in high-stress environments such as a cancer drop-in center. Researchers have determined that a balance of emotional care for oneself and empathetic connection is imperative in such settings. In the absence of this balance, providers become prone to emotional exhaustion, which decreases the level of patient care. To surmount this challenge requires continued investment in personal welfare as well as professional obligation. Thus, the integration of emotional intelligence into history taking health history not only enhances patient communication but also guarantees the sustainability of clinicians' engagement in spite of emotionally charged interactions, hence leading to better patients' health outcomes (Figure 3.10).

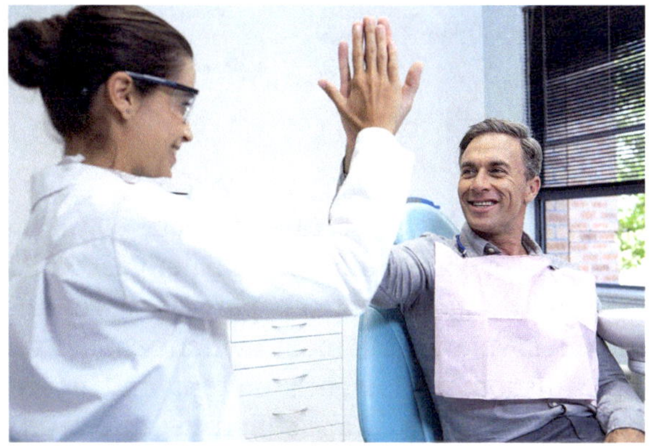

Figure 3.10. Building rapport with patients.

Source: https://cdn.todaysrdh.com/wp-content/uploads/2018/10/dental-hygiene-patient-rapport-rdh.jpg?strip=all&lossy=1&ssl=1.

Test Your Knowledge

1. What communication strategies can a nurse use to elicit complete and accurate information from patients during history taking?
2. How can active listening and open-ended questions improve the quality of information gathered in a health history?

3.4. Common Challenges in Health History Taking

Learning Outcome

1. Patient reluctance to share information;
2. Language and cultural barriers;
3. Time constraints in clinical settings.

One of the most important aspects of taking health history is its inherent challenges, which may significantly impact patient care and outcomes. Among the most evident challenges is the discomfort of both patient and health practitioner in raising sensitive questions, particularly related to sexuality. The majority of medical residents have identified inadequate training on how to handle such questions as a major reason for not wishing to discuss such topics within consultation. This discomfort tends to arise due to an insufficiency of skills and knowledge necessary for successful sexual history taking, as indicated in recent literature. Therefore, practitioners tend to forego the eliciting of important patient information that would be useful in making diagnoses and establishing treatment, thus compromising the quality of care. Overcoming these obstacles is key to advancing a more comprehensive and holistic process of health history taking, ultimately leading to greater patient trust and involvement in their own care (Bogaert et al., 2025). Aside from individual discomfort, there are also a number of biases that create a major obstacle in effective health history taking. Concerns such as religion, ethnicity, age, and gender can adversely impact the provider style and patient willingness to disclose vital information. For instance, certain biases may lead healthcare providers to make assumptions regarding patients based on their background rather than engage in open, objective discourse. This may lead to complete assessments being hindered and to misdiagnoses or treatment errors. Also, material concerns such as time constraints within busy clinical settings can exacerbate these biases by prompting health professionals to rush history-taking processes. Enhancing overall quality of health histories requires that programs be implemented targeting eradication of such biases along with effective communication skills among health providers (Bogaert et al., 2025). Incorporation of technology in healthcare practice has emerged as an effective way to combat some of the drawbacks associated with taking health history. Application of chatbots and artificial intelligence-based tools offers new answers to the history-taking process. Utilizing automated questions, such platforms can potentially improve patient engagement and augment data collection effectiveness, addressing time constraints for health care professionals. Systematic review has shown that chatbots enable accurate retrieval of information while guaranteeing a higher level of patient satisfaction. However, in order for such technology to be effective, there must be careful design so that ease of use and data protection are guaranteed without sacrificing the empathetic interaction necessary in the patient-physician relationship. Continued studies into the ability of chatbots and emotional intelligence are still required to make the most of them in modern healthcare environments, including in the field of health history taking.

3.4.1. Patient Reluctance to Share Information

Patient hesitation to share information when taking health history can significantly undermine the quality of care obtained. It is usually brought about by various personal, cultural, and system barriers that make it difficult for patients to identify with health professionals. Individuals may be afraid of exposing intimate information because they do not want to be judged or stigmatized, particularly for issues related to mental health, drug use, or sexual history. Also at stake is the problem of trust;

patients may not be willing to offer complete information if they perceive that providers lack an open ear or understanding mind. Since it has been established in research that increased inter-professional collaboration is essential for successful primary care delivery, communication among healthcare teams may have a direct impact on a patient's willingness to share significant health information, and also affect the overall outcome of treatment (Bond et al., 2014). Patient demographics also significantly affect willingness to disclose information about health. Specific ethnic and racial groups can also exhibit greater hesitancy on the basis of history of discrimination in healthcare settings. For instance, research has found differences in infant birth outcomes for Black/African Americans and Hispanic/Latinos in the US and how historical negative interactions with healthcare generate suspicion and hesitancy in seeking providers (Bryan et al., 2016). As have been reported by study participants, even with optimum quality care, these experiences were marred by perceived impersonality. These sentiments can perpetuate barriers to appropriate communication, eventually discouraging comprehensive health history taking and limiting the providers ability to deliver customized care. To avoid these situations, healthcare providers must work towards establishing a space of trust and openness. Efforts like intentionally encouraging patient dialogue and cultural competency expression are effective in enhancing quality communication. Skills training to improve interpersonal relationships among health care professionals can serve as a gateway to facilitating better relations with patients and deterring reluctance to share personal health information. Institutional guidelines should also evolve to address systematic types of barriers so that the health care environment is more inclusive and welcoming. By the shift from a one-size-fits-all to a more personalized interaction model, patients can be enabled to openly disclose their health histories, eventually obtaining improved health outcomes and an improved patient experience (Bond et al., 2014) (Figure 3.11).

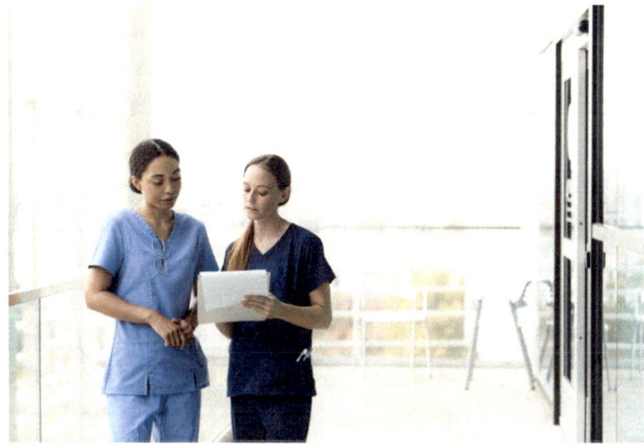

Figure 3.11. Patient reluctance to share information.

Source: https://medtrainer.com/wp-content/uploads/2021/06/image-blog-sharing-patient-information.png.

3.4.2. Language and Cultural Barriers

Language and cultural barriers are the major problems in the taking of health history, which can negatively impact the quality of the patient care. Effective communication between the healthcare provider and the patient is necessary for proper diagnosis and treatment. In the event of language differences, then patients cannot explain their symptoms or concerns clearly, and thus there can be misunderstandings by the healthcare providers. Cultural background also plays a very critical role as patients will hold contrasting beliefs about health, illness, and methods of treatment. These are obstacles that could deprive healthcare providers of a complete understanding of a patient's health history and therefore jeopardize clinical outcomes, as well as patient confidence. There are jarring contrasts across the means by which patients travel through healthcare systems due to such cultural and language barriers. For instance, the population members from linguistically diverse populations are likely to face obstacles in accessing life-sustaining healthcare information, which can discourage them from seeking the needed medical attention. This is most applicable in the environments wherein medical terminology and the healthcare system are predominantly constructed using a specific cultural lens. Here, the minority population members become victims of an added effect, leading to disparities in health outcomes. Sound strategies, such as the use of interpreters and culturally competent care, are crucial to fixing these issues. Health care organizations need to be aware of and address these barriers so that all patients can receive equal and high-quality care. Furthermore, the public health impact of language and cultural barriers starts to have broader ramifications beyond individual patient visits. Studies indicate that miscommunication leads to unsafe healthcare, aggravates conditions, and causes additional risk of harmful occurrences. Public health initiatives must address linguistic diversity in order to effectively disseminate important health information, particularly during emergencies or public health emergencies. Furthermore, understanding the cultural factors affecting health beliefs can optimize outreach activities, such as fostering confidence and cooperation between healthcare systems and individuals within communities. As our population becomes more diverse, language and cultural differences are not only helpful to address but are essential to improving overall health outcomes and promoting health equity for communities.

3.4.3. Time Constraints in Clinical Settings

In clinical practice, precious time has a calamitous impact on the quality of health history taking and thus on patient care. Physicians might be overwhelmed with tasks like managing patients' burdens, performing diagnosis tests, and communicating with clinical teams. Such competing demands could turn into hurried interactions with patients, compromising the thoroughness of health history assessments. The challenges that come with time shortages not only lead to insufficient data collection but also risk overlooking vital patient information. Research on medical residents established that one of the key hindrances to effective sexual history taking was insufficient time, among other inadequate skills and knowledge, making it challenging to commence such interactions (Bogaert et al., 2025). This background identifies the strong imperative to control time in clinical practice to maximize the quality of history taking of health. Furthermore, pressures of time can establish an environment under which health care providers are prone to employ heuristics or to shortcutting history-taking practice. These approaches may help deal with current patient needs but often shortchange complete assessments. Pressure to perform in tight time frames can make both the patients and providers anxious, particularly when discussing sensitive topics. The study referred to above points out the uneasiness as an indicator of how time pressures heighten prejudice on grounds of age, gender, or culture, further degrading the quality of the communication in the discussion of the health histories (Bogaert et al., 2025). This pressure creates a vicious cycle where hurried interactions result in poor patient histories, these in turn contributing to less-than-ideal treatment plans. Training and system modification permitting increased interaction in taking patient history independent of time pressure thus becomes a necessity for healthcare facilities. In emergency medicine, the pressure of time is even more important due to the acuity of the cases encountered. The urgency to make timely decisions must be balanced by providers with the challenge of communicating effectively with disadvantaged groups such as Deaf and Hard of Hearing patients. In a study of emergency medicine settings, researchers determined that these time pressures and inaccessibility of communication tools regularly disrupted meaningful interaction with Deaf patients, contributing to health care disparities among this group. This scenario also demonstrates that restrictions are multifaceted and impact not just procedural efficiency but even the quality of care being provided to vulnerable groups. To further improve health history taking in the time-pressed context, future training programs should incorporate interventions to assist in improving communication skills, foster cultural sensitivity, and develop effective workflows that do not involve sacrificing intensive patient interaction (Figure 3.12).

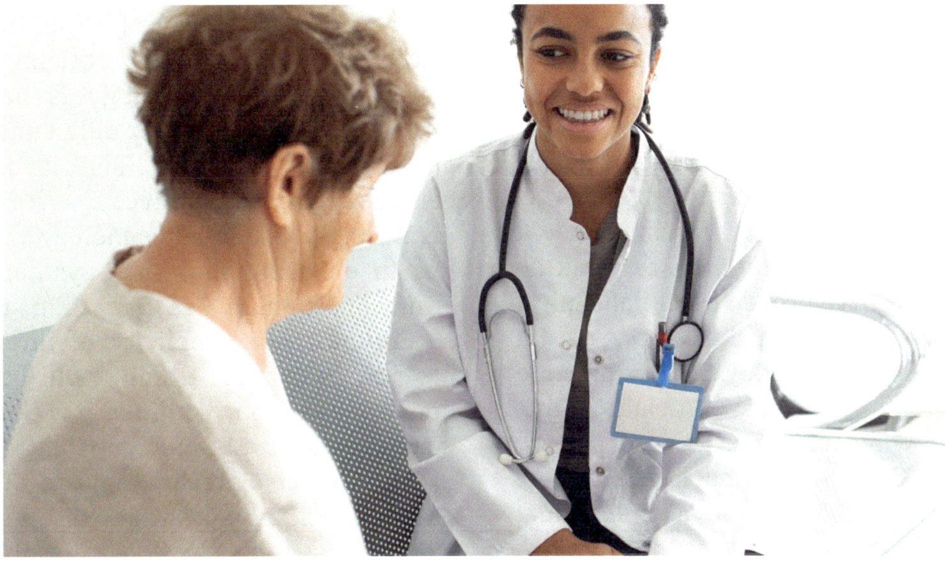

Figure 3.12. Time constraints in clinical settings.

Source: https://media.licdn.com/dms/image/v2/D4E12AQET8sKmQzngww/article-cover_image-shrink_720_1280/article-cover_image-shrink_720_1280/0/1737389356265?e=2147483647&v=beta&t=2oXIiZfBfDmBlwzQ_i5xQ05wnphICNEgtEXl7ZDYsiI.

Test Your Knowledge

1. What are the common barriers that can prevent patients from providing accurate or complete health histories?
2. How can language, cultural differences, or patient anxiety impact the effectiveness of health history taking?

3.5. Role of Technology in Health History Taking

Learning Outcome

1. Electronic health records (EHR);
2. Telehealth and remote consultations;
3. Mobile health applications.

Technology application in the taking of health histories has the ability to enhance significantly the speed and quality of gathering patient information. Computer-aided history-taking systems (CAHTS) have proven essential clinical practice tools, which enable clinicians to obtain patient histories more quickly. Studies indicate that the systems can save clinicians' time, ultimately allowing for more focused patient care. Besides, CAHTS have been effective in obtaining sensitive information such as sexual history and drug use that patients do not volunteer during usual interviews. Except for their advantages, there is limited utilization of CAHTS primarily for the application of traditional pen-and-paper methods and data security reasons. To effectively integrate CAHTS into everyday healthcare, there is a need for a shift in research, policy, and practice to overcome these obstacles and highlight the value of integrating technology in health history taking (Anandan et al., 2011). Just as important is the application of computer decision-support software (CDSS) within telephone triage, where technology supports healthcare providers in efficiently managing interactions with patients. This approach allows remote triaging by nurses, with optimal allocation of face-to-face appointments. With the use of CDSS, systematic structuring of patient information is facilitated, allowing for maximum capability to register and analyze various patient symptoms correctly. The dynamic interaction between the nurses and the patients becomes complex, as nurses need to manage both the technical interface and empathic communication. Evidence has indicated that nurses must learn advanced skills to reconcile the clinical expectations imposed by CDSS with the unique needs of patients during triage consultations. This requires professional training balancing technical proficiency with quality patient interactions to provide safe and effective patient care (Barnes et al., 2014). Amidst the background of evolving healthcare settings, where technology is harmonizing with history-taking, it not only enhances data-gathering efficiency but also favors patient-centered process delivery. With clinicians increasingly reliant on technology, the challenge lies in ensuring that such systems augment clinical judgment rather than undermine it. Emphasizing simplicity of interfaces and providing adequate training will be crucial in bolstering clinician confidence with using these instruments. Furthermore, ongoing surveillance of the impact of technology on outcomes in patients will be essential. Resolution of the advantages and issues surrounding the use of technology in history taking in health will inform future progress in such a way that these technologies advance process efficiency and emphasize patient interaction and care quality (Anandan et al., 2011; Barnes et al., 2014) (Figure 3.13).

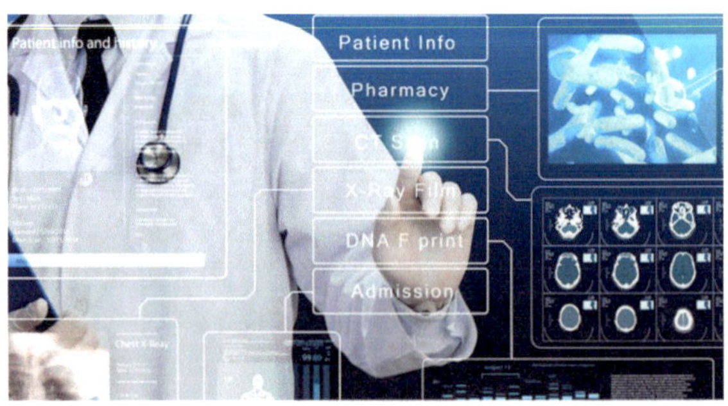

Figure 3.13. Role of technology in health history taking.

Source: https://www.gigadocs.com/blog/wp-content/uploads/2019/12/blog2-768x404.jpg.

3.5.1. Electronic Health Records (EHR)

The adoption of Electronic Health Records (EHR) has revolutionized health history taking in its very essence, promoting the quality of data acquisition and patient care. EHR systems allow healthcare professionals to capture patient information, including demographics, medical history, medications, and interventions with meticulous detail. This detailed record-keeping enables more standardized and efficient data capture, which translates into a strong basis for clinical decision-making. With EHRs, clinicians can readily access a patient's history of health, leading to enhanced diagnostic accuracy and tailored treatment regimens. The standardization in EHR format also minimizes data entry inconsistencies and thus increases the validity of medical records, perhaps even reducing the possibility of medication errors. All these are heavily in consonance with today's emphasis on patient-centered care that focuses on the role of valid history taking in delivering quality care. Aside from boosting data quality and accessibility, EHRs facilitate improved healthcare professional-to-professional communication necessary for quality history taking. With an EHR system, medical information can be readily accessed by any person authorized to engage in a patient's care, allowing coordinated and collaborative health care. This interconnectivity comes in handy for patients with complex histories of many conditions or multiple healthcare providers because it avoids fragmented care. By importing data from various specialties and making all healthcare teams cohesive, EHRs play a crucial role in mitigating the risk of omitted information while performing health history interviews. In addition, features such as allergy alerts and drug interactions facilitate a safer prescribing process since it is evidence of the direction toward a more proactive process in dealing with patient outcomes. Despite the numerous advantages, deployment of EHRs has numerous challenges that are most likely to impact the effectiveness of taking health history. Robust training programs play a significant role in ensuring a guarantee that practitioners will be proficient in managing EHR systems. Practitioners cannot work on these complex systems confidently if they are not adequately trained, and hence it is likely to introduce incomplete or inaccurate health histories. In addition, issues such as interoperability among heterogeneous EHR systems can hinder seamless sharing of patient information, thus complicating health history assessments. Not only does the fragmentation affect patient safety, but it may also result in inefficiency within healthcare centers because providers must access various systems to obtain comprehensive patient history. With these issues, ongoing investment in EHR technology and education, along with a dedication to developing standardization protocols that enhance overall efficacy in health history taking in the practice environment, is needed.

3.5.2. Telehealth and Remote Consultations

Telehealth and distant consultations have also become a very important part of contemporary healthcare service delivery, especially considering the current pandemic worldwide. These modalities enable the interaction between health professionals and their patients without requiring physical proximity, so that a wide array of services consisting of diagnosis, treatment, and monitoring is provided. This shift to virtual care has also highlighted the importance of good health history taking since medical professionals need to acquire in-depth details from patients in electronic form. Traditional methods of taking health history may not be directly applicable to remote environments, so techniques need to be modified which focus on crystal clear communication and empathy. The use of technology, such as video consultations, has been shown to enhance patient engagement and aid in more accurate historical data, leading ultimately to better patient outcomes through informed clinical decision-making (Alan et al., 2024). Despite the seemingly telehealth advantages, issues remain present within remote consultations that must be addressed to make easier health history taking possible. Providers may be faced with technical quality, confidentiality, and the intangible character of virtual communication that can render it challenging to assess patients' conditions. For example, performing physical exams is significantly limited in a remote environment, which compels health practitioners to delve deeper into patients' verbal reports and symptom self-reporting. Besides, as would be pointed out by research, the reluctance on the part of practitioners to be less confident about their ability to perform full examinations even when they are not physically present in the premises continues. Hence, developing the capacity of healthcare professionals to conduct virtual consultations is vital for resolving the above-stated problems and improving the accuracy and completeness of health histories gathered in remote areas (Alan et al., 2024). In addition, global discussion on telehealth also highlights the need to regularly monitor and renew remote consultation practice. In South Korea, for example, there has been massive discussion regarding the adoption and regulation of telemedicine, and this brought out a broader issue regarding the structure of healthcare delivery systems and the potential socio-economic disparity exacerbated by telehealth practice. Although telehealth is capable of bridging gaps in access to care, particularly in underserved or rural settings, it is essential to establish effective frameworks that guarantee quality and equitable outcomes. As highlighted within existing literature, further enhanced understanding of the strengths and limitations of telehealth will contribute to more effective incorporation into traditional models of healthcare. Regulatory support and cross-disciplinary collaboration is crucial in streamlining these remote practices, so that obtaining health history remains robust and effective regardless of the consultancy mode (Figure 3.14).

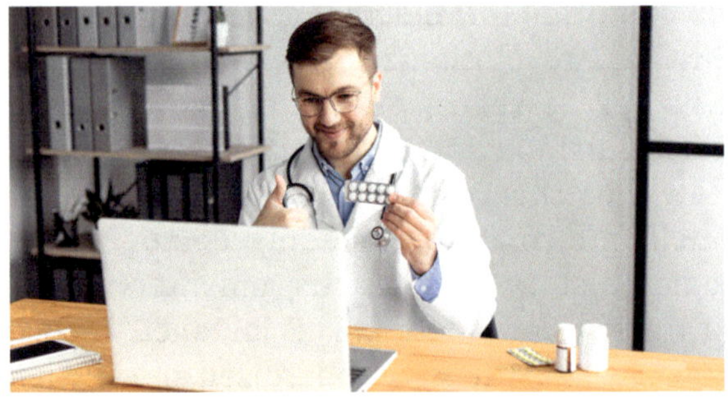

Figure 3.14. Telehealth and remote consultations.

Source: https://www.infovision.com/sites/default/files/styles/default/public/images/blogs/2024-07/Telemedicine.png?itok=drpo3pIa.

3.5.3. Mobile Health Applications

Introduction of mobile health (mHealth) apps has significantly transformed the practice of health history taking with the introduction of new data-collecting ways and patient participation. The apps enable patients to input their health information themselves, which is a more dynamic and individualized means of documenting health history. By facilitating self-reported data entries, mHealth applications have the ability to increase the validity of patient history because patients enter current information regarding their symptoms, medications, and lifestyle factors. importantly, through the development of deep learning models like YoloTR and YoloMBTR, it is now possible to identify ocular surface predictors of eye health more accurately, demonstrating the potential of mobile platforms to obtain invaluable health data in an orderly manner. This shift to self-reporting and real-time data processing supports the need to integrate technology into traditional healthcare processes, ultimately enhancing the overall reliability and availability of health information. Moreover, the use of artificial intelligence in mHealth applications supports their utility in history taking. Advanced AI processes can handle patient inputs, identify patterns, and pose questions to users that may be of clinical relevance in order to foster a better understanding of a patient's health status. In studies on the use of chatbots in taking medical history, it is indicated that chatbots as conversational agents are effective in improving patient engagement. As evidenced in systematic reviews, chatbots enhance the efficiency of data gathering as well as provide a 24/7 means for patients to ask advice about their condition (Hindelang et al., 2024). Apart from making history taking easier, the innovation also allows patients to become more active agents in their care, thereby maximizing patient satisfaction and outcomes. In spite of the wide range of benefits that mHealth apps provide in taking the health history, there are some challenges that still need to be overcome. Data security, privacy, and ethical problems need to take priority in order to promote patient trust and readiness to participate with these electronic tools. In addition, reliance on user-provided data and AI computations undermines the completeness and precision of the captured history, as argued in literature against AI-based diagnosis from user input alone (Wang et al., 2025). In order to integrate mHealth apps effectively into practice, there must be an equilibrium between robust technology backbones and empathetic patient-clinician relationships. Future studies would be focused on calibrating this software so that they not only incorporate comprehensive health histories but also develop an atmosphere conducive to patient dignity and confidentiality.

Test Your Knowledge

1. How can electronic health records (EHRs) enhance the efficiency and accuracy of health history documentation?
2. What are the potential benefits and drawbacks of using telehealth platforms for conducting patient health histories?

3.6. Ethical Considerations in Health History Taking

Learning Outcome

1. Patient confidentiality and privacy;
2. Informed consent;
3. Cultural sensitivity and respect.

Health history taking is a process that involves a complex interplay of ethical guidelines central to ensuring patient welfare and fostering trust in the healthcare environment. Confidentiality lies central to these ethical issues as patients must feel at ease in knowing that their personal health information will not be revealed and is only available to those who are in authority. This assurance promotes openness, whereby patients can divulge pertinent information concerning their condition without worrying about being condemned or their privacy breached. Ethical principles call for health professionals to be silent on patient matters because any deviation from practicing this principle would not only jeopardize patient trust but could have a negative impact in the delivery of care. Without appreciation and respect for these ethical guidelines, the impact of health history taking can be significantly diminished, both clinically and in terms of patient satisfaction. Informed consent, together with confidentiality, is another key ethical concern of health history taking. Patients must be informed, completely, about the purpose and significance of the information collected. This includes not only verbal explanations by healthcare professionals but also ascertaining the patient's comprehension of the potential risks and benefits of disclosing confidential information. Informed consent is greater than legal adherence; it is the ethical responsibility of healthcare professionals to facilitate patients under their care. By creating room for questioning and illumination, practitioners can ensure patients' autonomy while forming a partnership in the process of healthcare. These practices not only respect the right of the patient to self-determination but also create a trusting partnership among providers and patients. The ethical ramifications of health history taking also reach out to considerations of cultural competence and sensitivity. Health practitioners are required to recognize and accept the multiple backgrounds of their patients, which can influence their perceptions regarding health, disease, and revelation. Practitioners can cross obstacles, which could hinder effective accurate and comprehensive taking of health histories, by embracing cultural competence. This calls for understanding patients beliefs, values, and practices, which can influence patients' willingness to provide lucid and comprehensive information during health assessment. Moreover, including patient representatives and feedback mechanisms can work to systematically enhance the ethical quality of health history taking in alignment with the highest possible standards of ethics. By way of a culturally competent practice, physicians not only enhance the reliability of health histories, but also tackle overall healthcare ethics climate, as in programs described by (Bell et al., 2016; Plante et al., 2018).

3.6.1. Patient Confidentiality and Privacy

Confidentiality and patient's privacy are of utmost concern in today's healthcare setting, especially when taking the health history. Confidentiality ensures that the patient will feel comfortable in sharing sensitive information, which is a prerequisite for accurate diagnosis and proper treatment. The ethical obligation to protect patient information comes from a deep respect for the harm that can be caused by unauthorized disclosure, e.g., the risk of stigmatizing patients or avoidance of necessary medical treatment. This ethical foundation is not only important for patient trust but also a legal requirement for laws such as the Health Insurance Portability and Accountability Act (HIPPA), which calls for strict guidelines on how to manage and disseminate individual health information. Thus, healthcare providers must navigate these complexities in order to uphold both ethical codes and legal requirements successfully. The introduction of technological innovation such as virtual clinical trials raises the possibilities and pitfalls to maintaining patient confidentiality. Virtual trials offer a cost-saving approach for engaging patients through the internet, thus minimizing geographic barriers and allowing wider participation, in effect, democratizing clinical research (Andrews et al., 2017). However, the nature of these trials taking place online raises serious issues regarding informed consent and maintaining confidentiality. With sensitive information publicized online, there is increased risk of breaches, which do not maintain patient confidentiality and trust. Healthcare providers thus have to exercise caution, with robust cybersecurity measures and constructing elaborate consent procedures. The delicacy of balancing the exploitation of the advantages of modern technology with the demands of confidentiality is a significant challenge in the pursuit of ethical delivery of healthcare during the digital age. Moreover, the concept of ambivalence towards digital health reveals the intricate dynamics of patient privacy within the modern-day healthcare environment. Patients are often confronted with conflicting opposites on the ease of handling digital devices and having access to data risks (Darking et al., 2018). For instance, although others might appreciate the immediacy of contact offered by mobile health apps, they simultaneously have apprehension over security of their personal health data. This ambivalence is indicative of the need for healthcare professionals to converse with patients about their privacy matters in a manner that it will develop an environment where patients are assured to express their desires and apprehensions. These dilemmas not only enhance patient-clinician relationships but also inform the design and implementation of digital health interventions, ultimately balancing technological innovation with ethical norms of patient confidentiality and privacy (Figure 3.15).

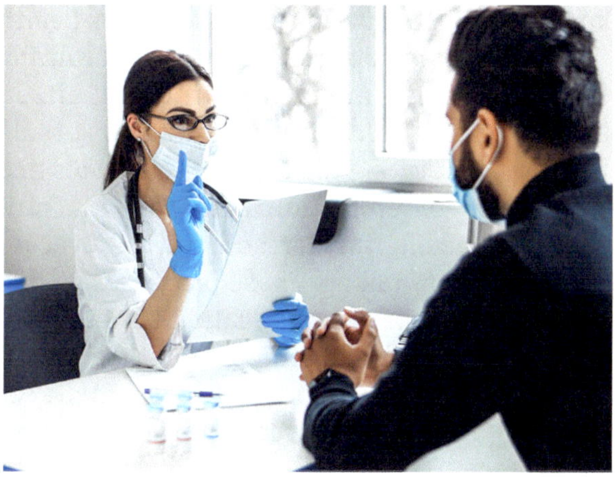

Figure 3.15. Patient confidentiality and privacy.

Source: https://tego.com.au/wp-content/uploads/2022/12/Patient-confidentiality-and-privacy.jpg.

3.6.2. Informed Consent

Informed consent is a core ethical principle in healthcare practice, especially in health history taking. The process goes beyond the act of getting a signature; it involves ensuring that patients receive sufficient information regarding their condition, the suggested interventions, as well as any risks and benefits involved. Good communication is particularly crucial in this field, as a healthcare professional must be able to express complex information in terms that the patient can comprehend at his level of knowledge. Otherwise, patients won't make informed decisions about their care, which can lead to complaints of suspicion or dissatisfaction with their practitioners. Moreover, the absence of this fundamental component may result in legal repercussions for the provider in case of disputes over the patient's consent, thereby highlighting the necessity of robust informed consent measures in health history taking. Beyond individual decisions, the consequences of informed consent extend to public health as a whole, affecting it as well. When patients take an active part in their own health care decision-making through provision of informed consent, they are more likely to adhere to prescribed prevention and treatments. Patient involvement is particularly relevant in interventions like rapid diagnosis testing of malaria. Here, health workers must deal with priority integration of patient-centered care that will facilitate informed consent, so that patients can understand the rationale for testing and treatment procedures. The PRIME study shows this need, revealing that although there was an awareness of the use of rapid diagnostic tests among health workers, there are issues with incorporating patient-centered practices within the restrictions, showing a gap that affects the effectiveness of interventions to improve patient outcomes via informed consent and relational engagement (Namagembe et al., 2017). Informed consent also has a close association with ethical challenges concerning patient autonomy and shared decision-making. In terms of treatment of chronic diseases like Charcot neuroarthropathy, the process of informed consent is all the more important. Patients who have long-term courses of treatment require lengthy discussions about options, and information on the meaning of agreement to enter new studies that can alter their treatment scenario is most paramount. By interacting with patients in an open and communicative manner about their condition, potential interventions, and the use of technology such as Magnetic Resonance Imaging to their treatment, healthcare providers can more readily facilitate autonomous decision-making (Mcinnes et al., 2020). This enables patients to be more empowered in their own care, which may ultimately lead to improved health outcomes and greater satisfaction with the healthcare experience in general. Therefore, informed consent transcends the documentary form, in that it describes the very nature of patient-centered care provision.

3.6.3. Cultural Sensitivity and Respect

Effective health history taking is not only technical skill, but also a large measure of cultural insight and respect. It is only when a person recognizes that patients come from diverse backgrounds, beliefs, traditions, and values that it is possible to establish a trusting relationship. Cultural sensitivity allows providers to approach each patient as a unique individual whose unique context will be a significant determinant of his/her health behaviors and requires. This validation promotes an honest exchange in which patients are respected and listened to, finally leading to better health outcomes. A culturally competent framework provides the opportunity to determine potential barriers to care, such as differences in language or cultural misconceptions regarding health and illness. Thus, the inclusion of cultural respect during the early stages of health history taking can enhance patient engagement and encourage compliance with medical recommendations. Furthermore, medical professionals must intentionally practice reflection in order to become more culturally competent. By examining their own biases and understanding the ways in which their culture influences them, providers are best able to navigate the nuances brought by a diverse patient base. Individual development as well as healthier interactions with patients of various backgrounds are the outcomes of reflective practice. In this model, health practitioners need to familiarize themselves with commonly accepted cultural practices and beliefs because they have the potential to impact perceptions of health and health choice. For example, an understanding of specific health-oriented cultural rituals may inform the best method of communication for each patient. Through the synthesis of these understandings with clinical expertise and policy from the institution, health history taking is kept respectful and culturally competent, enhancing the individualized patient care experience (Windecker et al., 2014). Incorporating the utilization of tools like interpreters or education materials that are culturally specific further adds to the process of health history taking. These processes enable the overcoming of communication barriers and the provision of sharing important information in accuracy and respect. Employment of culturally attuned resources has the potential to enhance patient understanding of both their health conditions and therapies, hence promoting adherence to recommended health regimens. Moreover, cultural competence instruction should form part of professional medical training. Such instruction prepares future health professionals to grasp and value the rich tapestry of cultural diversity defining their patient population (Chan et al., 2013). By translating these principles into practice, clinicians can achieve a standard of care that is not merely clinically appropriate but also culturally validating and, in the end, helping to create a more equitable health system.

Test Your Knowledge

1. How can healthcare professionals ensure patient confidentiality while collecting sensitive health information?
2. What ethical issues may arise if a patient is unwilling or unable to provide a full health history, and how should they be addressed?

SUMMARY

The art of taking health histories is fundamental to the practice of competent patient care and clinical decision-making. Not only is it a part of medical assessment but it also assists in the deeper understanding of a patient's unique health experience. Good health histories enable health care professionals to craft individualized treatment plans and minimize the likelihood of misdiagnosis as well as improve outcomes for patients. The incorporation of advanced tools such as Computer Interpretable Guideline Models (CIGMs) provides this process more strength with the availability of systematic approaches for invariant clinical guideline compliance. The application of context-dependent task ontologies (CTOs) reveals the practicability of embedding technology in taking the health history with a positive effect on clinician-patient interaction and offering pertinent and useful data (Ciccarese et al., 2004). Also, the use of innovative pedagogy, such as that of Virginia Commonwealth University, prioritizes interdisciplinary learning in health taking history. Incorporating humanities into medical education allows prospective healthcare providers to build observing skills within a non-clinical setting, such as an art gallery, which can be transposed to enhanced empathy and communication skills with patients. This integrated approach not only guarantees that students are exposed to clinical data but also that they learn essential soft skills, which are integral to the understanding of the human condition. Thus, integrating a range of pedagogical methods can help develop a more integrated picture of health history taking and its relevance in clinical practice, improving the overall education of medical students (Fuqua et al., 2012). Finally, the insistence on taking health history highlights the ongoing necessity for continuous progress in clinical practice and education. As healthcare continues to evolve, the adoption of evidence-based practice and interprofessional collaboration will be vital to equipping practitioners to manage complex patient histories. Defending health history taking as standardized yet responsive through technological advances and innovative educational methods will have a wide impact on the quality of care for patients. Clinicians and educators both must consider innovations that not only streamline the taking of health histories but also enhance the relationship between patient and provider. Finally, with focused efforts in the evolution of these processes, the medical community can shift toward more patient-oriented models of care, where technical skill and emotional intelligence are equally emphasized within clinical settings.

In health history taking, it is important to identify the multifaceted nature of patient assessments. Health history taking is not just systematic collection of medical and biological details but also includes the emotional and psychological status of patients. Such a level of questioning allows practitioners to identify potential risks and tailor individual care plans. The subtleties of medical history are highlighted by research on nonsteroidal anti-inflammatory drugs (NSAIDs), which emphasize the importance of an individualized process in measuring use of medication and risk factors. An instrument created for measurement by a multidisciplinary team identified important quality measures, both technical and interpersonal care elements. This entire system substantiates the integration of patient's own opinion into health history taking, which ultimately reinforces the validity of the assessments and the quality of care given to patients. Equally as important is the role of physical therapists in health history taking, as with conditions like VTE. The American Physical Therapy Association established clear clinical practice guidelines that assist therapists in identifying and intervening with patients at risk for or diagnosed with lower extremity deep vein thrombosis (LE DVT). The published literature systematic review that informed these guidelines supports the argument that extensive health history taking is crucial to the achievement of optimal patient outcomes. By employing action statements rooted in evidence-based practice, physical therapists optimize their decision-making capacities, and that further contributes to the prevention, diagnosis, and treatment of VTE and LE DVT. It thereby clearly indicates how the incorporation of meticulous health history into the therapeutic process can contribute to the reduction of long-term complications and promote patient care. Finally, but not least importantly, the importance of interdisciplinary collaboration in health history taking cannot be overemphasized. Evaluation of a patient's health history calls for coordination of efforts from a number of healthcare providers, each contributing their particular expertise toward gaining a full understanding. A collaboration of data from rheumatologists, nurse specialists, pharmacists, and physical therapists presents an ideal model for patient care that encompasses not just the immediate clinical presentation but also more universal social and behavioral factors affecting health. As demonstrated by the NSAID quality care index, bringing together the diverse range of opinions can help bridge gaps and tailor intervention to maximize patient engagement and safety. A more focused approach to health history taking with interdisciplinary support enhances overall quality of care, therefore establishing the argument that one needs to know a patient's history in order to be effective in providing care.

KEY TERMS FROM THIS CHAPTER

- Biographical Data
- History of Present Illness
- Surgical History
- Social History
- Allergies
- Review of Systems
- Lifestyle Factors
- Nutritional History
- Chief Complaint
- Past Medical History
- Family History
- Medication History
- Immunization History
- Functional Assessment
- Psychosocial History
- Sexual History

CRITICAL THINKING QUESTIONS

1. **Which of the following is the primary purpose of taking a health history?**
   a. To perform physical examination
   b. To identify patient health problems and risks
   c. To prescribe medications
   d. To schedule laboratory tests
2. **When collecting a patient's health history, which type of information is considered subjective?**
   a. Blood pressure readings
   b. Patient's description of pain
   c. Laboratory results
   d. X-ray findings
3. **The "COLDSPA" mnemonic is used in health history taking. What does the "D" stand for?**
   a. Diagnosis
   b. Duration
   c. Dosage
   d. Description
4. **Which of the following is an example of a past medical history question?**
   a. "When did your symptoms start?"
   b. "Do you have any chronic illnesses?"
   c. "Do you exercise regularly?"
   d. "Are you experiencing any pain right now?"
5. **Effective health history taking requires which of the following communication skills?**
   a. Active listening and open-ended questions
   b. Giving advice immediately
   c. Using only medical terminology
   d. Avoiding eye contact

Short Answer Questions

1. What is the primary purpose of obtaining a health history from a patient?
2. List the key components of a comprehensive health history.
3. How does a nurse differentiate between a "chief complaint" and a "present illness"?
4. Why is it important to ask about family medical history during health assessment?
5. What types of questions are considered open-ended versus closed-ended, and when is each used in health history taking?

Answer to Critical Thinking Questions

1. (b) 2. (b) 3. (b) 4. (b) 5. (a)

REFERENCES

1. Alzheimer's Association. (2023). 2023 Alzheimer's disease facts and figures. *Alzheimer's & Dementia, 19*, 1598–1695. https://doi.org/10.1002/alz.13016 (accessed on 16th July 2025).
2. Anandan, C., Car, J., Liu, J., Majeed, A., et al. (2011). Computer-assisted history-taking systems (CAHTS) in health care: Benefits, risks and potential for further development. https://core.ac.uk/download/130975127.pdf (accessed on 16th July 2025).
3. Andrews, L., Franco, A., Kostelecky, K., Spritz, R., et al. (2017). Virtual clinical trials: One step forward, two steps back. https://core.ac.uk/download/128127841.pdf (accessed on 16th July 2025).
4. Arthur, V., Griffiths, P., Jobanputra, P., Pugh, T., et al. (2005). Quality of care for NSAID users: Development of an assessment tool. https://core.ac.uk/download/pdf/19357.pdf (accessed on 16th July 2025).
5. Auerbach, A., Bachman, B., Baer, T., Benaroia, M., Bowling, B., Bruce, M., Bulpitt, C., et al. (2017). Computer-assisted versus oral-and-written history taking for the prevention and management of cardiovascular disease: A systematic review of the literature. https://core.ac.uk/download/151170821.pdf (accessed on 16th July 2025).
6. Auten, B., Frese, E. M., Hillegass, E., Puthoff, M., et al. (2016). Role of physical therapists in the management of individuals at risk for or diagnosed with venous thromboembolism: Evidence-based clinical practice guideline. https://core.ac.uk/download/213061294.pdf (accessed on 16th July 2025).
7. Barnes, H., Bateson, A., Boyd, J., Bunn, F., Campbell, S., Coiera, E., et al. (2014). The impact of using computer decision-support software in primary care nurse-led telephone triage: Interactional dilemmas and conversational consequences. https://core.ac.uk/download/29111138.pdf (accessed on 16th July 2025).
8. Bell, D., Kuo, S., Marvin, V., Poots, A., et al. (2016). Applying quality improvement methods to address gaps in medicines reconciliation at transfers of care from an acute UK hospital. https://core.ac.uk/download/77011330.pdf (accessed on 16th July 2025).
9. Bogaert, E., & Roels, R. (2025). Sexual health in patient care: Shortcomings in medical training and experienced barriers in sexual history taking. *BMC Medical Education, 25*. https://www.semanticscholar.org/paper/67f953fb225a1913081b87cb171e7a20a7a28dca (accessed on 16th July 2025).
10. Bond, A., O, A. S., Draper, K., Tirodkar, M., & Gourevitch, R. (2014). Overcoming challenges to teamwork in patient-centered medical homes: A qualitative study. https://core.ac.uk/download/75780924.pdf (accessed on 16th July 2025).
11. Bryan, J. K., D'Angelo, K. A., & Kurz, B. (2016). Women's experiences with prenatal care: A mixed-methods study exploring the influence of the social determinants of health. https://digitalscholarship.unlv.edu/cgi/viewcontent.cgi?article=1425&context=jhdrp (accessed on 16th July 2025).
12. Burcham, W. K., Gitter, B. D., Moser, E. A., Romito, L., et al. (2019). Analyzing medication documentation in electronic health records: Dental students' self-reported behaviors and charting practices. https://core.ac.uk/download/299809053.pdf (accessed on 16th July 2025).

13. Cameron, S. C., & Roberts, K. P. (2015). Observations from Canadian practitioners about the investigation and prosecution of crimes involving child and adult witnesses. https://core.ac.uk/download/143690113.pdf (accessed on 16th July 2025).

14. Chan, A. W., Tetzlaff, J., Gøtzsche, P. C., Altman, D. G., Mann, H., Berlin, J. A., Dickersin, K., et al. (2013). SPIRIT 2013 explanation and elaboration: Guidance for protocols of clinical trials. *BMJ, 346*, e7586–e7586. https://doi.org/10.1136/bmj.e7586 (accessed on 16th July 2025).

15. Chastain, A. M. (2019). Patient and provider perspectives on sexual history taking during gynecological care: A pilot study in an academic family medical setting in New York City. https://academicworks.cuny.edu/cgi/viewcontent.cgi?article=1039&context=sph_etds (accessed on 16th July 2025).

16. Ciccarese, P., Kumar, A., Piazza, M., Smith, B., et al. (2004). Context-based task ontologies for clinical guidelines. https://core.ac.uk/download/131212561.pdf (accessed on 16th July 2025).

17. Cook, T., & Inglis, P. (2008). Understanding research, consent and ethics: A participatory research methodology in a medium secure unit for men with a learning disability. https://core.ac.uk/download/4146674.pdf (accessed on 16th July 2025).

18. Corigliano, S. (2017). Devotion and discipline: Christian yoga and the yoga of T. Krishnamacharya. https://core.ac.uk/download/212824412.pdf (accessed on 16th July 2025).

19. Corvini, M., Cox, K., O'Neil, M., Ryer, D., et al. (2018). Addressing childhood adversity and social determinants in pediatric primary care: Recommendations for New Hampshire. https://core.ac.uk/download/215540986.pdf (accessed on 16th July 2025).

20. Dai, M., Liu, D., Liu, M., Zhou, F., Li, G., Chen, Z., Zhang, Z., et al. (2020). Patients with cancer appear more vulnerable to SARS-CoV-2: A multicenter study during the COVID-19 outbreak. *Cancer Discovery, 10*, 783–791. https://doi.org/10.1158/2159-8290.cd-20-0422 (accessed on 16th July 2025).

21. Darking, M., Henwood, F., & Marent, B. (2018). Ambivalence in digital health: Co-designing an mHealth platform for HIV care. https://core.ac.uk/download/286356547.pdf (accessed on 16th July 2025).

22. De Bienassis, K., Esmail, L., Lopert, R., & Klazinga, N. (2022). The economics of medication safety. *OECD Health Working Papers*. https://doi.org/10.1787/9a933261-en (accessed on 16th July 2025).

23. Deale, A., Heyting, A., Komaroff, A., Strauss, A., Wearden, A., Zigmond, A., Wearden, A. J., et al. (2006). Fatigue Intervention by Nurses Evaluation–The FINE Trial. A randomized controlled trial of nurse led self-help treatment for patients in primary care with chronic fatigue syndrome: Study protocol. [ISRCTN74156610]. https://core.ac.uk/download/52846.pdf (accessed on 16th July 2025).

24. Dwivedi, Y. K., Hughes, L., Baabdullah, A. M., Ribeiro-Navarrete, S., Giannakis, M., Al-Debei, M. M., Dennehy, D., et al. (2022). Metaverse beyond the hype: Multidisciplinary perspectives on emerging challenges, opportunities, and agenda for research, practice and policy. *International Journal of Information Management, 66*, 102542–102542. https://doi.org/10.1016/j.ijinfomgt.2022.102542 (accessed on 16th July 2025).

25. Escota, G., & Melia, M. T. (2020). The struggling infectious diseases fellow: Remediation challenges and opportunities. https://core.ac.uk/download/322802240.pdf (accessed on 16th July 2025).

26. Evans, D. (2009). Mental health nurse prescribing: Challenges in theory and practice. https://core.ac.uk/download/1654275.pdf (accessed on 16th July 2025).

27. Ferrari, R., Rosano, G. M. C., & Spoletini, I. (2020). Living with stable angina: Patients' pathway and needs in angina. https://core.ac.uk/download/322366758.pdf (accessed on 16th July 2025).

28. Fuqua, E. (2012). Art and the human condition: Incorporating visual analysis of artworks into an undergraduate pre-medicine curriculum. https://core.ac.uk/download/51291422.pdf (accessed on 16th July 2025).

29. Ge, Y., Jetty, R., Newhook, D., Webster, R., Mills, A., McCann, V., Trincao-Batra, S., et al. (2021). 136 Characterizing the medical and social complexity of Inuit children, youth, and their families from Nunavut who access care at an urban tertiary level pediatric hospital-A retrospective chart review of an Inuit child health clinic. *Pediatrics & Child Health*. https://www.semanticscholar.org/paper/2731e2522c229953192e98c45f538a8eaf9753a5 (accessed on 16th July 2025).

30. He, Z., & Ke, Y. (2023). Challenge and future of cancer screening in China: Insights from esophageal cancer screening practice. *Chinese Journal of Cancer Research, 35*(6), 584–594. https://www.semanticscholar.org/paper/162caba3184287e9da0409a030e37f6472dea96b (accessed on 16th July 2025).

31. Hindelang, M., Sitaru, S., & Zink, A. (2024). Transforming health care through chatbots for medical history-taking and future directions: Comprehensive systematic review. *JMIR Medical Informatics, 12*. https://www.semanticscholar.org/paper/8b7d4cb903fa0c692adbbf4eed645b003361f253 (accessed on 16th July 2025).

32. Höpfl, F., & Schellhorn, M. (2025). Balancing innovation and trust: Assessing artificial intelligence's role in medical history taking and physician perspectives on patient care. *Design+*. https://www.semanticscholar.org/paper/63c99f5f87643c53f0d994f32e4d32bae79eaf08 (accessed on 16th July 2025).

33. Hudson, N., McKivett, A., & Paul, D. (2018). Healing conversations: Developing a practical framework for clinical communication between Aboriginal communities and healthcare practitioners. https://core.ac.uk/download/213607715.pdf (accessed on 16th July 2025).

34. Iroegbu, B. (2016). A phenomenological assessment of factors that affect medication adherence among hypertensive Nigerian immigrants. https://core.ac.uk/download/129532354.pdf (accessed on 16th July 2025).

35. Johnson, L., Smetana, S., Hall, W., Weaver, A. D., & Rotoli, J. (2025). Dos and don'ts of taking care of deaf patients. *Journal of Education & Teaching in Emergency Medicine, 10*, L1–L8. https://www.semanticscholar.org/paper/949a01476656fc016fc18f1b6e5877ed418416d9 (accessed on 16th July 2025).

36. Koch, L., & Stemerding, D. (1994). The sociology of entrenchment: A cystic fibrosis test for everyone? https://core.ac.uk/download/pdf/11456324.pdf (accessed on 16th July 2025).

37. Kwon, I. H. (2015). High time to discuss future-oriented telemedicine. *Healthcare Informatics Research, 21*, 211, 212. https://www.semanticscholar.org/paper/82f0d000075662134a0cb03b33e35607c79cbaae (accessed on 16th July 2025).

38. Lyon, T. D. (2002). Applying suggestibility research to the real world: The case of repeated

questions. https://core.ac.uk/download/62568574.pdf (accessed on 16th July 2025).

39. Mallia, P. (2015). Point-of-care genetic counselling: Should family physicians counsel patients on genetic testing and screening? https://core.ac.uk/download/46603085.pdf (accessed on 16th July 2025).

40. McInnes, A., Zigmond, A., Armstrong, D., Sinacore, D., Charcot, J., Labovitz, J., et al. (2020). A randomized feasibility study of serial magnetic resonance imaging to reduce treatment times in Charcot neuroarthropathy in people with diabetes (CADOM): A protocol. https://core.ac.uk/download/305118534.pdf (accessed on 16th July 2025).

41. Melchert, T. P., & Meyer, L. (2011). Examining the content of mental health intake assessments from a biopsychosocial perspective. https://core.ac.uk/download/213064254.pdf (accessed on 16th July 2025).

42. Namagembe, A., Mbonye, A. K., Cundill, B., Maiteki-Sebuguzi, C., Nabirye, C., Chandler, C. I. R., et al. (2017). The impact of an intervention to introduce malaria rapid diagnostic tests on fever case management in a high transmission setting in Uganda: A mixed-methods cluster-randomized trial (PRIME). https://core.ac.uk/download/81670433.pdf (accessed on 16th July 2025).

43. Placido, D., Yuan, B., Hjaltelin, J. X., Zheng, C., Haue, A. D., Chmura, P. J., Yuan, C., et al. (2023). A deep learning algorithm to predict risk of pancreatic cancer from disease trajectories. *Nature Medicine, 29*, 1113–1122. https://doi.org/10.1038/s41591-023-02332-5 (accessed on 16th July 2025).

44. Plante, S. (2018). An inpatient rehabilitation interprofessional care pathway for traumatic hip fracture: A pilot quality improvement project. https://core.ac.uk/download/215520988.pdf (accessed on 16th July 2025).

45. Priyadarshini, R., Eerike, M., Varatharajan, S., Ramaswamy, G., Raj, G. M., Cherian, J., Rajendran, P., et al. (2024). Assessing the efficacy of the ARMOR tool–based deprescribing intervention for fall risk reduction in older patients taking fall risk–increasing drugs (DeFRID Trial): Protocol for a randomized controlled trial. *JMIR Research Protocols, 13*. https://www.semanticscholar.org/paper/ec9c47f7afa9c2e5e160e750c303f43eb1a682ef (accessed on 16th July 2025).

46. Szymanski, T. L. (2002). The fit of Certified Disability Management Specialists' (CDMS) knowledge domains with Minnesota's Qualified Rehabilitation Consultants' (QRCs') competencies. https://core.ac.uk/download/5066221.pdf (accessed on 16th July 2025).

47. Taylor, A. D., Connolly, J., & Pearce, C. (2024). A rural doctor's telehealth training program during the COVID-19 pandemic. *Rural and Remote Health, 24*(1), 8032. https://www.semanticscholar.org/paper/e37c46c6a5f08f76c72c8abcf09e99fa52d88043 (accessed on 16th July 2025).

48. Ulischenko, I. A., Dmitriyev, A., Gudkov, R. A., & Pak, V. I. (2022). Clinical and statistical characteristics and risk factors in children with bronchial asthma having comorbid pathology. *Nauka Molodykh (Eruditio Juvenium)*. https://www.semanticscholar.org/paper/b09f9c09b6aabecc20882055049c989f8f3f4db4 (accessed on 16th July 2025).

49. Visseren, F. L. J., Mach, F., Smulders, Y. M., Carballo, D., Koskinas, K. C., Bäck, M., Bénétos, A., et al. (2021). 2021 ESC guidelines on cardiovascular disease prevention in clinical practice. *European Heart Journal, 42*, 3227–3337. https://doi.org/10.1093/eurheartj/ehab484 (accessed on 16th July 2025).

50. Wang, M., Pan, Y., Jiang, X., Lin, Z., Liu, H., Liu, Y., Cui, J., et al. (2025). Leveraging artificial intelligence and clinical laboratory evidence to advance mobile health applications in ophthalmology: Taking the ocular surface disease as a case study. *iLABMED*. https://www.semanticscholar.org/paper/6a4fa24aacd54bf455a40bbd76824cdf095c3ec9 (accessed on 16th July 2025).
51. Watts, J. H. (2008). Emotion, empathy and exit: Reflections on doing ethnographic qualitative research on sensitive topics. https://core.ac.uk/download/1590.pdf (accessed on 16th July 2025).
52. Windecker, S., Kolh, P., Alfonso, F., Collet, J. P., Cremer, J., Falk, V., Filippatos, G., et al. (2014). 2014 ESC/EACTS guidelines on myocardial revascularization. *European Heart Journal, 35*, 2541–2619. https://doi.org/10.1093/eurheartj/ehu278 (accessed on 16th July 2025).
53. Zhou, J., Liu, L., Xue, P., Yang, X., & Tang, X. (2020). Mental health response to the COVID-19 outbreak in China. *American Journal of Psychiatry, 177*, 574–575. https://doi.org/10.1176/appi.ajp.2020.20030304 (accessed on 16th July 2025).

TECHNIQUES OF PHYSICAL EXAMINATION

4

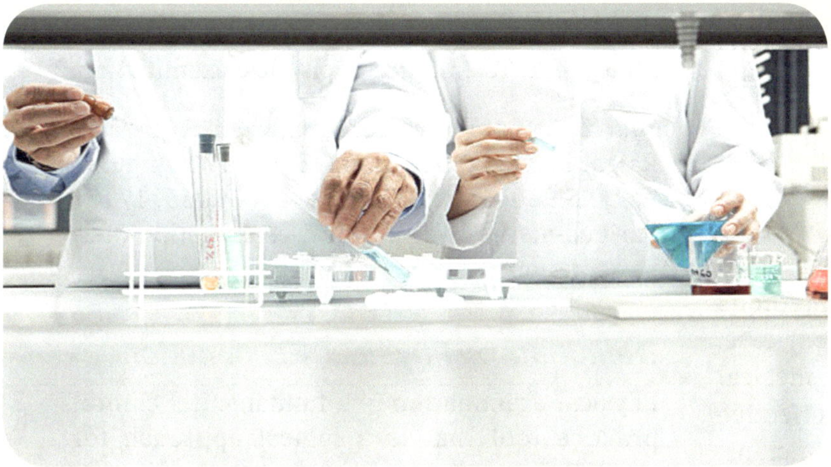

LEARNING OBJECTIVES

After studying this chapter, you will be able to:

1. Discuss about inspection;
2. Define palpation;
3. Describe percussion;
4. Explain about auscultation;
5. Identifu the special tests;
6. Explore the documentation.

Introduction

The initial phase of any clinical encounter is paramount in determining the success of follow-up tests and treatment. Physical exam techniques are the foundations of healthcare professionals, enabling them not only to obtain valuable information but also to establish a therapy relationship with patients. Such effective communication methods should be added at this point since they can be very advantageous towards facilitating increased patient engagement and better health outcomes. Research identifies that clinicians who adopt full strategies towards patient interaction, i.e., shared decision making and motivational interviewing, are able to use more patient engagement, thereby becoming an integral part of their healthcare process (Elwyn et al., 2018). This trend towards patient-focused care is increasingly regarded as an essential component of effective clinical practice. In addition, advancements in physical examination techniques involve traditional techniques alongside more contemporary innovations that aim to increase the diagnostic scope. Owing to advances in technology, incorporation of decision-support systems into clinical assessments can raise the efficiency and effectiveness of physical examinations. For instance, studies have examined the potential for computer decision-support software (CDSS) to be utilized by nurses in triage situations, demonstrating both its potential benefits and the challenges it introduces in the presence of patients (Barnes et al., 2014).

Nurses who possess sophisticated tools must manage patient communication tactfully even when using these tools, hence pointing towards the need to respond to an equilibrium between technical competencies and clinical acumen. These subtleties underscore the importance of continuous training and adaptation in physical examination methods to meet the evolving demands of patient care. Ultimately, a proper introduction to physical exam techniques sets the stage for effective encounters between patients and clinicians. It constitutes understanding the physiological aspects of exams as well as the psychological aspects of interacting with patients.

As healthcare delivery shifts toward more holistic, multidimensional care, the practices employed during physical exams also need to change in reaction to stay aligned with these innovations. Through emphasis on patient activation and engagement, medical practitioners can become more sophisticated in their examination techniques, ultimately producing improved health outcomes and patient satisfaction. This congruence not only honors ideals of patient-centered practice but also prepares practitioners for the complexities of modern clinical practice, where empirical evidence and human relatedness intersect (Figure 4.1).

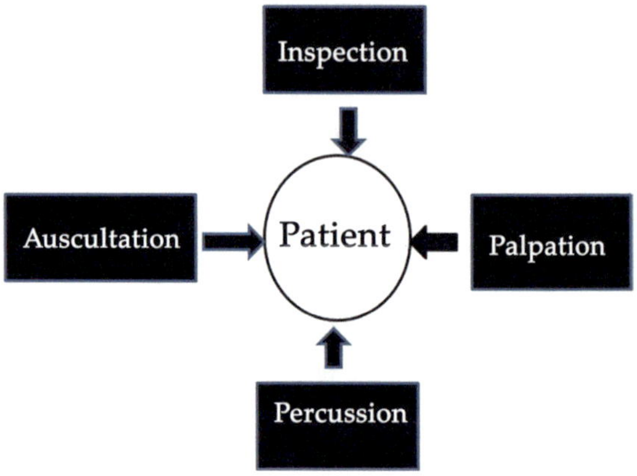

Figure 4.1. Techniques of physical examination.

Source: https://www.researchgate.net/profile/Rajani-Singh-4/publication/336531710/figure/fig1/AS:960055897776139@1605906571717/Various-methods-of-physical-examination-of-a-patient.png.

Definition of Physical Examination

Physical examination is a fundamental clinical practice tool that is a logical approach for assessing an individual's overall state of health. Physical examination is a process of employing a set of methods for obtaining general information regarding an individual's physical condition. Physicians usually employ visual inspection, palpation, percussion, and auscultation in this multi-dimensional evaluation. Each of these processes allows physicians to gather useful information, leading to improved diagnosis and treatment plans. Furthermore, the value of thorough physical examination transcends simple identification of physical status; it includes the development of a trusting relationship between patient and caregiver. Such trust is precious as it facilitates open discussion about health concerns, resulting in fuller evaluations and comprehensive care. Practically speaking, the term physical examination tends to broaden in usage by the inclusion of various techniques of diagnosis to complement traditional methods. For instance, in combination with the utilization of physical examination skills, the advances in technology have included imaging techniques and laboratory studies as part and parcel of the examination procedure. Whereas these newer technologies can impart precise information, they cannot be applied in place of, but as an addition to, the traditional physical examination. For example, evaluation of fever of unknown origin (FUO) in children emphasizes the importance of a focused history and thorough physical examination, which may provide a clue of considerable significance to the underlying etiology. Therefore, the physical examination remains a pillar of diagnostic thinking, essential for an objective approach to patient care (Fiordelisi et al., 2023). Moreover, the success of a physical examination greatly relies on the ability of the clinicians to synthesize the information gathered through observation and palpation. Synthesis is critical, particularly when presented with complex medical presentations, where the nuances of a patient's physical status can direct differential diagnosis and ensuing management strategies. An appropriately conducted examination not only discloses overt and palpable evidence of disease but also heightens the clinician's clinical acumen, which guides them through the diagnostic maze. Practitioners are therefore encouraged to continually enhance their examination skills through practice and education, such that the physical examination is envisioned as an indispensable tool for clinical assessment. Within the frame of new approaches and greater emphasis on wholistic care, the physical examination remains a traditional and important part of sound practice (Kitsiou et al., 2013).

Importance in Clinical Practice

In healthcare practice, the physical examination skills are a requirement for successful diagnosis and successful treatment planning. Competent physical examination skills enable healthcare practitioners to gather critical information regarding the health status of a patient through observation, palpation, percussion, and auscultation. The integrated approach underscores the necessity not only to apply diagnostic imaging and laboratory results, but to integrate physical assessments that inform clinical thinking. Sound examination proficiency facilitates the clinician's ability to differentiate signs and symptoms, and thus better understand the status of a patient. Prioritization of physical examination competencies may lead to early detection of health issues, eventually improving patient satisfaction and outcomes. Fostering trust and rapport between patients and healthcare professionals is another critical element of physical examination skills in clinical practice. When a clinician administers a thorough, respectful physical examination, not only is accurate evaluation made simpler, but also sends the message to the patient that his or her health matters. Such a visit will allay patient fear, as they are active participants in their care process. Furthermore, practitioners who demonstrate competence in physical exam facilitate a healthy care environment conducive to patient cooperation. The. ability to perform a successful examination fosters patient confidence, particularly when dealing with sensitive issues or symptoms. Grace et al. (2016) highlights the way peer physical examination perceptions reinforce respect and empathy for each other, enhancing the clinician-patient relationship. The. effects of successful physical examination skills extend beyond individual patient visits and have implications for healthcare education and practice in general. As highlighted by Grace et al. (2016), peer physical examination by osteopathy students is an effective pedagogical approach that prepares the skills of students before practice with real patients. The model facilitates the acquisition of required competencies in a controlled environment, hence reducing anxiety and improving mastery of skills. It underscores the need to incorporate such approaches in medical curricula to prepare future practitioners in good time. In addition, this learning focus can foster professionalism via self-assessment and feedback, eventually leading to enhanced clinical practice. Excellent physical examination skills are thus essential not only for patient care but also for developing an educated and competent healthcare workforce that is capable of delivering quality services (Figure 4.2).

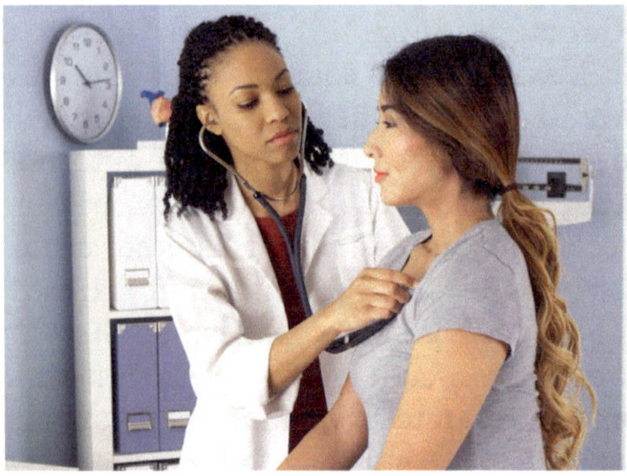

Figure 4.2. Clinical practice of physical examination.

Source: https://assets.contenthub.wolterskluwer.com/api/public/content/9721dd0920e940adb8291187198bfd44?v=3b68598d.

Overview of Techniques to Be Discussed

An adequate understanding of the techniques of physical examination is essential to facilitate healthcare providers to conduct effective patient examinations. In this essay, some basic techniques that form the foundation of the physical examination will be discussed. These techniques include inspection, palpation, percussion, and auscultation, which all contribute greatly to collecting information required for diagnosis and treatment. Inspection is the method of observing patients carefully for physical presentations of illness so that clinicians can form early hypotheses regarding a patient's status. Palpation, utilizing touch to assess structures beneath the skin, provides additional light regarding abnormalities. Percussion and auscultation also offer unique insights, assisting in organ function and pathology assessment. Together, these techniques form an overall strategy through which clinicians may accurately communicate with their patients and form competent clinical decisions. The application of sophisticated imaging techniques in physical examination has assumed a greater importance in contemporary healthcare. Ultrasound, X-ray, and magnetic resonance imaging (MRI) are examples of techniques through which internal structures' normal anatomy and trauma can be observed in detail. The application of ultrasound, for instance, facilitates real-time imaging and evaluation of soft tissues and organs, which assists in improving the accuracy of diagnosis. X-rays, on their part, allow for an insight into the skeletal framework, helping in the identification of fractures and degenerative processes. MRI has changed the ability to assess intricate soft tissue disorders, hence improving the diagnostic abilities of practitioners. As more of these newer imaging modalities are used, they not only aid in complementing the findings of physical examination but also help in arriving at a more definitive diagnosis and contribute greatly to patient management and treatment planning. The application of several techniques for physical examination emphasizes the importance of ongoing education and training for healthcare workers. As scholars advocate for interdisciplinarity in addressing healthcare, integrating sustainable practices in medical education systems is more important. Aligning sustainable development principles, particularly in Technical and Vocational Education Training (TVET) programs, supports the establishment of such techniques. As future medical professionals educated in traditional and innovative examination methods, education institutions are capable of valuable contributions to the general health agenda. Evidence indicates that despite sustainable ideas becoming increasingly prominent in healthcare training, their integration into curricula effectively is missing. One of the aims of this essay is not just to extend on the procedures of physical examination but also to pose questions on how future practice can be transformed to prepare health practitioners more suitably to address the needs of a constantly evolving health landscape, thereby bringing medical examination and sustainable practice together.

4.1. Inspection

Learning Outcome

1. Visual assessment of the patient;
2. Importance of body language and posture;
3. Use of tools in inspection (e.g., otoscope, ophthalmoscope).

Inspection is the foundation of physical examination that makes it possible for healthcare providers to acquire crucial visual information about a person's general health and pathologies. In this method, physicians examine the patient in a structured way, analyzing various physical attributes like skin color, body posture, and ambulation. The visual assessment makes it possible for clinicians to identify abnormalities or evidence of disease early, which can contribute significantly to accuracy during diagnosis. For instance, in skin illness, color change or lesions can suggest underlying systemic disease. In addition, careful inspection of anatomic areas, such as the joints or abdomen, can exhibit signs of inflammation or asymmetry, prompting further evaluation and intervention. By developing a fine sense of detail, healthcare providers can apply inspection to build a comprehensive picture of their patient's overall health and become a key component in correct diagnosis and patient care. Moreover, the role of inspection is not merely observing but requires contextual integration and a reflective interpretive process. Practitioners should integrate observation findings with knowledge of presenting symptoms and medical history. It is essential to build this combined perception, especially in complex cases where transient signs can be easily overlooked. For example, pediatric examinations need to know about developmental milestones, which are likely to impact interpretation. Apart from that, as exemplified in reports of child protection issues in health care facilities, scheduled inspection routines may reveal potential risks or abuse in clinical environments (Kendrick et al., 2000). Such instances prove that providing an environment for open and honest communication with patients and their families ultimately results in improved quality and safety in care.

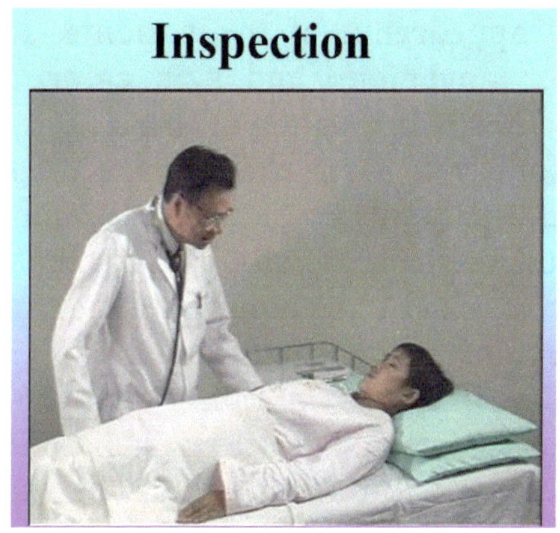

Figure 4.3. Inspection of physical examination.

Source: https://images.slideplayer.com/26/8633631/slides/slide_5.jpg.

Finally, good inspection is not only a matter of practitioners competence but also the calibration of training staff who work with patient care. While initial training in inspection practice is of prime importance, ongoing training and adherence to reflective practice must lie at the core of maintaining high standards. Research has indicated that merely providing training is not likely to provoke long-term changes in behavior; improvement in staff attitudes and performance is equally highly important (Campbell et al., 2013). This is evidence for the necessity of continuous professional development, as well as support mechanisms that allow staff to improve their observational abilities. Through the cultivation of an excellence culture in inspection practice, patient outcomes can be enhanced and firmness towards safety and well-being strengthened, thereby lessening the chances of physical examination practices not realizing their intent (Figure 4.3).

4.1.1. Visual Assessment of the Patient

Visual observation of the patient is a fundamental physical examination technique, which is the initial patient-clinician contact. The method involves observing closely the general appearance of the patients, such as posture, movement, and skin color, among others. Visual observation of these signs allows practitioners to form preliminary judgments about the patients physical and psychological condition. For instance, stooping or limping gait in a patient can be symptomatic of neurological or musculoskeletal complications. Moreover, alterations in skin coloration—jaundice, pallor, or cyanosis—can be the only sign of underlying systemic complications that must be explored. Thus, a thorough visual examination provides not just decisive diagnostic evidence but also guides further assessments and intervention planning. Besides the identification of physical characteristics, the visual examination allows clinicians to closely examine a patient's emotional state and mental conditions. Facial expression, eye contact, and body postures can provide invaluable information regarding a patient's psychological condition. An example would be a patient who fails to make eye contact, who may either present signs of depression or anxiety that need careful assessment beyond the body. These behaviors can also be utilized as indicators of discomfort or distress, and professionals can utilize an integrated physical and emotional cues observation to tailor their evaluation and create a more coordinated plan of management. Successful communication and rapport establishment form the foundation for this two-pronged approach to patient compliance and satisfaction. Visual assessment techniques are of primary importance in conditions that have a direct effect on mobility and function, such as cited in specific groups of patients, for instance, those with Parkinson's Disease. The postural instability, the hallmark symptom of this illness, can be visually assessed to ascertain how much it affects daily activities and general quality of life. Both spatial-temporal gait parameters and visual assessment are useful tools to clinicians for judging disease progression and treatment effect, such as the intervention of dance therapy, which has been reported to improve gait and balance in the affected patients (Agnetti et al., 2012). Moreover, a careful visual inspection assists in the early detection of complications such that intervention can be initiated in a timely manner specific to the individual patient. Consequently, the visual assessment not only adds physical impairment information but also improves informed decision-making throughout the patient's care pathway (Akyol et al., 2019) (Figure 4.4).

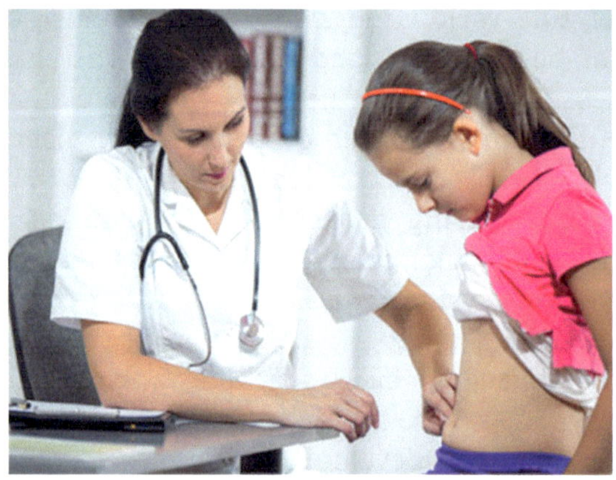

Figure 4.4. The visual assessment of the patient.

Source: https://nityanandaclinic.co.in/images/demo/diagnostic/physical.jpg.

4.1.2. Importance of Body Language and Posture

In physical examination skills, the significance of body posture as well as body language cannot be overemphasized. Health professionals utilize considerable non-verbal cues in establishing rapport with their patients as well as in expressing empathy. The orientation of a practitioner in terms of his or her position toward the patient may influence the latter's comfort and cooperativeness in information disclosure. For instance, standing with an open posture, as signaled by uncrossed arms and a forward lean, communicates attentiveness and receptivity, encouraging patients to communicate their concerns in a non-confrontational environment. This enhances the therapeutic alliance, which is of prime importance for sound diagnosis and treatment planning. In addition, the interaction between clinician and patient body language contributes to the diagnostic process itself. In conducting an examination of patients, clinicians often conduct what might be described as "communicative body work." It is not simply a question of verbal exchange but also one of embodied interaction between patient and clinician, with the result of configuring a diagnostic space that extends beyond physical examination. Observations suggest that the way that clinicians communicate themselves through their own body is of significant importance to the diagnosis outcome, as it creates an environment where both contribute to the interpretation of the patient (Buscher et al., 2015). Thus, the necessity for sensitivity to body language extends beyond relational purposes and becomes firmly embedded in clinical practice and diagnosis. Moreover, posture affects not just clinician-patient relationships but also clinician self-perception and confidence. Body language projecting confidence will tend to make practitioners appear competent and, in turn, can make patients feel at ease during examinations. This is particularly important in careers requiring intricate evaluations, e.g., those of neurological conditions, where familiarity with body responses can lead to improved outcomes. As highlighted in cerebral palsy intervention literature, successful physical examination is founded on a firm premise of mutual comprehension facilitated by body language (Bowers et al., 2009). Such evidence records bidirectional body language as a key component of successful physical examination that enhances clinician ability and patient experience.

4.1.3. Use of Tools in Inspection (e.g., Otoscope, Ophthalmoscope)

Physical examination in medicine includes the utilization of medical instruments to facilitate correct diagnosis and treatment. An ophthalmoscope and an otoscope help medical practitioners view inner structures that could not otherwise be accessed. The otoscope, which helps in viewing the ear canal and tympanic membrane, allows practitioners to diagnose conditions like otitis media or earwax blockage. By illuminating the ear canal and expanding the field of view, the instrument increases the clinician's chance to make informed decisions based on what can be visualized of pathology. Careful scrutiny is important because early detection of ear pathology may significantly influence patient prognosis and inform guided intervention. Similarly, the ophthalmoscope plays a critical role in ocular structural assessment, especially the retina, optic disc, and vascular anatomy. This instrument plays a pivotal role in the identification of eye conditions such as diabetic retinopathy, glaucoma, and macular degeneration. With an ophthalmoscope, clinicians are able to carry out a thorough assessment of the condition of the eyes, thereby being able to identify early detection and intervention of potentially vision-threatening diseases. The ability to image the posterior eye segment without invasion allows understanding of systemic diseases that manifest in the eye, highlighting the interconnectedness of body systems as identified in recent studies on how systemic health affects ocular outcomes (Edison et al., 2020). Furthermore, the integration of technological advancements in examination tools significantly enhances the accuracy of physical examinations. Equipment is continuously being upgraded to incorporate digital imaging and improved optics, which offer clearer imaging and improved diagnosis. For instance, modern ophthalmoscopes will often feature digital interfaces allowing for enhanced visualization and documentation of findings. Improved optics not only allow the practitioner to view finer detail but also facilitate enhanced patient education and involvement during consultations. With medicine becoming more and more accepting of emerging technologies, the correct application of these machines even more so emphasizes the importance of high standards in physical examination techniques so that health practitioners can provide well-versed and integrative care (N/A, 2020) (Figure 4.5).

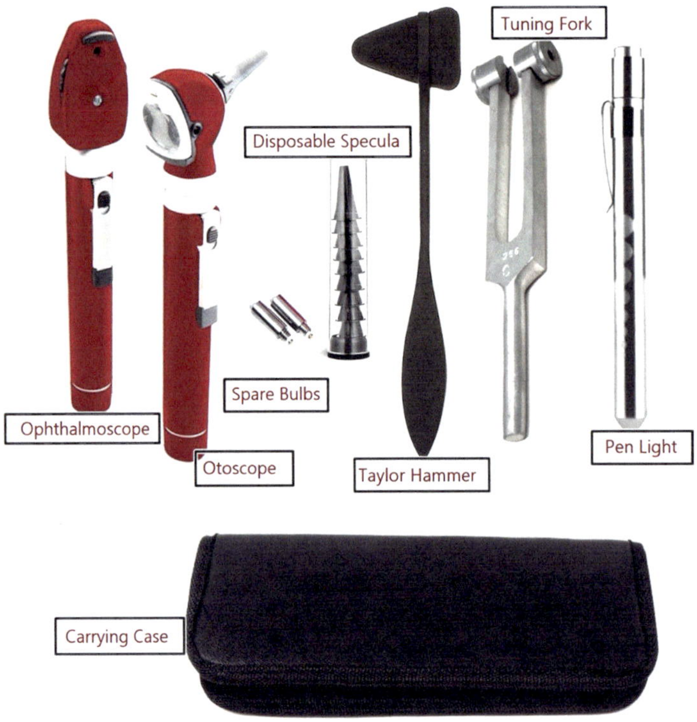

Figure 4.5. Tools in inspection.

Source: https://i.ebayimg.com/images/g/Ar8AAOSwibNhN40i/s-l1200.jpg.

Test Your Knowledge

1. What key observations should a nurse make during the inspection phase of a physical assessment?
2. How can subtle changes in a patient's appearance provide important clues about their health status?

4.2. Palpation

Learning Outcome

1. Techniques for effective palpation;
2. Areas commonly assessed through palpation;
3. Importance of patient comfort during palpation.

Palpation is a key technique in the clinical practice of physical examination whereby medical practitioners can gain critical information about a patient's status through the use of touch. Not only is this method beneficial in the assessment of physical evidence, but it also enhances the rewarding interaction between clinician and patient to form an important rapport that helps ensure successful diagnosis. During a palpation examination, healthcare professionals are taught to notice variation in texture, temperature, and pain upon palpation of various regions, such as the abdomen, lymph nodes, or musculoskeletal tissues. While performing the method, the clinician will typically have to employ both sensitivity and methodical reasoning in order to interpret appropriately and make valid conclusions regarding a patient's health status. Its efficacy is also underscored by its employment across multiple medical specialties, underpinning clinical decisions and directing additional inquiry. Sports medicine, for instance, relies significantly on palpation as a means of diagnosing muscle trauma or arthropathy, allowing the physician to identify focal tenderness indicative of underlying problems. Second, its utility is to specialties such as urology and gynecology, where knowledge of pelvic floor dysfunction becomes critical in the treatment of patients. Present treatment regimens are more geared toward an integrated examination approach, which balances palpation with other forms of physical exam. By doing so, clinicians are better equipped to construct a more thorough picture of a patient's condition, lending credence to a continuing education and training in palpation skills as health care changes. In addition, the need for standardized terms for palpation and related practices cannot be more critical. The recent report by the International Urogynecological Association and the International Continence Society highlights the need for definitions in female pelvic floor dysfunction, as compared to how agreement-based terminology helps clinical practice. By converging contributions from various specialties—physiotherapy, neurology, urology, and nursing—the initiative intends to impart a common understanding to practitioners. The establishment of such uniform terms not only makes multidisciplinary team communication easier but also assists research and development of palpation techniques. With healthcare moving towards evidence-based practice, the integration of detailed palpation procedures in conjunction with standardized models will be the cornerstone in achieving improved patient outcomes and enhancing medical science (Abramov et al., 2016; Pace et al., 2012) (Figure 4.6).

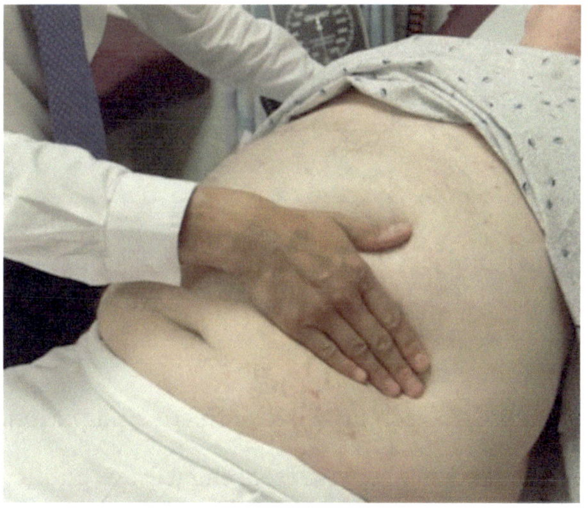

Figure 4.6. Palpation of physical examination.

Source: https://cloudfront.jove.com/files/media/science-education/science-education-thumbs/10143.jpg.

4.2.1. Techniques for Effective Palpation

Accurate palpation skills are an important part of conducting sufficient physical examinations, allowing practitioners to assess underlying tissues and identify concealed dysfunctions. The palpation method involves applying accurate hand positions in order to gather information on soft tissues, organs, and musculoskeletal integrity. Technique starts with the creation of a relaxed and comfortable environment for the patient, both relaxed and in the correct position. This facilitates accessibility in addition to reducing tension in muscles, ultimately maximizing the provider's capacity for evaluating anatomical structures beneath the skin.

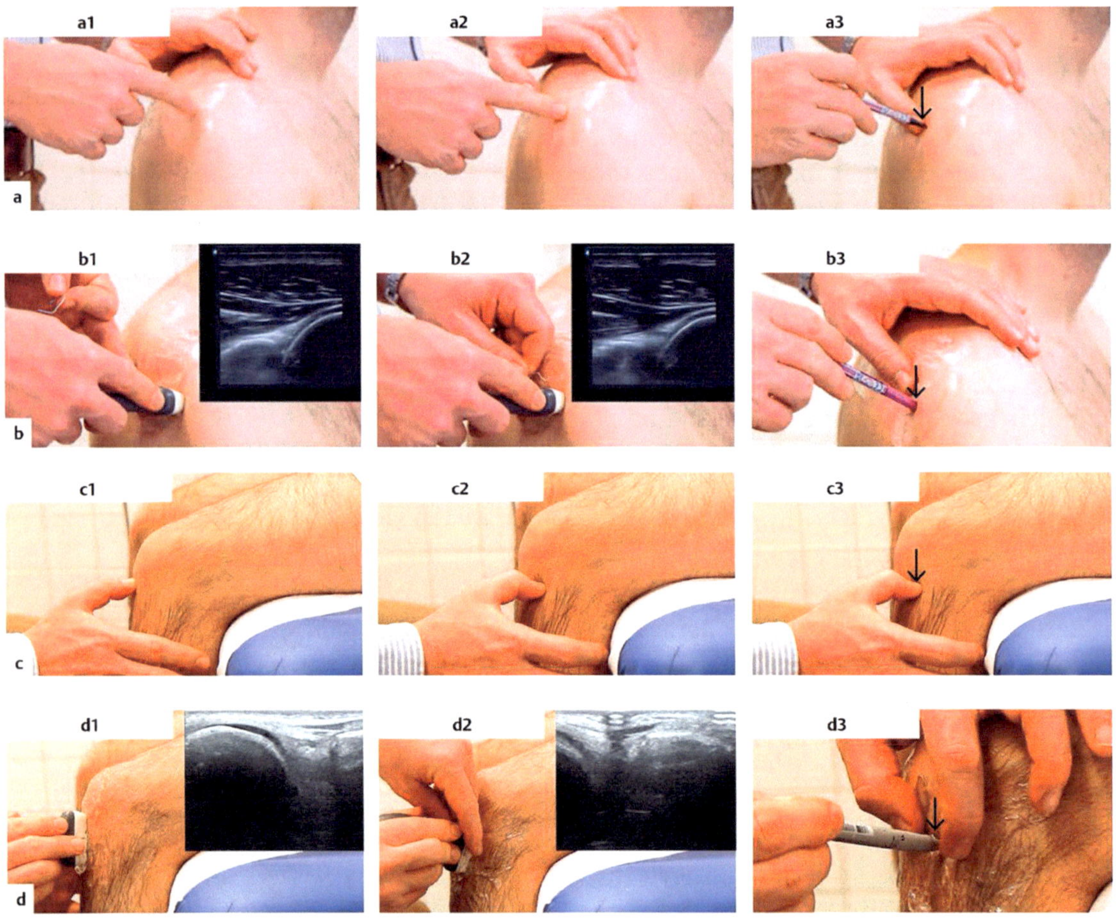

Figure 4.7. Techniques for effective palpation.

Source: https://www.researchgate.net/publication/379569364/figure/fig2/AS:11431281243847599@1715732280939/PalpMethod-a-c-and-SonoMethod-b-d-for-determining-the-optimal-access-points-to-the.jpg.

The application of different levels of pressure is also necessary, as light palpation can evaluate superficial landmarks, while more forceful techniques may be needed to detect deeper layers and yield critical information that may determine treatment. The inclusion of specific palpation techniques, such as trigger point release, enhances the effectiveness of physical examinations. An excellent example involves the application of dry needling, which treats myofascial trigger points, particularly in myofascial pelvic pain (MFPP) (Katzman et al., 2012). Dry needling involves the insertion of a fine needle into the trigger point, which produces a neural twitch response that eases tension and promotes range of motion. By integrating dry needling with routine palpation, practitioners may not only identify tender points but also provide some immediate effect. Furthermore, understanding the subtleties of muscle anatomy by palpation may facilitate accurate assessment of the location of trigger points, and thus the value of an integrative practice incorporating assessment and treatment. The diversity of skills involved in effective palpation underscores the importance of ongoing education and training for healthcare professionals. It takes more than one practice session and a sound understanding of anatomical landmarks, neuromuscular physiology, and the principles of therapeutic intervention to master palpation skills. Workshops, simulated practice, and case study discussion are good options for training necessary skills. In addition, interdisciplinary exchange of experiences and expertise on palpation techniques between providers is likely to promote the understanding of such conditions as MFPP, leading to enhanced patient care (Kotze et al., 2019). Lastly, integration of advanced palpation techniques in physical examination contributes significantly to patient care outcomes, enabling providers to make accurate diagnoses and to tailor treatment interventions appropriately (Figure 4.7).

4.2.2. Areas Commonly Assessed Through Palpation

Palpation is a basic physical assessment method by which physicians are capable of gaining important information about a patient's anatomical organs and conditions. Prolific in abdominal assessments, palpation allows clinicians to identify the point of tenderness, rigidity, or mass. For instance, identification of hepatomegaly, where palpation is utilized to press deeply into the right upper quadrant to palpate for the edge of the livers. By systematic palpation of the abdomen and by noting any aberrant findings, the clinician can make hypotheses regarding potential underlying pathologies such as liver pathology or gastrointestinal blockages. Palpation as a component of routine examination protocols is not simply a matter of tradition but improves the accuracy of diagnosis by producing subjective data to augment objective data, as in later studies on abdominal evaluation techniques. Beyond palpation of the abdomen, palpation is also essential in musculoskeletal assessment to assist in detecting soft tissue lesions and joint effusions. Professionals will palpate major muscle groups, joints, and bony prominences to assess for abnormal enlargement, tenderness, or deformity that would be suggestive of conditions like arthritis or muscle pull. For instance, a swollen knee may have palpation of the region around the patella to assess joint effusion as other local heat or tenderness is being identified. This tactile assessment gives the tools to include various forms of musculoskeletal examination and therefore enhance clinical decision-making. Furthermore, a profound knowledge of anatomy in a normal situation is needed, as contextual palpation application indicates, which enables professionals to become sensitive to deviations from predicted findings. Moreover, certain areas, such as the thyroid gland and lymph nodes, also need accurate palpation during physical examination. Palpation of the thyroid involves assessment for asymmetry, hypertrophy, or nodularity indicative of goiter or malignancy pathologies. Likewise, lymph node examination, particularly from regions like the cervical, axillary, and inguinal nodes, can reveal signs of infection, malignancy, or systemic illness. As an example, lymphadenopathy has a frequent correlation with infectious etiology or malignancies and therefore is a crucial clue for diagnosis. Informed discussion of these regions is supported by the necessity for standardized terminology and clear recommendations, as perceived in reports pertaining to conservative management of various health conditions, which optimize practitioners' appreciation of normal and abnormal observations—demonstrating the worth of palpation as a core method in physical examination techniques (Figure 4.8).

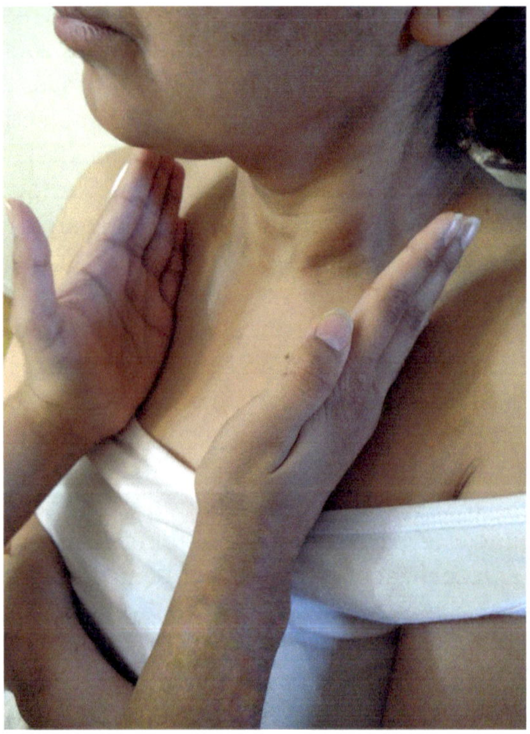

Figure 4.8. Areas commonly assessed through palpation.

Source: https://pressbooks.library.ryerson.ca/ippa/wp-content/uploads/sites/114/2020/11/IMG_20201101_0842576-01-768x1024.jpeg.

4.2.3. Importance of Patient Comfort During Palpation

The value of patient comfort while palpating cannot be overstated in the topic of physical examination techniques. Palpation, a sense-based measurement technique utilized by healthcare professionals to analyze various physical conditions, inherently entails some level of nearness and trust between the clinician and patient. Since patients feel comfortable, they are relaxed as well and thus allow better assessment. On the other hand, anxiety or tension will result in tension in the muscles, obscuring the clinician's vision of subtle pathology. Thus, establishing a secure and soothing environment prior to palpation maximizes diagnostic effectiveness, proving that patient comfort has a direct influence on clinical outcome in this useful examination tool. Additionally, knowing the patient's own perception of comfort with palpation is crucial, as proven by recent experiments with chiropractic students. Findings show that while most are accepting of peer physical examinations, there were some young female students who reported being very uncomfortable, particularly for exposure and examination by the opposite sex (Ardakani et al., 2022). This discomfort highlights the need for healthcare providers to be attuned to the psychosocial factors that may impact patient comfort levels during examination. Resolution of such issues not only makes for a more helpful clinical interaction but also establishes trust, which is essential to effective patient-provider relationships. Integration of patient-centered processes into palpation training, therefore, becomes an indispensable part of health education and practice. The importance of comfort in patients extends beyond single tests; it affects compliance of patients with medical treatment and satisfaction with care in general. When patients are relaxed and treated in a respectful manner, they tend to be forthcoming, which is fundamental in obtaining a thorough medical history and conducting effective exams. For instance, pain associated with palpation techniques can lead to resistance from patients, which eventually leads to aversion to necessary care (Campbell et al., 2014). Hence, the emphasis on comfort in palpation not only is ethically correct but also a sensible issue to be of practical concern which can have an impact on more favorable patient outcomes as well as the general quality of healthcare delivery. Recognition and rectification of discomfort-causing issues will still lead the way to the future of physical examination procedures down more compassionate and effective lines.

Test Your Knowledge

1. How does palpation help in assessing underlying structures such as organs, muscles, and lymph nodes?
2. What techniques can be used to ensure palpation is both safe and effective for the patient?

4.3. Percussion

Learning Outcome

1. Definition and purpose of percussion;
2. Techniques for different body areas;
3. Interpretation of percussion sounds.

Among the skills of physical examination, percussion is a valuable tool for doctors. It is a method in which the body is struck over specific locations to create sounds that may provide useful information regarding what lies beneath. The sounds created may vary significantly based on tissue density and composition. For example, the dull note may refer to fluid or mass presence, and resonance refers to the presence of air, such as in healthy lung tissue. Mastering percussion techniques is not only important in disease diagnosis but also in guiding future inquiry, ultimately optimizing patient care outcomes. Hence, the integration of strong physical assessment skills into nursing programs is essential because physical assessment skills have a direct relationship with practitioners' capability to deliver quality care in different clinical settings (Brembo et al., 2023). Moreover, technology-facilitated learning can contribute significantly towards increasing the efficacy of percussion. Existing literature reveals that nursing students can benefit significantly in terms of building confidence in physical assessment skills by leveraging digital tools. For instance, the Suite of Mobile Learning Tools has been viewed in a favorable manner for helping nursing students become proficient in basic concepts related to percussion and other assessment skills. The tools contribute towards the consolidation of theoretical knowledge while providing practical models which are accessible for students to refer to during clinical rotations. Enhanced proficiency in physical assessment skills like percussion is of paramount importance in that it contributes towards the basis of person-focused care. Thus, technology interventions are able to facilitate improved learning outcomes and ultimately improved patient assessments, affirming the need for continued innovation in nursing education methods (Brembo et al., 2023). Incorporation of percussion into routine practice both enhances clinical competency and warrants collaboration among healthcare professionals. To develop a well-rounded strategy, interdisciplinary cooperation can enhance patient evaluations by combining the information obtained with percussion with other types of testing such as auscultation and palpation. For instance, percussion evidence in the case of lung sounds may be combined with auscultation techniques to enable a better understanding of pulmonary diseases. As healthcare continues to progress, the need for nursing students to establish competent core competencies such as percussion is greater than ever. Emphasizing these core competencies ensures a well-prepared workforce that can meet patient care complexities, thereby identifying the necessity of integrating stringent physical assessment training into nursing curricula (Figure 4.9).

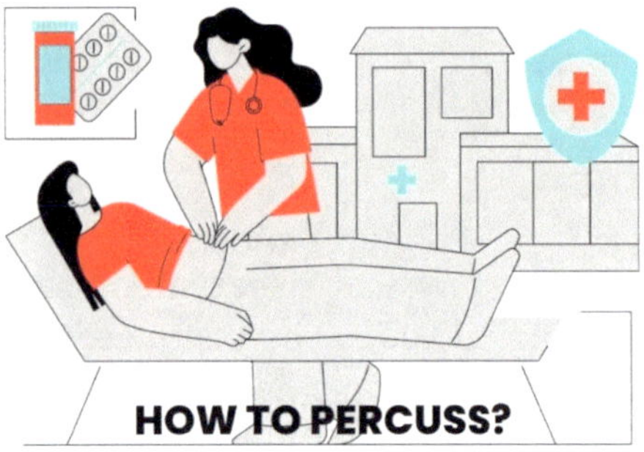

Figure 4.9. Percussion method of clinical examination.

Source: https://medicosage.com/wp-content/uploads/2023/10/PERCUSSION-METHOD-OF-CLINICAL-EXAMINATION-1-e1697810610892.webp.

4.3.1. Definition and Purpose of Percussion

Percussion is a central technique in the overall category of physical examination and is employed primarily to assess underlying structures of the body. By causing the surface of the body to impact by fingers or an instrument, doctors produce sound waves that enable them to check for the dullness or resonance of tissues. The technique is a non-invasive method that is employed to acquire essential information, in the majority of instances preceding diagnosis by revealing abnormality inside the internal organs. The ultrasound sound is utilized in order to distinguish between varying consistencies of tissues, namely air-filled tissues as well as solid tissues, thereby providing information critical for accurate medical analysis. For this reason, knowing the function and role of percussion is important for medical professionals because it becomes an essential part of their assessment skills and clinical judgment. In practice, percussion can reflect a person's health status in many instances. In some respiratory exams, for instance, abnormal sounds on percussion may indicate pneumonia or pleural effusion. The tone and pitch of the sounds produced are understood by medical practitioners to determine whether there is fluid, air, or an obstruction in specific areas and thus to perform a focused analysis of the patient's condition. Percussion is also applied in the examination of the abdomen to determine organ size and detect fluid collections or masses. The versatility of method highlights its clinical importance, being amenable to application across a wide variety of different diagnoses ranging from respiratory disease to gastrointestinal disorder, and hence affirming its place as a resource in the clinician's toolbox. Lastly, the significance of percussion transcends immediate diagnostic benefit in generating an appreciation of patient physiology. The sound output obtained through percussion acts as an adjunct form of information, complementing visual and touch results from a physical examination. In accordance with the topics of contemporary medical training, the practice of percussion on a daily basis promotes an integrated form of patient assessment leading to timely interventions and better patient outcomes. The acquisition of proficiency in this skill, among others, is thus important for healthcare providers who aim to deliver quality care. With systematic training and practice, clinicians will be in a position to fully leverage the power of percussion in an effective manner, so it contributes significantly to the intricate diagnostic and patient care process (Hadraba et al., 2018; Khomazyuk et al., 2019).

4.3.2. Techniques for Different Body Areas

It is important in clinical examination to use techniques appropriate to different regions of the body in order to enhance diagnostic accuracy. For instance, abdominal examination uses a stepwise approach that includes inspection, auscultation, percussion, and palpation. These techniques all provide essential information regarding the underlying pathosis. Inspection allows for visual inspection for contour and movement, while auscultation allows for bowel sound recognition and vascular pathology. Together, percussion tells the density of underlying tissue, and palpation evaluates organ size and texture. By using these maneuvers in conjunction with one another, health practitioners can detect conditions like organ enlargement or accumulation of fluid that would not be immediately evident by sight. While evaluating the pelvic region, the use of specific techniques such as the identification of myofascial trigger points is significant in the diagnosis of myofascial pelvic pain (MFPP). MFPP has been noted as a significant cause of chronic pelvic pain that is often not a consideration in clinical assessment. Myofascial trigger points within the pelvic floor musculature are diagnosed, and these trigger points refer pain to the surrounding regions. Myofascial trigger point release, biofeedback, and electrical stimulation are some of the methods by which it can be treated effectively. In addition, an interdisciplinary team approach becomes paramount in detection and management of MFPP, offering integrative care and improved patient outcomes (Katzman et al., 2012). Respiratory examination of the upper body also requires a discerning application of physical exam techniques. Effective assessment begins with observation of respiratory rate, rhythm, and effort, then auscultation for the identification of abnormal lung sounds such as wheezing or crackles. Percussion can also be employed to define the site of dullness or hyper-resonance, which can indicate disease states like pneumonia or pleural effusion. Also, the use of techniques beneficial in managing the anxiety frequently caused by respiratory distress is of particular interest. It is evident from patient experience that access to applicable coping assets is central to recovery and management, and this emphasizes the intersection of psychological care and physical assessment (Fletcher et al., 2008). Through such methods, healthcare professionals are not only able to identify physical states but also facilitate an integrationist patient care (Figure 4.10).

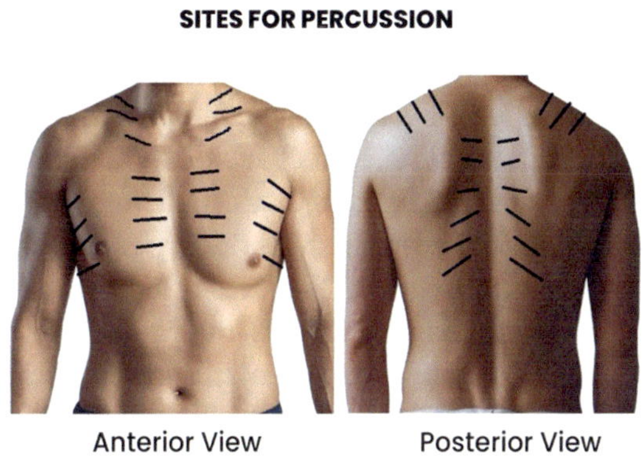

Figure 4.10. Percussion of techniques for different body areas.

Source: https://encrypted-tbn0.gstatic.com/images?q=tbn:ANd9GcS34Tl6XYo8H95MXuIkONBDPHNHhfqNFknk8Q&s.

4.3.3. Interpretation of Percussion Sounds

Percussion sounds interpretation is a simple physical examination method that provides critical information about the state of a patient's anatomical structures. Through percussion, medical professionals tap parts of the body with their fingers, and they produce sounds whose characteristics are relative to the density and composition of the underlying tissue. The various percussion notes, e.g., tympanic, dull, or resonant sounds, are able to provide information on various pathological states. For instance, resonant sounds will generally be connected with healthy lung tissue, while dullness can signal the presence of fluid or solid masses, such as in pleural effusion or hepatomegaly. The specific appreciation of such sounds is critical for clinicians because it is helpful in differentiating normal from abnormal findings in a variety of thoracic and abdominal investigations, thus dictating further diagnostic and therapeutic management. According to the underlying principle of percussion, there is a need to highlight the clinical application of the technique. In the case of ascites or abdominal distension assessment, the clinician can ascertain a shifting dullness by percussion that correlates with the movement of the fluid within the peritoneal cavity. This can be further verified by imaging techniques and biochemical ascitic fluid analysis, which allows clinicians to classify the underlying causation of the condition. Besides, percussion is not only limited to the thoracic and abdominal cavities but is also effective in evaluating the size and position of the heart, where changes in sound may reflect structural change or pericardial effusion. Thus, the incorporation of percussion sounds in an amplified physical examination optimizes the precision of diagnosis and improves patient care management plans (Scott et al., 2021). Overall, percussion sound interpretation is a dynamic skill that easily intersects with evidence-based practice and clinical decision-making. With specialization in this method, healthcare professionals are capable of obtaining crucial information about a patient's health condition as they ensure the importance of appropriate physical assessment in clinical practice. As recognized by several systematic reviews, the use of non-pharmacological interventions like education programs aimed at enhancing examination skills can be an element in improved patient care outcomes (Abraha et al., 2017). Thus, ongoing education and training in the clinical skill of percussion, along with the integration of technology and clinical guidelines, is critical to enhancing future healthcare practitioners' assessment abilities and enhancing patient outcomes. An understanding of percussion not only has diagnostic uses, but also educates the clinicians about their patient base, building trust and better communication within the therapeutic relationship.

Test Your Knowledge

1. How does percussion help in determining the size, density, and location of internal organs?
2. What differences in percussion sounds indicate normal versus abnormal findings in the thorax or abdomen?

4.4. Auscultation

Learning Outcome

1. Equipment used for auscultation (e.g., stethoscope);
2. Types of sounds assessed (e.g., heart, lung);
3. Importance of quiet environment during auscultation.

Auscultation, one of the key physical examination skills, refers to the activity of listening to a patient's internal sounds, generally with the use of a stethoscope. Clinicians utilize this method in order to assess the functional characteristics of organ systems, such as the cardiovascular and respiratory systems. By identifying those that are out of the ordinary, such as heart murmurs or abnormal breath sounds, clinicians can learn about potential underlying conditions. For example, the prevalence of systolic ejection murmurs in boxer dogs as reported in cardiac auscultation studies justifies the role of experience to detect low-intensity murmurs (Höglund et al., 2007). Such findings justify the importance of auscultation not only in humans but also in veterinary medicine, where diagnosis is reliant on similar auditory assessments. Precision of auscultation is enhanced by frequent practice and exposure to normal and abnormal auscultations. Certain techniques can be used to optimize precision of auscultation results. For instance, body position can impact the sounds heard; supine or lateral recumbent may produce auscultation results different from sitting or standing position. Additionally, the clinician's ability to perceive variations in sound intensity and character can be enhanced with the aid of additional diagnostic apparatus, i.e., echocardiography. Utilizing contemporary techniques, e.g., time-frequency analysis for murmurs differentiation, demonstrates how traditional auscultation may evolve along with advancements in technology (Höglund et al., 2007).

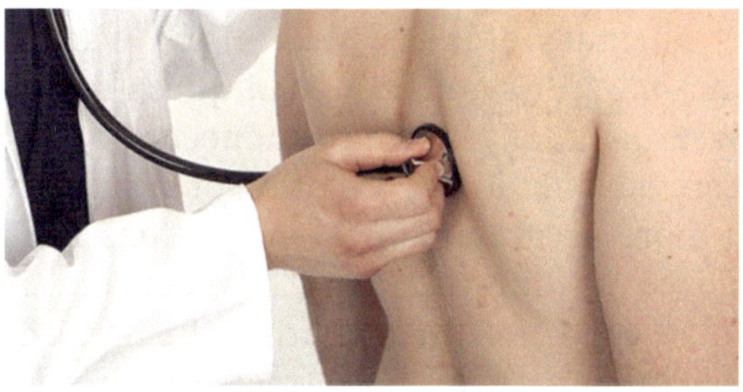

Figure 4.11. Auscultation in physical examination.

Source: https://www.littmann.in/wps/wcm/connect/047766ca-fe36-4e0a-ae58-094e7eda2e51/content-columns-540-resources-auscultation-tips-patient-in-a-medical-exam.jpg?MOD=AJPERES&CACHEID=ROOTWORKSPACE-047766ca-fe36-4e0a-ae58-094e7eda2e51-mF9uh8G.

Thus, while auscultation is a timeless skill, its effectiveness relies on the practitioner's training as well as on the techniques applied during examination. Apart from its application in cardio and respiratory tests, auscultation also plays a critical role in the diagnosis of pulmonary conditions. As noted in recent studies, auscultation techniques play an important role in the detection of pulmonary edema—a condition well known recently as a significant perioperative complication, where their quick detection largely depends on high sensitivity and specificity inherent in the auscultatory process in order for practitioners to act quickly. Moreover, auscultation complements imaging modalities by giving real-time feedback about lung function that can guide subsequent diagnostic maneuvers. Through observation of trends over time, auscultation is even useful in assessing the patient's response to treatment, further cementing its position as a useful element of the entire arsenal of physical examination techniques (Figure 4.11).

4.4.1. Equipment Used for Auscultation (e.g., Stethoscope)

Auscultation, a very important component of physical examination, has significant reliance on sophisticated apparatus such as the stethoscope, a very valuable tool for doctors. It facilitates identification of various body sounds that are of immense importance in interpreting the respective physiological conditions of patients. The stethoscope is used primarily to hear heart sounds, lung sounds, and bowel sounds, all of which are significant in diagnosing potential medical issues. Not only the design and construction of the stethoscope, but also the skill and proficiency of the doctor performing the examination, contribute to making the examination effective. Therefore, knowing the types and characteristics of auscultation equipment is important for effective assessment and efficient management of patients. Unamplified and amplified stethoscopes are the two categories of stethoscopes available in the market. Unamplified stethoscopes, even though being simple in design with clear sound transmission, are still used because of their consistency in clinical application. In contrast, amplified stethoscopes benefit hearing-impaired practitioners or those requiring more auditory discrimination in noisy environments. It has been found that the associated sound pressure levels produced by such a device can substantially vary, impacting their diagnostic value. The choice between unamplified and amplified stethoscopes can decide not only the quality of auscultation performed but also the entire efficacy of the physical examination process. Moreover, the experience and training of the examiner also play a crucial role in the efficacy of auscultation. Research indicates that the experience of clinicians enhances their skills for detecting and interpreting faint heart murmurs (Höglund et al., 2007).

Inconsistency of these murmurs can render auscultation difficult; therefore, clinicians must develop their hearing through repeated practice and training. New diagnostic techniques, such as time-frequency analysis, have been explored as adjunctive approaches to complement the conventional auscultation (Höglund et al., 2007). Therefore, while the stethoscope remains a vital instrument, the clinician's skill and continuous adaptation to evolving technology are also essential to the success of the physical examination technique (Figure 4.12).

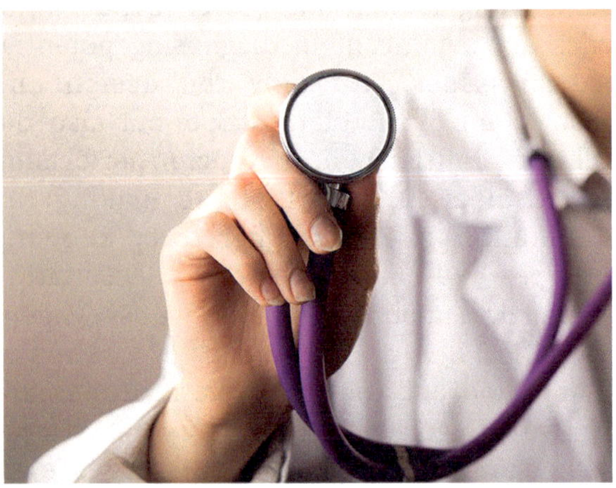

Figure 4.12. Equipment used for auscultation.

Source: https://media.post.rvohealth.io/wp-content/uploads/2020/08/Auscultation-732x549-thumbnail.jpg.

4.4.2. Types of Sounds Assessed (e.g., Heart, Lung)

The sounds elicited on physical examination are critical indicators of the physiological mechanisms underlying, such as the cardiovascular and respiratory systems. The heart sounds, for instance, are critical to the diagnosis of valvular heart disease, in which the clinician listens to faint sounds related to the opening and closing of heart valves. Systolic ejection murmurs caused by turbulence in left ventricular outflow tract are a significant auscultatory clue. It is notable that the prevalence of such murmurs can vary between populations, as in studies on boxer dogs where the murmur intensity was highly variable. Using more advanced techniques, such as echocardiography linked to phonocardiography, a more advanced interpretation of such sounds and more accurate clinical evaluations can be achieved by differentiating between multiple cardiac conditions, illustrating the wealth of information that can be extracted with careful auscultation (Höglund et al., 2007). More than heart sounds, lung sound evaluation provides critical information regarding pulmonary health. The character of the breath sounds, such as wheezes, crackles, and rhonchi, provides a diagnostic model for conditions like asthma, pneumonia, and chronic obstructive pulmonary disease. When inspected during a physical examination, identification of abnormal lung sounds usually warrants further research, due to their presence in relation to the respiratory system's function. Wheezing, for example, usually signifies airway obstruction or inflammation, leading the clinician to suspect the possibility of conditions such as bronchial constriction. Recent research indicates that systematic lung sound assessment can greatly enhance patient outcomes, especially in the case of chronic respiratory diseases. Therefore, these auditory evaluations play a central role in making accurate diagnoses and framing treatment plans, highlighting the importance of auscultation in patient management (Cruz et al., 2015). The addition of advanced methodologies in heart and lung sound evaluation enhances the efficacy and precision of physical examination techniques. For example, the application of time-frequency analysis and measures of complexity to cardiac auscultation has been encouraging in identifying subtle differences in physiological conditions. These advances are able to facilitate heart murmur interpretations for healthcare professionals and ultimately decide on pathological status, as found in recent studies. Also, ongoing development of patient-specific measures of outcome in respiratory physiotherapy underlines the necessity of individually tailored interventions based on precise auditory feedback. The techniques point to a continued need for adaptation and learning in the clinic, where advancing technology and greater understanding of sound parameters can aid more efficient patient management strategies. Through diligent examination of sounds, clinicians can not only identify but also anticipate potential health problems, and this supports the prime position of physical examination techniques in modern healthcare.

4.4.3. Importance of Quiet Environment During Auscultation

An ideal environment is critical during auscultation in physical examination since correct interpretation of body sounds can directly impact diagnostic findings. Externally interfering noise may mask subtle auditory cues that medical staff desire to evaluate, hampering them from distinguishing between normal and abnormal states. This is particularly critical in settings such as pediatric examinations, where features of benign heart murmurs and those that foretell heart disease can be challenging to distinguish. The requirement for a noise-free environment highlights the necessity of removing auditory distractions to enable a proper assessment of sounds crucially associated with cardiac and respiratory processes (Canha et al., 2008). Thus, health practitioners must emphasize more on building the acoustically conducive setting to enhance their clinical assessment skill, ultimately leading to improved patient outcomes. Beyond the reduction of background noise, auscultation also relies significantly on the providers' capacity to concentrate and become completely engaged in listening to the patient's physiological sounds. This relationship between tranquil surroundings and increased focus can't be asserted too categorically, as clarity of mind needs to happen if correct interpretation is to take place. Stressful settings or hectic clinical settings provide a condition of chaos as electronic equipment, talk, and activity distract from the provider's attention, leading to potential misinterpretations. In addition, a tranquil setting provides relaxation for both clinician and patient, eliminating fear and allowing for a more in-depth assessment (Bivens et al., 2025). This prioritization of creating a quiet setting is not a voluntary choice but rather a vital aspect of the diagnostic process, highlighting the necessity for health care providers to actively design their exam rooms with acoustical goals in mind. In certain medical environments, such as neonatal intensive care units (NICUs), the impact of a quiet setting extends beyond auscultation to encompass general health results. The literature suggests that ambient noise levels in clinical environments not only affect diagnostic precision but also the general quality of recovery and patient care (Bivens et al., 2025). With the understanding of the integral role of sound in body sound reception and interpretation, healthcare professionals can cultivate an environment that fosters enhanced clinical interactions. Application of sound-reducing technologies and optimal spatial design practices can significantly improve auscultation accuracy and efficiency and ultimately improve patient outcomes. Ultimately, a self-awareness of the need for a quiet environment for auscultation is fundamental to ensuring standards of physical exam technique and quality healthcare provision.

Test Your Knowledge

1. How does auscultation assist in evaluating heart, lung, and bowel sounds during a physical assessment?
2. What are common errors to avoid when performing auscultation to ensure accurate findings?

4.5. Special Tests

Learning Outcome

1. Overview of common special tests (e.g., reflex tests);
2. Indications for using special tests;
3. Interpretation of results from special tests.

Special tests are a critical part of the physical examination methods, acting as a complementary tool to the healthcare practitioners in the evaluation of certain conditions or injuries. Special tests, particular to the examination of various anatomical structures, aid in the comprehensive evaluation and diagnosis of patients. Special tests aid health professionals in recognizing the presence of pathologies such as injury to a ligament, tendonitis, or various musculoskeletal disorders. For instance, the Lachman test is often employed to evaluate the integrity of the knee's anterior cruciate ligament (ACL) in order to help determine imaging or surgical need. As a result, appropriate application of these tests enhances the clinician's capacity to formulate informed treatment plans based on accurate diagnoses, an essential component in patient care. Special examinations require not only technical proficiency but a keen sense of pathology and anatomy as well. The interpreter must have the ability to put the findings that have been created by these examinations into the general clinical picture of the patient's presentation. The Neers test and Hawkins-Kennedy test are important in diagnosing impingement syndromes of the shoulder, for example. But the results must correlate with patient history, symptom patterns, and results of the full examination to enable the right diagnosis. Misinterpretation of such tests will result in misdiagnosis, potentially jeopardizing patient safety and outcomes. Special tests therefore must be employed judiciously, and the necessity for rigorous training and continuous education for the health workers. Furthermore, application of special tests shifts with developing technologies and progressing research. Other imaging modalities, such as ultrasound and MRI, provide additional information verifying or defining results of special tests.

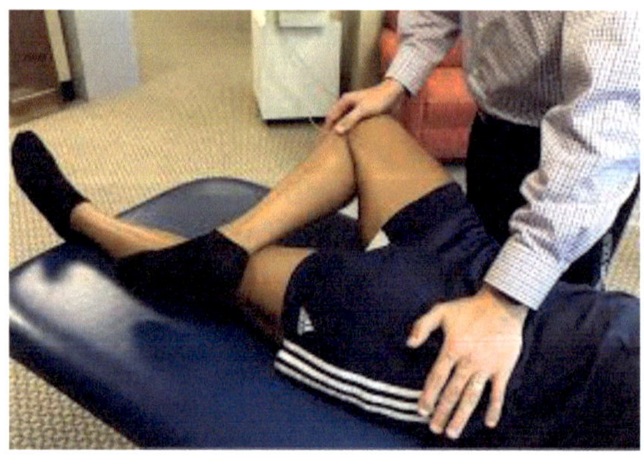

Figure 4.13. Special tests of physical examination.

Source: https://www.sportsmedreview.com/wp-content/uploads/2022/11/demonstration-of-the-FABER-test.png.

Through the combination of traditional testing with new imaging technologies, diagnosis and treatment planning are addressed from different planes. A report summarizing some scientific and technical papers highlights that special tests remain a key research and development priority area in the discipline, as evident through ongoing studies examining ways to improve their specificity and validity (N/A). On the other hand, the interactive nature of special tests highlights their contribution towards evidence-based practice across physical examinations (Kitsiou et al., 2013). With advancing medical practice, practitioners should be up to date with developments that could affect the selection and interpretation of special tests (Figure 4.13).

4.5.1. Overview of Common Special Tests (e.g., Reflex Tests)

In the physical exam, special tests are a critical component in assessing neurological function and one of the most common used is reflex tests. Reflex tests, such as the patellar reflex and Achilles reflex, are utilized to assess the integrity of specific neurological pathways. Upon striking a tendon by a clinician, the muscle contraction that follows permits the clinician to obtain extremely valuable information with regards to the sensory as well as motor components of a reflex arc. For instance, hyperactive patellar reflex can be observed in upper motor neuron damage, whereas reduced response is suggestive of lower motor neuron injury. Through systematic assessment of these reflexes, clinicians can gain information regarding underlying neurological disease, which assists in the formulation of a differential diagnosis and guides further evaluative action. Another important category of special tests includes provocation tests that assess joint function and stability, particularly in orthopedic examination. These exams, such as Lachman test for the integrity of ACL or McMurray maneuver in meniscal injuries, provide specialized evaluation of musculoskeletal structures. Abnormal findings in these tests are generally consistent with specific types of injury and assist in the diagnosis of issues such as ligamentous injury or meniscal lesion. However, it should be understood that although these exams can indicate possible pathologies, their sensitivity and specificity are variable. Thus, clinicians need to put the test findings into the broader clinical perspective, patient history and imaging studies being taken as adjunct data in order to understand the patient's condition fully. Ultimately, utility of special tests is not only applied to standard reflex testing but also to more subtle testing such as the Concealed Information Test (CIT). Though the CIC is most commonly associated with lie detection, its scientific approach can bring complexity to the research of neurological process and response. In the clinical setting, specialized tests like the CIT need to be handled carefully due to risks of false positives and false negatives. For example, though the structure of the CIT can have substantial effects when conditions are optimal, practitioners must avoid misinterpreting results. This test sensitivity emphasizes the necessity of situating such tests in a holistic investigative context so that proper conclusions are drawn from both mental and physical responses observed in the course of examination (Meijer et al., 2014) (Figure 4.14).

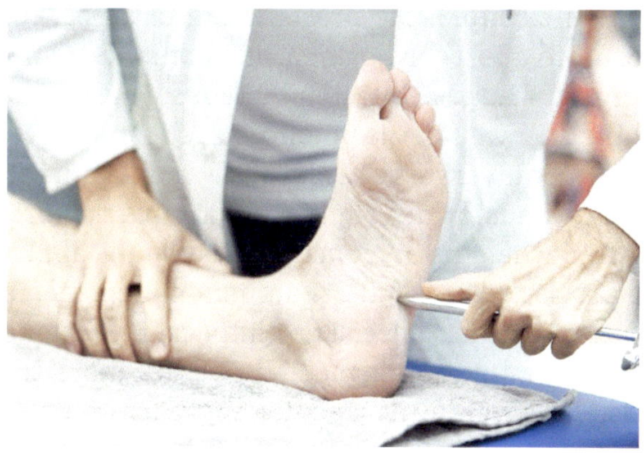

Figure 4.14. Reflex tests.

Source: https://external-content.duckduckgo.com/iu/?u=https%3A%2F%2Fwww.atlantabrainandspine.com%2Fwp-content%2Fuploads%2F2022%2F02%2FiStock-472064219-1024x683.jpg&f=1&nofb=1&ipt=0d5c9c770853390923790ebf69e1efbd6a99a49d56345defd754981b7d2cd74a.

4.5.2. Indications for Using Special Tests

Special tests are a part of the physical examination process, weighing clinical assessment and diagnostic strategy. The greatest need for special tests is to diagnose or exclude specific conditions based on presenting complaints in a patient. For instance, orthopedic special tests are very helpful to evaluate musculoskeletal injuries and provide precise feedback that helps guide treatment decisions. They are specially designed to pinpoint precise components of a joint or muscle so that clinicians can differentiate between differential injuries or conditions. The rational use of these examinations is hence paramount, as they are based on the use of the clinician's judgment as well as test specificity in enhancing the reliability of diagnosis, ultimately leading to better clinical decisions. In addition to diagnosis, special tests also help in guiding future interventions and management plans. A key to their use is to be found in the finessed intuition they provide as to the degree and nature of the injury or disease in question. To put an example: the presentation of a positive result to a test for ligament instability not only helps to diagnose but simultaneously makes the clinician aware of the potential need for surgical treatment versus conservative management. These kinds of discrimination are particularly crucial when the outcome is based on the ability to precisely ascertain the amount of damage. In such cases, then, special test implications extend far beyond mere diagnosis and determine the patient's overall therapeutic approach, serving as a map to effective clinical management. In addition, the integration of special tests in the physical examination procedure also emphasizes the need for a thorough assessment of the overall health status and functional capability of the patients. Indications for their use become even more significant in complicated cases where involvement of more than one system is possible. For instance, the presence of systemic states may complicate the understanding of the meaning of local symptoms, hence necessitating the use of special tests to rule out the differential diagnosis. In doing so, the ability to utilize focused assessments will lead to the identification of underlying states not readily apparent. Therefore, special tests become a critical physical examination tool that equips the clinician with the power to perform advanced assessment that informs diagnosis as well as treatment strategies (Kitsiou et al., 2013; Virginia Commonwealth University, 2018).

4.5.3. Interpretation of Results from Special Tests

Special test findings analysis is a key component of physical examination technique in the clinical environment. Special tests are designed to assess specific functions or states, providing valuable information that can impact diagnosis and treatment options. For instance, in musculoskeletal evaluations, some tests can distinguish among various types of injuries or conditions based on patient response to unique maneuvers. The credibility of these tests also relies heavily on the clinician's expertise in anatomy and biomechanics, as well as the nuances of presenting complaints. If the clinician is not adequately knowledgeable about these issues, the clinician will inevitably misread the results, which may lead to incorrect conclusions and potentially harmful clinical interventions. In the realm of best patient care, special test outcomes are frequently read concurrently between medical providers. The results can be important points of reference in patient management; thus, collaboration between several stakeholders, such as other professionals, including radiologists and physical therapists, can enhance diagnostic precision. Proper clarification of test results, and their implications, enhances a multi-disciplinary environment conducive to the patient's overall healthcare experience. Application of uniform protocols for test interpretation also can help achieve consistency and objectivity within the clinical setting, enabling a shared understanding of best practices among providers. Furthermore, application of advances in research using technology and evidence-based practice also can help augment interpretation of special test results. As diagnostic tools continue to advance, clinicians must keep pace with the latest research to provide interpretations that are compatible with current standards. The pursuit of accreditation, for instance, by agencies such as the American College of Radiology, depicts the resolve to continue to improve patient outcomes through standardized models of care. The long process of gaining accreditation gives healthcare institutions the blueprints through which they may review and refine their examination protocols. Hence, reporting the outcomes of special tests not only signifies the professional acumen of the clinician but also reflects the dedication of the institution towards delivering high-quality patient care in accordance with emerging clinical guidelines and standards (Kitsiou et al., 2013; Manigold et al., 2019) (Figure 4.15).

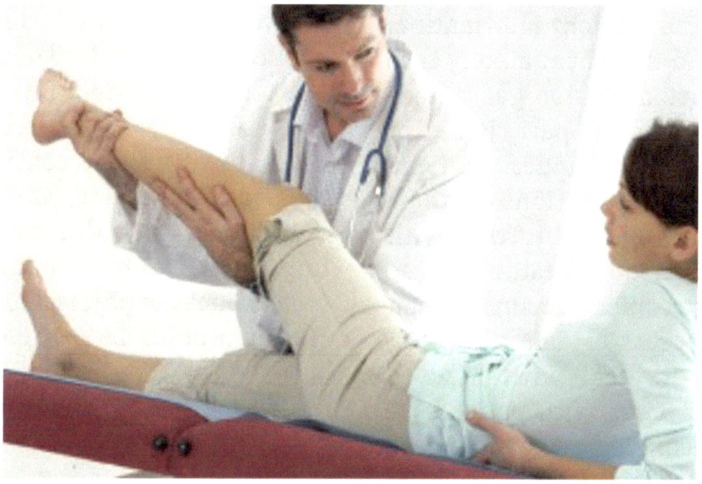

Figure 4.15. Interpretation of results from special tests.

Source: https://corechiropractic.net/wp-content/uploads/2013/06/orthopedic_examination.jpg.

Test Your Knowledge

1. What is the purpose of performing special tests during a physical assessment, and how do they aid diagnosis?
2. How can specific orthopedic or neurological special tests help identify underlying musculoskeletal or nerve conditions?

4.6. Documentation

Learning Outcome

1. Importance of accurate documentation;
2. Components of a physical examination report;
3. Legal and ethical considerations in documentation.

Documentation is a central element of the physical examination skills, serving as the primary vehicle for the transfer of patient information, clinical information, and treatment among care providers. Effective documentation guarantees proper communication since all participants of the healthcare team come to understand the patient's status and any alterations in their care. The process is complicated further with the introduction of electronic health records (EHRs), which seek to streamline documentation and increase patient access to data. However, providers also have to deal with how to maintain the personal touch with patients as they also deal with technology. Thus, defining best practices of EHR usage is significant to enhance provider-patient communication and make documentation a reliable component of patient care (Leamon et al., 2016). Careful documentation is not just about documentation; it is an element of patient safety and quality care rendered. Sufficient and consistent records not only support clinical decisions but are also essential in legal cases as well as in quality assurance audits. Health professionals must be trained to document results in a full and accurate manner so that misinterpretation that could lead to unwanted outcomes is avoided. For this purpose, continuing education about documentation processes, especially related to EHR systems, is necessary for improving overall patient outcomes. With the advancement of healthcare, the role of documentation to support clinical practice can be regarded as a critical set of abilities that are nurtured by all professionals to promote effective communication and coordination of care by various healthcare teams (Virginia Commonwealth University, 2018). Good documentation practices also promote continuity of care, particularly in cases where the transitions are occurring among various healthcare settings. For instance, in the case of a patient being referred by a primary care doctor to a specialist, proper documentation is crucial to ensure that the specialist receives pertinent health information and past examination results. Smooth transfer of information minimizes the likelihood of redundancies in testing and facilitates informed decision-making. The application of standard documentation protocols and templates within EHR systems can enhance this efficiency across providers and settings. Ultimately, with the continued development of the health landscape, commitment to enhancing documentation practices will remain an important catalyst for improving the overall effectiveness of physical examination techniques (Leamon et al., 2016) (Figure 4.16).

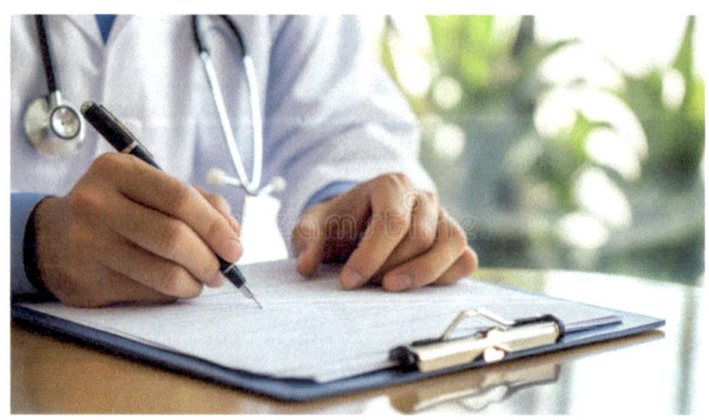

Figure 4.16. Documentation of physical examination.

Source: https://thumbs.dreamstime.com/b/doctor-writing-notes-clipboard-physical-examination-doctor-focused-writing-notes-clipboard-348084092.jpg.

4.6.1. Importance of Accurate Documentation

Accurate documentation is the cornerstone of physical examination because it serves as the foundation for patient care and informs clinical decision. Each physical examination yields critical findings which must be well documented in order to facilitate continuity of care and optimum communication among healthcare providers. As the healthcare environment continues to evolve towards electronic health records, providers must navigate the complexities of documentation in these computerized systems. The shift toward electronic documentation has necessitated a refinement of communication skills, so much so that practitioners must now be proficient in utilizing these devices effectively when communicating with patients. This has consequently introduced into practice emphasis on best practices regarding documentation, which can greatly affect the overall patient experience and reduce potential areas of error (Leamon et al., 2016). These records' accuracy impacts not just patient-by-patient results, but broader healthcare practice and policy. In addition, combining telehealth technology with the delivery of healthcare only adds to the imperative of detailed documentation in various healthcare settings. The larger number of practitioners who incorporate telehealth into their practice, the larger the imperative for accurate documentation. WoundView and other tools and applications illustrate technology's potential to facilitate documentation of physical exams, especially in more remote areas where physician access is sometimes less readily available. This technological development offers opportunities as well as challenges, however, for while it encourages expanded access to care, it also requires a commitment to thorough documentation processes. Through proper documentation throughout telehealth sessions, nurse practitioners and other health practitioners are able to enable precise assessments, enhance interdisciplinary communication, and provide assurance that patients receive coordinated care. The data gathered from such documented exchanges informs the healthcare system, emphasizing the need for constant improvement in documentation practices (Reimer et al., 2018). Moreover, the effect of good documentation extends beyond patient contacts and touches upon the integrity of the health system at large. Well-maintained records facilitate accountability, allowing healthcare professionals to track patient history, treatment outcomes, and results efficiently. This uniformity is crucial not only for immediate patient care but also for research and developing evidence-based practice. Through conscientious documentation of findings, clinical practices are helping to build an aggregate body of knowledge informing clinical guidelines and best practices. Incomplete or inaccurate documentation also has adverse repercussions, from patient safety issues to lawsuits against providers. Practitioners must then understand the significance of precise and meticulous documentation as an integral part of their exam techniques. This focus will ultimately enhance patient safety and the quality of care as well as promote a culture of accountability in healthcare (Leamon et al., 2016) (Figure 4.17).

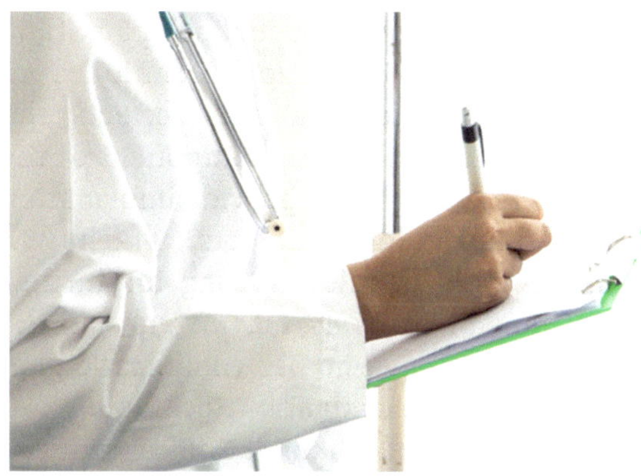

Figure 4.17. Accurate documentation of physical examination.

Source: https://lhatrustfunds.com/assets/uploads/_contentWidth/Website-Article-Documentation.png.

4.6.2. Components of a Physical Examination Report

The components of a physical examination report are essential in giving a general assessment of a patient's health. They typically begin with the patients history, such as the present illness, medical background, medications, and family illnesses. This first component not only assists in establishing rapport with the patient but also gives context for the clinicians subsequent observations and diagnosis. For instance, experience of previous procedures, such as total hip replacement, can guide follow-up examination techniques relevant to assessing the integrity and functionality of a joint. The interface of history taking and physical examination techniques is most critical in determining an appropriate diagnosis and treatment plan, emphasizing continuity care to which all patients are entitled, as illustrated in the comprehensive case report of an examination of aseptic loosening of a hip prosthesis (Baldacchino et al., 2012). Following the history, the actual physical examination is a systematic evaluation consisting of vital sign evaluation, overall appearance, and a specific examination of the relevant system. Physicians use various inspection, palpation, percussion, and auscultation techniques to acquire appropriate data that reflects the patient's health status. Each component of the examination is designed to provide information regarding physiological defects, which will help in directing decision-making for further investigations or referrals. For instance, in the instance of a patient who has complications in the hips, physical examination techniques can produce evidence of inflammation or reduced range of motion, and these are crucial in the diagnosis of conditions like osteoarthritis or infection. Thus, proper application of these examination techniques offers the cornerstones for good clinical reasoning and patient-centered care (Baldacchino et al., 2012). Documentation of results is a fundamental part of the physical examination report, making findings unambiguous and enabling continuity of patient care. Careful documentation of all observations that are obtained during the examination, both normal and abnormal findings, is required. There are various reasons for detailed recording: it serves as a legal record of the care administered, directs future clinical management decisions, and facilitates communication among multidisciplinary teams caring for the patient. In compounded cases such as pelvic floor dysfunction, consensus definition of the symptoms and the healing process can be particularly beneficial to concerted documentation and care coordination. Therefore, through proper documentation, medical professionals are capable of proving that every component of the physical examination is located within a comprehensive context of patient care, enhancing even further the quality and efficacy of the examination process.

4.6.3. Legal and Ethical Considerations in Documentation

Legal and ethical documentation guidelines are of utmost significance in the practice of physical examination and aim at safeguarding patient care as well as healthcare professionals' integrity. Accurate documentation not only serves legal requirements but also supports effective communication among multidisciplinary teams. Ethically, patient details must be documented accurately and comprehensively to provide continuity of care. These types of violations may lead to legal repercussions, for instance, malpractice claims or the imposition of regulatory penalties. Finally, confidentiality of patient records is required because their violation can destroy patient trust and safety. In documentation practice, seeking consent and establishing clear policies on how patient information is used are the essential aspects reinforcing both legal and ethical actions. In addition, the advancement of technology in the practice of healthcare documentation has necessitated the re-evaluation of ethical standards as to privacy and protection of data. With increased applications of electronic health records, physicians have to navigate a labyrinth of legislation that governs use of sensitive patient information. Features such as the Health

Insurance Portability and Accountability Act (HIPAA) underscore the necessity of good security measures as well as patient consent when handling documents. Moreover, ethical dilemmas would ensue when healthcare workers are pressured into recording information that doesn't always accurately represent the condition of a patient, which underlines the importance of integrity in record maintenance. Technological integration should therefore aim at enhancing accuracy and simplicity in documentation without compromising ethical practice, ultimately producing a more responsible and credible health system. Above all, the question is how documentation influences clinical judgment and patient outcomes. The ethical obligation of medical professionals is not merely one of adherence to policy and regulation; it involves the responsibility to provide quality care through careful documentation. Poor or missing records can lead to misdiagnosis or inappropriate use of treatment, compromising patient safety. There are legal implications as well if documentation is poor, which exposes health professionals to lawsuits. Moreover, different imaging technologies, symbolized by the use of Contrast Agents (CA), emphasize the need for accurate and appropriate documentation on the risks and benefits of each intervention. Last but not least, the interweaving of legal and ethical issues within documentation functions to enhance the quality of physical examination, while assuring that patient care is always at the very core of medical practice, guided by unyielding professionalism and ethical dedication.

Test Your Knowledge

1. Why is accurate and timely documentation of physical assessment findings critical in patient care?
2. How can standardized documentation improve communication among healthcare team members?

SUMMARY

The physical examination methods remain the core of clinical practice, particularly in the evaluation of diseases like pneumonia. The literature review conducted by Gennis et al. identifies the significance of various physical examination methods, with examples of findings such as rales and decreased breath sounds that have high sensitivity with pneumonia. The fact that they are crucial notwithstanding, is that physical examination alone cannot provide complete diagnostic confidence. As noted in the study, although rales are most useful in pneumonia diagnosis, their use alone through only examination techniques can lead to misdiagnosis. It is thus significant that other instruments such as chest radiographs are used in order to enhance successful patient management. This incorporation indicates the necessity for health practitioners to possess not just acute observing skills but also awareness of the limitation that comes with physical examination (Tordoff et al., 2018). In addition, the integration of physical exam skills into the curriculum is crucial in equipping competent healthcare professionals. As uncovered by the integrated consultation course studies, students benefit significantly through integrating theoretical knowledge into hands-on skills within simulated clinical environments. The transition from theory to clinical practice is a complex procedure that needs guided practice and ongoing feedback. Surprisingly, diminishing supervisory direction in this learning process promotes independence and critical thinking. However, there is a need to balance increasing student responsibility to prevent overloading them with additional tasks to heighten feelings of incompetence or anxiety in clinical environments. Accordingly, educational programs should include systematic teaching approaches that increasingly develop students' abilities to render them competent to solve real clinical problems (Derese et al., 2014). Ultimately, the union of effective physical examination skills and comprehensive education systems has a significant impact on effective patient care. As the future of healthcare is developed, building practitioners able to utilize these skills is of utmost concern. The findings of the systematic review of pneumonia diagnosis and the integrated consultation course both speak to the significance of these skills in producing competent clinicians who are able to offer quality medical care. By placing proper instruction in physical exam skills and providing practical exposure at an early point in medical school, health schools can prepare the future doctors to accurately diagnose and treat patients and maintain the art and science of medicine (Derese et al., 2014; Tordoff et al., 2018).

The physical examination methods form the cornerstone of the diagnostic process as the foundation for clinical thinking. They are focused on a systematic approach that values completeness and accuracy. Inspection, palpation, percussion, and auscultation are widely used by medical professionals in certain purposes and methods. Inspection is a visual assessment of the patient to detect abnormalities, while palpation is the examination by hand to obtain information about structures deep inside, such as texture, warmth, and tenderness. Clinicians can detect signs that might be present in medical conditions by using these methods together. Besides, proper use of these techniques relies on a discriminating level of understanding of the patient's environment and the numerous variables that may impact their physical health, as illustrated by how practitioners take the correct information during exams (Mutawa et al., 2015). The capacity of the practitioners to analyze and interpret data acquired from physical examinations is also key in maintaining clinical precision in diagnoses. For example, percussion techniques can help to determine fluid or mass in specific regions of anatomy and thus put into the limelight potential issues to be investigated further. Similarly, auscultation can provide significant clues regarding cardiovascular or respiratory status by identifying abnormal cardiac or pulmonary sounds that denote underlying pathophysiology. Employed together, these techniques enhance the practitioners capability to gather comprehensive data, which not only yields information for immediate clinical decision-making but also for extended care planning. As emphasized by existing research in the clinical practice, developing such skills is indispensable for clinicians to adapt the evolving healthcare needs and improve patient outcomes (Fletcher et al., 2008). Furthermore, the use of advanced technologies in traditional physical examination techniques represents a revolutionary shift in the medical practice. With increasing progress in the field of healthcare, telemedicine and online assessment technologies facilitate a more interactive and dynamic examination process. These advances allow real-time data exchange and enhance practitioners ability to access information on patient conditions. For example, application of cell phone-based health applications for remote monitoring of patients symptoms has been observed to complement physical examination processes with high efficiency. Nevertheless, practitioners must still be proficient in fundamental examination skills because the techniques provide context information in grasping technology-based data and patient care as a whole. Therefore, with the evolving character of healthcare, the integration of traditional techniques and innovations is a necessity (Mutawa et al., 2015).

KEY TERMS FROM THIS CHAPTER

- Inspection
- Palpation
- Percussion
- Auscultation
- General Survey
- Vital Signs
- Head-to-Toe Assessment
- Focused Assessment
- Light Palpation
- Deep Palpation
- Direct Percussion
- Indirect Percussion
- Diaphragm (of stethoscope)
- Bell (of stethoscope)
- Observation
- Palmar Surface

CRITICAL THINKING QUESTIONS

1. **Which sequence of techniques is commonly used during an abdominal examination?**
   a. Inspection → Palpation → Percussion → Auscultation
   b. Inspection → Auscultation → Percussion → Palpation
   c. Percussion → Auscultation → Palpation → Inspection
   d. Auscultation → Inspection → Percussion → Palpation
2. **Which physical examination technique is primarily used to assess the size, shape, and consistency of organs?**
   a. Inspection
   b. Palpation
   c. Percussion
   d. Auscultation
3. **Percussion during a physical exam is used to determine:**
   a. Heart rate and rhythm
   b. Sound, density, and location of underlying structures
   c. Skin texture and temperature
   d. Patient's pain level
4. **Auscultation is best described as:**
   a. Listening to internal body sounds using a stethoscope
   b. Feeling body parts with hands to detect abnormalities
   c. Tapping on the body to elicit sounds
   d. Observing the patient for visible signs
5. **Which of the following is an example of inspection during a physical examination?**
   a. Listening to lung sounds
   b. Observing a rash on the patient's arm
   c. Palpating the abdomen for tenderness
   d. Percussing the chest to detect fluid

Short Answer Questions

1. What are the four primary techniques used in a physical examination, and in what order are they generally performed?
2. Explain the purpose of inspection during a physical assessment. What should a nurse observe?
3. How is palpation used to assess the body, and what are the differences between light and deep palpation?
4. Describe the technique of percussion and its clinical significance.
5. What information can auscultation provide, and which organs or systems are typically assessed this way?

Answer to Critical Thinking Questions

1. (b) 2. (b) 3. (b) 4. (a) 5. (b)

REFERENCES

1. Abraha, I., Rimland, J. M., Trotta, F., Dell'Aquila, G., Cruz-Jentoft, A. J., Petrović, M., Guðmundsson, A., et al. (2017). Systematic review of systematic reviews of non-pharmacological interventions to treat behavioral disturbances in older patients with dementia. The SENATOR-OnTop series. *BMJ Open, 7*, e012759–e012759. https://doi.org/10.1136/bmjopen-2016-012759 (accessed on 16th July 2025).
2. Abramov, Y., Almeida, F. G., Berghmans, B., Bo, K., et al. (2016). An International Urogynecological Association (IUGA)/International Continence Society (ICS) joint report on the terminology for the conservative and nonpharmacological management of female pelvic floor dysfunction. https://core.ac.uk/download/293861075.pdf (accessed on 16th July 2025).
3. Agnetti, V., Aiello, E., De Natale, E., Deriu, F., et al. (2012). Effects of dance therapy on balance, gait and neuro-psychological performances in patients with Parkinson's disease and postural instability. https://core.ac.uk/download/16749566.pdf (accessed on 16th July 2025).
4. Akyol, M. U., Alden, T. D., Amartino, H., Ashworth, J., et al. (2019). Recommendations for the management of MPS VI: Systematic evidence- and consensus-based guidance. https://core.ac.uk/download/323074857.pdf (accessed on 16th July 2025).
5. Al Mutawa, A., Andriotis, P., Backes, M., Barghouthy, N., Chung, H., Do, Q., Enck, R., et al. (2015). Conceptual evidence collection and analysis methodology for Android devices. http://arxiv.org/abs/1506.05527 (accessed on 16th July 2025).
6. American Psychological Association, & Melchert, T. P. (2018). Professional practice guidelines for occupationally mandated psychological evaluations. https://core.ac.uk/download/231843503.pdf (accessed on 16th July 2025).
7. Ardakani, E. M., Beynon, A. M., Losco, B., Théroux, J., et al. (2022). Exploring 1st- and 2nd-year chiropractic students' willingness and attitudes toward peer physical examination. https://core.ac.uk/download/543488072.pdf (accessed on 16th July 2025).
8. Assaad, S., Friedman, M. B., Kratzert, W. B., Perrino, A. C., et al. (2018). Assessment of pulmonary edema: Principles and practice. https://core.ac.uk/download/145643671.pdf (accessed on 16th July 2025).
9. Barnes, H., Bateson, A., Boyd, J., Bunn, F., Campbell, S., Coiera, E., et al. (2014). The impact of using computer decision-support software in primary care nurse-led telephone triage: Interactional dilemmas and conversational consequences. https://core.ac.uk/download/29111138.pdf (accessed on 16th July 2025).
10. Biggins, S. W., Angeli, P., García-Tsao, G., Ginès, P., Ling, S. C., Nadim, M. K., Wong, F., et al. (2021). Diagnosis, evaluation, and management of ascites, spontaneous bacterial peritonitis and hepatorenal syndrome: 2021 practice guidance by the American Association for the Study of Liver Diseases. *Hepatology, 74*, 1014–1048. https://doi.org/10.1002/hep.31884 (accessed on 16th July 2025).
11. Bivens, K. M. (2025). A history of rhetoric, sound, and health and healing. https://core.ac.uk/download/637931273.pdf (accessed on 16th July 2025).
12. Bowers, R., Ross, K., & ISPO (Funder). (2009). A review of the effectiveness of lower limb orthoses used in cerebral palsy. https://core.ac.uk/download/9024488.pdf (accessed on 16th July 2025).

13. Brembo, E. A., Byermoen, K. R., Egilsdottir, H. Ö., Eide, H., et al. (2023). Factors associated with changes in students' self-reported nursing competence after clinical rotations: A quantitative cohort study. https://core.ac.uk/download/646135988.pdf (accessed on 16th July 2025).
14. Buscher, M., Callon, M., Gardner, J., Goodwin, D., Henke, C. R., Jutel, A. G., Keating, P., et al. (2015). Corporal diagnostic work and diagnostic spaces: Clinicians' use of space and bodies during diagnosis. https://core.ac.uk/download/29140424.pdf (accessed on 16th July 2025).
15. Campbell, L. (2014). "MacGyver-meets-Dr. Ruth": Science journalism and the material positioning of Dr. Carla Pugh. https://core.ac.uk/download/213068873.pdf (accessed on 16th July 2025).
16. Campbell, M. (2013). Staff training and challenging behavior: Who needs it? https://core.ac.uk/download/9821909.pdf (accessed on 16th July 2025).
17. Canha, J., Castela, E., Dinis, A., Martins, A., et al. (2008). Innocent heart murmurs. https://core.ac.uk/download/61497247.pdf (accessed on 16th July 2025).
18. Cartocci, G., Fineschi, V., Frati, P., Guglielmi, G., et al. (2017). The choice of gadolinium-based contrast agents: A radiologist's responsibility between pharmaceutical equivalence and bioethical issues. https://core.ac.uk/download/153367327.pdf (accessed on 16th July 2025).
19. Chmela, O. (2015). Different imaging techniques for investigation of treatment effects on various substrate surfaces. https://core.ac.uk/download/30277444.pdf (accessed on 16th July 2025).
20. Cruz, J., Jácome, C., Marques, A., Oliveira, A., et al. (2015). Outcome measures for respiratory physiotherapy in cystic fibrosis–Challenges and advances. https://core.ac.uk/download/322424867.pdf (accessed on 16th July 2025).
21. Derese, A., Sutter, C., Ilgen, D., Jacobson, D., Pendleton, D., Widyandana, D., Edelson, D. C., et al. (2014). Managing the complexity of doing it all: An exploratory study on students' experiences when trained stepwise in conducting consultations. https://core.ac.uk/download/55843932.pdf (accessed on 16th July 2025).
22. Dunnington, J. A. (2017). Acoustical properties of amplified and unamplified stethoscopes when examining typical body sounds. https://core.ac.uk/download/236621129.pdf (accessed on 16th July 2025).
23. Edison, C. C. (2020). The design and application of a decision-making process for identification of critical curricular variables which affect optimal application of CAI in a baccalaureate school of nursing. https://core.ac.uk/download/344444036.pdf (accessed on 16th July 2025).
24. Elwyn, G., Fisher, E., Mishra, M. K., Rodriguez, H., et al. (2018). How do healthcare professionals working in accountable care organizations understand patient activation and engagement? Qualitative interviews across two time points. https://core.ac.uk/download/323081191.pdf (accessed on 16th July 2025).
25. Fiordelisi, A., Resti, M., Stinco, M., Trapani, G., et al. (2023). Update on fever of unknown origin in children: Focus on etiologies and clinical approach. https://core.ac.uk/download/610297807.pdf (accessed on 16th July 2025).
26. Fletcher, P. C., Schneider, M. A., & Snider, H. (2008). Mind over matter: A qualitative examination of the coping resources used by women with cancer. https://core.ac.uk/download/143689565.pdf (accessed on 16th July 2025).

27. Grace, S., & Vaughan, B. (2016). Perception of peer physical examination in two Australian osteopathy programs. https://core.ac.uk/download/77983046.pdf (accessed on 16th July 2025).

28. Hadraba, D., Jelen, K., Koucky, V., Lopot, F., et al. (2018). Functional lung examination in diagnostics of asthma and its phenotypes. https://core.ac.uk/download/322437794.pdf (accessed on 16th July 2025).

29. Höglund, K. (2007). Systolic ejection murmurs and the left ventricular outflow tract in boxer dogs. https://core.ac.uk/download/11695170.pdf (accessed on 16th July 2025).

30. Jaat, N., Kamaruddin, R., Khalid, A., Mohamed, N., et al. (2017). A document analysis of the visibility of sustainability in TVE teacher education programmed: The case of a Malaysian HEI. https://core.ac.uk/download/19451574.pdf (accessed on 16th July 2025).

31. Katzman, W. B., & Pastore, E. A. (2012). Recognizing myofascial pelvic pain in the female patient with chronic pelvic pain. https://core.ac.uk/download/305124272.pdf (accessed on 16th July 2025).

32. Kendrick, A., & Taylor, J. (2000). Hidden on the ward: The abuse of children in hospitals. https://core.ac.uk/download/9015509.pdf (accessed on 16th July 2025).

33. Khomazyuk, T. (2019). Propaedeutics of internal medicine. Collection of clinical lectures: The educational and visual guide: In two parts. Part 1. https://core.ac.uk/download/346618368.pdf (accessed on 16th July 2025).

34. Kitsiou, A., Caforio, A. L. P., Porta-Sanchez, A., Vahanian, A., Iung, B., Carrera, C., Szymanski, C., et al. (2013). ESC core curriculum for the general cardiologist (2013). https://core.ac.uk/download/55756305.pdf (accessed on 16th July 2025).

35. Kotze, K. (2019). The pairing of trigger points dry needling with rehabilitation techniques. https://core.ac.uk/download/213463742.pdf (accessed on 16th July 2025).

36. Leamon, A. E. (2016). The electronic health record scorecard: A measure of utilization and communication skills. https://core.ac.uk/download/79664897.pdf (accessed on 16th July 2025).

37. Manigold, R. (2019). ACR accreditation for Utah Valley Hospital's radiation oncology center. https://digitalscholarship.unlv.edu/cgi/viewcontent.cgi?article=4649&context=thesesdissertations (accessed on 16th July 2025).

38. McClave, L. M. (2015). RN-BSN program: On-demand, online, competency-based modules. https://core.ac.uk/download/217256941.pdf (accessed on 16th July 2025).

39. Meijer, E. H., & Verschuere, B. (2014). What's on your mind? Recent advances in memory detection using the concealed information test. https://core.ac.uk/download/55798501.pdf (accessed on 16th July 2025).

40. N/A. (2020). *Optics in Our Time*. https://core.ac.uk/download/478097922.pdf (accessed on 16th July 2025).

41. N/A. (2025). *Aerospace Medicine and Biology: A Continuing Bibliography with Indexes, Supplement 165, March 1977*. https://core.ac.uk/download/pdf/42879072.pdf (accessed on 16th July 2025).

42. N/A. (2025). *Aerospace Medicine and Biology: A Continuing Bibliography with Indexes, Supplement 144*. https://core.ac.uk/download/pdf/42887122.pdf (accessed on 16th July 2025).

43. Pace, O. (2012). Complementary and alternative medicine: Facts and figures (Part I). https://core.ac.uk/download/46603042.pdf (accessed on 16th July 2025).
44. Reimer, N., & Shelton, A. (2018). Telehealth wound applications: Barriers, solutions, and future use by nurse practitioners. https://core.ac.uk/download/228066223.pdf (accessed on 16th July 2025).
45. Steerforth, D., & Van Winden, S. C. L. (2018). Development of clinical sign-based scoring system for assessment of omphalitis in neonatal calves. https://core.ac.uk/download/151393668.pdf (accessed on 16th July 2025).
46. Tordoff, A., & Williams, L. A. (2018). Community-acquired pneumonia in adults: Diagnostic reliability of physical examination techniques and their teaching in academia. https://core.ac.uk/download/214175121.pdf (accessed on 16th July 2025).
47. Vella Baldacchino, A., & Vella, C. (2012). Hip arthroplasty. https://core.ac.uk/download/46603939.pdf (accessed on 16th July 2025).
48. Virginia Commonwealth University. (2018). *Virginia Commonwealth University Professional Bulletin*. https://core.ac.uk/download/215485746.pdf (accessed on 16th July 2025).

GENERAL HEALTH SURVEY AND VITAL SIGNS IN NURSING

5

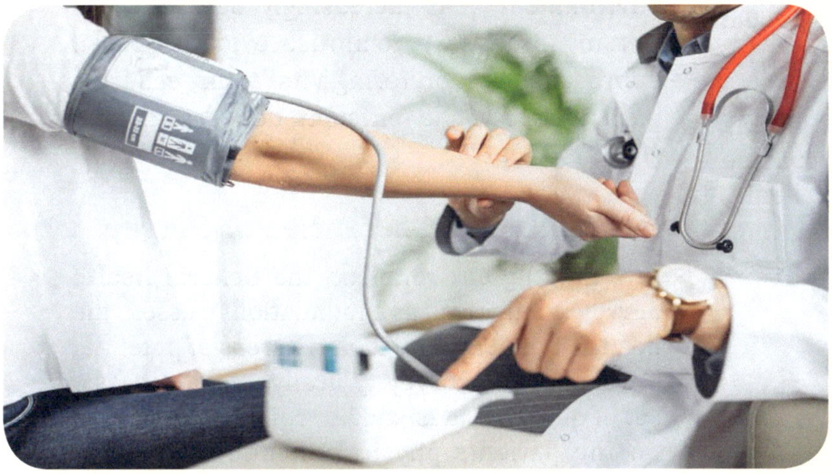

LEARNING OBJECTIVES

After studying this chapter, you will be able to:

1. Identify the purpose of the general health survey;
2. Describe the components of the general health survey;
3. Detailed understanding vital signs;
4. Explain the techniques for measuring vital signs;
5. Explore the interpretation of vital signs;
6. Define the role of nursing in health surveys and vital signs.

Introduction

In medical care, punctuality and reliability of monitoring vital signs are crucial elements of effective nursing practice. Temperature, pulse, respiratory rate, and blood pressure are some of the vital signs that are crucial indicators of a patient's health status. Nurses stand in the middle of monitoring these signs because they play a central role in availing baseline information that influences clinical decision-making. However, monitoring techniques for vital signs have, in the past, relied on expert opinion without empirical support, leading to heterogeneity in practice within clinical settings. This incongruity can lead to misinterpretation of an early indicator of patient deterioration or unnecessary consumption of resources, thus making the introduction of evidence-based, but adaptable, protocols that are tailored to individual patient needs, hence enhancing quality of care within nursing institutions, an imperative. In order to more fully appreciate the complexity of monitoring vital signs, it is important to more comprehensively understand the overall context of the general health survey. Surveys obtain demographic information, health status, and availability of care in order to assist in the direction of public health efforts and to improve patient care planning. For instance, a recent article emphasized the frustration expressed by parents and pediatricians alike regarding currently existing wired vital signs monitoring in neonatal intensive care settings. The research found that more than half of the parents complained that wired systems hindered skin-to-skin care and total bonding, substantiating the necessity for creative solutions that balance patient comfort with precise monitoring (Senechal et al., 2025). Thus, assessment of current practices, coupled with findings obtained from general health questionnaires, may guide the creation of more efficient monitoring protocols to cater to different patients' needs.

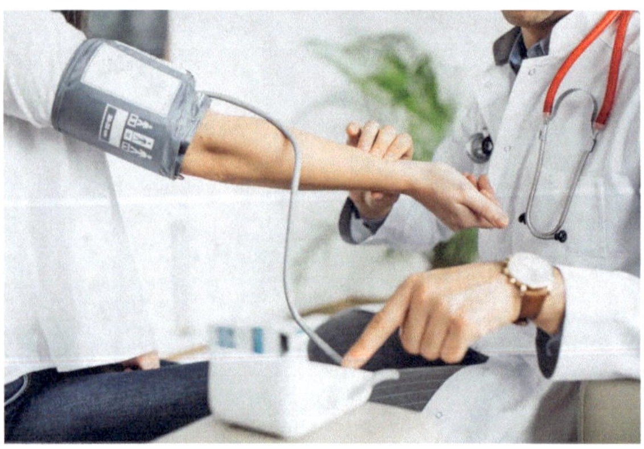

Figure 5.1. General health survey and vital signs in nursing.

Source: https://health-e.in/wp-content/uploads/2023/03/7-Vital-Signs-to-Monitor-Regularly.webp.

Moreover, equilibrium of the level of observation that is enough but not more than necessary can create an optimized climate for healthcare. Current literature reports that vital sign monitoring in most instances happens more often than necessary for stable patients and may divert important nursing resources (Briggs et al., 2024). Accordingly, guidelines that connect observation frequency with patient risk stratification need to be established in order to enhance patient outcomes overall without compromising quality care. By employing the National Early Warning Score system, nursing policy can be tailored to discriminate between high- and low-risk patients, thereby optimizing the allocation of nursing time and resources. With ongoing revolution in the healthcare environment, it is increasingly necessary for nursing practice to embrace evidence-based approaches to monitoring vital signs, ensuring patient safety and efficient delivery of care (Figure 5.1).

Definition of General Health Survey

In a nursing environment, the General Health Survey is employed as a foundation to assess the health of patients and identify areas of potential problems. The survey typically encompasses a set of questions designed to collect information on the patients physical, mental, and social welfare. By getting an entire picture of a patient's condition, the General Health Survey allows the identification of risk factors, chronic conditions, and other determinants of health deserving of examination or treatment. Additionally, it is a vehicle through which important vitals can be put into a larger picture of health. As healthcare providers strive to deliver comprehensive care, incorporation of such surveys into routine assessments is increasingly being seen as critical to informing successful nursing practices and interventions, ultimately enhancing patient outcomes and easing greater health management practices (Stoutenberg et al., 2017). The utility of the General Health Survey is also improved when administered alongside assessment of vital signs. Vital signs—biologic indicators of physiological function—are included among them and include recordings of heart rate, blood pressure, respiratory rate, and temperature. They are essential in the clinical setting since they provide immediate information regarding a patients current health status and direct impact on immediate care needs decisions. When General Health Survey data are compared with vital signs, nurse practitioners can further understand underlying disease states or emerging complications. This blend of objective and subjective data creates a solid basis for assessment of patients, promoting evidence-based practice in care that can adapt to the subtlety of individual health needs. Proper use of both vital signs and the survey thus promotes not just timely intervention, but also the development of customized health management plans (Stephen et al., 2016). In practice, the General Health Survey and the vital signs overall are a dynamic nursing assessment duo that fosters an understanding among patients and health care providers. The survey enables patients to voice their health problems and health aspirations, thereby establishing a teamwork-based care environment. If heard and interpreted, the extent of patient involvement in health care is likely to enhance, with enhanced compliance with health care plans and preventive interventions. This combined evaluation approach also can identify health behavior trends that may need greater education or intervention. With better patient-provider communication and a fuller picture of a patient's health status, nurses are better positioned to be advocates for their patients' needs and values. Through this, the General Health Survey, together with vital signs, is a vital component of enhancing quality nursing care and adopting a patient-centered healthcare model (Stoutenberg et al., 2017).

Importance of Vital Signs in Nursing

In nursing practice, accurate measurement of vital signs is a critical element of healthcare effectiveness as well as patient safety. The body's usual physiological processes, the vital signs, are temperature, pulse, respiration, and blood pressure. Keeping them under observation from time to time enables nurses to identify any possible health issue early, thereby preventing complications through early interventions. For example, a sudden rise in temperature will indicate infection, whereas pulse or blood pressure variations will portend deteriorating condition of a patient. With a numeric account of the state of health of a patient, essential signs are extremely helpful in clinical decision-making and constitute basic components of a general health examination. Therefore, nurses must be properly trained to take and interpret vital signs because the latter is directly associated with improved patient outcomes and quality of care in general. Additionally, vital signs serve as important indicators for determining treatment regimen effectiveness. In many cases, medical practitioners implement specific interventions—such as medication or lifestyle adjustment—that can have an effect on a patient's vital statistics. Repetition of these signs is being constantly observed to check whether the therapeutic aims are being met. For instance, if an individual is under antihypertensive medication, repeated measurement of blood pressure is done to measure their effectiveness. Additionally, as cited in recent health publications, there is a need to keep a comprehensive understanding of body wellness, considering the fact that an estimated 80% of US adults and adolescents are insufficiently active, affecting further their own health status (Katrina et al., 2018). Therefore, ongoing vigilance in tracking key indicators allows nurses to make quick alterations of care plans, ensuring maximum patient handling throughout the treatment process. The use of technology in nursing interventions has also propelled the importance of monitoring vital signs. Advanced medical equipment and electronic health records (EHRs) provide means of easily gathering and evaluating the vital statistics, enabling nurses to act quickly on changes in a patient's status. For example, electronic blood pressure cuffs and pulse oximeters are now routine equipment, allowing rapid and accurate readings. Furthermore, EHRs can provide alerts automatically, informing medical personnel of important changes in vital signs, which need to be addressed urgently. As such, this convergence of technology, nursing, and patient care best represents a contemporary health system where proactive monitoring has direct bearing on enhanced clinical decision-making and patient safety. As delineated in clinician well-being literature, it is increasingly important that healthcare facilities prioritize systems and processes for ensuring continuous monitoring of important signs in patient encounters (Charlene et al., 2020). Ultimately, these technologies emphasize that vital signs are not merely numbers; they are an integral part of understanding a patient's trajectory of health and making nursing decisions (Figure 5.2).

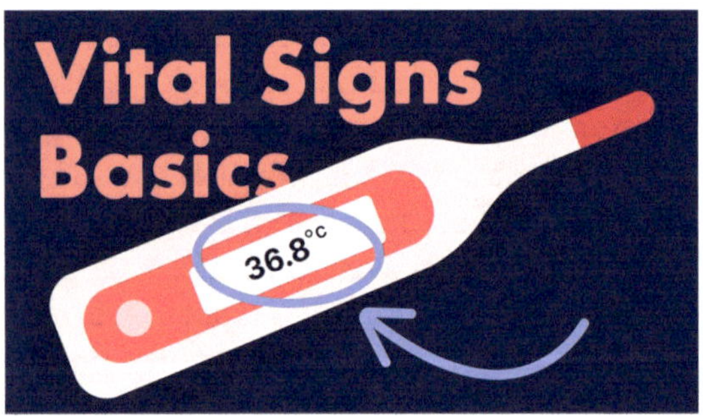

Figure 5.2. Vital signs in nursing.

Source: https://ausmed-images.s3.ap-southeast-2.amazonaws.com/ausmed.com/ausmed-articles/20190912_cover_V2.jpg.

5.1. Purpose of the General Health Survey

Learning Outcome

1. Assessing patient health status;
2. Identifying risk factors;
3. Establishing baseline data.

General Health Survey is a central tool in the practice of nursing that provides essential information for both healthcare decision-making and policy health. By systematic collection of data related to health among different populations, the survey facilitates healthcare providers to establish the health status, needs, and risk factors of various populations. Importantly, its application allows designated healthcare interventions aimed at optimizing individual and population health effects. Also, by integrating data on vital signs, the survey enables nurses to identify significant trends that may be an early indication of emerging health crises or issues requiring immediate attention. In return, the General Health Survey demonstrates a preventive approach to health care, emphasizing prevention and early intervention, thereby leading to improved patient outcomes and satisfaction. In addition to supplying patient care on an individual basis with information, the General Health Survey assists in reacting to broader health system problems. The information gathered through the survey can be employed for epidemiological analysis, monitoring trends in chronic conditions, and assessing the effectiveness of public health measures. For instance, outcomes of typical omitted nursing care items, such as observation of vital signs and emotional support, can have a direct impact on nursing practices and resource consumption in healthcare. As has been shown by recent studies, the relationship between nurses' mental well-being and omitted care highlights systematic support in healthcare facilities as a primary concern (Jeong et al., 2023). When nurses are in a better position to manage their workload and mental health, patient care is also significantly improved, as this indicates the broader implications of the survey findings. Further, technological development has altered the scope of operations and efficiency of the General Health Survey. With the integration of wearable devices and remote monitoring technology, medical information can be collected in real-time, enhancing timeliness and accuracy of patient assessment (Kseniia et al., 2023). These advanced technologies facilitate

24-hour monitoring of vital signs, allowing for timely clinical intervention in accordance with patient condition changes. In particular, the incorporation of interactive questionnaires and mobile applications motivates increased patient engagement and adherence to treatment plans by engaging them actively in self-care. As healthcare continues to evolve, understanding the intention and worth of the General Health Survey is imperative in ongoing nursing practice development, formation of a culture of anticipatory care, and, ultimately, enhanced health outcomes at multiple levels (Figure 5.3).

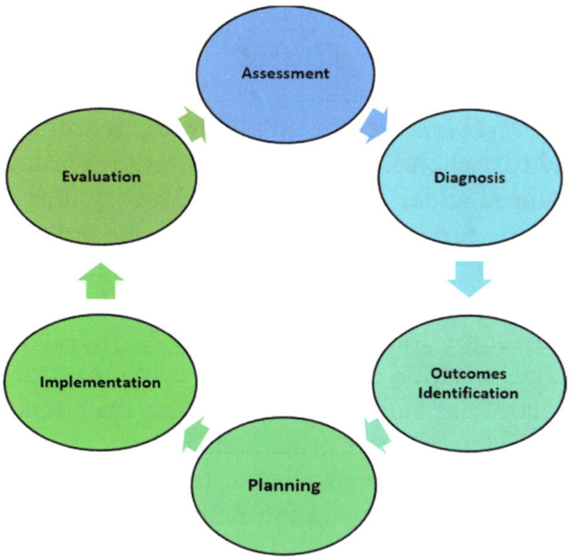

Figure 5.3. Purpose of the general health survey.

Source: https://wtcs.pressbooks.pub/app/uploads/sites/29/2020/08/unnamed-1.png.

5.1.1. Assessing Patient Health Status

The holistic process of assessment of patient health status is a significant aspect of nursing practice and the foundation of effective delivery of care and clinical decision-making. The process usually begins with obtaining subjective data, including the patient's own description of health occurrence, symptoms, and lifestyle. By questioning the patients about their medical history and their specific complaints, nurses can gain useful information that directs their knowledge of the patient's individual situation. Furthermore, combining objective data, such as vital signs including blood pressure, heart rate, and temperature, with subjective findings offers empirical evidence for the measurement of health status. Therefore, the combination of subjective and objective data improves the validity of measurements of health status, guiding nurses in creating effective interventions that respond to the demands and expectations of patients. During recent years, the use of systematic methods such as triage has gained more attention among nursing professionals, particularly in emergency and acute care departments. The triage system is developed to prioritize patients based on the severity of their illness in order to enable healthcare professionals to use resources effectively in stressful situations. Research has shown that, even though Indonesia has established a triage system, its implementation is still uneven compared to worldwide standards and is typically incomplete without obligatory frameworks such as re-triage and sound analysis of primary and secondary processes. As has been indicated by contemporary research, the strengthening of these triage processes is essential to advancing the effectiveness of patient management and reducing waiting times in health centers. Thus, the enhancement of the triage process will not only enhance the quality of patient care but is also essential to advancing the professionalization of nurses in policy-making and emergency response measures (Morphet et al., 2016). Educational activities aiming to enhance the competence of medical providers in the assessment of the state of health are equally critical in this domain. Existing evidence highlights the need for interprofessional learning that equips professionals from various professions, including medicine, nursing, and pharmacy, with necessary knowledge and skills for the comprehensive assessment of patients. For instance, a field study involving medical students demonstrated there to be significant improvements in their confidence level, attitudes, and clinical skill after they were taught specially structured curricula regarding children's oral health. The findings indicated there to be a positive correlation between enhanced knowledge and clinical skill, highlighting the critical significance of structured training towards attaining competence in patient examination. These educational programs not just make the next providers equipped to fill individualized health requirements efficiently, for example, children's oral health care, but also make the healthcare environment more collaborative, which impacts patient outcomes immensely in the end (Niranjan et al., 2020) (Figure 5.4).

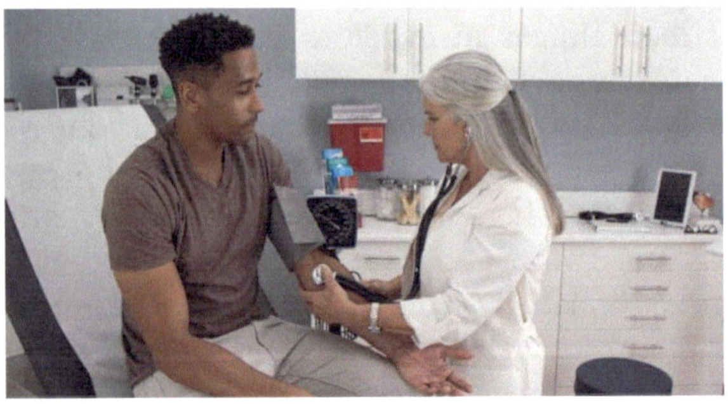

Figure 5.4. Assessing patient health status.

Source: https://patientbetter.com/wp-content/uploads/2024/05/health-status-768x402.jpg.

5.1.2. Identifying Risk Factors

It is essential to recognize risk factors in the nursing environment in order to enhance patient outcomes as well as avoid harm. Risk factors may be viewed within various domains, including biological, behavior, and environmental determinants. Biologically, the health status of a patient may be greatly affected by factors such as age, sex, and comorbidities. Behaviorally, smoking, physical inactivity, and poor diet similarly play a strong role in chronic disease risk. Such are the complexities that necessitate an integral general health evaluation that enables nurses to evaluate patients holistically, thereby informing targeted interventions that directly manage implicated risks. The significance of ascertaining such factors justifies the nursing contribution to preventive medicine and chronic disease management, emphasizing an anticipatory as opposed to a reactive approach in the clinical setting. Aside from that, accurate identification of the risk factors is at the heart of monitoring vital signs, which are also ultimate predictors of health status. Abnormal or elevated vital signs have a tendency to mirror the underlying influence of these risk factors, guiding clinical judgment in patient assessment. For instance, fever and tachycardia in post-operative patients may denote surgical site infection, a complication of several risk factors entailing wound dressing and care choice. According to current literature, nuanced understanding about such correlations allows for early intervention by nurses, reduction of morbidity, and maximization of recovery periods. Effective measurement of vital signs linked to risk factors, therefore, makes a critical contribution to evidence-based practice decisions, which underpins the nursing professions key role in maintaining patient safety and quality care provision. Interprofessional working also improves the ability to identify and address risk factors effectively. Interdisciplinary approaches leverage team members' different knowledge, which provides improved accuracy and information to health assessment. For instance, organizations such as the National Board of Certification and Recertification for Nurse Anesthetists undertake projects with an emphasis on simulation training to avoid the identification of what clinical practices practitioners require to re-enter practice. The consensus reached through such collaborative effort not only validates significant risk indicators but also stimulates continued enhancement of clinical assessment methodologies. Through the facilitation of team-based approaches anchored in sound risk factor identification, health care settings are better able to foresee patient needs and promote overall outcomes in practice environments (Figure 5.5).

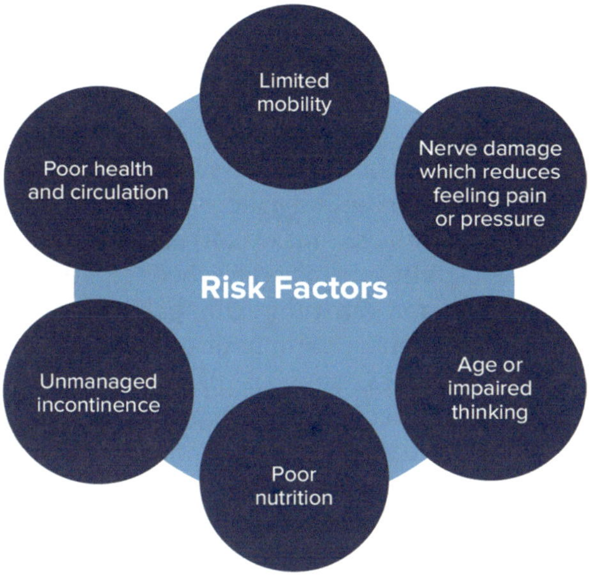
Limited mobility
Poor health and circulation
Nerve damage which reduces feeling pain or pressure
Risk Factors
Unmanaged incontinence
Age or impaired thinking
Poor nutrition

Figure 5.5. Identifying risk factors within the nursing.

Source: https://external-content.duckduckgo.com/iu/?u=https%3A%2F%2Fwww.activehealthcare.co.nz%2Fwp-content%2Fuploads%2F2023%2F06%2FACT0293-Aged-Care-LinkedIn-Image-Risk-factors-v2-1024x1024.png&f=1&nofb=1&ipt=09e139625a7cb877d82b645f59b7b2db415cadab687e813ed367258a3a7905ec.

5.1.3. Establishing Baseline Data

In nursing practice, baseline data establishment is an integral part of the health assessment and a point of reference against which future changes in health are compared. Baseline data offer an integrated picture of a person's health status before interventions or treatment take place. Through systematic gathering of baseline information such as vital signs, medical history, and lifestyle, nurses are able to see what current health problems and areas for monitoring or intervention exist. This initial information is necessary not just for individual patient care, but also for aggregating health data on a more population-based public health level, thereby making possible trend identification and resource planning. Lastly, good baseline data collection informs immediate nursing practice and future strategic healthcare planning. To set baseline data effectively, the application of standard tools and techniques is essential. Implementation of technologies like remote monitoring systems can significantly help make processes related to data gathering reliability and timeliness more efficient. For instance, projects like the Health Buddy Patient Telemonitoring Program that was showcased by Cook County Health and Hospitals illustrate how technology is important in gathering the information on health in real time.

These advanced systems not only allow the effective tracking of life-critical indicators but also facilitate the immediate follow-up of patients who have shown any concerning patterns. Since baseline data is richer and more intricate, it also provides opportunities for personalized healthcare practices adapted to the needs of individual patients. In considering the relevance of baseline data in nursing, it is inherent to note its place within evidence-based practice and continuous quality improvement. In delineating a firm foundation of data, practitioners are able to tackle outcome measurement and apply findings to enhance patient care methods. Further, ongoing testing of clinical practice, such as in research involving simulation for nurse anesthetists, helps to legitimate the real-world relevance of baselines drawn from clinical practice (Heyes et al., 2018). The ongoing process of data collection and evaluation helps nurses with evidence-based decision-making about patient care, so that the method is not merely reactive but proactive in disease prevention and improving health. In so doing, the practice will continue to evolve, developing environments that prioritize quality care and patient safety.

Test Your Knowledge

1. Why is conducting a general health survey important in establishing a patient's baseline health status?
2. How does a general health survey help in identifying potential health risks and planning care?

5.2. Components of the General Health Survey

Learning Outcome

1. Patient history and demographics;
2. Review of systems;
3. Physical examination.

The General Health Survey is an essential element of nursing practice because it is a needed guide for the gathering of comprehensive information regarding patient health. Its primary purpose is to ascertain various areas of health like the medical history of the patient, medications, and way of life. These all present a full picture of the patient, which enables the nurses to understand the patient's health more vividly and identify any existing or possible health problems. A thorough health survey is particularly important in nursing since it constitutes the basis of effective care planning and intervention. Moreover, the general health survey encourages a multidisciplinary approach that enables nurse-patient communication, which lies at the core of developing a trustworthy therapeutic relationship. Furthermore, the data gathered from the survey comes a significant way in encouraging a patient-centered care model, enhancing overall patient outcomes as well as satisfaction. During the conduct of a General Health Survey, certain elements take precedence for successful data gathering. Basic vital signs such as temperature, pulse, respiratory rate, and blood pressure are essential barometers of a patient's health status and physiological well-being. They offer live data that can pinpoint important shifts in a patient's status, prompting immediate intervention where required. Also, assessing body mass index (BMI) and nutritional status is significant since these bear significant implications for general health, particularly in the management of chronic diseases. Patients' health behaviors, such as physical activity, smoking, or alcohol consumption, can also direct health education and promotion, which are essential aspects of nursing practice. These elements, when made part of the General Health Survey, allow nurses to formulate personalized care plans addressing some of the patient's needs and health problems. In addition, the General Health Survey must integrate psychosocial and environmental factors influencing the patients' health. Questions regarding family history, social support networks, and mental state can uncover underlying influences that can affect the patient's well-being. Recognizing these factors not only allows for the evaluation but also reveals the possibilities of interventions that promote physical and emotional health. As a case in point, understanding the environmental condition in which a patient lives can help in recognizing possible treatment obstacles and adherence. Secondly, integrating patient education with the survey process can enhance health literacy, and patients become empowered with knowledge that they require in order to manage their health effectively. It is therefore the General Health Survey that becomes a valuable tool in nursing, weaving elements of physical, psychological, and social well-being to formulate a complete picture of the patients' needs and fostering an anticipatory approach to nursing care (Figure 5.6).

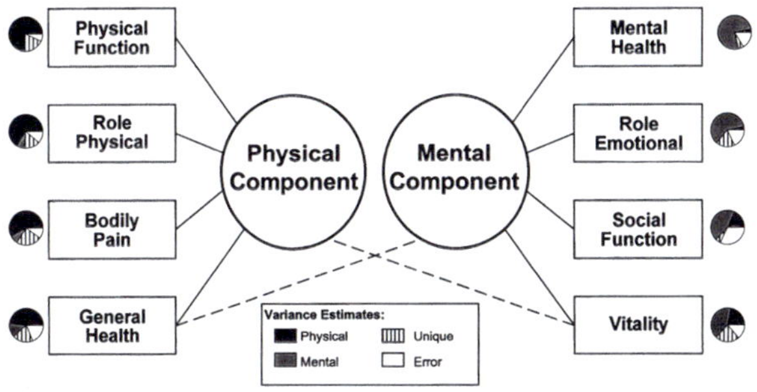

Figure 5.6. Components of the general health survey.

Source: https://www.researchgate.net/publication/248320488/figure/fig2/AS:888553068310531@1588858968514/SF-36-scales-measure-physical-and-mental-components-of-health-Source-Ware-Kosinski.ppm.

5.2.1. Patient History and Demographics

Patient demographics and patient history are significant in the case of nursing, particularly when conducting general health questionnaires and monitoring vital signs. Patient demographics, including gender, age, and medical history, are major predictors of health outcomes and can have a broad impact on nursing care plans. Physiological changes by way of aging, for instance, may dictate shifts in vital sign standards, necessitating specific assessment based on individual patient profiles. Further, demographic factors can impact the transmission of certain health conditions. An appreciation of such factors, therefore, enables nurses to offer more effective and personalized care regimes based on the personal history and context of their patients, thereby enhancing the quality of healthcare delivery. Further, a patient's history of past events can reflect habits of comorbidities that are essential in formulating and managing health conditions. For example, understanding past illnesses such as hypertension or diabetes can both influence the urgency and type of interventions that a nurse may employ during health screenings. In one cross-sectional study of nurses' understanding of COVID-19 management, it was observed that healthcare workers' education and experience have significant effects on their attitude towards infection control (Ali et al., 2025). These findings identify the importance of nurse education that involves the use of patient demographic information, as a key element, in preparing for healthcare crises. Accordingly, comprehensive knowledge of patient history becomes crucial for nurses to deliver the best possible care and to facilitate successful interventions in dynamic healthcare settings.

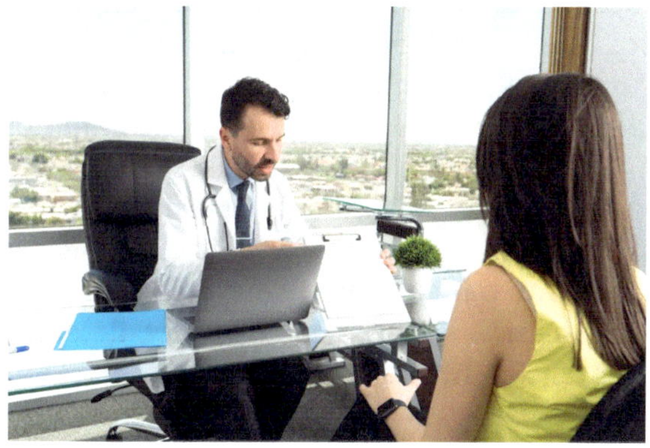

Figure 5.7. Patient history and demographics.

Source: https://www.imagnumhealthcare.com/img/content/patient-demographic-entry-services-content.webp.

Successful collection of patient history can also enhance the validity of vital sign monitoring and overall health checks. As a case in patient data analyses, awareness of the relationship between demographic data and clinical outcomes can lead to enhanced prevention and intervention approaches. For instance, fall risk analyses for postoperative patients indicate that age, history of previous falls, and medication consumption have been key in the direction of clinical practices (Chen et al., 2025). By incorporating demographic data into regular assessments, nurses can more effectively recognize risk populations, thus preemptively instituting preventive measures to decrease negative outcomes. Ultimately, the integration of patient history and demographics not only informs clinical decision-making but also facilitates a comprehensive approach to nursing care that prioritizes patient well-being and safety (Figure 5.7).

5.2.2. Review of Systems

The Review of Systems (ROS) is part of the overall assessment of general health and a core element of nursing evaluations. Its systemic process allows caregivers to gain expansive data about the body systems of patients, emphasizing potential areas of concern not readily apparent with a physical examination. Through the review of various systems (i.e., cardiovascular, respiratory, neurological, and gastrointestinal), nurses are able to emphasize integrative patient care. This comprehensive assessment not only enables early detection of potential health concerns, but also aids in clinical decision making. It is through a systematic ROS that helps in the creation of accurate patient histories, which are pivotal in determining effective care plans formulated around the individual's special needs and concerns that are emphasized through holistic nursing practices. Telehealth has grown more relevant in the process of augmenting the Review of Systems process, particularly with the advent of recent technological advancements and the ongoing impacts of the COVID-19 pandemic. As healthcare providers initiated remote sites, the ROS had to be adjusted to accommodate remote evaluations without being less rigorous and accurate. The shift also introduced solitary challenges, like the necessity to present effective communication to garner expansive feedback from patients who may be unwilling to share personal health information in a virtual environment. Insights by Susie et al. (2020) showcase the ongoing evolution of telehealth practice and its relevance in specialties, further highlighting the need for nurses to alter their assessment measures in concert with the changes in healthcare delivery. Using digital technology ensures a high priority always given to patient care and safety even when physically remote. Additionally, integrating the Review of Systems into routine nursing screenings closely aligns with upcoming trends in patient-centered models of care. Patient involvement in the ROS process promotes a sense of belonging and ownership in health decision-making, a foundational factor in adherence to treatment guidelines. Nurses have a central role to play in facilitating this discussion, ensuring patients value the relevance of system-specific questions to their overall health state. Through open-ended questioning and active listening, healthcare practitioners are able to elicit information with subtle differences that can be extremely useful therapeutically. Thus, as practice and education in nursing embrace the practice of patient-centered care, the ROS remains a vital tool in empowering patients and optimizing health outcomes, consistent with evidence reported by Charlene et al. (2020) (Figure 5.8).

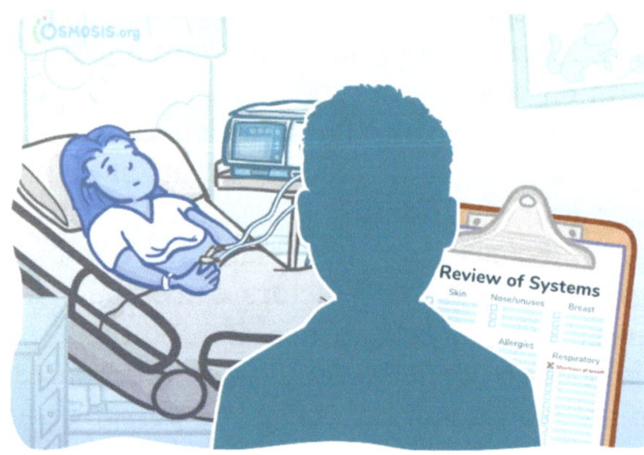

Figure 5.8. The review of systems (ROS).

Source: https://www.osmosis.org/blog/wp-content/uploads/sites/2/2024/08/78.png.

5.2.3. Physical Examination

Physical examination is an integral component of overall health screening in nursing, providing valuable information regarding the overall state of patients' health. Through systematic evaluation procedures, nurses can identify abnormalities, monitor current health states, and evaluate the effectiveness of treatment measures. Physical exams consist of various assessments, including monitoring vital signs, which are fundamental indicators of physiological condition. These indications, such as heart rate, blood pressure, respiratory rate, and temperature, provide baseline data and alert healthcare professionals to potential health issues. In addition, regular physical monitoring and screenings have been found to influence the health behavior of nursing staff positively, as demonstrated in studies indicating greater probabilities of adopting routine health habits among staff members in health-promoting hospitals compared to staff members in non-health-promoting hospitals (Chen et al., 2023).

When performing a physical assessment, nurses are required to use a systematic process that involves observation, palpation, percussion, and auscultation. All these methods are necessary for obtaining comprehensive information regarding the physical condition of the patients. Observation includes scrutinizing the patients appearance, mobility, and attitude, which gives preliminary indications regarding their state of health. Palpation and percussion yield information about structures beneath, while auscultation allows the nurse to identify organ system function, particularly cardiovascular and respiratory systems.

Together, they present an entire picture of the patients state of health. Also, the importance of quality of life for health, particularly in middle-aged populations, shows how extensive assessment gives targeted nursing interventions in responses to physical and psychological determinants of wellness (Sohn et al., 2020). Incorporation of the findings of physical checks into a composite health questionnaire is required by the work of interprofessional health teams that enhances the quality of care for patients. Regular physical check-ups and health screenings can lead to early diagnosis of risk factors and chronic conditions that are treatable with proactive management and intervention strategies. For instance, adherence to cancer screening guidelines can be significantly higher among the nursing staff working in health-promoting environments, demonstrating how institutional culture could spur more positive health behaviors (Chen et al., 2023). The physical examination, therefore, not only turns into a diagnostic tool but advances the fringes of health promotion, thereby finding a place within the paradigms of nursing practice for advancing preventative care and integrated patient health management. The role of the nurse, therefore, exceeds immediate clinical assessment, including the broader picture of holistic health promotion in healthcare provision (Figure 5.9).

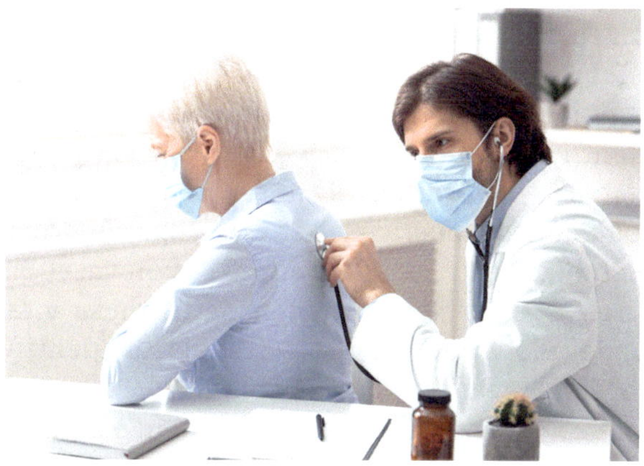

Figure 5.9. Physical examination.

Source: https://external-content.duckduckgo.com/iu/?u=https%3A%2F%2Fwww.doforms.com%2Fwp-content%2Fuploads%2F2020%2F10%2Fannual-physical-exam-checklist.jpg&f=1&nofb=1&ipt=390e0ce78b18a1994bd9463de144a7a2df81b72818aea7e803c2baf8e1888b90.

Test Your Knowledge

1. What key elements are typically assessed during a general health survey, and why is each significant?
2. How do observations of physical appearance, mobility, and behavior contribute to a comprehensive health survey?

5.3. Understanding Vital Signs

Learning Outcome

1. Definition and importance;
2. Key vital signs: Temperature, pulse, respiration, blood pressure;
3. Normal ranges and variations.

Vital signs are core measures of a patient's physiological status and are essential in the evaluation of overall health in nursing practice. These measures usually consist of body temperature, heart rate, respiratory rate, and blood pressure. All of these parameters offer individual information regarding the functioning of the body, allowing nurses to identify potential health problems early. For instance, a significantly increased heart rate could reflect underlying distress, while abnormal blood pressure could reflect cardiovascular disease. Continuous monitoring of these vital signs allows health professionals to identify baseline measurements, which makes it easier to recognize variations from a patient's optimal condition and thereby improve patient care outcomes.

Apart from that, identifying and interpreting the abnormalities assist nurses in introducing timely interventions, which in emergency situations where seconds make a difference could be vital. It requires not just capability but also understanding of how to interpret differences in the reading of vital signs to have a comprehensive understanding of them. Age, activity, and basic medical conditions could dramatically affect vital signs. For example, in conducting a health screen, a nurse will need to consider the ways that anxiety may influence the heart rate of a patient or fever raises the temperature of the body. This kind of background information is especially important when caring for populations with widely different baseline vital signs due to age or comorbid disease. Besides, continuing training and continuing professional development courses are essential, as they equip nurses with the up-to-date practices and technologies in vital sign monitoring, inculcating a culture of accuracy and precision in patient assessment. Additionally, the integration of triage procedures into nursing facilitates the effective management of patients' vital signs in high-traffic environments, such as emergency departments. Research has also indicated that effective triage protocols not only make patient management easier but also play an essential role in prioritizing the levels of medical priority according to the urgency reflected in vital signs (Morphet et al., 2016). In Indonesian hospitals, for example, the triage system is still immature; therefore, formalizing nurses' roles in policy formation is critical in promoting such systems. Second, this approach also involves working with families, particularly in pediatrics, where understanding a child's baseline and potentially challenging behaviors can assist in ensuring that their vital signs are properly interpreted within context (Johnson et al., 2013). Such collaborative approaches enhance the ability to provide relevant and timely care, ultimately providing improved patient outcomes (Figure 5.10).

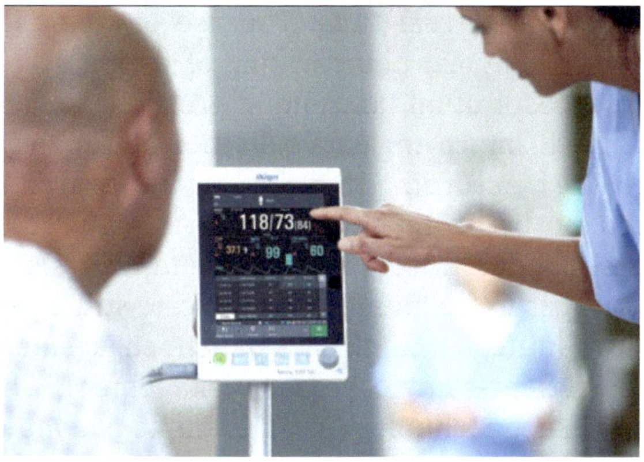

Figure 5.10. Understanding vital signs.

Source: https://external-content.duckduckgo.com/iu/?u=https%3A%2F%2Fcentersurgentcare.net%2Fwp-content%2Fuploads%2F2024%2F05%2FUnderstanding-Vital-Signs_-A-Comprehensive-Guide-from-Centers-Urgent-Care.png&f=1&nofb=1&ipt=bb4ec0d4b50514f43b8d060df20f48a86ec6d453ebbfd3d769c012fc8c07105b.

5.3.1. Definition and Importance

The principle of general health surveys is critical in nursing practice as it serves as a critical tool in assessing the overall condition of individuals' health and populations. The surveys are specifically designed to obtain extensive information on various health indicators, including behavioral, physical, and emotional factors that contribute to health outcomes. This information helps the nurses identify vulnerable populations and develop suitable interventions to promote healthier living. Besides, integrating health survey results into clinical practice encourages enhancing the ability to monitor health behavior trends and outcomes, resulting in quality nursing care effectiveness. With the passage of time as data are piled up, nurses can utilize this data to drive policy change and public programs that advocate for public health. The need for these comprehensive evaluations justifies their function in directing evidence-based nursing care plans aimed at meeting the diverse needs of patients (Stoutenberg et al., 2017). Vital signs are major constructing blocks of patient evaluations in nursing and are crucial indicators of physiological status. These measurable values—temperature, pulse, respiratory rate, and blood pressure—are direct measures of a patient's health and helps in the identification of possible complications in the process of care. Regular monitoring of the vital signs by nurses helps them establish baselines for patients, making it possible to identify deviations from normal that may be related to underlying health complications at an early stage. Regular monitoring of vital signs not only enhances patient safety but also helps enhance effective communication within healthcare teams. In this context, the addition of information from general health surveys can also further contribute towards the knowledge of a patient's health profile by associating vital signs with general trends in health and lifestyle. This holistic approach ultimately supports more focused and effective care planning to respond to individual patient needs (Stephen et al., 2016). This dialogue between general health questionnaires and vital signs underscores the importance of an integrated approach to nursing practice. The two complement each other to present a more comprehensive representation of a patient's wellbeing and health status, contributing to improved diagnosis and more tailored interventions. Health surveys can render risk factors such as inactivity and nutritional deficiencies visible, which can impact vital signs and overall state of health. For instance, identification of the correlation between physical activity and cardiovascular well-being, as underscored by relevant study literature, can guide nursing practice in encouraging patients toward lifestyle change. By integrating overall health data and technological physiological testing, nurses not only improve individual patient outcomes but also help guide broader public health initiatives that promote optimal community health. Therefore, integration of tools is imperative for nursing professionals who are dedicated to promoting health equity and maximizing health outcomes for populations with varying characteristics (Stoutenberg et al., 2017).

5.3.2. Key Vital Signs: Temperature, Pulse, Respiration, Blood Pressure

Monitoring critical vital signs—temperature, pulse, respirations, and blood pressure—is the basis of patient assessment and management in nursing practice. These readings provide significant information about a patients physiologic state and serve as early indicators of improvement or deterioration in health. For instance, changes in temperature may signal infection or the onset of inflammation, and changes in pulse rates may indicate cardiac disease or systemic distress. Accurate measurement and interpretation of these critical signs enable nurses to make informed decisions regarding intervention strategies and the need for further diagnostic testing, thereby enhancing patient outcomes through timely medical intervention. Respiratory rates also give important information about lung function and overall oxygenation status. An elevated respiratory rate may indicate hypoxia or distress and is a call to immediate attention and potentially intervention. Combined with pulse oximetry, the monitoring of oxygen saturation, clinicians can have a comprehensive view of the respiratory efficacy of a patient. Blood pressure, the second important parameter, helps in the monitoring of cardiovascular health. Fluctuations in blood pressure can alert nurses to impending complications, such as hypertensive emergency or shock, thereby guiding the direction of therapy that is paramount to patient stabilization and recovery. Advances in recent health technology have enabled the incorporation of artificial intelligence into monitoring devices for these critical signs. Artificial intelligence-based remote patient monitoring (RPM) systems, as reported in the literature, are transforming the manner in which nurses monitor and react to vital signs in real time. The use of wearable devices supports the tracking of temperature, pulse, respiration, and blood pressure around the clock, improving data collection and analysis accuracy. According to the latest health trends outlined by health innovations, AI can predict potential health setbacks via trend analysis of vital signs to facilitate preventive care strategies. These strategies emphasize patient engagement and patient-centric health management. The use of such technology is an example of a move towards increasingly dynamic nursing practice focused on early intervention and holistic patient care, which is essential in dealing with chronic diseases and enhancing general health outcomes (Patel et al., 2021; Shaik et al., 2023) (Figure 5.11).

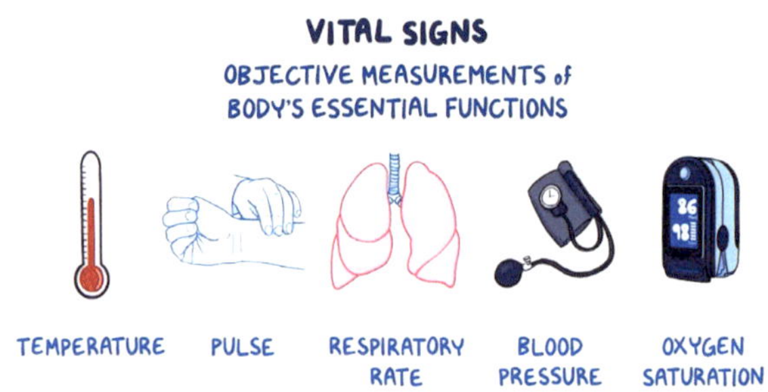

Figure 5.11. The assessment of key vital signs.

Source: https://external-content.duckduckgo.com/iu/?u=https%3A%2F%2Fosmose-it.s3.amazonaws.com%2FkSOCH_1HS6CEFndpPgtzkRoOSbe5N8OG%2F_.jpg&f=1&nofb=1&ipt=45cfc8a4f97acc70100fe8b78e98230bda01c0085122eaa2743fcb1f93c59f88.

5.3.3. Normal Ranges and Variations

In nursing and general health questionnaires, it is important to understand normal ranges and variation of vital signs in order to make a correct assessment and plan of care for the patient. The four vital signs that are utilized as valuable indicators of physiological status and health are body temperature, heart rate, respiratory rate, and blood pressure. Normal ranges will vary from individual to individual based on his or her age, sex, and overall health status. For instance, resting heart rate at 60 to 100 beats per minute is typical in adults, but the range can be expanded or contracted in specific populations, such as trained athletes or children. Knowledge of these variations is important for nurses so that they do not make erroneous interpretations that lead to inappropriate interventions or clinical errors (Karen et al., 2023). Thus, a sharp awareness of normative data provides nursing professionals the authority to identify anomalies in due time. Variations in vital signs are not exclusively physiological; extrinsic factors like environmental conditions, stress, or even cultural routines influence them as well. For example, blood pressure readings can be affected by the position of the patient at the time of measurement—sitting, standing, or recumbent may result in varying readings. Also, anxiety or distress may temporarily elevate heart and respiratory rates, and thus the readings of the vital signs collected may not accurately reflect the patient's baseline. Research has revealed that discrepancies in clinical coding, such as under-recording of Long COVID, influence detection of vital sign abnormality in some groups (Abbasizanjani et al., 2023). Therefore, it is of utmost importance that nursing professionals put vital sign measurements into the greater context of each patient's unique situation to offer a holistic and individualized care. Accurate interpretation of vital signs and understanding normal ranges of vital signs enable enhanced clinical judgment and patient safety. Further, deviation from the normative values necessitates further investigative studies in order to uncover subclinical illness or acute processes. For instance, enduring hypertension is a manifestation of cardiovascular risk, and persistent low body temperature may be a sign of hypothermia or systemic infection. Nurses play an integral role in monitoring, documenting, and reporting these changes in vital signs to interdisciplinary care teams. Appropriate use of telemedicine, as demonstrated in the recent evidence, demonstrates that quality care can be provided remotely without diminishing patient satisfaction or experience of empathy (Karen et al., 2023). This system not only attends to the immediate clinical needs but also focuses on the necessity for normal values and ranges in significant signs in order to promote enhanced overall patient outcomes and access.

Test Your Knowledge

1. What are the primary vital signs, and why are they considered essential indicators of health?
2. How can changes in vital signs reflect the onset or progression of disease?

5.4. Techniques for Measuring Vital Signs

Learning Outcome

1. Equipment used in vital sign measurement;
2. Proper techniques for accurate readings;
3. Common errors in measurement.

Accurate assessment of vital signs is critical in nursing practice, as it provides valuable information regarding a patient's physiological status. The parameters for the assessment of vital signs are typically the assessment of temperature, pulse, respiratory rate, and blood pressure. These measures serve as baseline data on health status and enable nurses to detect early warning signs of deterioration or improvement in a patient's condition. For instance, temperature measurement can identify febrile responses that are indicative of infection, while pulse rate can identify cardiovascular status. In addition, the vital signs need to be taken systematically and uniformly in order to ensure that any changes seen are because of true physiological changes and not due to variations in style of measurement. Employing overall strategies for precise and timely measurements enhances overall patient care and assists in developing a quality nursing diagnosis and course of action. Other than fundamental techniques, more advanced technologies are increasingly utilized to enhance the precision and efficiency of acquiring vital signs. Devices such as automatic blood pressure monitors, pulse oximeters, and digital thermometers have revolutionized nursing practice by reducing the level of human interaction and accelerating monitoring. These technologies enable continuous or remote monitoring that can be extremely useful in the management of critical care patients that require constant monitoring. Pulse oximetry is one such example, which provides instant oxygen saturation measurement and is priceless in assessing respiratory function.

The incorporation of such advanced equipment into clinical practice is a testament to their utility in maximizing patient benefits through timely intervention on the basis of vital sign data. These advances represent a step forward in tapping into technology-based tools to complement traditional nursing practices in the measurement of vital signs. Equally significant is the significance of healthcare personnel responsibility in the interpretation and response to changes in vital signs. Nurses must be highly qualified not just to take vital signs but also to critically analyze the data collected. They should have an understanding of normal values, the implications of deviations, and interventions in clinical practice to practice nursing effectively. Empirical evidence attests that attitudes of nurses towards monitoring vital signs are crucial in their performance when taking the parameters. For instance, research indicated the necessity of ongoing education to increase nurses' knowledge on ailments like neonatal sepsis, which underscores the significance of observing vital signs in determining early pathological alterations (Abdullah et al., 2019).

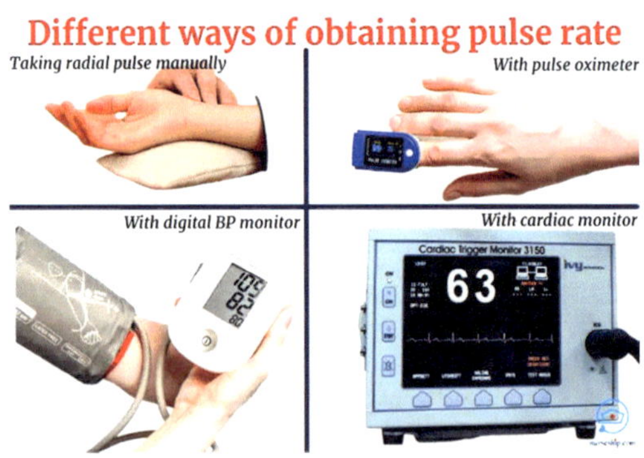

Figure 5.12. Techniques for measuring vital signs.

Source: https://external-content.duckduckgo.com/iu/?u=https%3A%2F%2Fnurseship.com%2Fwp-content%2Fuploads%2F2021%2F04%2FDifferent-ways-of-obtaining-pulse-rate-400x267.png&f=1&nofb=1&ipt=9995c8cf4fa92620db59c33295807f64159df92f9d6db91c45673507fd330c65.

As healthcare continues to evolve, the means of assessing vital signs also have to undergo changes in association with continuous professional development to guarantee high standards of patient care in nursing (Figure 5.12).

5.4.1. Equipment Used in Vital Sign Measurement

Measurement of vital signs is a central aspect of nursing practice predicated heavily on specialized equipment to determine accuracy and dependability. Key equipment includes sphygmomanometers for blood pressure measurement, thermometers to determine temperature, and stethoscopes to utilize in auscultation. The sphygmomanometer, with many instances supplemented by a digital display, provides medical professionals precise determinations of blood pressure, which are crucial in-patient assessment. Thermometers, in turn, both analog mercury ones and digital ones, assist nurses in measuring body temperature, which is essential for diagnosing fever or hypothermia. Stethoscopes, necessary for respiratory and cardiac examinations, enable nurses to hear heartbeats and lung sounds, making it possible to detect abnormalities in their early stages. The efficiency of such equipment underscores their utility in a broad health survey, where the vital signs are important indicators of a patient's general state of well-being and potential medical needs. Among developments in vital sign measuring instruments, technologically sophisticated ones such as automatic vital sign monitors are notable. They integrate various functionalities, measuring blood pressure, heart rate, respiratory rate, and temperature in one machine. This not only offers time-saving advantages but also enhances reading accuracy by minimizing human error. Through the use of automated monitors, nurses can efficiently acquire vital signs, making patient assessments detailed but fast. Further, these devices generally integrate with electronic health record systems, allowing real-time data updating and patient safety improvement through increased monitoring. These technological developments are at the forefront of current practice in healthcare and represent a paradigm shift to a more efficient and integrated approach to patient observation and vital sign monitoring as part of integrated nursing assessment to enable best health outcomes. The impact of reliable vital sign measuring devices extends beyond individual patient care in that it reaches public healthcare quality and safety programs as a whole. For example, initiatives like the VAs National Center for Patient Safety emphasize the importance of accurate vital sign monitoring as a measure in preventing adverse events related to patient care. By using systematic approaches and promoting a safety culture, health care organizations aim to reduce complications, errors, and mortality due to health care. The accurate and consistent monitoring of vital signs is a critical piece to the achievement of these objectives, as nurses rely on quality data to make evidence-based practice decisions. These efforts not only ensure conformity to quality requirements but also promote overall patient safety, demonstrating that equipment used in the measurement of patients' vital signs is essential not only to nursing practice but to healthcare systems as a whole, enabling providers to deliver improved quality care for patients (Chase et al., 2011; Heyes et al., 2018).

5.4.2. Proper Techniques for Accurate Readings

Accurate measurement of vital signs is central in nursing because it is a key constituent of assessing the state of a patient's health. The method employed while taking vital signs—temperature, pulse, breathing, and blood pressure—vitally influences the accuracy of data obtained. To illustrate, the utilization of calibrated and working equipment is paramount. Nurses need to be instructed in proper use of thermometers, sphygmomanometers, and pulse oximeters, all of which are to be tested and calibrated for accuracy at regular intervals. Environmental factors such as noise, temperature variability, and patient position may also have an undesirable impact on readings. The use of standardized techniques, for example, the use of a single hand in taking the pulse and positioning the patient in physical and emotional relaxation, enhances the accuracy of the readings. This diligence is a sign of professionalism as well as adherence to the best practices in nursing. Secondly, the incorporation of technology is the main contributing factor in providing accurate readings when performing health assessments. The advent of the Internet of Things (IoT) has introduced new methods of monitoring vital signs, providing real-time information that can potentially enhance patient care outcomes. Advanced wearables with sensor capabilities can transmit continuous health information, not just help nurse assessment but also instigate a proactive approach to treating the patient. As stated, "the rapid expansion of Internet of Things (IoT) technology in recent years has enabled connections of numerous smart things and sensors and generated seamless data exchange" (Dang et al., 2019). Due to the use of these technological advancements, nurses can get more precise readings, thus making interventions on time. However, nurses also need to be sensitive to concerns regarding privacy and security involved in using networked devices for patient data protection and adherence to regulations that govern health technology. Lastly, documentation and communication are of the greatest significance in recording vital signs. Nurses must document all findings accurately in the patients electronic medical record (EMR) for maintaining continuity of care. Misdocumentation or miscommunication of critical signs can produce severe health repercussions. Adherence to systematic reporting processes and abbreviations ensures effective communication and interpretation of vital sign information by all members of the healthcare team. Also, the European Stroke Organization (ESO) puts significant emphasis on the significance of integrated care and communication measures that describe the stroke management under an organized strategy and comprises observation of vital signs as an essential part of patient assessment (Norrving et al., 2018). Overall, proper documentation combined with accurate readings helps not just to improve patient outcomes but also creates a robust platform for further research and nursing practice policy development (Figure 5.13).

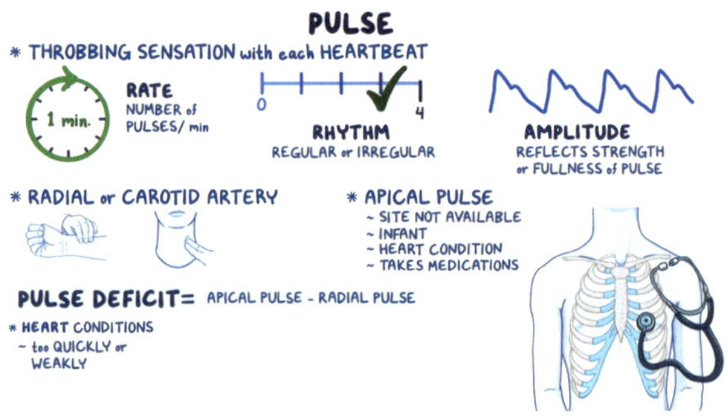

Figure 5.13. Proper techniques for accurate readings vital signs.

Source: https://external-content.duckduckgo.com/iu/?u=https%3A%2F%2Fosmose-it.s3.amazonaws.com%2FtONNyMrRTMKfa75o4SnBsg6SSDGtREh7%2F_.jpg&f=1&nofb=1&ipt=40c3d6c27460d010b5b3df890450f321d91970cedf135fabd97b649b6399f814.

5.4.3. Common Errors in Measurement

Accurate measurement of vital signs is a necessary component in nursing that can be an integral contributor to patient outcomes. Common errors in measurement often result from human variables like variability in technique, inconsistency in training between workers, and distraction in the environment of a hospital. For instance, manual observation to take temperature, pulse rate, blood pressure, and other vital signs is susceptible to discrepancy if taken under a state of urgency or in the absence of standards of procedure. Discrepancies in such measures can lead to biased patient data, hence misdiagnosis or inappropriate treatment. It is crucial that the loopholes be identified to minimize errors in standardization procedures and training so that reliability in taking vital signs is enhanced. Technology. It is playing an increasingly important part in rectifying common measurement errors encountered in nursing practice. Contemporary innovations such as computerized data entry systems and wearable health monitoring devices have transformed the manner in which vital signs are monitored and recorded. For instance, a study identified the usefulness of an intelligent crowd isolation medical observation management system using wireless telemetry in gathering vital sign data in real time. This process greatly reduced the percentage of error that is associated with traditional approaches, and it demonstrated that these technologies could identify anomalies that would go unreported in manual readings. The application of such new technologies not only increases precision but also allows medical practitioners to focus more on patient care than paperwork, hence increasing patient outcomes and the efficiency of healthcare delivery. Besides, nursing workload of manual data entry has been identified as a major source of measurement errors that compromise patient safety. A recent attempt to automate data entry processes in electronic health records (EHRs) discovered that these innovations are able to reduce errors by up to 20% to almost 0%. Through releasing nurses from time-consuming data entry, automation increases their ability for hands-on patient care, leading to improved job satisfaction and performance. Interweaving streamlined processes via automated devices not only facilitates timely and accurate documentation of vital signs but also supports a culture that is centered on quality care. As more advanced nursing practice emerges, it is essential to embrace technology as a means of overcoming typical measurement errors and facilitating safe, effective healthcare services (Bauer et al., 2019; Sun et al., 2022).

Test Your Knowledge

1. What are the proper techniques for accurately measuring temperature, pulse, respiration, and blood pressure?
2. How can patient positioning or external factors affect the accuracy of vital sign measurements?

5.5. Interpretation of Vital Signs

Learning Outcome

1. Recognizing abnormal findings;
2. Correlating vital signs with patient conditions;
3. Clinical decision-making based on vital signs.

The analysis of vital signs is a core element of nursing care, and it is an integral part of patient assessment and monitoring. Blood pressure, heart rate, respiratory rate, temperature, and oxygen saturation are the vital signs that offer valuable information regarding an individual's physiological status. In practice, the nurses are not only required to measure these signs but also interpret and compare data against patients' overall state of health. For instance, changes in blood pressure and heart rate might be indicative of pathologies or acute diseases that require immediate treatment. The knowledge of the manner in which different critical signs interact can enhance clinical decision-making, allowing nurses to set priorities well and respond to changes in patients' status rapidly, as proposed in recent research emphasizing the places of vital signs in nursing assessments. Also, the incorporation of technology in interpreting vital signs presents a number of emerging areas in healthcare services. Deep learning algorithms are among the new developments that have significantly improved the precision of forecasting nursing needs from vital sign data. Studies that employed deep learning models have shown that recurrent neural networks (RNN) and long short-term memory (LSTM) models are more precise than regression models in predicting patient needs and consequently enabling a more anticipatory nursing practice.

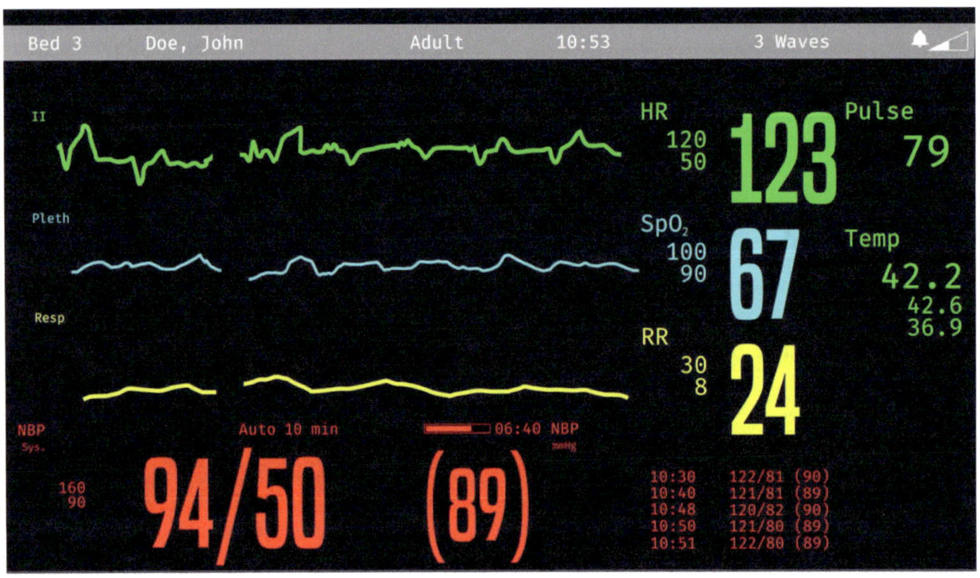

Figure 5.14. Interpretation of vital signs.

Source: https://external-content.duckduckgo.com/iu/?u=https%3A%2F%2Fhealthjade.com%2Fwp-content%2Fuploads%2F2018%2F12%2Fvital-signs.jpg&f=1&nofb=1&ipt=68e75d1c805faf5dd5a4d2bff281d0c4c9d10bdf45b54ce0fe085c0ff69ca1eb.

These technologies not only enhance predictive capability but allow for real-time monitoring of vital signs, supporting timely intervention. Nurses who have the ability to interpret these complex datasets can enhance patient management, particularly in high-acuity settings where abrupt physiological alteration is the norm (Mihirette et al., 2025). The applications of actual interpretation of vital signs are not only to individual patient management but also to guide broader public health interventions. Vital signs data can be aggregated to identify trends and patterns in larger populations, which in turn can lead to improved healthcare outcomes at a community level. As an example, monitoring vital signs in specific populations can identify correlations with public health conditions, such as how environmental influences affect breathing rates or temperature trends during flu season. Further, more analysis functions can incentivize resource allocation and direct preventive care decisions. Since nurses employ advanced means of interpreting vital signs, they can contribute to the generation of nursing practice knowledge, eventually yielding an integral health management system in the community (Mihirette et al., 2025) (Figure 5.14).

5.5.1. Recognizing Abnormal Findings

The assessment of abnormal findings on a general health survey and check of vital signs is essential in nursing practice. It is the responsibility of the nurse not only to observe physiological markers but also to assess these results in the context of patients' overall well-being. Abnormal findings can often be indicative of serious pathology or emergent health crises, necessitating urgent further investigation or intervention. For instance, an elevated heart rate, tachycardia, could indicate a variety of conditions from dehydration to anxiety, or serious cardiovascular disease. Therefore, thorough understanding of the norms and variability of vital signs is essential for proper clinical judgment (Forster et al., 2022). Moreover, recognition of abnormal findings is complemented by conceptual frameworks and protocols that guide nursing evaluations. Evidence-based interventions often include evidence-based early recognition protocols for physiological deterioration. The use of tools such as Observation Response Charts can help nurses observe systematically for signs and record trends in vital signs, allowing for early response to indicators of distress. This systematic surveillance facilitates intervention strategies that have the potential to avert adverse outcomes, particularly in risk populations. For instance, the deployment of specific criteria for escalating care based on important sign abnormality can enhance patient safety and leads to that, as research identifies, improved mental health decline identification on general wards and systematic interventions to such results (Elfeshawy et al., 2022). Secondly, the necessity of repeated practice adaptation and training also underscores the importance of detecting unusual results. Increasing times and changing faces of healthcare also necessitate that nurses be updated with latest information on population-related risk factors and pathological presentations. Repeated training can aid in developing the skill of healthcare professionals in detecting subtle variations in vital signs, fostering a proactive and watchful culture of care. This view is not only important for patient care at the level of the individual but also for guiding broader public health initiatives, such as preventing choking trauma among children. The incorporation of educational strategies addressing recognition of atypical results is therefore necessary within nursing education and continuing professional education (Forster et al., 2022).

5.5.2. Correlating Vital Signs with Patient Conditions

Good practice nursing greatly relies on the accurate measurement and interpretation of vital signs since they are highly significant markers of a patient's status. Temperature, pulse, respiration rate, and blood pressure are some of the vital signs that give very serious pointers to physiological changes and the body's response to illnesses. For instance, increased heart rate may be a sign of fever or dehydration, while hypertension may be a precursor to severe health conditions such as cardiovascular disease. The understanding of these associations allows the nurses to intervene timely and enhance patient outcomes. Besides, abnormal patterns in vital signs will often necessitate further investigation, so clinicians are able to identify the underlying medical conditions that are not yet apparent from symptomology alone, allowing them to treat the patient early and, in the process, avert further decline in patient well-being. The significance of mental health in vital signs cannot be underestimated, particularly in nursing practice. There is evidence to show a strong relationship between mental illness, such as depression and anxiety, and alterations in vital signs. For example, individuals with depressive states have alterations in heart rate variability and blood pressure that reflect heightened stress responses and possibly delayed opportunity for care due to emotional stress on healthcare providers. Including mental health consideration in assessment of vital signs is in line with growing recognition of holistic care in the nursing profession. Thus, by taking into consideration and addressing both patients' and nurses' mental health, healthcare systems can create a better supportive environment for effective patient healing and care and obtain the optimal health outcomes (Jeong et al., 2023). With the evolving nursing practice, the application of technology in monitoring vital signs has been revolutionary, especially in patient involvement and precision of data. Bringing in digital platforms for monitoring health has allowed real-time checking of vital signs with instant responses to life-threatening shifts in patient conditions. This technology has also been realized in the treatment of older persons, whose vital signs can reveal medical conditions that are connected with mental health. Electronic platforms not only enhance the precision of monitoring vital signs but also open opportunities for patients to act as custodians of their health by using self-monitoring strategies. Moreover, they provide valuable data that can be employed to identify trends and relationships to mental health, which hastens the development of interventions specifically aimed at improving general patient outcomes (Chan et al., 2024). In this way, vital signs play a role that goes beyond a mere numerical form, but instead serve as an essential part of whole person care for nurses (Figure 5.15).

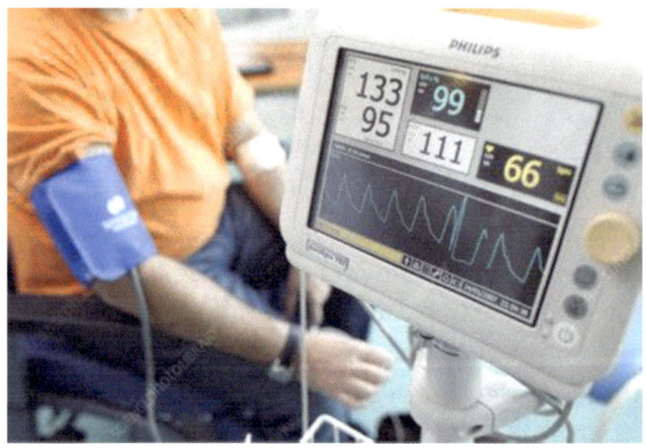

Figure 5.15. Correlating vital signs with patient conditions.

Source: https://external-content.duckduckgo.com/iu/?u=https%3A%2F%2Ftse4.mm.bing.net%2Fth%2Fid%2FOIP.5xL0ILJHE5mT9kkdi3DP6gAAAA%3Fpid%3DApi&f=1&ipt=fb331e044f44090826113ed772f837eaade5c882c58addad033c4031d7a8bf25.

5.5.3. Clinical Decision-Making Based on Vital Signs

Nursing clinical decision-making is greatly reliant on the interpretation of vital signs, which are determinants of a patient's physiological status. Heart rate, blood pressure, respiratory rate, temperature, and oxygen saturation are obtained to assist clinicians in assessing health status, identifying problems, and making decisions about treatment. These vital signs must be interpreted correctly; deviations from normal measures may signify acute or chronic conditions that require interventions in a timely manner. For instance, an elevated heart rate would be an indicator of impending shock or dehydration and would necessitate fluid resuscitation in the hospital setting as soon as possible. In addition, incorporating vital sign data into electronic health records encourages a dynamic process of review, wherein nurses are able to correlate vital sign changes with patient outcomes for enhanced clinical decision-making (Charlene et al., 2020). Effective interpretation of vital signs in nursing practice is not only necessary for immediate direct care of patients but also for facilitating patient safety overall. Nursing policies normally give significant importance to regular observation and documentation of vital signs, especially in critical care environments where trends from minute to minute can critically affect patient planning. Instructive clinical decision-making involves using such readings to develop evidence-based practice protocols tailored to the needs of each patient. For nurses, this is what leads to interpreting readings between changes in vital signs to determine when to escalate care or to employ other preventative interventions, thereby decreasing risk for complications and improving patient outcomes (Stephen et al., 2016). This practice highlights the critical role of vital signs in informing clinical activities within a nursing context. Additionally, the integration of technology into vital sign monitoring has transformed clinical decision-making, providing real-time information that improves situational awareness in nursing. With the introduction of wearable sensors and remote monitoring technologies, clinicians are now able to monitor vital signs constantly, thus adding a safety layer and instant feedback. These advances enable proactive interventions; rather than holding off for scheduled evaluations, nurses can intervene immediately upon alterations in a patient's condition the moment they occur. This timeliness is particularly beneficial in acute conditions were having the ability to react immediately could be the difference between life and death. Lastly, the judicious application of vital signs, augmented by technology, enhances the effectiveness of decision-making and enables the delivery of quality patient care (Charlene et al., 2020).

Test Your Knowledge

1. How can normal versus abnormal vital sign readings guide clinical decision-making?
2. What patterns in vital signs might indicate acute or chronic health conditions?

5.6. Role of Nursing in Health Surveys and Vital Signs

Learning Outcome

1. Responsibilities of nurses in patient assessment;
2. Documentation and reporting;
3. Patient education and communication.

The nursing role in health examination and observation of vital signs is most important in the whole process of patient care. Nurses are the frontline caregivers who, besides assuming control over health condition through systematic examination, also interpret key information on vital signs such as heart rate, blood pressure, and respiratory rates. Regular monitoring allows the nurses to detect deviations from baseline measures of health and act accordingly on alterations in a patient's condition. Utilization of today's technology, e.g., wearable sensors for remote monitoring, has also enhanced the nurse's capacity to conduct health surveys efficiently. These innovations enable sustained data collection, which can be invaluable in managing chronic illnesses, as exposed by studies showing correlations between physical activity in patients and measures of vital signs (Kseniia et al., 2023). Such types of innovation highlight the significance of nursing in taking advantage of health surveys to tailor patient-focused interventions. Moreover, the practice of nursing entails massive responsibilities that are quite beyond mere data collection. As frontline health workers, nurses translate survey data and interview patients to help understand their health issues in a complete way. This involves not only monitoring vital signs but also educating patients on their health and what the gathered data entails. When conducting health surveys, nurses create an environment that encourages open communication, enabling patients to express symptoms and concerns that may not be indicated through numbers alone. This nurse-patient relationship can improve adherence to treatment protocols and lifestyle modifications. Where health workforce gaps are prevalent, such as in Pakistan, the impact of educated nurses offering quality care is all the more significant. Addressing these issues in the workforce is essential in order to ensure effective health surveys and improving health outcomes (Hassan, 2023). Moreover, the assessment and analysis of essential signs are significant components of nurse examinations employed to inform clinical decisions. Through meticulous recording of vital signs and health survey findings, nurses play a large role in detecting nascent threats to patient health early enough to avoid adverse occurrences. Through the use of established nursing protocols, accuracy and consistency of assessment is ensured.

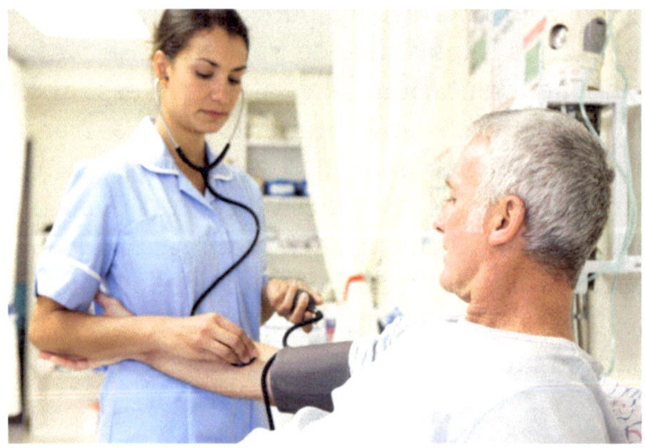

Figure 5.16. Role of nursing in health surveys and vital signs.

Source: https://external-content.duckduckgo.com/iu/?u=https%3A%2F%2Fwww.oncologynurseadvisor.com%2Fwp-content%2Fuploads%2Fsites%2F13%2F2020%2F07%2Fhypertension_G_105692049-860x573.jpg&f=1&nofb=1&ipt=82d606f9cdb18e07a7162f33757b1f1dd3331c2697d094e67fb61818e04daca7.

In chronic disease care, constant monitoring through health questionnaires allows for dynamic adjustment of treatment protocols through real-time evidence. This being forward-looking allows not only for patient safety but for a holistic understanding of individual health trends over time as well. The intersection of intelligent monitoring technologies, as proven in existing studies, points to the central role nursing plays in patient care consistency and, ultimately, the need for nursing in health questionnaires and intelligent monitoring of vital signs (Kseniia et al., 2023) (Figure 5.16).

5.6.1. Responsibilities of Nurses in Patient Assessment

Nurses' functions in patient assessment are critical to the provision of effective delivery of health care and optimal patient outcomes. Their foremost task is the conduct of comprehensive assessments of health, such as taking and processing vital signs. By doing so, not only do they establish a baseline for each patient, but also, they can identify any deviation from normal parameters, which may indicate underlying issues with their health. Through a variety of assessment techniques such as observation, palpation, and auscultation, nurses gather valuable information that guides clinical decision. Besides, the assessments must include mastery of the patients history, environmental, and social factors in order to enhance the quality and relevance of information gathered. These thorough patient evaluations are central to the implementation of timely interventions, thus directly affecting the course of care and general patient health outcomes, especially in more complex cases (Susie et al., 2020). In addition to conducting physical examinations, nurses also play a significant role in monitoring patients' reactions to care and treatment. Continual observation of vital signs including blood pressure, heart rate, and temperature gives nurses feedback on the status of the patients and assists in detecting trends that can be utilized to foretell deterioration or improvement. Modern healthcare systems incorporate more use of technology, and nurses must learn to use electronic health records and telehealth systems to document and evaluate patient information efficiently (Margaret et al., 2018). These instruments not only enable effective communication with other healthcare providers but also enhance patient involvement through the provision of real-time information regarding their health. In addition, nurses must maintain elaborate records of their assessment as well as encounter with patients, as these data are invaluable in the provision of continuity of care, maintaining regulatory requirements, and facilitating interdisciplinary coordination.

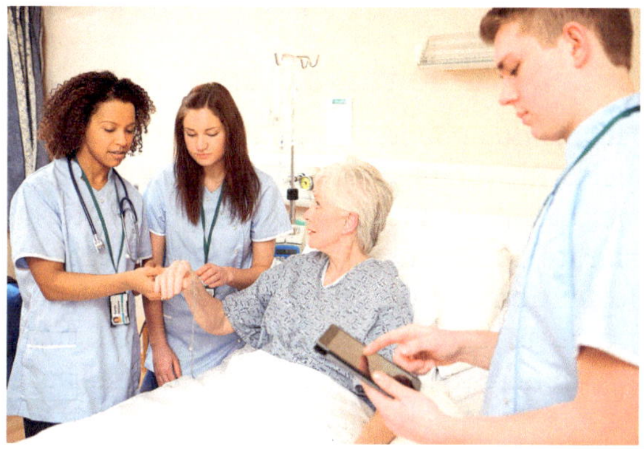

Figure 5.17. Responsibilities of nurses in patient assessment.

Source: https://external-content.duckduckgo.com/iu/?u=https%3A%2F%2Fblogs.biomedcentral.com%2Fon-medicine%2Fwp-content%2Fuploads%2Fsites%2F6%2F2023%2F09%2Fnursing-assessment.jpg&f=1&nofb=1&ipt=7c8350d366dacaf022bbeda819542bac262235c66e239b53cb3b017aba7ed45c.

Finally, nurses' patient assessment functions are more than data collection; they involve communication and patient education to increase patient understanding of their health condition. Nurses ought to present assessment findings to patients in an understandable and acceptable manner, establishing a trusting relationship with patients who will be encouraged to participate in their care. This training is paramount, especially when discussing the need for monitoring the essential signs and being in a position to recognize the signs which require urgent intervention. Nurses are also in charge of care coordination among various healthcare professionals, with the team members being sufficiently informed regarding the assessments of the patients to administer holistic care (Susie et al., 2020). Lastly, the multifaceted role of nurses in patient assessment is not merely clinical competence but also patient advocacy in an empathetic manner, which is key to achieving high-quality health outcomes (Figure 5.17).

5.6.2. Documentation and Reporting

Accurate documentation and reporting are key aspects in nursing, particularly in the case of general health surveys and vital sign monitoring. Accurate documentation ensures that patients' information is well recorded, and continuity of care is established, enabling healthcare practitioners to make informed decisions based on concrete data. It is not merely taking the vital signs such as pulse, blood pressure, respiratory rate, and temperature but interpreting them in relation to the overall status of the patients. By carefully documenting these vital signs, nurses can identify patterns or trends, which are essential in making interventions in a timely manner. Besides, in-depth reporting promotes accountability in practice nursing and is a legally binding document, therefore protecting the patient and the health worker in the event of conflicts or questions regarding decisions reached in the clinic. No less important is documentation use for assessment and remediation of broader health concerns. For example, ongoing tracking of physical inactivity is very important in comprehending its role in chronic diseases as well as general morbidity in the population. Systematic health surveys allow for data collection that reflects trends in physical activity and health behavior, laying the groundwork for future interventions. Outcomes of such surveys indicate the pressing public health issue of physical inactivity, which, as outlined by Stoutenberg et al. (2017), is responsible for significant health threats and cost burdens. Nurses also play a significant role here by being very careful about patient history associated with lifestyle and exercise, thereby helping in the building of tailored health promotion interventions that can be disseminated on both community and individual levels. Good documentation practice is directly linked to improved patient outcomes and good decision-making in nursing environments. Integrating structured documentation equipment and electronic health records can potentially facilitate the acquisition of necessary data, such as the psychosocial aspects of care such as distress (Michelle et al., 2019). The emphasis on psychosocial care demonstrates the importance of understanding the emotional and psychological well-being of a patient as important as recording physical parameters of health. With the adoption of methodical approaches to documentation, healthcare professionals are able to offer comprehensive reporting that not only complies with regulations but also facilitates an integrated comprehension of patient well-being, leading ultimately to improved care outcomes and patient satisfaction.

5.6.3. Patient Education and Communication

Effective communication and patient education are crucial aspects of nursing, particularly when it comes to the general health survey and vital sign monitoring. Nurses are the focal point of connection between patients and the healthcare system, bringing clinical knowledge and communication together to improve comprehension. Throughout a general health survey, nurses need to effectively and clearly state information in a manner that allows patients to fully comprehend their state of health. This encompasses not only the transmission of medical information but also management of patients' feelings, concerns, and questions. Having the capacity to create a supportive context reinforces patients' self-efficacy, which ultimately has the effect of leading to better compliance with treatment protocols and more active participation in their care decisions, with significant implications for patient outcomes. The complexities of contemporary healthcare require individualized communication strategies to address specific patient needs. In a time of increased patient activation, health literacy has become a pillar of effective communication. Nurses must assess every patient's health literacy, and adjust teaching methods, accordingly, focusing on simple language, visual aids, and teach-back to ensure understanding. By means of alternative means of communication, nurses can better prepare patients to manage their health issues and understand how vital signs fit into the big picture of health. By such a focus on individualized communication, the barriers to effective learning are dismantled, and all patients receive equal support and resources for making intelligent health decisions. Furthermore, technology integration in health care presents worthy challenges and opportunities for patient education. Telehealth and digital technologies enable the extension of nursing reach to patients outside clinical settings, allowing continuous interaction and education. Patient portals and mobile health applications provide continuous communication and access to critical health information. Nurses play a key role in guiding patients through such online materials, educating them on the significance of their vital signs and follow-up treatment as advised by the health questionnaire. As healthcare continues to evolve with more developments, patient education and communication will remain important, ensuring nursing professionals can effectively advocate for their patients and address their care (Hassan, 2023; N/A, 2023).

Test Your Knowledge

1. How do nurses use general health surveys and vital signs to assess patient needs and prioritize care?
2. What responsibilities do nurses have in monitoring, documenting, and responding to changes in vital signs?

SUMMARY

In assessing the important function of vital signs in nursing, it is essential to understand that their regular checking is called for in diagnosis and management of patient health. The evidence provided in studies affirms the requirement for tailored monitoring protocols in accordance with the risk factors of individual patients. Increased monitoring of vital signs in high-risk patients not only enables early intervention but also merits enhanced clinical outcomes. Overall, the general conclusion that current protocols are prone to lead to over-monitoring in stable patients indicates the need for reassessment to optimize resource use in healthcare settings. Consequently, a more prudent approach towards the measurement of vital signs might promote improved nurse-patient relationships without sacrificing effective utilization of healthcare resources, as evident in implementation proposals made upon current studies (Briggs et al., 2024). Second, the intersection of monitoring of vital signs and effective discharge planning presents questions regarding the complexity challenging nursing professionals. General wards and intensive care units are exposed to enhanced pressures that require a bifocal strategy for patient safety and use of resources. Admission and discharge principles come to be essential in ensuring continuity of care, often under threat from systemic shortcomings. Analyzing the degree to which the practices of current discharge are influenced by observations of vital signs supports the elaboration of likely barriers to be overcome in enhancing patient flow. Stakeholder recommendations highlight the importance of standardized processes and increased interdisciplinary communication as essential principles to optimize patient transitions, ultimately substantiating the argument for extensive monitoring protocols extending beyond immediate clinical settings (Hiller et al., 2024). Finally, reconceptualizing vital signs monitoring in nursing is not merely the technical process of measurement but also the organizational factors as a whole that contribute to enhancing patient care. By following evidence-based protocols that respond to patient-specific requirements, healthcare practitioners can deal with risks of deterioration more efficiently while offering comprehensive nursing care. The data gathered from observational studies and stakeholders emphasize the importance of a balanced approach that saves resources but maximizes safety. In the future, efforts should go towards cooperative structures that facilitate inter-disciplinary interaction, thereby ensuring the healthcare team members are well-suited to meet changing patient needs. This holistic plan ultimately serves towards the realization of the two-fold aim of clinical excellence and resource efficiency in nursing practice (Briggs et al., 2024; Hiller et al., 2024).

Effective assessment of health status in nursing heavily depends on ongoing observation of vital signs and comprehensive health questionnaires. Vital signs, which consist of measures such as heart rate, blood pressure, temperature, and respiratory rate, are essential signs of the patient's physiological status. Through systematic collection and analysis of these parameters, nurses are empowered to detect possible health concerns at an early stage, enabling timely interventions that can enhance patient outcomes. Additionally, incorporation of technology into these processes, as noted in upcoming frameworks, enables increased precision and efficiency. The evolution towards intelligent systems, utilizing wireless telemetry and big data platforms, is a classic example of how contemporary nursing practices can be evolved to extend better care and monitoring for patients. There exist tremendous variations in the healthcare practices utilized in various countries, particularly with regard to patient transfers from nursing homes to hospitals. In a comparative study, the occurrence of such transfers was much higher in German homes for the elderly compared to Dutch ones, which signals that different healthcare systems are to blame for varying ways of treating patients. General practitioners' contribution in such transfer decisions was observed to be rather different; they are less involved in Germany than in the Netherlands, where older care doctors play a more focal role in ensuring adequate patient transfers. These observations remind us that the healthcare systems need to be explored as to how they assist patient care paths, thus influencing the effectiveness of nursing interventions and overall healthcare outcomes (Fassmer et al., 2024). COVID-19 pandemic has underscored the vital necessity of effectively monitoring significant indicators during isolation and medical observation, respectively. New technology opens up new avenues to complement traditional procedures; intelligent wearable devices, for instance, provide real-time monitoring essentially replacing human assessment that may have risks related to neglect. A recent trial indicated that using a technology of this type would be capable of 100% sensitivity and specificity in the recognition of abnormal body temperatures, outperforming the manual method. Not only does this new technology increase the accuracy of monitoring, but it also adheres to infection control practices by minimizing direct contact between patients and healthcare personnel. Hence, adopting such advancements is an imperative step towards enhanced patient safety and quality of care in nurse settings, best observed in high-risk environments such as hospitals and nursing facilities (Sun et al., 2022).

KEY TERMS FROM THIS CHAPTER

- General Appearance
- Posture
- Hygiene
- Vital Signs
- Pulse
- Blood Pressure
- Pain Assessment
- Weight
- Body Build
- Gait
- Level of Consciousness
- Temperature
- Respiration
- Oxygen Saturation
- Height
- Body Mass Index (BMI)

CRITICAL THINKING QUESTIONS

1. **What is the primary purpose of a general health survey?**
   a. To diagnose a specific disease
   b. To gather initial information about a patient's overall health status
   c. To prescribe medications
   d. To perform a laboratory test
2. **Which of the following is considered a vital sign?**
   a. Height
   b. Blood pressure
   c. Weight
   d. Level of education
3. **A patient's temperature is 101.4°F (38.6°C). How is this classified?**
   a. Hypothermia
   b. Fever (Hyperthermia)
   c. Normal
   d. Hypotension
4. **Which method of measuring pulse provides information about the rate, rhythm, and strength of the heartbeat?**
   a. Auscultation
   b. Palpation
   c. Inspection
   d. Percussion
5. **When assessing blood pressure, the first Korotkoff sound represents:**
   a. Diastolic pressure
   b. Systolic pressure
   c. Mean arterial pressure
   d. Pulse pressure

Short Answer Questions

1. What is the purpose of a general health survey in nursing practice?
2. List the components typically assessed in a general health survey.
3. Why is observing a patient's overall appearance important during a health survey?
4. How can a nurse assess a patient's mental status as part of a general survey?
5. What are the normal ranges for adult vital signs, including temperature, pulse, respiration, and blood pressure?

Answer to Critical Thinking Questions

1. (b) 2. (b) 3. (b) 4. (b) 5. (b)

REFERENCES

1. Abbasizanjani, H., Bedston, S., Robinson, L., Curds, M., & Akbari, A. (2023). Clinical coding of long Covid in Wales: A cohort study of 3.5 million people using linked health and demographic data. *International Journal of Population Data Science, 8*. https://www.semanticscholar.org/paper/ed980c6e679591b54b50b6e3e240b2888a8be086 (accessed on 16th July 2025).
2. Abdullah, K., & Atrushi, A. (2019). Knowledge, altitude and practice of nurses towards neonatal sepsis in Duhok Governorate. *The Journal of The University of Duhok*. https://www.semanticscholar.org/paper/f447749c99e798b06d667452450bdfeee1c49f6e (accessed on 16th July 2025).
3. Ali, I., Khan, M. A., Naz, S., Rafiq, U., Naseem, N., & Ali, I. (2025). Knowledge, attitude, and practices among staff nurses in a tertiary health care hospital towards COVID-19 in Karachi, Pakistan. *Journal of Medical & Health Sciences Review*. https://www.semanticscholar.org/paper/c867bf0fed81dfda5a589a12704dcbc5f1ca43e3 (accessed on 16th July 2025).
4. Baek, Y., Han, K., Jeon, E., & Yoo, H. (2024). Prediction of nursing need proxies using vital signs and biomarkers data: Application of deep learning models. *Journal of Clinical Nursing*. https://www.semanticscholar.org/paper/89415029e06ced4dad51675c331086e451c38505 (accessed on 16th July 2025).
5. Bauer, J., John, E., Wood, C. L., Plass, D., & Richardson, D. (2019). Data entry automation improves cost, quality, performance, and job satisfaction in a hospital nursing unit. *JONA: The Journal of Nursing Administration, 50*, 34–39. https://www.semanticscholar.org/paper/57a361aae6b70edbf5423549966912f1f39289a5 (accessed on 16th July 2025).
6. Bergerød, I. J. (2021). Quality and safety in hospital cancer care: A mixed methods study of next of kin involvement. https://www.semanticscholar.org/paper/e21de40b58a6e368a70529f7e25ca7bd513ffa1c (accessed on 16th July 2025).
7. Briggs, J., Kostakis, I., Meredith, P., Dall'ora, C., Darbyshire, J., Gerry, S., Griffiths, P., et al. (2024). Safer and more efficient vital signs monitoring protocols to identify the deteriorating patients in the general hospital ward: An observational study. *Health and Social Care Delivery Research, 12*(6), 1–143. https://www.semanticscholar.org/paper/794f06e0583f77b87a7ca3e6a77f0df6cbb047b6 (accessed on 16th July 2025).
8. Chan, S., Kwan, R., Ng, F., Lau, B. H. P., & Chan, A. (2024). S17: The translation of digital technology to promote mental health of older adults. *International Psychogeriatrics, 36*, 28–32. https://www.semanticscholar.org/paper/65875783d522573db4a14206c325e65ec3c5d00b (accessed on 16th July 2025).
9. Chase, D., & McCarthy, D. (2011). Advancing patient safety in the U.S. Department of Veterans Affairs. https://core.ac.uk/download/75777631.pdf (accessed on 16th July 2025).
10. Chen, H. H., Lai, J. C. Y., Chiou, S., Huang, N., & Chien, L. (2023). The effect of hospital-based health promotion on the health practices of full-time hospital nurses: A cross-sectional study. *Scientific Reports, 13*. https://www.semanticscholar.org/paper/977b4b7ca649fe1f47a4257fc19a5461856d622a (accessed on 16th July 2025).
11. Chen, Y. H., Luo, X. Y., Chang, C. H., Kuo, C. T., Shih, S. J., Chang, M. Y., Weng, M. R., et al. (2025). Post-surgical fall risk prediction: A machine learning approach for spine and lower extremity procedures. *Frontiers in Medicine, 12*. https://www.semanticscholar.org/paper/191c7f55841e789e5f9a0598e360f3a81c3c7712 (accessed on 16th July 2025).

12. Dang, L. M., Piran, M. J., Han, D., Min, K., & Moon, H. (2019). A survey on internet of things and cloud computing for healthcare. *Electronics, 8*, 768–768. https://doi.org/10.3390/electronics8070768 (accessed on 16th July 2025).
13. Dewey, C. M., Hingle, S., Goelz, E., & Linzer, M. (2020). Supporting clinicians during the COVID-19 pandemic. *Annals of Internal Medicine, 172*, 752–753. https://doi.org/10.7326/m20-1033 (accessed on 16th July 2025).
14. Elfeshawy, R., El Sobky, F., Mohamed, F., & Darweesh, H. (2022). Effect of health education program-based on a health belief model on mothers' knowledge and practices regarding choking prevention and management for their children. *Tanta Scientific Nursing Journal*. https://www.semanticscholar.org/paper/276aafc4639746b91f79f8f93b2957d329309ab8 (accessed on 16th July 2025).
15. Fassmer, A., Zuidema, S., Janus, S. I. M., & Hoffmann, F. (2024). Differences in emergency department visits and hospitalization between German and Dutch nursing home residents: A cross-national survey. *European Geriatric Medicine, 15*, 787–795. https://www.semanticscholar.org/paper/e731624aac91d371bd0c44f98a200d5f7794a8f0 (accessed on 16th July 2025).
16. Forster, J., Coventry, A., & Daniel, C. (2022). Optimizing the response to mental health deterioration: Nurses' experiences of using a Mental Health Observation Response Chart. *International Journal of Mental Health Nursing*. https://www.semanticscholar.org/paper/46f8fad3ec23a9525367b5f619e238512c69dec3 (accessed on 16th July 2025).
17. Hassan, S. M. A. (2023). Nursing shortage in Pakistan. *NURSEARCHER (Journal of Nursing & Midwifery Sciences)*. https://www.semanticscholar.org/paper/953f75757c6fcb3f2489dc4496fb4af53faf41dc (accessed on 16th July 2025).
18. Heyes, M. E., Muckler, V. C., Schnitzen, L., Starr, L., et al. (2018). Recertification and reentry to practice for nurse anesthetists: Determining core competencies and evaluating performance via high-fidelity simulation technology. https://core.ac.uk/download/213088562.pdf (accessed on 16th July 2025).
19. Hiller, M., Burisch, C., Wittmann, M., Bracht, H., Kaltwasser, A., & Bakker, J. (2024). The current state of intensive care unit discharge practices–Results of an international survey study. *Frontiers in Medicine, 11*. https://www.semanticscholar.org/paper/a16e856630b323b1c24cac66baf3315651619325 (accessed on 16th July 2025).
20. Jeong, Y. M., & Chang, H. E. (2023). Depressive symptoms and missed nursing care among clinical nurses: A cross-sectional survey. *Journal of Korean Academy of Fundamentals of Nursing*. https://www.semanticscholar.org/paper/b4306037ffe2f895a7ab9a9cef8e06dbcd5f1360 (accessed on 16th July 2025).
21. Johnson, N. L., & Rodriguez, D. (2013). Children with autism spectrum disorder at a pediatric hospital: A systematic review of the literature. https://core.ac.uk/download/213081757.pdf (accessed on 16th July 2025).
22. Kruk, M. E., Gage, A., Arsenault, C., Jordan, K., Leslie, H. H., Roder-DeWan, S., Adeyi, O., et al. (2018). High-quality health systems in the Sustainable Development Goals era: Time for a revolution. *The Lancet Global Health, 6*, e1196–e1252. https://doi.org/10.1016/s2214-109x(18)30386-3 (accessed on 16th July 2025).
23. Lew, S. Q., Wallace, E., Srivatana, V., Warady, B. A., Watnick, S., Hood, J., White, D. L., et al. (2020). Telehealth for home dialysis in COVID-19 and beyond: A perspective from the

American Society of Nephrology COVID-19 Home Dialysis Subcommittee. *American Journal of Kidney Diseases, 77*, 142–148. https://doi.org/10.1053/j.ajkd.2020.09.005 (accessed on 16th July 2025).

24. McClave, S. A., Taylor, B., Martindale, R. G., Warren, M., Johnson, D. R., Braunschweig, C., McCarthy, M. S., et al. (2016). Guidelines for the provision and assessment of nutrition support therapy in the adult critically ill patient. *Journal of Parenteral and Enteral Nutrition, 40*, 159–211. https://doi.org/10.1177/0148607115621863 (accessed on 16th July 2025).
25. Mihirette, S., Cal, E. D. L., Tan, Q., & Sedano, J. (2025). Cross-contextual stress prediction: Simple methodology for comparing features and sample domain adaptation techniques in vital sign analysis. *Applied Intelligence, 55*, 420. https://www.semanticscholar.org/paper/5446862c7fcdeab6e2d87cb67246e536a25c2514 (accessed on 16th July 2025).
26. Morphet, J., Plummer, V., & Rochana, N. (2016). Triage process in emergency departments: An Indonesian study. https://media.neliti.com/media/publications/155129-EN-triage-process-in-emergency-departments.pdf (accessed on 16th July 2025).
27. N/A. (2013). Complex care management program overview–Technology. https://core.ac.uk/download/71362337.pdf (accessed on 16th July 2025).
28. Niranjan, R. (2020). Pediatric dental education improves interprofessional healthcare students' clinical competence in children's oral health assessment. https://core.ac.uk/download/294626429.pdf (accessed on 16th July 2025).
29. Norrving, B., Barrick, J., Dávalos, A., Dichgans, M., Cordonnier, C., Guekht, A., Kutluk, K., et al. (2018). Action plan for stroke in Europe 2018–2030. *European Stroke Journal, 3*, 309–336. https://doi.org/10.1177/2396987318808719 (accessed on 16th July 2025).
30. Ousey, K., & Roberts, P. (2013). Understanding effective management of postoperative wounds. https://core.ac.uk/download/13641332.pdf (accessed on 16th July 2025).
31. Patel, V., Chesmore, A., Legner, C., & Pandey, S. (2021). Trends in workplace wearable technologies and connected-worker solutions for next-generation occupational safety, health, and productivity. *Advanced Intelligent Systems, 4*. https://doi.org/10.1002/aisy.202100099 (accessed on 16th July 2025).
32. Piercy, K. L., Troiano, R. P., Ballard, R., Carlson, S. A., Fulton, J. E., Galuska, D. A., George, S. M., et al. (2018). The physical activity guidelines for Americans. *JAMA, 320*, 2020–2020. https://doi.org/10.1001/jama.2018.14854 (accessed on 16th July 2025).
33. Proceedings of the 2022 CANO Conference. (2023). *Canadian Oncology Nursing Journal*. https://www.semanticscholar.org/paper/0dea9a631f308dc8dea1f3b3d231a47713a68edd (accessed on 16th July 2025).
34. Riba, M. B., Donovan, K. A., Andersen, B. L., Braun, I., Breitbart, W., Brewer, B. W., Buchmann, L., et al. (2019). Distress management, version 3.2019, NCCN clinical practice guidelines in oncology. *Journal of the National Comprehensive Cancer Network, 17*, 1229–1249. https://doi.org/10.6004/jnccn.2019.0048 (accessed on 16th July 2025).
35. Senechal, E., Radeschi, D. J., Kearney, R. E., Shalish, W., & Sant'Anna, G. M. (2025). Parents and health care providers' perspectives on vital signs monitoring technologies in the neonatal intensive care unit: An international survey. *American Journal of Perinatology*. https://www.semanticscholar.org/paper/f3cf3cd327d51df26ce04bd665d1406e17f67ea6 (accessed on 16th July 2025).

36. Shaik, T., Tao, X., Higgins, N., Li, L., Gururajan, R., Zhou, X., & Acharya, U. R. (2023). Remote patient monitoring using artificial intelligence: Current state, applications, and challenges. *Wiley Interdisciplinary Reviews: Data Mining and Knowledge Discovery, 13*. https://doi.org/10.1002/widm.1485 (accessed on 16th July 2025).

37. Shubina, K. M., Mishlanov, V. J., Nikitin, I. G., Bekker, K. N., Emelkina, V. V., & Shubin, I. V. (2023). The role of subjective and objective criteria in the assessment of the state of patients with bronchobstructive diseases in remote monitoring conditions. *The Bulletin of Contemporary Clinical Medicine*. https://www.semanticscholar.org/paper/31b507e566ad22a84c6624d213c50e9aace03e94 (accessed on 16th July 2025).

38. Sohn, J., & Chang, H. (2020). Effects of health-related perception, physical activity practice rate and stress on health-related quality of life for middle-aged women: Based on the Seventh Korea National Health and Nutrition Examination Survey (KNHSNES ?-3), 2017, Korea Centers for D. *Medico-Legal Update, 20*, 261–266. https://www.semanticscholar.org/paper/ee78f27890fd331b50eb9013a978109e0da7e7af (accessed on 16th July 2025).

39. Stoutenberg, M., Shaya, G. E., Feldman, D., & Carroll, J. K. (2017). Practical strategies for assessing patient physical activity levels in primary care. *Mayo Clinic Proceedings Innovations Quality & Outcomes, 1*, 8–15. https://doi.org/10.1016/j.mayocpiqo.2017.04.006 (accessed on 16th July 2025).

40. Sun, W., Wang, C., Sun, J., Miao, Z., Ling, F., & Wu, G. (2022). An intelligent medical isolation observation management system based on the internet of things. *Methods of Information in Medicine, 61*, 155–166. https://www.semanticscholar.org/paper/fff7ae084b895d09171dbb6b33488654d438c888 (accessed on 16th July 2025).

41. Truitt, K. A., Arumaithurai, K., & Young, N. (2023). Patient satisfaction and perception of physician empathy in outpatient community general neurology telemedicine. *Telehealth and Medicine Today*. https://www.semanticscholar.org/paper/3bd9005de7d7c2d69c19b57e6b3c218a0e21b748 (accessed on 16th July 2025).

42. Wilson, R., Godfrey, C., Sears, K., Medves, J., Ross-White, A., & Lambert, N. (2015). Exploring conceptual and theoretical frameworks for nurse practitioner education: A scoping review protocol. *The JBI Database of Systematic Reviews and Implementation Reports, 13*, 146–155. https://doi.org/10.11124/jbisrir-2015-2150 (accessed on 16th July 2025).

SKIN, HAIR, AND NAILS ASSESSMENT IN NURSING

6

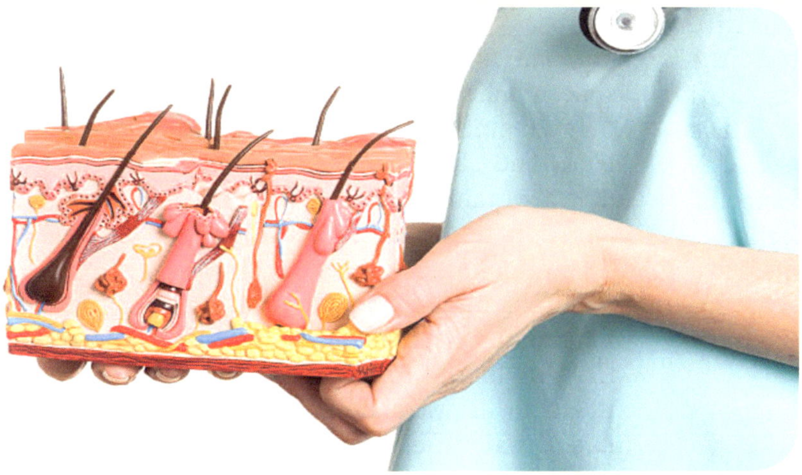

LEARNING OBJECTIVES

After studying this chapter, you will be able to:

1. Define anatomy and physiology of skin;
2. Discuss about hair assessment;
3. Explain nail assessment;
4. Describe assessment techniques;
5. Identify cultural considerations;
6. Explore documentation and communication.

Introduction

The assessment of skin, nails, and hair is a valuable component of practice nursing and is an integral component of patient assessment. Only with a detailed knowledge of these areas can nurses recognize healthcare problems that would otherwise be unapparent because findings in the skin often indicate systemic illness. For instance, changes in skin color, texture, or integrity may portend diabetes or inflammatory illnesses. Therefore, a comprehensive assessment involves both palpation and visual observation for data gathering on patients overall wellbeing. As noted in the nursing education guide, the use of culturally-responsive approaches in this practice allows nurses to modify their assessment technique, thereby acknowledging various practices of health and beliefs that can influence patient care interactions and outcomes (Accettola et al., 2023). In addition, converting theoretical know-how to practical skill sets is of the highest significance for health assessment specialized nursing students. The practical guidelines facilitate the ability of nursing students to sharpen clinical judgment skills so that they can determine signs of clinical deterioration effectively. For example, with the skin examination, hair, and nails, students can interpret findings like hair loss or lesions in the context of a patient's current health status as part of their medical history. The integrative approach enables improved nursing graduates who can make informed decisions, prioritize, and ultimately contribute to improved patient health outcomes and safety (Accettola et al., 2023). Modules that provide tutorial aids and interactive clinical training significantly contribute to the learning process of the students, equipping them with the devices they will have in their future nursing careers. Apart from general knowledge of the skin, hair, and nails examination, specific training on infection control and disinfection is necessary, particularly within the perioperative setting. Good skin disinfection practices are sound infection control measures, just like strict evaluations in operating rooms.

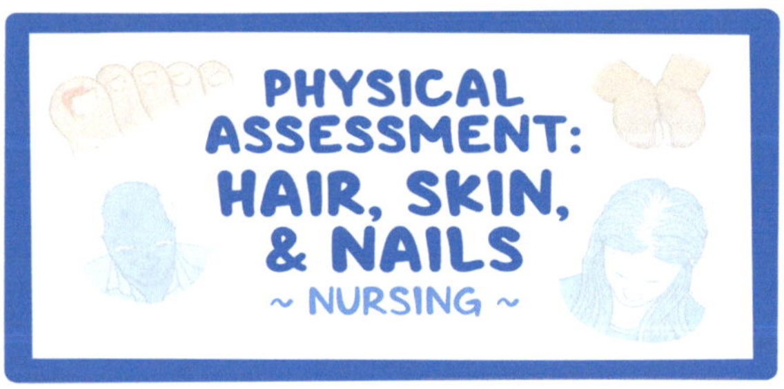

Figure 6.1. Physical assessment – skin, hair, and nails.

Source: https://external-content.duckduckgo.com/iu/?u=https%3A%2F%2Fosmose-it.s3.amazonaws.com%2Fid-KyPkXSP24fh42yA0sXGI3SSC7xKzq%2F_.jpg&f=1&nofb=1&ipt=a6bf671e562dc6431132b3fa8bf301a7f95fd106f10eb556b5004edc2e39b5a9.

Production of instructional materials such as education posters not only supports learning for nursing students but also serves as valuable tools for healthcare workers to enforce safe clinical standards. With the move towards practice-oriented applications of theory in nursing education, it is important that future nurses are skilled in analyses of skin, hair, and nails, and particularly with their implications for general health as well as safety guidelines. This initial knowledge eventually helps nurses to provide better patient care in diverse healthcare scenarios (Figure 6.1).

Importance of Skin, Hair, and Nails Assessment in Nursing

Skin, hair, and nail examination is an essential aspect of nursing because these aspects are most likely the initial reflection of a patient's overall health and status. The skin, being the body's largest organ, reflects internal physiological condition and can be indicative of various systemic conditions. Altered color, temperature, or texture of the skin, for instance, can point to metabolic disease, autoimmune disorders, or infection. Identification of the changes enables nurses to act in a timely fashion, which can make great differences to patient outcomes. Routine assessment also offers a baseline for every patient, enabling more efficient monitoring of changes over the long term. This is a practice that not only enhances the nurses clinical decision-making but one that enables a more thorough view of patients health status, supporting the important place of skin, hair, and nails assessment within nursing. Also to be noted is the assessment of nails and hair, which may offer valuable information regarding a patient's nutritional condition and health. For example, brittle nails reflect deficiency of major minerals or vitamins, while hair loss may be a sign of underlying processes like hormonal imbalance or autoimmune disorders. Furthermore, some forms of hair loss can suggest different etiologies and require different intervention methods. By measuring such attributes, nurses can examine not only immediate health problems but also long-term hazards that may influence the patients' quality of life. Such measurements result in a holistic understanding of the status of the patients, allowing the nurses to start individualized health education interventions, critical in the prevention of personal hygiene and skin disease, as noted in the findings of Akrom et al. (2019). Finally, the role of thorough examination of skin, hair, and nails extends beyond straightforward clinical outcomes to encompass the psychosocial realms of patient care. Appreciation of the interactive nature of somatic symptoms and mental status is critical, especially when conditions like systemic lupus erythematosus (SLE) tend to present with painful cutaneous complaints that impact health-related quality of life (HRQoL) (Aggarwal et al., 2012). Patients who encounter visible alterations in their hair or skin usually suffer from increased depression and anxiety, further aggravating their general well-being. Nurses can help by attending to these issues through compassionate evaluations so that they can offer emotional support and formulate well-rounded care plans in the hope of enhancing their mental and physical well-being. Thus, the nursing assessment of skin, hair, and nails is at the core not only of the process of diagnosing disease states but also of promoting holistic care that recognizes the full spectrum of patient need.

Overview of Assessment Techniques

An adequate skin, hair, and nail assessment is a crucial requirement for nurses as it provides significant information regarding the overall health status of a patient. There are various approaches used to determine these aspects, beginning with close visual inspection. This initial inspection allows the medical practitioner to identify abnormalities in the form of coloration, lesions, or texture alterations, which can be an indication of any underlying health problems. For instance, cyanosis is an indicator of hypoxia, while jaundice is a sign of liver compromise. Palpation comes in after visual inspection as part of the technique that helps to check temperature, moisture, and turgor of the skin, which are also significant indicators of hydration and levels of circulation. These thorough checks help nurses establish a baseline of health and determine any deviation that necessitates investigation or demand for immediate intervention. Inclusion of the patient history in the diagnosis process maximally enhances the understanding of possible dermatologic or systemic conditions. Data on prior medical history, such as any dermatologic disease, allergic conditions, or surgeries, may provide information that will aid in the interpretation of the physical examination. Family history of dermatologic diseases may provide information regarding genetic predisposition, which may render people vulnerable to some diseases. Discussion with patients about their hair and nail conditions is also capable of disclosing behavioral patterns, such as hair-pulling and nail-biting, as repetitive habits that must be resolved through nursing interventions. The example of the evidence of body-focused repetitive behavior disorders, as mentioned in recent studies, sheds light on the importance of thorough assessment of nail and hair conditions alongside their psychological counterparts (Houghton et al., 2015). This multi-faceted approach captures the integration of physical and mental well-being in integral patient care. The use of audiovisual methods in the education for personal hygiene is also able to further enrich nursing evaluation methods. As noted by current evidence, effective health education raises awareness and boosts knowledge of practice regarding personal hygiene in different populations, including disabled children (Akrom et al., 2019). These new methods not only aid in enhancing patient understanding but also assist in the reinforcement of regular skin, hair, and nail examinations. In this regard, the use of technology can assist in the delivery of proper care practices and warning signs through self-assessment. Thus, applying educational strategies alongside conventional assessment techniques has the promise of active patient participation in health through enhanced outcomes by shared responsibility for compliance and consequent awareness. Integrating these strategies, nurses are in a position to optimize practice by realizing holistic assessment of skin, hair, and nails that enables informed individualized patient care (Figure 6.2).

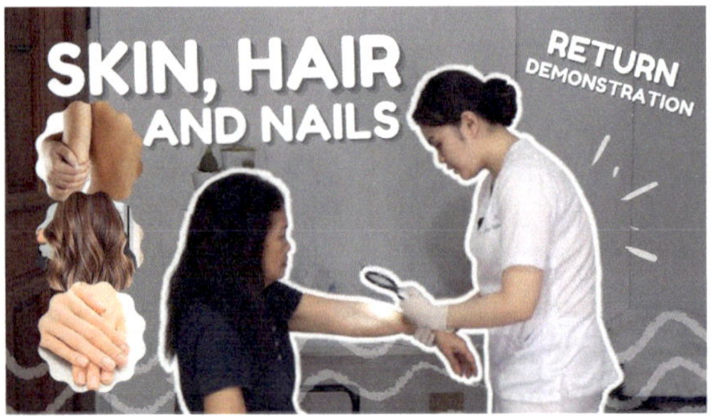

Figure 6.2. Skin, hair, and nails assessment.

Source: https://i.ytimg.com/vi/cgaJ0MOLDX0/hq720.jpg?sqp=-oaymwEhCK4FEIIDSFryq4qpAxMIARUAAAAAGAElAADIQj0AgKJD&rs=AOn4CLCN7FXPmw6r9nI0akLpejNYCUCOcg.

Relevance to Patient Care and Diagnosis

A thorough inspection of the nails, hair, and skin is essential in quality patient care and diagnosis, as integumentary structures mirror underlying diseases. The largest organ is the skin, and while it serves as a barrier, it also functions as a sign of systemic disease. Systemic lupus erythematosus (SLE), for instance, can be manifested as cutaneous signs with more impact on a patient's quality of life. Studies indicate that the most unpleasant of SLE symptoms are musculoskeletal pain, discomfort, and fatigue, and that there is strong correlation between the symptoms and health-related quality of life (HRQoL) scores (Aggarwal et al., 2012). Thus, a detailed assessment that also assesses skin manifestations can help clinicians obtain valuable information regarding patient conditions that require immediate intervention and treatment. In addition to skin assessment, hair and nail evaluation is an important aspect of nursing care that affects diagnosis and patient outcome. Abnormal hair texture or hair loss may be indicative of nutritional deficiencies or endocrine dysfunction, while changes in the nails, such as color alteration or pitting, may be a reflection of underlying systemic disease, including autoimmune disease or fungal infection. These physical signs can guide the nurses' assessment process, enabling earlier identification of potential health issues. Furthermore, identification of interrelationships between nail and hair disease and systemic symptoms can enable patients to be more aware and engaged in their care. For instance, patient education about the significance of nail health as an indicator of overall well-being generates greater awareness and anticipatory healthcare behaviors, ultimately translating into improved health outcomes.

The value of thorough skin, hair, and nail examinations transcends diagnosis; it encompasses the formulation of tailored care plans intended to address the unique requirements of each patient. Effective nursing interventions are largely contingent on data collected through these examinations, which allows for focused therapeutic interventions aimed at the alleviation of symptoms and control of chronic diseases. For example, recognition of the impact of symptoms like pain or fatigue on the performance of a patient may lead to interventions to address symptom management and improved HRQoL, particularly in long-term illnesses like SLE (Bortolotto et al., 2012). Such a method not only puts a huge focus on patient-centered care but also guarantees that the nurses are equipped to adapt their methods as per the dynamic needs of their patients, thereby providing holistic and efficient nursing care that focuses on physical as well as emotional comfort.

6.1. Anatomy and Physiology of Skin

Learning Outcome

1. Structure of the skin layers;
2. Functions of the skin in the body;
3. Common skin conditions and their implications.

The anatomy and physiology of the skin are integral to understanding its role in disease and health. The largest organ of the body, the skin has three primary layers: epidermis, dermis, and subcutaneous tissue. The epidermis is protective and largely composed of keratinocytes, which secrete keratin—a key protein that protects the skin. Beneath the epidermis is the dermis, which contains the blood vessels, nerve endings, and connective tissue that provide structural support and nutrients. The subcutaneous tissue, composed primarily of fat and connective tissue, keeps the skin in place over the underlying structures as well as providing insulation for the body and a store of energy. An understanding of all these layers and their functions is valuable to nursing assessments, as changes or abnormalities in skin structure may be associated with underlying illness.

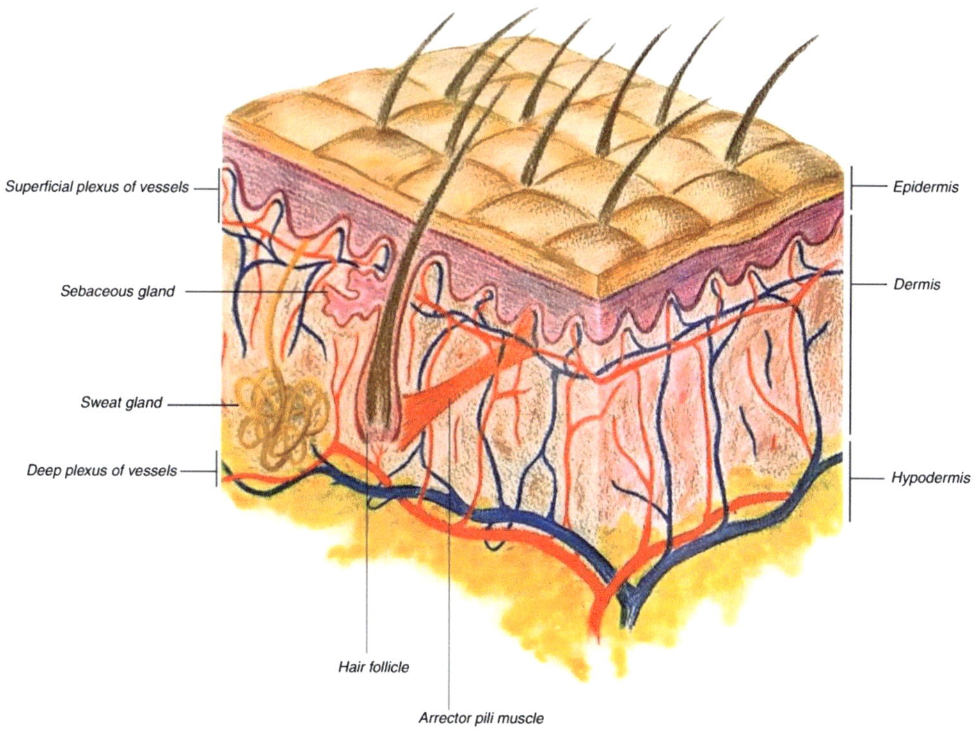

Figure 6.3. Anatomy and physiology of skin.

Source: https://media.springernature.com/lw685/springer-static/image/chp%3A10.1007%2F978-3-319-78310-9_2/MediaObjects/426858_1_En_2_Fig1_HTML.png.

Familiarity with the skin's physiology also encompasses its essential functions in thermoregulation, sensation, and immunological activity. The skin maintains body temperature through mechanisms like sweat production and dilation or constriction of blood vessels. Besides, it has a network of sensory receptors to detect peripheral stimuli so that pain, temperature, and touch can be felt. Sensory input is a significant element in clinical exams since changes in sensation can reveal neurological or systemic disease. The skin likewise plays an important role in the immune system and is a first line of defense against invading pathogens. The presence of Langerhans cells, which reside in the epidermis, allows the skin to react immunologically. A perception of the interactions of these physiological processes assists nurses in assessing patients' general state and predicting potential complications. Skin assessment in practice is more than a check of superficial observation; it requires knowledge of basic anatomy and physiology as determinants of clinical judgment and intervention.

The skill of recognizing signs of skin integrity, such as lesions, rashes, or changes in color and temperature, is important in recognizing various health conditions. For instance, conditions such as psoriasis, eczema, or infection may manifest in the form of some alterations in the skin. Further, assessments that involve hair and nails can provide some insight into systemic health issues, as these structures reflect the overall condition of body health. Through the integration of skin anatomy and physiology with clinical assessment tools, patients can be made safer and improved health outcomes can be achieved, maximizing a patient-focusing strategy to care (Accettola et al., 2023; Nursing, 2020) (Figure 6.3).

6.1.1. Structure of the Skin Layers

The skin, which is the largest body organ, is composed of three major layers: dermis, epidermis, and subcutaneous tissue. The outermost layer, which is the epidermis, plays a critical role in protecting the body from external hazards such as pathogens, UV radiation, and chemicals. Comprising predominantly keratinocytes, the epidermis is of different thickness levels depending on where it is situated on the body. It is not just a mechanical barrier but also participates in the immune response through its resident immune cells, which are capable of recognizing and responding to possible threats. This information is essential to the nursing professionals who assess skin integrity and health for the presence of injury or disease because it describes the structure and function of the epidermis and guides effective intervention plans and patient safety. Beneath the epidermis is the dermis, a thick layer of structural support and elasticity for skin. The dermis is formed from connective tissue, blood vessels, and specialized structures like hair follicles and sweat glands.

This layer is also filled with collagen and elastin fibers, which are what gives the skins flexibility and resilience. Dermal layer is also core to thermoregulation and feeling as it houses nerve endings that respond to touch, pressure, and pain. The nurses must remember these dermal features when conducting skin examination because changes in the texture, turgor, or temperature of the skin can be indicative of underlying medical conditions or systemic disease. The vast understanding of the dermis enables nurses to evaluate and manage skin conditions, ultimately resulting in enhanced patient care. Finally, the subcutaneous tissue, or hypodermis, is a skin-deep interface with deeper structures that harmonizes skin wellness and the functioning of the entire body. This tissue consists primarily of adipose tissue, which insulates, stores energy, and cushions muscles and bones that lie beneath it.

The subcutaneous layer also contains larger vessels and nerves, which contribute to total skin wellness as well as systemic function. In clinical nursing, awareness of the hypodermis and its role is essential, especially during assessments for weight disorders, pressure ulceration, or in patients with compromised vascular status. Effective nursing assessment of the skin, hair, and nails requires an understanding of all skin layers as this will inform abnormality and undertake appropriate interventions that improve skin integrity and patient welfare (Accettola et al., 2023; Chukwu et al., 2018) (Figure 6.4).

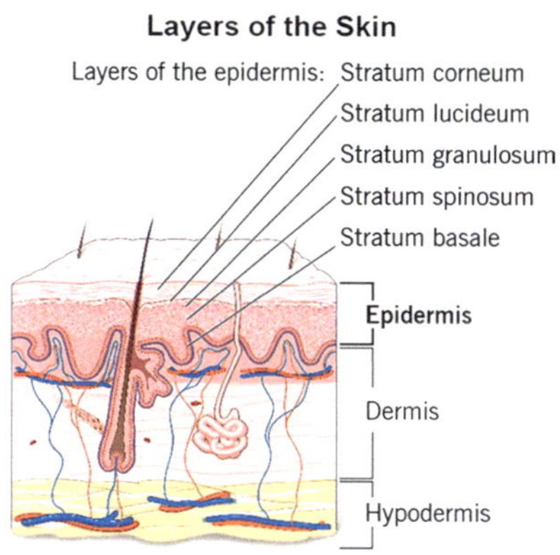

Figure 6.4. Structure of the skin layers.

Source: https://my.clevelandclinic.org/-/scassets/images/org/health/articles/21901-epidermis.

6.1.2. Functions of the Skin in the Body

The skin is also a barrier that protects the body from outside aggressions, including pathogens, UV radiation, and physical trauma. The organ is composed of multiple layers, each contributing to its protective role. Its outer layer, the epidermis, is home to keratinocytes that produce keratin, a protein that hardens the skin but keeps water trapped inside. Further, melanocytes in this layer confer pigmentation that offers a degree of protection against damaging UV radiation.

Maintaining homeostasis also requires a healthy skin barrier to regulate fluid balance and protect underlying tissues from dehydration and infection. Knowledge of the protective mechanisms of the skin is fundamental in the practice of nursing, since compromised skin integrity subjects patients to increased susceptibility to infections and other clinical problems, particularly in vulnerable groups such as the elderly and chronically ill patients (Nolan et al., 1997). In addition to its protective roles, the skin also plays a significant role in thermoregulation. The hypothalamus, which monitors body temperature, works together with the skin's blood vessels and sweat glands to attain thermal homeostasis. When the body gets hotter, skin blood vessels expand (vasodilation), allowing increased blood flow and increased heat loss through evaporation of sweat. During cold temperatures, blood vessels tighten up (vasoconstriction) to reduce blood flow to save body heat.

This thermoregulatory function is particularly crucial during nursing assessments since alterations in body temperature can be indicative of underlying medical pathology. For instance, the patient's cold clammy extremities might signify shock or hypoglycemia, whereas excessively warm extremities can indicate infection or fever (Atkinson et al., 2013). The skin is also a body sense organ, which allows it to respond to the stimuli in the environment with an arrangement of nerve endings within its layers. Sensory receptors, present there, perceive touch, temperature, pressure, and pain and transmit crucial feedback to the central nervous system. Sensory input is significant for protective reflexes and allows an individual to react promptly to hazardous situations. For nurses, a careful inspection of a patient's skin integrity and sensitivity can give important information about neurological and general health. Results outside of the norm, such as loss of sensation and altered skin texture, can be indicative of potential nerve damage or other systemic issues, and reinforce the importance of assessing skin as part of complete patient care (Nolan et al., 1997) (Figure 6.5).

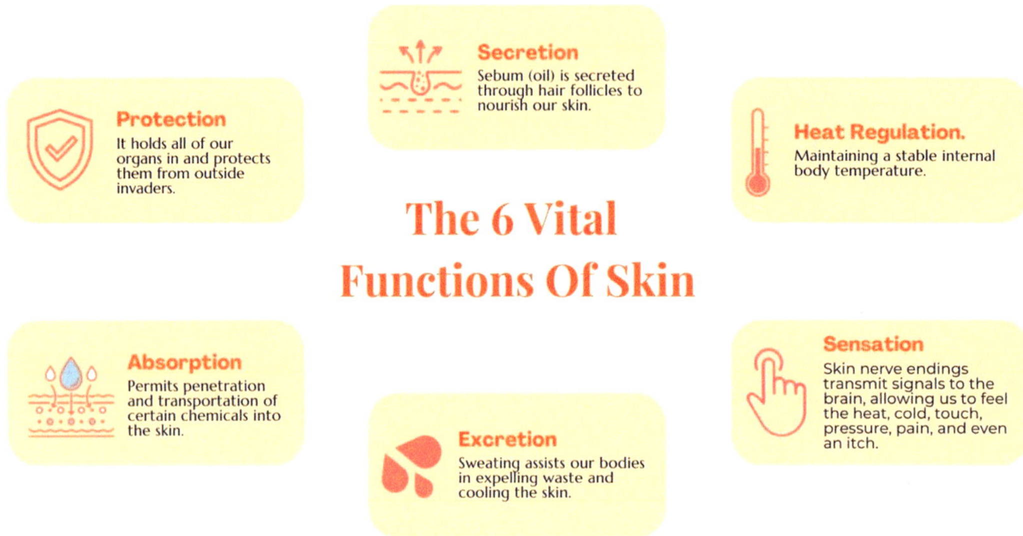

Figure 6.5. Functions of the skin in the body.

Source: https://www.glowsthetics.com/cdn/shop/articles/The-6-Vital-Functions-Of-Skin-1-1536x864.jpg?v=1696989887.

6.1.3. Common Skin Conditions and Their Implications

Skin condition assessment is a critical aspect of the nursing practice with significant implications for patient care. The common skin diseases such as eczema, psoriasis, and acne not only have physical consequences on people but also result in psychological distress and social stigmatization. Eczema, which results in dry and inflamed skin, can lead to discomfort and compromised quality of life due to its chronic nature. Similarly, psoriasis, an autoimmune disease, is expressed as red, scaly plaques that are painful to the touch and psychologically distressing and frequently cause patients to feel isolated. Acne, prevalent among teenagers and young adults, also has the ability to highly disrupt self-concept and body image, essential considerations in assessment and treatment planning by nurses. Awareness of these conditions and their broader influence allows nurses to provide holistic care and support to patients. Nursing input towards the management of common dermatological conditions extends beyond treatment; it also involves patient education and psychosocial support. For instance, advance knowledge regarding the provocation and treatment of conditions like eczema and psoriasis has the potential to empower patients to be more proactive in taking care of themselves. In addition, nurses are expected to confront lifestyle modifications, i.e., the consumption of dietary supplements, which have become progressively well-liked during the last few years. Dietary supplements have become progressively well-liked, increasing concerns about whether they work and whether or not they can produce unwanted side effects, particularly in patients with cutaneous diseases (Djaoudene et al., 2023). Thus, the nurses' job is to guide patients through the evidence-based paths, ensuring they make decisions based on safe practice principles in managing their skin.

Second, the implications of skin disease create particular difficulties for the nursing profession, particularly in developing holistic care strategies addressing both the physical and emotional aspects. Skin diseases like acne and psoriasis carry not only clinical issues, but also significant psychological concerns, which are indicative of the necessity for an interdisciplinary treatment approach. Integration of mental health measures into routine skin assessment could enhance patient outcomes overall since most of these patients struggle with the social implications of their dermatoses (Gefen et al., 2022). By this, the nurses must facilitate open communication; to introduce trust and understanding in order to address the emotional load these disorders pose on patients. By championing a balanced skin examination procedure that combines medical treatment, lifestyle counseling, and psychosocial support, the nurses manage to improve the quality of life of the patients with common skin disorders.

Test Your Knowledge

1. What are the primary functions of the skin, and how do they contribute to overall health?
2. How do the layers of the skin (epidermis, dermis, subcutaneous) differ in structure and function?

6.2. Hair Assessment

Learning Outcome

1. Types of hair and their characteristics;
2. Common hair disorders and their significance;
3. Techniques for assessing hair health.

The assessment of hair in holistic nursing assessment is part and parcel to be able to determine potential health issues and improving patient health. Hair assessment is not only an assessment of the physical condition of the hair, such as texture, distribution, and cleanliness, but overall scalp health. Detailed observation can reveal conditions such as alopecia, fungal infection, or dermatological disease. Moreover, patients hair health will provide clues to nutritional health as well as general health. Data acquired through evaluation of hair can guide nurses when it comes to offering integrative care, as hair usually signals the individual's general physiological status and may even influence psychological status, as well. Hence, thorough evaluation of hair offers precious data about the health of a patient that cannot be overlooked in practice nursing. It cannot be overemphasized that culturally-sensitive practice is vital in hair assessment. Variations in hair types and styles among ethnic groups call for an inclusive policy that is sensitive to each patient's background. An understanding of diverse beliefs about hair grooming and treatment by different cultures facilitates nurses' ability to create personalized care plans that are in line with patients' beliefs and values. In providing care, it is essential that nurses do not jump to conclusions from a patient's hair type and, instead, practice open communication on issues of hair. This interaction not only enhances trust but also quality and comfort of care provided. Enhancing cultural competence in hair evaluation ensures nursing practice as just and responsive, resulting in patient satisfaction and health outcomes (Accettola et al., 2023). In addition, hair assessment can become an integral part of identifying systemic diseases that require further study. For instance, certain textures of hair, regions of hair loss, or unusual textures may indicate nutritional deficiencies or endocrine imbalances that should be treated urgently. Hair care evidence-based guidelines can assist nurses in making the correct assessments and recommendations. Furthermore, the psychological consequences related to hair health—i.e., issues which exist as a consequence of hair loss or scalp diseases—can reinforce a nurse's empathetic care ability. Nurses must also stay up-to-date on recent developments within hair health and personal grooming tendencies that can have an effect on patient attitudes and choices. In aggregate, an evidentiary-based assessment process that is culturally sensitive and comprehensive will improve nursing procedures pertaining to hair examination and support patient-centered care (Fonseca-Miranda et al., 2012) (Figure 6.6).

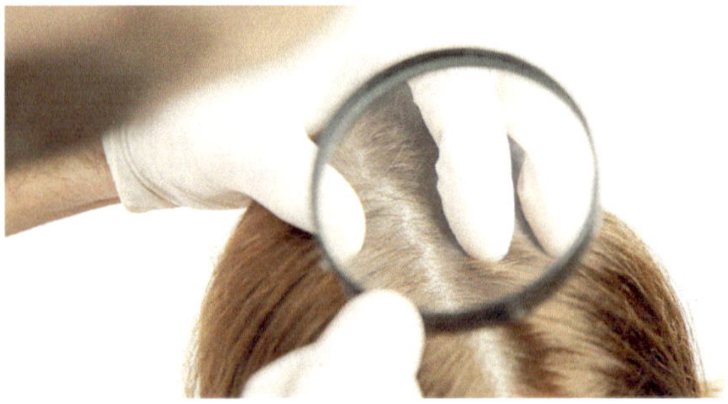

Figure 6.6. Hair assessment.

Source: https://reviveclinic.com/wp-content/uploads/2020/03/Scalp-and-hair-analysis.jpg.

6.2.1. Types of Hair and Their Characteristics

Identifying the types of hair is significant in nursing work since hair is not only a beauty aspect but also a significant indicator of overall health and well-being. Human hair can be classified into three general categories: lanugo, vellus, and terminal hair. Lanugo is the fine, soft hair that everyone has in the womb during pregnancy, which warms and protects them. It usually clears up prior to birth but is seen in newborns. The vellus hair, or peach fuzz, is the soft, fine hairs that cover most of the body and help with thermoregulation. Terminal hair is coarser and pigmented and appears in areas such as the scalp, armpits, and pubic area and is influenced by changes in hormones. All forms of hair contain hair characteristics that determine individualized assessment and intervention in nursing. Besides mere classification, the quality of hair also plays a role based on genetic and environmental factors. Hair texture, density, and orientation may vary significantly among individuals, which may lead to differences in clinical nursing assessments. In disease conditions such as alopecia or trichotillomania, hair loss may reveal underlying psychological or physiological states. Patterns of hair loss may be utilized as indicators for diagnostics, guiding nursing care towards holistic interventions. Further, some environmental determinants such as nutrition, toxin exposure, and grooming patterns affect hair conditions, and hence, a holistic approach must be followed in assessment. Recognition of these characteristics helps the nurses provide focused teaching and interventions, e.g., discussions regarding hair care, prevention, and the psychosocial implications of hair loss or change. Understanding the structure and purpose of different types of hair is also crucial in nursing practice and affects patient education regarding scalp and skin conditions. Besides providing insulation, hair protects the skin from UV rays and minor cuts. Hair health, particularly terminal hair, has a strong relationship with the functioning of sebaceous glands that secrete sebum which lubricates and defends hair follicles. Any straying from the hair growth or appearance can show possible changes such as hormonal imbalances or nutritional deficiencies. For instance, oversimplification or dryness can indicate underlying health problems, including metabolic disorders or dehydration. An entire assessment of hair type and characteristics, thus, significantly enhances nursing exams of skin integrity and overall health, guiding effective nursing interventions and supporting patient health (Banta-Wright et al., 2000; Houghton et al., 2015) (Figure 6.7).

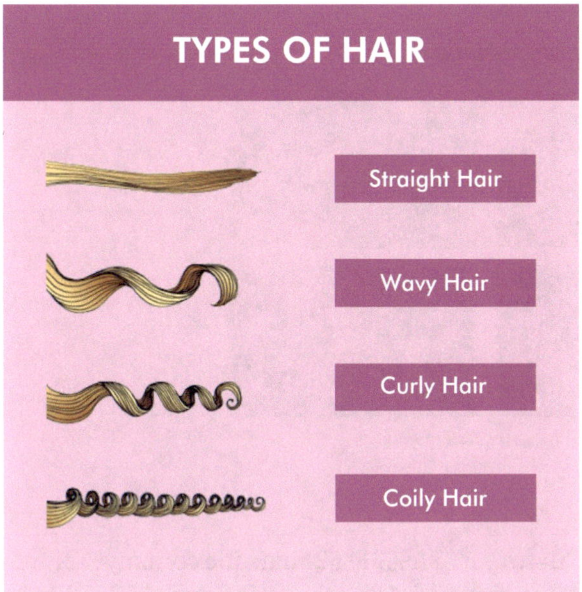

Figure 6.7. Types of hair and their characteristics.

Source: https://blog.paulayoung.com/wp-content/uploads/2023/01/types-of-hair.jpg.

6.2.2. Common Hair Disorders and Their Significance

It is essential that nursing professionals learn about common hair diseases since they influence patients' general health and well-being. Hair loss disorders such as alopecia areata and androgenetic alopecia are the most prevalent in clinical practice. Alopecia areata, an acute condition of hair loss caused by an autoimmune condition, causes psychological distress and reduced self-esteem in victims. On the other hand, androgenetic alopecia, otherwise referred to as male or female pattern baldness, tends to occur gradually and can affect a person's sense of self. Due to this, diagnoses of these disorders allow nurses to create appropriate educational materials and therapeutic practices based on each patient's unique situation, promoting an integrated system of care and promoting psychological health and physical welfare. Besides alopecia, scalp and hair shaft malformations must also be kept in mind by nursing personnel. Trichotillomania, or the condition of compulsive hair pulling, is one disorder that best represents the psychological complexity of hair diseases. Nurses must remain attuned to the clinical manifestation of such disorders so as to facilitate early intervention and treatment of subjects suffering from underlying mental illnesses.

Besides, hair disorders like seborrheic dermatitis and psoriasis are capable of creating a lot of distress as well as impacting a patient's quality of life. By systematically assessing such disorders, nurses are able to initiate appropriate treatment and counsel patients regarding management interventions. The holistic intervention showcases the immense role of nursing in the treatment of the physical symptoms as well as the emotional impact of hair disorders. The significance of proper diagnosis and treatment of hair disease extends beyond the individual patient into more universal concerns of public health. Conditions such as head lice infestation are a vector for transmission in public places, like schools, and can cause a domino effect of anxiety between parents and educators. Intervention at the school level has been shown to enhance understanding of personal hygiene, with an emphasis on why hair health education should be incorporated into community health programs (Accettola et al., 2023).

Moreover, understanding hair disorders offers an opportunity to advocate for early intervention and preventive care, thereby preventing potential complications. Such a proactive approach not only enhances patient care on an individual level but also augments better health outcomes on a community level. Overall, an assessment of hair disorders is a significant part of nursing care, enhancing patient integrative care and public health literacy (Figure 6.8).

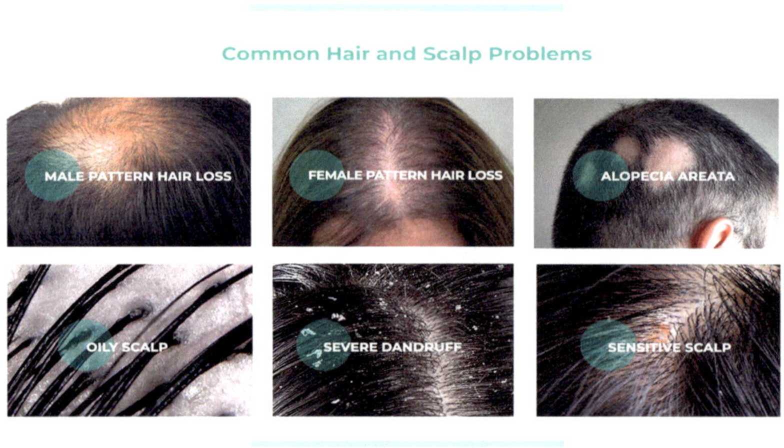

Figure 6.8. Common hair disorders.

Source: https://external-content.duckduckgo.com/iu/?u=https%3A%2F%2Fhairdoc.com.my%2Fwp-content%2Fuploads%2F2020%2F07%2FHair-Issue_Banner.jpg&f=1&nofb=1&ipt=bff2053c785e9b22b55e99291dec89d6057f4a08d186660e162d096d7977bddf.

6.2.3. Techniques for Assessing Hair Health

Assessing the health of hair is a multifaceted process that entails both observational techniques and clinical findings. Visual inspection is one of the first processes in the assessment of the health of hair, by which clinicians are able to view signs of possible pathology such as thinning of the hair, brittleness, or abnormal hair shedding. Examining the quality, texture, and pattern of hairs on the scalp can give clues to the overall health of the individual, which may be determined by a combination of issues such as diet, genetic predisposition, and environmental influences. Additionally important to the assessment is the health of the scalp in general; dandruff or psoriasis, for instance, may influence the quality and development of hair. With a systematic visual inspection, nurses can gather vital information to guide further inquiry or intervention measures to improve hair well-being. The addition of haptic data can complement hair well-being assessment, reporting on hair resistance and strength. Techniques such as the pull test, where a small section of hair is gently pulled to record the resistance of the hair and the extent of the loss, can indicate the stage and type of loss of hair, whether temporary or persistent. Also, examining the elasticity of the hair strand and if it returns to its original shape when stretched can serve as a useful diagnostic tool. Other assessments can include measuring the moisture levels of the scalps, as hair that is soaked in water will appear healthier and stronger than dry hair that is brittle. Such tactile methods combined with visual inspections present a comprehensive method of hair evaluation in nursing practice. Intervention strategies based on the findings of the assessment can be developed to correct the recognized hair-associated health issues. For instance, educational preparation of nurses in the areas of adequate hygiene and care practices, according to health education policy, is greatly essential in maintaining hair health. Implementing personalized hair management practices, such as the application of restorative products or change of diet to enhance nutrients, can best solve issues that patients might experience with their hair. In addition, therapeutic interventions that treat root psychologic issues, including body-focused repetitive behavior disorders (BFRBDs) such as trichotillomania, will be required for certain patients because these issues will foster hair health issues. In working in an integrated manner to combine assessment methods with evidence-based treatments, nurses can actually play a valuable role in improving hair health in their patients (Akrom et al., 2019; Houghton et al., 2015) (Figure 6.9).

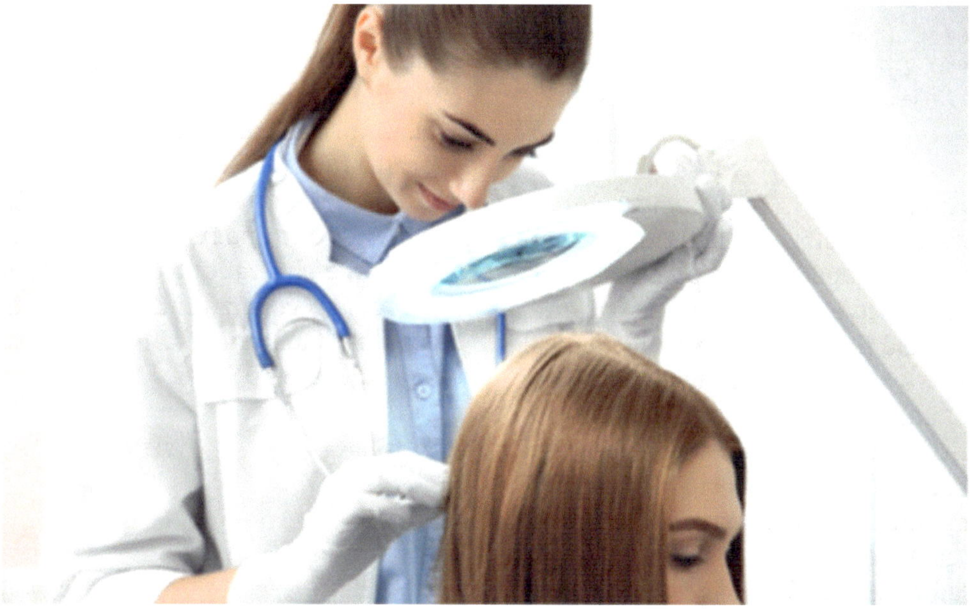

Figure 6.9. Techniques for assessing hair health in nursing.

Source: https://external-content.duckduckgo.com/iu/?u=http%3A%2F%2Fwww.allthingsmindful.org%2Fwp-content%2Fuploads%2F2021%2F04%2Fhair-assessment.jpg&f=1&nofb=1&ipt=b5a1b7509d3129739f3ad320b23e884e76aa77fd54e5144d50a8db0546583cea.

Test Your Knowledge

1. What characteristics of hair should be evaluated during a physical assessment, and why?
2. How can changes in hair texture, distribution, or growth indicate underlying health issues?

6.3. Nail Assessment

Learning Outcome

1. Anatomy of the nail structure;
2. Common nail abnormalities and their meanings;
3. Importance of nail assessment in overall health.

Nail evaluation is also a key component of the complete skin, hair, and nails evaluation in nursing. This aspect of the assessment provides informative data about a patients general health and potential underlying medical illnesses. Nurses should gradually examine the color, shape, and texture of the nails because these qualities can provide indication of systemic processes like anemia, lung illness, and even malnutrition. For instance, clubbing of the nails may point to chronic hypoxia, and spoon-shaped nails may be suggestive of iron-deficiency anemia. These signs are important to recognize early on so that intervention may be initiated, which can lead to more integrated healthcare management, ultimately enhancing patient outcomes. The nails also serve as a good indicator of hygienic habits and personal behaviors that can potentially compromise a patient's health. Nail biting behavior can lead to infections and serve as an indicator of anxiety or stress, and so it needs to be treated with a multi-modal treatment. There has also been exploration of the correlation between nails and behavior under body-focused repetitive behavior disorders (BFRBDs), with individual behavior therapy proving to be effective in treating nail biting problems (Houghton et al., 2015). Identifying these dynamics can help nurses deliver holistic care that transcends the physical expression of disease, taking into account the psychological aspects of nail integrity. Identification of these behaviors can initiate discussions on treatment and coping strategies for the patient through careful nail exams. In conclusion, integrating culturally informed approaches to nail assessment is essential to nursing practice. The worth of diverse backgrounds can impact the understanding and treatment of nail health in diverse populations. The multicultural awareness provides a judgment-free environment that allows patients to speak freely about their nail health. In line with the principles of health promotion, this thoughtful and embracing practice enhances the overall effectiveness of nursing interventions and assessments (Accettola et al., 2023). It treats various determinants of nail health not only to improve clinical outcomes but also to allow patients to recognize and prioritize their health, ultimately facilitating a more holistic nursing care (Figure 6.10).

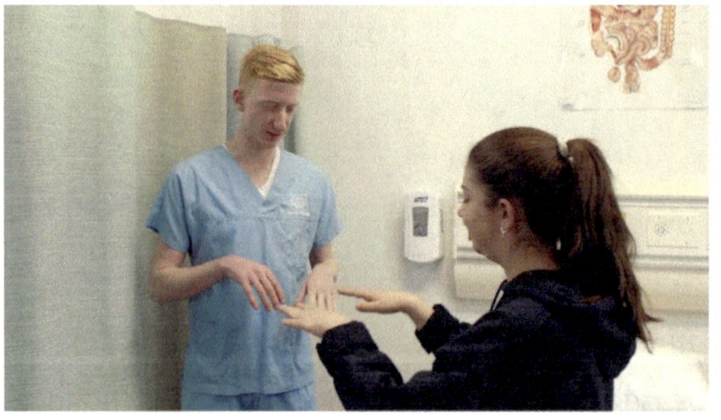

Figure 6.10. Nail assessment in nursing.

Source: https://i.ytimg.com/vi/CXGN89Bkl-0/maxresdefault.jpg.

6.3.1. Anatomy of the Nail Structure

Anatomy of the nail structure is important in the overall assessment of skin, hair, and nails in clinical assessment. Nails are predominantly composed of keratin, a tough protein that provides them with strength and elasticity. Every nail possesses several important structures like the nail plate, nail bed, cuticle, and lunula, which have various functions. The nail plate is the outer part of the nail, visible and enclosing the underlying tissue, while the nail bed contains the nerve endings and blood supply that provides the nourishment to the nail. The cuticle, the thin skin at the base of the nail, acts as an infection barrier. Finally, the lunula, the white crescent-shaped structure at the base of the nail, is engaged in nail growth and development. Identification of these structures is vital for nurses conducting nails' assessment of structure and correlation with overall health. Assessment of the nail structure helps medical practitioners identify a number of possible conditions of health. For instance, a change in nail color, texture, or shape could reflect underlying medical conditions. A pale-colored nail may reflect anemia, while a blue nail could reflect absence of oxygen. Besides, ridging or pitting of the nail surface may suggest skin conditions such as dermatitis or psoriasis. Physical examination findings from detailed examination of the nails may provide valuable information about a patient's internal status. Nurses are asked to pay attention to these findings as part of their course material, and they can be the deciding factor in early treatment and diagnosis. Given the complex interaction between hair, skin, and nails, it is a comprehensive examination that falls within holistic health care for clients, which requires nursing practice expertise. As an education component of nursing, the inclusion of knowledge about nail anatomy in the nursing curriculum is essential in producing competent practitioners. As noted in open education resources, it is essential for nursing professionals to have knowledge of the physical changes of aging and the nail and skin changes when attending to patients with different patient populations. For instance, the aging process brings about thinning and fragility of the nails, and there must be a change in care for older adults. Cultural nail care aspects, such as behaviors that have an effect on nail health and beauty, also emphasize the use of a culturally-sensitive approach. Engaging students with interactive clinical judgment skills can enhance their capacity to assess and manage specific states of nails, ultimately improving patient outcomes in nursing practice (Accettola et al., 2023; Allen et al., 1994) (Figure 6.11).

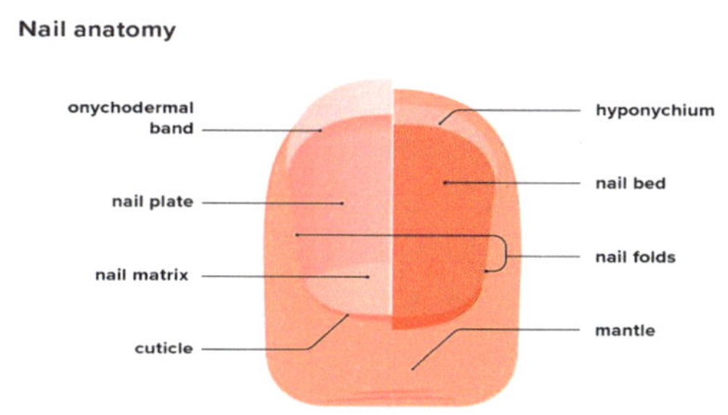

Figure 6.11. Anatomy of the nail structure.

Source: https://media.post.rvohealth.io/wp-content/uploads/sites/3/2024/11/3598932-nail-anatomy-1024x736.png.

6.3.2. Common Nail Abnormalities and Their Meanings

Nail abnormalities are also extreme indicators of underlying health issues and therefore are a mandatory area of focus for nurses in their patient assessments. Yellowing or darkening of the nails is one of the most common nail abnormalities and may be a sign of respiratory illnesses or infections. A yellow discoloration, for instance, may indicate a fungal infection such as onychomycosis, particularly in diabetic or immune-compromised individuals. Moreover, white nails with a blackened nail bed, a condition known as Terrys nails, can be linked to systemic illness such as liver disease or congestive heart failure. With close observation and assessment of such changes, nurses can provide early interventions and referrals, ultimately leading to improved patient outcomes. Observation of structural abnormalities such as clubbing and spoon nails is another crucial element of nail examination. Clubbing, characterized by enlargement of the fingertips and downward curvature of the nails, seems to point to chronic hypoxia and is often found in lung cancer or pulmonary disease. By contrast, spoon nails, or koilonychia, are concave and can signal iron deficiency anemia or generalized diseases. In a clinical setting, these are a complete patient history and might necessitate additional testing. Awareness of the significance of these changes in form enhances the ability of nurses to provide holistic care taking into account the patients' overall health problems. Ridges or lines on the nails can also give clues to the state of health of a person. For example, Beaus lines—horizontal indentations in the nail—can be a sign of severe illness or stress, indicating interruptions to nail growth that are typical of acute conditions like infection or general illness. Nevertheless, vertical ridges, commonly known as onychorrhexis, may be a feature of aging or malnutrition. A complete assessment of these conditions is crucial because they cannot only be a marker of bodily health but psychological health as well, particularly for patients concerned with appearance. Recognition and comprehension of the clinical indicators enable nurses to become more caring and responsive in-patient care, ultimately enhancing overall healthcare management (Howard-Ruben et al., 2014; Namwong et al., 2014) (Figure 6.12).

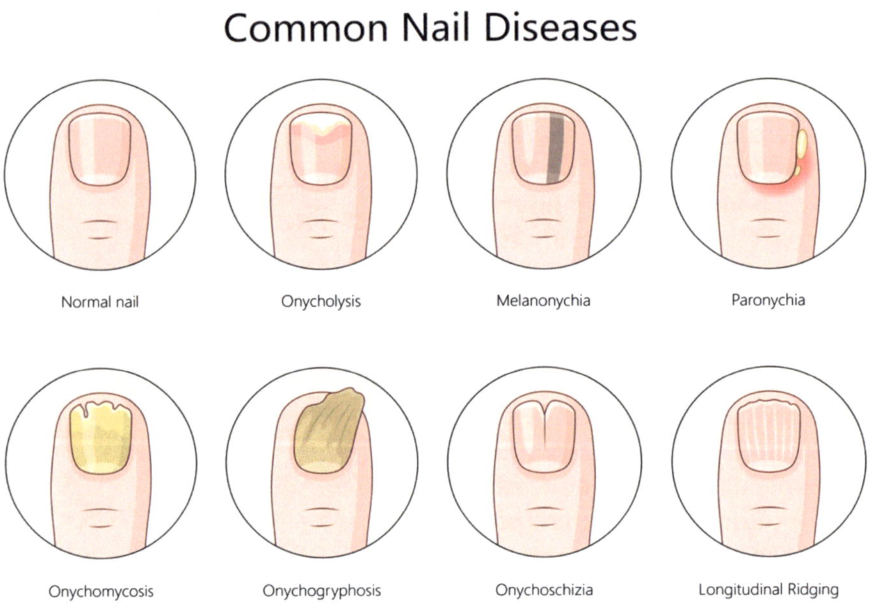

Figure 6.12. Common nail abnormalities.

Source: https://thumbs.dreamstime.com/b/common-nail-diseases-conditions-diagram-medical-nail-diseases-including-onycholysis-melanonychia-paronychia-onychomycosis-358873768.jpg9.

6.3.3. Importance of Nail Assessment in Overall Health

Nail analysis is a significant aspect of determining overall health because nails can be employed as a marker for systemic medical conditions. Nails may mirror medical status, nutritional health, and toxin exposure and thus become an indispensable component of patient assessments in nursing practice. Nail alterations, such as color changes, thickening, or change in shape, may reflect many health conditions, ranging from infections and circulatory problems to even systemic diseases like diabetes or renal disease. From the routine assessment of nails while evaluating health, nurses identify an early indicator of a potential health condition and request further investigation or refer appropriately. Such an anticipatory approach not only enhances the quality of care given to patients but also promotes holistic methods of assessment that consider physical signs to be markers of broader health status. In addition, specific observations in relation to nail condition have been linked to conditions that may have a significant effect on people's quality of life. For instance, a study among renal transplant patients revealed a high prevalence of skin and nail diseases, such as onychogryphosis and onychocryptosis. These findings demonstrate the importance of nail assessment in the detection of complications arising from comorbidities that typically are present with chronic illness. Through the research of scientists, precise examination of the nails can detect patterns recognized to be associated with underlying illness complications, hence enabling more targeted healthcare intervention. This underlines the importance of nursing professionals and students being competent in the identification of nail abnormalities as part of their universal assessment toolkit because it is directly correlated with optimal patient outcomes and health equity promotion. Moreover, observations in nails convey more than bodily health indicators; they give information regarding patients' lifestyle and psychosocial quality of life. Poor nail health can potentially impair self-esteem and body image, leading to potential social withdrawal or psychological distress. Nurses hence must approach nail assessment with sensitivity to the intricate role nails play in an individual's sense of self and welfare. Emphasizing culturally-sensitive approaches, as elucidated in teaching materials like that conducted by Accettola et al. (2023), can help nursing practitioners adjust assessment techniques towards embracing the diversity of patient needs. By integrating nail assessment into general nursing practice, practitioners can facilitate holistic care that addresses physiological and psychosocial components of health, ultimately enhancing patient-oriented outcomes and satisfaction.

Test Your Knowledge

1. What key features of nails are assessed to determine overall health, and what do they reveal?
2. How can nail abnormalities such as clubbing or brittleness provide clues about systemic diseases?

6.4. Assessment Techniques

Learning Outcome

1. Visual inspection methods;
2. Palpation and its role in assessment;
3. Use of diagnostic tools in skin, hair, and nails assessment.

During practice in nursing, techniques for skin, hair, and nail assessment in the evaluation of integumentary system abnormality or disease are central to ensuring holistic care to the patient. Visual examination is the beginning of the assessment, which allows nurses to identify abnormalities or signs of diseases of the integumentary system. Thorough inspection includes noting color changes, abnormal texture, and the presence of lesions or any other abnormality. Observations built from visual assessment can suggest hidden systemic conditions or localized issues. For instance, pigmentation can present symptoms of circulatory disorders or skin diseases, underlining the importance of learning nurses to recognize these essential signs. Competent visual assessment, alongside a sufficient knowledge base in skin pathology, can significantly aid in enhancing patient outcomes and informing related interventions, ultimately reiterating the importance of sufficient assessing strategies within nursing practice. Palpation is also an important evaluation technique that assists in complementing visual examination when assessing nails, hair, and skin. Palpation is a tactile technique employed to assess texture, temperature, wetness, and turgor, which are good indicators of a patient's hydration level and health. Dryness of the skin, for example, may represent dehydration or a dermatologic process, while over-wetness might suggest hyperhidrosis or infectious process. This palpation examination can reveal more subtle changes not observable by visual examination alone. Furthermore, nurses must also examine the hair for distribution and texture, as abnormalities in these may reflect nutritional imbalance or endocrine disturbances. Also, observing nails for brittleness or color change can provide information regarding systemic health disturbance and, therefore, palpation is an invaluable tool in the nurse's tool kit. The inclusion of instructional materials and participation of patients in the assessment of nails, hair, and skin is particularly significant in promoting health awareness and hygiene practice. Effective health education methods, including audiovisual aids, have been effective in improving patients' understanding of personal hygiene and skin care. Such educational interventions are crucial for both healthy and disabled individuals since studies have demonstrated that health education is highly effective in improving knowledge regarding personal hygiene practice (Akrom et al., 2019). Under the concept of body-focused repetitive behavior disorders, including trichotillomania and nail biting, nurses can initiate specific psychological interventions grounded on the basis of findings during assessment, educating patients about the effects of these behaviors on skin integrity and general well-being (Houghton et al., 2015). By incorporating methods of assessment with health education, nurses are able to encourage the culture of proactive care of the nails, hair, and skin, and finally improved patient outcomes and quality of life (Figure 6.13).

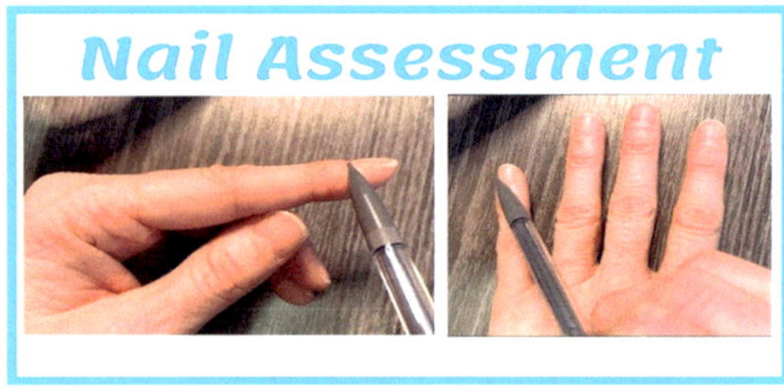

Figure 6.13. Nail assessment techniques.

Source: https://i.ytimg.com/vi/kSARLuC7vzo/mqdefault.jpg.

6.4.1. Visual Inspection Methods

Visual assessment techniques in nursing practice are simple evaluation tools used for observing the skin, hair, and nails. The evaluation process begins with a systematic investigation, which allows medical practitioners to identify abnormalities or changes that are indicators of underlying health issues. Nurses acquire skills to monitor key features such as skin color, texture, and integrity, as well as the condition of the hair and nails. These visual cues not only signal the physical status of a patient but are capable of signaling potential problems with systemic disease too. For instance, pallor signals anemia, and cyanosis is the harbinger of respiratory issues. Moreover, the emphasis on culturally competent techniques also means that nursing assessments are sensitive to variation in skin color and type, which enhances the quality of care and health promotion in multiculturally diverse populations (Accettola et al., 2023). The eye test in dermatological assessment works beyond observation; it requires a discerning eye and good judgment. Adequate eye checks are critical to clinical decision-making because they enable nurses to recognize patterns and irregularities that are not yet obvious as clinical presentations. For instance, conditions such as eczema or psoriasis can frequently be diagnosed by visual signs like scaling and erythema. Visual examination skills are also of the same significance in the evaluation of hair and nails, where alopecia or onychomycosis is diagnosed from visible signs that can be observed on inspection. Therefore, the inclusion of visual examination skills in nursing curricula allows students to learn the skills necessary for efficient assessment of patients, eventually allowing for effective and safe care to be provided (Mehrtash et al., 2024). In addition, the inclusion of interactive clinical judgment practice in nursing study materials emphasizes the importance of honing visual observation skills. By employing nursing students in real-life settings mirroring actual assessments, educators can make their students confident and precise in such key skills. By these methods of education, not only is the prioritization ability of the learners enhanced, but it is also ensured that they are in a position to respond instantly to any indication of health deterioration. Cultural competence also comes to the forefront of the effectiveness of visual inspection skills since it allows nurses to notice and understand the diverse presentations of the skin, hair, and nails among diverse populations. A sound basis in visual inspection skills thus improves nursing practice and maintains the commitment to providing equal health outcomes for all patients (Accettola et al., 2023).

6.4.2. Palpation and Its Role in Assessment

Palpation as an underlying component of physical assessment performs a vital role in skin, hair, and nail examination in nursing. Palpation is a manual technique that allows the examiner to obtain important information utilized for the identification of abnormalities or pathological conditions. By manipulation of the skin and deeper tissue, nurses are able to evaluate texture, temperature, moisture, and tenderness. For instance, skin palpation may reflect evidence of dehydration and inflammation, while assessment of nails may reflect systemic diseases like clubbing or cyanosis. Additionally, nurses are also able to feel slight variations in subcutaneous tissue and muscle tone as well as possess a greater overall understanding of a patient's health. Use of palpation in conjunction with other evaluation procedures enhances clinical judgment, and therefore clinical decision-making, in patient care, particularly among populations of diversity where culturally targeted strategies are vital to effective assessment (Accettola et al., 2023). Additionally, the use of palpation is essential in the evaluation of the skin and its appendages as part of the comprehensive nursing assessment. These assessments not only look at surface characteristics but also query for underlying tissue status, therefore offering valuable clues about a patient's general condition. As an example, an astute nurse may palpate for lymphadenopathy when assessing skin lesions, and it may be evidence of underlying infections and malignancies. Further, the technique allows for scalp and hair assessment to detect scalp conditions or irregularities in hair texture, which may suggest nutritional deficiency or skin conditions. This would call for skill and knowledge, pointing once more towards education and practice in honing palpation skills by nurses. Through this skill, students acquire the ability to synthesize evidence into usable care plans that eventually enhance patient outcomes and safety (Luca et al., 2014). Its application during the assessment process is particularly crucial in nursing education because it provides a platform for clinical practice. By promoting awareness of how to correctly use this ability, nursing educators enable students to be prepared with the skills needed to conduct intricate and sophisticated assessments. Adding palpation to nursing education promotes awareness of clinical judgment models that maintain patient care as the foremost consideration. Educators can also utilize simulation and interactive training drills to reinforce these skills so that they can practice in a safe environment before taking their skills to work on patients. Therefore, the ability to perform palpation successfully not only adds to the student's set of skills but also leads to improved clinical judgment that can make a significant contribution to the health outcome for all types of patient populations. Finally, learning about palpation reiterates the value of tactile examination skills so that graduating nurses are well-positioned to fulfill the complex needs of their patients (Accettola et al., 2023) (Figure 6.14).

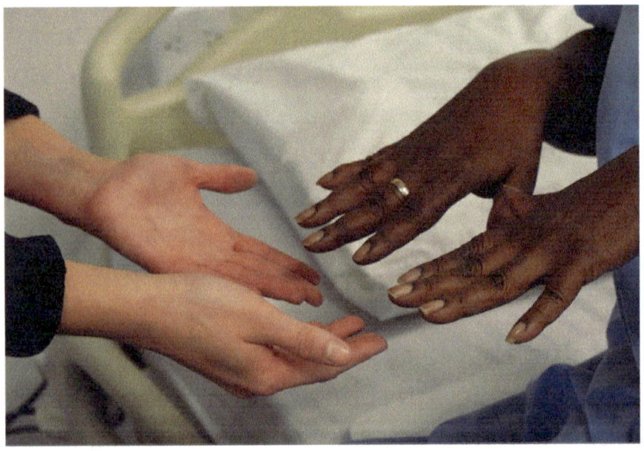

Figure 6.14. Palpation and its role in assessment.

Source: https://pressbooks.library.torontomu.ca/assessmentnursingmain/wp-content/uploads/sites/421/2022/12/DSC00122-scaled-1.jpg.

6.4.3. Use of Diagnostic Tools in Skin, Hair, and Nails Assessment

Skin, hair, and nail examination in nursing interventions is necessary for the identification of various conditions impacting health. The application of diagnostic tools efficiently allows nurses to conduct thorough evaluations that transcend physical examinations. For instance, devices such as dermatoscopes allow one to view skin lesions at a microscopic level, thereby enhancing the distinction between malignant and benign tumors. Furthermore, skinfold calipers can measure subcutaneous fat, helping to assess nutritional status, while tools like Wood's lamp can detect fungal infections or pigmentation disorders. These instruments are vital in fostering a proactive approach to patient care, allowing healthcare professionals to identify issues early. This initial diagnosis is especially crucial in disadvantaged populations where there may be restricted access to specialized dermato-logical care and where nurses tend to be the first contact when it comes to detecting dermatological conditions (Accettola et al., 2023).

In addition to traditional approaches like medical history taking and physical examination, the integration of technology has revolutionized dermatological diagnosis. Teledermatology, on the other hand, allows nurses to utilize computerized images and patient files to obtain expert opinion from specialists over distance, widening the reach of expert evaluation. This advancement is not just critical for improving patient outcomes but also for timely interventions, which could stop further complications. Furthermore, mobile apps now assist nurses in recording and monitoring skin diseases over time, making it easier to observe change and act on it. Placing a high value on education regarding these instruments ensures that nursing professionals are up to date with the use of advanced technology. Ongoing training increases their diagnostic proficiency, hence improving patient management outcomes in skin, hair, and nail examinations (Waller et al., 2015).

For maximal effectiveness of such diagnostic devices, there must be an overall strategy founded on patient history and psychosocial factors. Skin, hair, and nail disorders often reflect systemic disorders, and ascertaining these relationships is most critical in nursing diagnosis. For instance, changes in the growth patterns of the hair or texture of the nails may reflect hormonal or metabolic disorders. Therefore, relating diagnostic equipment with comprehensive patient histories adds to a comprehensive evaluation. Nurses can utilize diagnostic tool results to inform patient discussions about their health behavior, lifestyle, and environmental exposures, thus enhancing health literacy. The multidimensional profile facilitates the establishment of therapeutic alliances and patient activation of the care processes, ultimately leading to improved health outcomes (Accettola et al., 2023).

Test Your Knowledge

1. What techniques are used to assess the skin, hair, and nails, and how do they ensure accurate findings?
2. How can inspection and palpation be combined to detect abnormalities in skin, hair, or nails?

6.5. Cultural Considerations

Learning Outcome

1. Variations in skin, hair, and nails across different ethnicities;
2. Impact of cultural practices on assessment;
3. Importance of cultural competence in nursing.

Culture plays an important role in nursing assessment, particularly when evaluating the nails, hair, and skin. Cultures influence how people perceive their skin health, their grooming, and what beauty is. Nurses must consider these cultural spectacles during history taking from patients since there are people who may have certain rituals or products essential for their hair and skin. For example, there are societies where cosmetic product use is a normal part of life, and there are others that emphasize minimalist approaches. Understanding and valuing these practices can assist in an improved nurse-patient relationship, such as better communication and trust. Through the delivery of culturally competent care, nurses can personalize assessment and interventions and thereby maximize health outcomes and make patients feel valued and understood. Evaluation of skin disease in culturally diverse individuals requires that nurses keep themselves abreast of the prevalence and presentation of different dermatoses among different ethnic groups. Certain skin illnesses are endemic to particular groups and therefore need modified assessment procedures. For instance, individuals with darker pigmentation have different presentations for the same pathology, e.g., keloids or disorders of skin color. Since diabetes rates are rising among populations, with the projection that maybe up to 30% of diabetic patients will have skin problems at some stage, nurses need to modify protocols to meet these specific challenges (David et al., 2021). By incorporating cultural elements into such assessments, nurses can effectively anticipate and manage the skin complications posed by chronic diseases. Similarly, cosmetic use and its health impacts need to be considered in the context of culture when assessing skin, hair, and nails. In the case of different ethnicities, different mind sets regarding the utilization of cosmetic products influence not only their utilization but even their side effects. Evidence has indicated that there is extensive use of cosmetics by some groups, particularly women, but not much about potential health hazards of using such products (Hasan et al., 2020). Nurses are in the best position to educate patients on cosmetic skin problems and encourage informed choices. Awareness programs can be developed to combat these issues based on safe practices and the importance of making individuals aware of the potential side effects of cosmetics. With the help of sensitive education in cultures, nurses can help individuals make appropriate choices in accordance with beliefs while protecting the skin.

6.5.1. Variations in Skin, Hair, and Nails Across Different Ethnicities

It is essential for nurses doing assessments to know the variations of skin, hair, and nails in different ethnicities since they have a potential to significantly influence both the appearance and health of an individual. Ethnicity tends to define some characteristics in these features; e.g., individuals of African descent are typically found to have tighter curly hair, while individuals of Asian descent can have straighter and shinier hair.

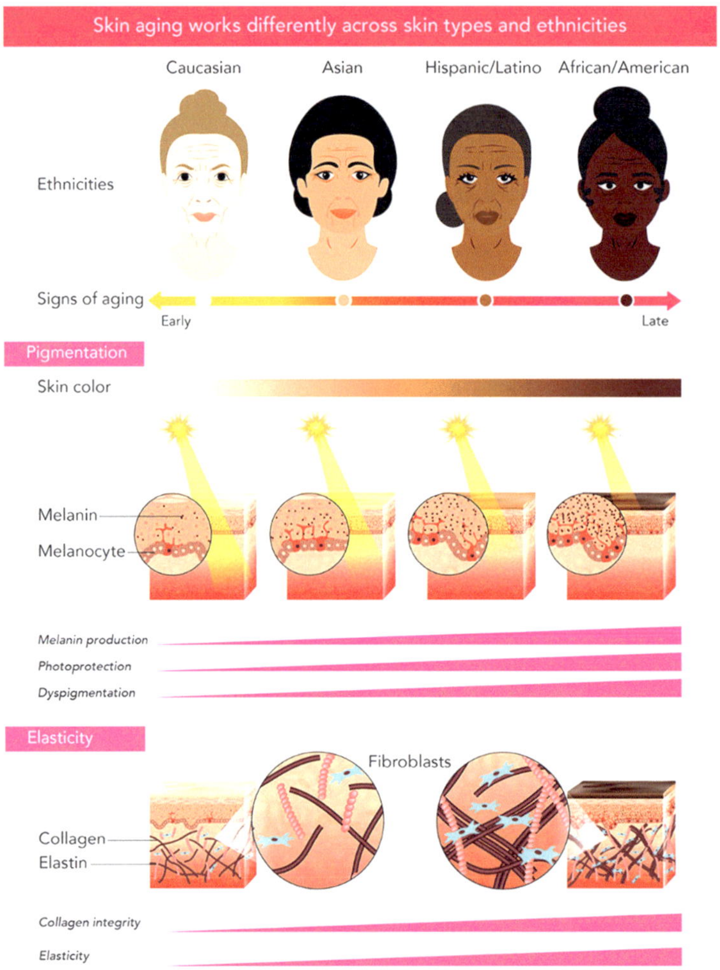

Figure 6.15. Variations in skin across different ethnicities.

Source: https://cosmeticsbusiness.com/article-image-alias/does-ethnicity-affect-how-our-skin-2.png.

Variations in hair texture can impact scalp care, grooming practices, and the health of the hair in general, and need to be considered in assessments. In addition, coloration of the skin is what is accountable for determining susceptibility to certain dermatologic diseases, such as hyperpigmentation in dark skin. Thus, with an appreciation of these differences comes not only better nursing assessment but also culturally responsive care that honors and respects unique health differences and brings individualized and appropriate intervention to all patients. Beyond the physiological, cultural importance of these differences is their direct impact on an individual's health experience and impression of treatment. For example, pale skin may be associated with increased vulnerability to skin cancers due to increased sensitivity to UV light, whereas dark skin offers some resistance but at the cost of delayed diagnoses of conditions such as melanoma. Nurses must be comprehensively trained in these variations so that they are able to communicate effectively with patients about their specific risk level and self-care behaviors. Significantly, culturally responsive nursing care can increase compliance and trust in treatment among patients because those who feel they are comprehended tend to engage in their health-care processes. Awareness of these differences is, therefore, fundamental to advocating for consistent health outcomes among populations with diverse differences while practicing holistic nursing care. Moreover, nail differences among different ethnic groups are also extremely important and cannot be overlooked in nursing exams. Nails may vary in thickness, shape, and growth patterns based on both genetic and environmental reasons, reflecting general health complications or dietary deficiencies. For instance, individuals of Asian ancestry are likely to have relatively wider nail beds, and individuals of African descent are more likely to have diseases such as onycholysis. Nurses can identify potential associated health complications specific to some populations based on knowledge of these variations. By assessing the status of skin, hair, and nails against ethnic origin, nursing professionals can identify early systemic illness and offer targeted education on preventive care. Last but not least, the use of this knowledge in nursing practice instills a climate of inclusiveness and personalized care for patients from different backgrounds because knowledge of the unique attributes of each individual significantly enhances overall health outcomes and patient satisfaction (Figure 6.15).

6.5.2. Impact of Cultural Practices on Assessment

Cultural beliefs play a very vital role in shaping what constitutes healthy or normal appearances, and healthcare providers must be well-informed of and consider these influences in assessments. For instance, patients from specific ethnic groups may have unique hair textures and skin types to be handled with up-to-date knowledge for assessment. This cultural nuance is not merely what underpins the physical examination but also patient-nurse interpersonal interaction since respect for convention may create trust and improve overall health care. Excellent nursing education, such as that provided by the instrument designed for use with undergraduate nursing students, prioritizes these culturally-sensitive practices as being at the heart of professional practice (Accettola et al., 2023). Besides, cultural attitudes typically inform practices concerning hair and skin care, and these may impact the outcomes of assessment. The majority of patients can have conventional treatments or have some skincare routines depending on their cultures, thus possibly influencing the condition of their skin and hair. For instance, the use of oils, herbs, or certain cleansing procedures alters the outlook of rashes or infections on the skin, and nurses should correctly interpret them in order to provide appropriate care. If nurses learn these customs, they will better be able to assess symptoms and make effective interventions for patient education and treatments. Thus, integrating cultural sensitivity into nursing assessments not only enhances clinical thinking but also produces the setting for patient-centered care on the basis of individual values and beliefs (Saqinah et al., 2024). Last but not least, the intersection of cultural practice and nursing assessments is the means to achieve equivalent health outcomes. Culturally sensitive practice enables nurses to observe diversity in patients' presentations and behaviors, which impacts clinical decisions directly. As the nursing field continues to recognize cultural competence, resources providing theoretical basis and practical application of culturally-sensitive assessment practices become invaluable. Such instructional focus equips prospective nurses with the competence to successfully prioritize care, ultimately meeting the unique needs of a diverse patient base. By cultivating sensitivity to skin, hair, and nails differences in cultures, nursing procedures can lead to improved patient satisfaction and health outcomes, validating the importance of a holistic approach in healthcare (Accettura et al., 2023).

6.5.3. Importance of Cultural Competence in Nursing

Cultural competence in nursing is essential to provide equitable and effective care, particularly while taking history of skin, hair, and nails. As diverse patients are now being received by healthcare providers, cultural beliefs, values, and practices about skin conditions are the most important to know. Cultural norms and societal expectations may affect patients' understanding of skin, hair, and nails. For instance, the definitions of certain skin diseases vary widely across cultures, and they can affect compliance of patients with treatment regimens. By cultural competence, nurses can tailor the assessment to account for such variation, thereby optimizing patient cooperation and results. Thirdly, culturally competent assessments bridge communication gaps, enhance trust, and pave the way for more effective therapeutic relationships, which are an essential aspect of nursing practice (Aggarwal et al., 2012). Furthermore, holistic skin, hair, and nails assessments involve comprehending how cultural factors influence health-related behaviors. Different ethnic groups possess unique characteristics concerning these assessments, such as hair texture or color differences in the skin. This understanding allows nurses to provide accurate assessments and not culturally influenced ones that will lead to misdiagnosis or inappropriate treatment. Moreover, cultural competence allows nurses to communicate with patients in a way that is respectful, recognizing, and affirming each individual's particular history and experience. Not only does this improve clinical outcomes, but patient satisfaction and overall improved healthcare experience result as well. Thus, cultural competency incorporation in nursing practice and education is a necessity to equip nurses with skills necessary to deal with the intricacies of skin, hair, and nails examinations (Aggarwal et al., 2012). Lastly, cultural competency importance transcends the single patient to encompass the entire healthcare setting. As health systems increasingly recognize the value of diversity, the integration of culturally competent care into the nursing practice ensures that healthcare is made available and accessible to all, fairly. The necessity of culturally competent care is particularly urgent in populations with inherent health disparities. In such situations, nurses must continue their education on cultural competence, ultimately translating this into their assessments and care plans. By doing so, they contribute to making a more welcoming health culture where diverse patients are given better understanding and respect. Not only does cultural competence enhance patient assessments but also creates a healthier population through ensuring health equity and improving the quality of care for diverse populations (Accettura et al., 2023) (Figure 6.16).

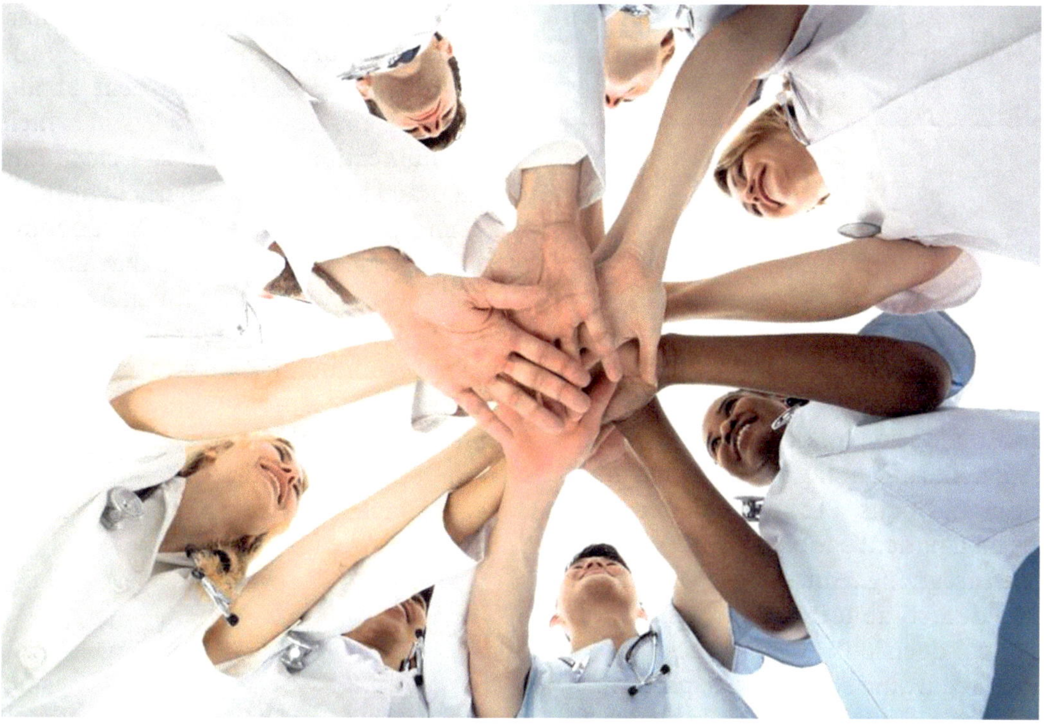

Figure 6.16. Importance of cultural competence in nursing.

Source: https://blog.diversitynursing.com/hs-fs/hubfs/culturalcompetence.jpg?width=1000&name=culturalcompetence.jpg.

Test Your Knowledge

1. How can cultural differences in skin color, hair type, or grooming practices influence assessment findings?
2. Why is it important to be culturally sensitive when evaluating and documenting skin, hair, and nail conditions?

6.6. Documentation and Communication

Learning Outcome

1. Best practices for documenting assessments;
2. Importance of clear communication with healthcare team;
3. Role of patient education in assessment findings.

Careful documentation and communication are essential elements in nursing hirsutism diagnosis of hair, skin, and nails. Proper documentation of findings on a patient's integumentary system enables the caregiving team to observe changes over time, detect abnormalities, and make correct clinical decisions. For instance, precise descriptions regarding skin lesions, patterns of hair loss, or nail shape can be quite insightful regarding intrinsic health status. Taking part in systematic documentation ensures legal compliance and ensures continuity of care, making all relevant patient information available to all team members. Furthermore, possessing sophisticated documentation tools, such as electronic health records (EHRs), facilitates communication by allowing timely updates and notifications regarding patient status. This emphasizes the significance of documentation as a collaborative tool, thereby improving patient outcomes and facilitating an integrated approach to nursing assessments across different healthcare settings. Incorporating evidence-based practice into documentation and communication practices further enhances the effectiveness of skin, hair, and nails assessment in nursing. As identified in nursing literature, utilization of standardized assessment tools and audit systems can promote homogenous data collection and interpretation by practitioners, and this will yield enhanced patient care. For example, utilization of an infection prevention quality audit tool in operating theaters not only promotes compliance but also enhances communication among multidisciplinary teams so that they are all well informed on infection control measures (Engelbrecht et al., 2017). This plan illustrates the ways in which formal communication channels can close knowledge and practice gaps, particularly in difficult clinical settings. Additionally, precise documentation enables timely interventions that allow the nurse to successfully advocate for their patient. Thus, evidence-based documentation approaches and proper communication are crucial to uphold nursing assessment standards and patient safety. Additionally, good documentation and communication in nursing create an environment that is conducive to professional development and mentorship.

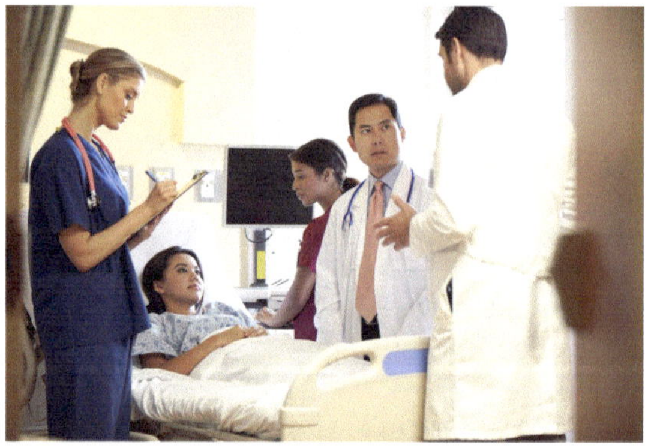

Figure 6.17. Documentation and communication in nursing.

Source: https://medcominc.com/wp-content/uploads/2019/12/doctors-nurse-patient-discussion.jpg.

The acquisition of such skills is emphasized particularly at the transition-to-practice stage for new nurses, who benefit from experience that enhances their assessment skills. Mentorship opportunities such as the Perioperative Orientation, Education, and Mentoring (POEM) program emphasize the importance of proper documentation and effective communication within the perioperative setting, circumventing common errors associated with discharge assessments and post-op care (Johnstone et al., 2016). Through organized direction and constructive criticism of documentation abilities, experienced nurses assist in the growth of their mentees as well as the enhancement of patient assessment and care quality in general. Finally, encouragement of good documentation and communication habits not only improves clinical practice but also facilitates professional development for nursing professionals, ultimately leading to quality patient care in the specialty of skin, hair, and nails examinations (Figure 6.17).

6.6.1. Best Practices for Documenting Assessments

An integrative approach to assessment documentation in nursing is necessary to ensure clear and consistent patient care, particularly for skin, hair, and nails assessments. Effective documentation not only documents the current status of a patient's condition but also serves as the basis for future clinical decision and intervention. Best practice demands that assessments are objective, utilizing standardized language and clear descriptions to document the findings. This creates an up-to-date record accessible to all members of the health care team. Where nursing staff assist with personal hygiene, as in bed bathing, note should be taken not only of the interventions performed, but also of the patient's response and any alterations observed in skin integrity that might suggest underlying generalized health problems (Downey et al., 2013). Furthermore, the incorporation of a systematic assessment documentation process enhances interprofessional communication. As a fundamental requirement of effective collaboration, healthcare professionals must understand other professionals' findings and conclusions concerning the patient's skin, hair, and nails. Specific findings such as rashes, lesions, or unexplained hair loss should be recorded in an orderly manner. This enhances mutual understanding among nurses, physicians, dietitians, and other professionals involved in the care of patients. Moreover, the application of visual aids or template assessment tools can enhance documentation to be more lucid and uniform in application. For instance, employment of a guided assessment tool would improve the acquisition of critical details of a nutrition-directed physical examination as emphasized in nutrition assessment training models (Tyler et al., 2017). Finally, engagement of patients in documentation of assessment can be very beneficial. Having the ability to elicit the patient's complaints regarding their skin, hair, and nails is not only empowering but also is one method of bringing to light necessary information that might not be so obvious to health professionals. Documenting must also reflect this patient involvement through consideration of their subjective accounts, which can better characterize their state of health than anything else. Therefore, best practices in patient care documentation consist of objective observation and subjective opinion, hence ensuring an all-inclusive approach for the best overall results. By encouraging proper communication and documentation skills, nursing practitioners are able to considerably enhance the quality of care provided in such as skin, hair, and nails assessment.

6.6.2. Importance of Clear Communication with Healthcare Team

Effective communication of the healthcare team is a foundation of providing quality patient care, particularly in conducting skin, hair, and nails examination among nursing. The process entails the coordination of various medical practitioners, including doctors, nurses, and dermatologists, who must harmonize their efforts to identify possible dermatological issues. Good communication ensures every team member knows their own role and the patient's special needs, which is essential for accurate assessments and care planning.

Misunderstandings or communication errors might lead to inconsistencies in patient assessments and cause missed diagnoses or inappropriate care plans. Therefore, emphasis on open communication fosters teamwork culture and accountability, which ultimately leads to improved patient outcomes in nursing practice. Furthermore, the significance of good communication does not stop at face-to-face patient assessment and continues to document and reporting. All medical professionals who participate in skin, hair, and nails assessment are required to document observations and findings thoroughly to achieve a seamless story in the patient's medical record. This facilitates continuity of care and allows follow-up caregivers to make decisions based on correct information. Inadequate reporting or poor documentation of findings can lead to lost nursing care, as is noted in research findings that examine the root causes of patient management gaps (Andersson et al., 2021).

By applying sound communication practices, healthcare teams are better placed to minimize the likelihood of errors and facilitate the exchange of all relevant information among members in a timely and comprehensive manner, ultimately leading to enhanced patient safety. Towards this end, the collaboration setting in nursing practice necessitates that all participants feel they are empowered to raise their observations and concerns regarding skin, hair, and nails observations. This ensures that a culture of embracing feedback is established and with the integration of diverse input into patient care. Frequent open communication between nursing professionals and experts not only enhances the credibility of observations but also enhances thoroughness in patient care. Through actually engaging in discussion regarding their observations, healthcare professionals draw upon a shared understanding of areas of concern and collaborate toward the best action. Intersubjectivity of this type is necessary to address the complexities involved in skin disease, making effective communication a necessary pillar of holistic nursing care to this region (Gefen et al., 2022) (Figure 6.18).

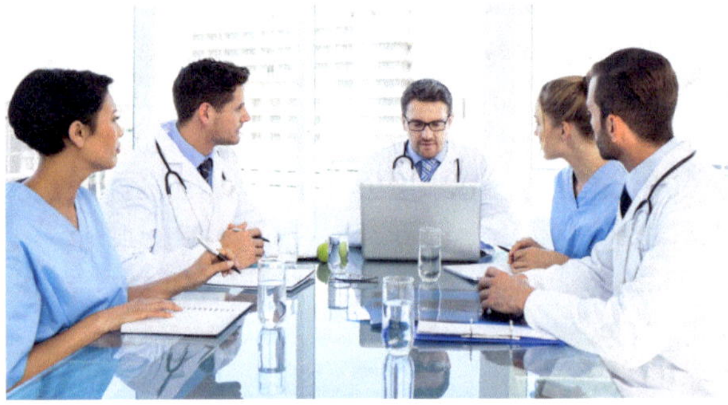

Figure 6.18. Importance of clear communication with healthcare team.

Source: https://www.sermo.com/wp-content/uploads/2023/02/effective-communication-img6-min-1050x555.jpg.

6.6.3. Role of Patient Education in Assessment Findings

Patient education is key to the results of skin, hair, and nail assessment findings in nursing practice. Effective patient education brings an informed environment where patients can perceive body changes that may suggest underlying conditions. With a lack of knowledge of normal and abnormal appearance or sensation, patients will miss indications of potential problems. For instance, by educating patients on how to screen themselves, nurses empower patients to report anomalies such as discoloration, lesions, or hair loss more effectively. This proactive engagement not only aids in the early detection of conditions but also enhances the nurse's ability to interpret findings comprehensively and accurately, resulting in improved patient outcomes and earlier interventions, especially in high-risk groups that may be more vulnerable to dermatological conditions. Moreover, patient education initiatives such as pamphlets and workshops can facilitate patient knowledge about self-care practices conducive to skin, hair, and nail health. A quality improvement project highlighting the importance of hygiene practices in minimizing surgical site infections demonstrated that even though healthcare workers use prophylactic practice, patients' compliance at home is necessary for efficacy (Hasan et al., 2018). By including patient education in their evaluations, nurses have the potential to make significant impacts on patients' behaviors with regards to skincare and hygiene after a procedure. When patients learn about how to preserve their skin's integrity and about early signs of infection or complications, they become more likely to follow the appropriate care guidelines, which eventually translates to improved surgical outcomes and decreased healthcare costs related to complication management. Incorporating culturally responsive practice in patient education is essential in effective nursing assessment and intervention. The use of inclusive resources that respond to varied populations ensures that all patients receive relevant information that suits their specific backgrounds, which could lead to increased understanding and adherence to health recommendations (Accettola et al., 2023). For example, patient education among various ethnicities and races involves the consideration of particular skin conditions prevalent among these communities, which may enhance the effectiveness of assessment findings. As soon as patients feel that attempts made are educational and respectful of who they are, they are more likely to communicate effectively with health providers. Ultimately, successful patient education can bridge health literacy gaps and maximize collaboration between patients and nurses, leading to improved health outcomes with skin, hair, and nail assessment.

Test Your Knowledge

1. How should findings from skin, hair, and nail assessments be documented to support continuity of care?
2. What communication strategies can nurses use to effectively report abnormal assessment findings to the healthcare team?

SUMMARY

The assessment of skin, hair, and nails is a significant component of nursing practice that demands a complete understanding of their contribution to overall health. These structures not only serve as protective coverings but also contain significant indicators of systemic disease that may be underlying. For the practicing nurse, observation of abnormalities such as color, texture, or changes in hair loss can indicate underlying pathology necessitating further assessment. An astute determination of these attributes becomes a priority in early diagnosis and treatment ultimately, resulting in enhanced patient outcomes in treatment. Second, integration of best practice evidence in skin, hair, and nails assessment can in fact enhance the quality of nursing care provided. As noted in most studies, for example, the importance of avoiding surgical site infection (SSI), education on hygiene and skin care among patients can go a long way towards enhanced health outcomes. For instance, measures such as preoperative education of patients on proper hygienic measures assist in equipping them with the knowledge to aid in their recovery, thereby reducing infection and complication rates (Hasan et al., 2018). Such education is important in instituting health literacy and establishing a collaborative relationship between healthcare workers and patients. Last but not least, theory-practice congruence in skin, hair, and nails assessment improves nursing practice and education. Utilized tools, such as preparing teaching materials on skin disinfection techniques, demonstrate the focus on holistic patient care (Ala-Luhtala et al., 2011). With increasing proficiency in utilizing assessment findings to support clinical interventions, nurses will be better equipped to advocate for the needs of patients and deliver tailored interventions. By prioritizing careful observation of skin, hair, and nails, nursing practitioners enhance their own practice while also contributing something worth returning to the wholeness of their patients' health.

The assessment of nails, hair, and skin is a highly significant component of nursing care because it is an important tool for gauging overall health and detecting possible medical conditions. The observation of the skin does more than inform us about hydration and circulation; it signals possible underlying conditions, e.g., infection or systemic disease. The intricacy that is involved in conducting meticulous assessments—ranging from visual inspection to palpation—heightens the requirement for nurses to develop keen observing skills. Second, there is new evidence highlighting the merit of optimizing assessment processes, especially in the operating room. This is evidenced through demonstration of how inefficient protocols for preparing the skin for surgery can lead to increased rates of surgical-site infection. Hence, access and quality of evidence-based protocols are core elements for patient safety and optimal nursing performance (Fonseca-Miranda et al., 2012). Nurses should also value the broader significance of physical assessments of the skin, hair, and nails beyond mere sensory information. Understanding the lived world of people, particularly elderly individuals, enriches the assessment process by allowing the care providers to reach the care table with compassion and sensitivity. The experiences of aging skin reflect deeper existential realities—patients are often confronted with strangeness while attempting to maintain their sense of self. Engaging with patients within the context of their experiences and incorporating their stories into care, nurses can make interventions more individualized to honor the patient's dignity and aid psychological health. Such holistic understanding leads to a nursing practice that recognizes patients as complete people rather than mere physical bodies essential to effective caregiving (Adam et al., 2018). Incorporating an integrative understanding of skin, hair, and nails leads nursing assessments beyond technicality, imparting emotional intelligence to clinical practice. For instance, discussion of skin integrity may serve as launching points to explore themes beyond, such as self-image, interpersonal relationships, and history. Nurses need to have discussions with patients that affirm emotional feelings regarding alterations in the body, resulting in a more holistic method of care. Second, strict adherence to evidence-based standards in both routine and specialty assessments not only reaffirms clinical information but also aligns nursing practice with contemporary standards of care. With these values, nurses are making a tremendous impact not only to the treatment outcome of individual patients but also to the general growth of the nursing profession, creating the demand for continuous enhancement and acquisition of skills in skin, hair, and nail assessment (Adam et al., 2018; Fonseca-Miranda et al., 2012).

KEY TERMS FROM THIS CHAPTER

- Epidermis
- Dermis
- Subcutaneous Tissue
- Sebaceous Glands
- Sweat Glands
- Melanin
- Pallor
- Cyanosis
- Jaundice
- Erythema
- Lesion
- Turgor
- Edema
- Alopecia
- Hirsutism
- Nail Clubbing

CRITICAL THINKING QUESTIONS

1. **Which of the following is the primary function of the skin?**
   a. Production of hormones
   b. Protection against infection and injury
   c. Filtration of blood
   d. Regulation of electrolytes
2. **During a skin assessment, a nurse notes a lesion with a circular shape and a raised border. This is most likely:**
   a. Macule
   b. Papule
   c. Nodule
   d. Ringworm (tinea corporis)
3. **Clubbing of the nails is commonly associated with which condition?**
   a. Hypothyroidism
   b. Chronic hypoxia or lung disease
   c. Iron deficiency anemia
   d. Diabetes mellitus
4. **Which of the following is an expected finding in aging skin?**
   a. Increased elasticity and turgor
   b. Thinner epidermis with decreased sebaceous activity
   c. Increased melanin production
   d. Rapid wound healing
5. **When assessing hair, a nurse finds patchy hair loss with brittle strands. This may indicate:**
   a. Fungal infection
   b. Poor nutrition or endocrine disorder
   c. Normal aging
   d. Excessive washing

Short Answer Questions

1. What are the primary functions of the skin in maintaining overall health?
2. List the key components of a complete skin assessment.
3. How can changes in skin color indicate underlying systemic conditions? Give examples.
4. What techniques are used to assess skin temperature, texture, turgor, and moisture?
5. Why is it important to examine the scalp and hair during a physical assessment?

Answer to Critical Thinking Questions

1. (b) 2. (d) 3. (b) 4. (b) 5. (b)

REFERENCES

1. Accettola, E., Bogdan, A., Callahan, S., Chawda, S., et al. (2023). Introduction to health assessment for the nursing professional: Part II. https://core.ac.uk/download/622362029.pdf (accessed on 16th July 2025).
2. Adam, S., Baker, A., Beeckman, D., Blume-Peytavi, U., Bullington, S., Carville, K., et al. (2018). A lifeworld phenomenological study of the experience of living within ageing skin. https://core.ac.uk/download/157860846.pdf (accessed on 16th July 2025).
3. Aggarwal, R., Almehed, K., Bauernfeind, B., Bjelland, I., Bombardier, C., Brennan, P., Moberg, C., et al. (2012). An exploration of patient-reported symptoms in systemic lupus erythematosus and the relationship to health-related quality of life. https://core.ac.uk/download/29017094.pdf (accessed on 16th July 2025).
4. Akrom, A., Erviana, E., Hidayati, T., Nurasa, N., et al. (2019). Health education improves behavior and self-efficacy on personal hygiene among children with intellectual disability. https://core.ac.uk/download/480549857.pdf (accessed on 16th July 2025).
5. Al Ghamdi, H. S., Abukhelaif, A. E. E., Croft, M., Yusif, M., Al Ghamdi, H. A., & Mangi, A. (2020). Assessment of prevalence, awareness and practices regarding cosmetics harmful effects among Saudi female university students of Albaha, Saudi Arabia. *Journal of Pharmaceutical Research*. https://www.semanticscholar.org/paper/ce87ee0a402d293156f8ba50a3de5a3043fee4ce (accessed on 16th July 2025).
6. Ala-Luhtala, J., & Kaasalainen, E. (2011). Surgical site skin disinfection: A desired guideline. https://core.ac.uk/download/38038366.pdf (accessed on 16th July 2025).
7. Allen, M. C. (1994). The normal physiological aspects of aging as they relate to nurse aid care. https://core.ac.uk/download/560696978.pdf (accessed on 16th July 2025).
8. Andersson, I., Bååth, C., Nilsson, J., & Eklund, A. (2021). A scoping review—Missed nursing care in community healthcare contexts and how it is measured. *Nursing Open, 9*, 1943–1966. https://doi.org/10.1002/nop2.945 (accessed on 16th July 2025).
9. Atkinson, P., Edmonds, B., Eve, F., Glazebrook, C., et al. (2013). Guideline for UK midwives/health visitors to use with parents of infants at risk of developing childhood overweight/obesity. https://core.ac.uk/download/18620563.pdf (accessed on 16th July 2025).
10. Balboa-Barreiro, V., Couceiro-Sánchez, E., García-Rodríguez, M. T., González-Martín, C., et al. (2023). Podiatric skin and nail involvement and biomechanical pathology in renal transplant recipients: Assessment of the foot as a contributing factor to their health. https://core.ac.uk/download/595770811.pdf (accessed on 16th July 2025).
11. Banta-Wright, S., & Campbell, J. (2000). Neonatal skin disorders: A review of selected dermatologic abnormalities. http://digitalcommons.georgefox.edu/cgi/viewcontent.cgi?article=1004&context=sn_fac (accessed on 16th July 2025).
12. Barratt, M., Bail, K., & Paterson, C. (2022). Children living with long-term conditions and their experiences of partnership in nursing care: An integrative systematic review. *Journal of Clinical Nursing, 32*, 3185–3204. https://doi.org/10.1111/jocn.16429 (accessed on 16th July 2025).
13. Bortolotto, L. A., Brunorio, L., Consolim-Colombo, F. M., Giribela, A., et al. (2012). Distances walked in the six-minute walk test: Suggestion of defining characteristic for the nursing

diagnosis ineffective peripheral tissue perfusion. https://core.ac.uk/download/268297821.pdf (accessed on 16th July 2025).

14. Chukwu, R., & Mankila, J. (2018). Dermatology nurses' job description: Literature review. https://core.ac.uk/download/161432240.pdf (accessed on 16th July 2025).

15. David, P., Yeola, M., & Ankar, R. (2021). Efficacy of nursing skin care protocol on prevention of skin related problems among newly diagnosed diabetic patients. *Journal of Pharmaceutical Research*. https://www.semanticscholar.org/paper/6791257a05249dd39bfbb25d0e7a5348a1f7e626 (accessed on 16th July 2025).

16. Dawnay, N., & Sheppard, K. (2023). From crime scene to courtroom: A review of the current bioanalytical evidence workflows used in rape and sexual assault investigations in the United Kingdom. *Science & Justice, 63*, 206–228. https://doi.org/10.1016/j.scijus.2022.12.006 (accessed on 16th July 2025).

17. Djaoudene, O., Romano, A., Bradai, Y. D., Zebiri, F., Ouchene, A., Yousfi, Y., Amrane-Abider, M., et al. (2023). A global overview of dietary supplements: Regulation, market trends, usage during the COVID-19 pandemic, and health effects. *Nutrients, 15*, 3320–3320. https://doi.org/10.3390/nu15153320 (accessed on 16th July 2025).

18. Downey, L., & Lloyd, H. (2013). Bed bathing patients in hospital. https://core.ac.uk/download/4147609.pdf (accessed on 16th July 2025).

19. Engelbrecht, L. (2017). The development of a comprehensive infection prevention quality audit tool for operating room theatres in a private health care environment. https://core.ac.uk/download/188769498.pdf (accessed on 16th July 2025).

20. Fonseca-Miranda, Y., Gama, Z. A. S., Peñalver-Mompeán, M. D., Saturno-Hernández, P. J., et al. (2012). Evaluación de la normalización de la preparación prequirúrgica en una red regional de hospitales. https://core.ac.uk/download/268297837.pdf (accessed on 16th July 2025).

21. Gefen, A., Alves, P., Ciprandi, G., Coyer, F., Milne, C., Ousey, K., Ohura, N., et al. (2022). Device-related pressure ulcers: SECURE prevention. Second edition. *Journal of Wound Care, 31*, S1–S72. https://doi.org/10.12968/jowc.2022.31.sup3a.s1 (accessed on 16th July 2025).

22. Hasan, M. (2018). Educational prevention program of surgical site infections at a metropolitan pediatric hospital. https://core.ac.uk/download/216990516.pdf (accessed on 16th July 2025).

23. Houghton, D. C., & Woods, D. W. (2015). Evidence-based psychosocial treatments for pediatric body-focused repetitive behavior disorders. https://core.ac.uk/download/213076990.pdf (accessed on 16th July 2025).

24. Howard-Ruben, J. A. (2014). The symptom experience of patients receiving epidermal growth factor receptor inhibitors. https://core.ac.uk/download/48610130.pdf (accessed on 16th July 2025).

25. Johnstone, E. M. (2016). Perioperative orientation, education, and mentoring (POEM) program. https://core.ac.uk/download/147835250.pdf (accessed on 16th July 2025).

26. Luca, A. (2014). Care management process in appendectomy nursing. https://core.ac.uk/download/236412577.pdf (accessed on 16th July 2025).

27. Mehrtash, M. (2024). Avoidant attachment, coping styles, and body image in adults with trichophagia and onychophagia disorders. https://core.ac.uk/download/616423931.pdf (accessed on 16th July 2025).

28. Namwong, T. (2014). Nursing practice guideline for foot care for patients with diabetes in Thailand. https://core.ac.uk/download/228192907.pdf (accessed on 16th July 2025).
29. Nolan, M. (1997). Gerontological nursing: Professional priority or eternal Cinderella? https://core.ac.uk/download/56526.pdf (accessed on 16th July 2025).
30. Nursing. (2020). *Nursing Student Handbook.* https://core.ac.uk/download/541430864.pdf (accessed on 16th July 2025).
31. Saqinah, A. W., & Hidayah, E. (2024). Menstrual education in improving women's health: Scientific and cultural perspectives. https://core.ac.uk/download/617858071.pdf (accessed on 16th July 2025).
32. Saranya, S. (2014). A comparative study to assess the effectiveness of laptop assisted teaching versus child-to-child approach regarding personal hygiene among school age children in selected corporation school at Choolai in Chennai. https://core.ac.uk/download/235669154.pdf (accessed on 16th July 2025).
33. Tyler, C. A. (2017). Incorporating simulations of the nutrition-focused physical exam into graduate-level dietetics curriculum. https://core.ac.uk/download/213424322.pdf (accessed on 16th July 2025).
34. Waller, T. (2015). Physical assessment of children with FASD: Evidence based practice. https://core.ac.uk/download/162578507.pdf (accessed on 16th July 2025).

HEAD, FACE, NECK, AND LYMPHATICS ASSESSMENT IN NURSING

7

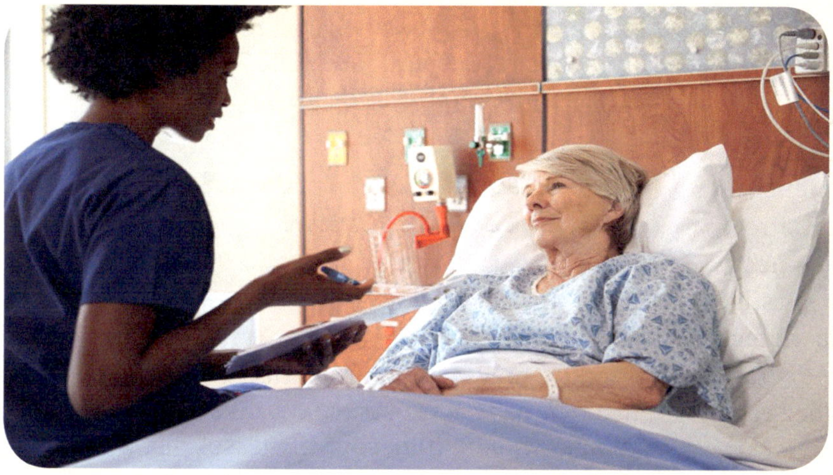

LEARNING OBJECTIVES

After studying this chapter, you will be able to:

1. Elaborate the anatomy of the head and neck;
2. Illustrate the assessment techniques;
3. Describe the common conditions and disorders;
4. Identify the cultural considerations in assessment;
5. Discuss about documentation and reporting;
6. Explore nursing interventions.

Introduction

In nursing, expert assessment of the head, face, neck, and lymphatics is critical in comprehensive assessment of a patient's overall health status. The assessment not only aids in identifying any potential medical conditions, but also serves as the foundation for effective diagnosis and treatment planning. The intricate anatomy of these regions demands keen insight into their structure and function. These are typically performed first by nurses; thus, it becomes their skill which is vital in the early detection of problems such as infection, tumors, or systemic disease. Nurses utilize keen observation and palpation to gain critical information which contributes to a patient's medical record and information about the trajectory of their health, and hence enhance the interdisciplinary care provided to them. The relationship of the lymphatics with the face, neck, and head defines a broad variety of clinical implications. With the knowledge of the complexity of this anatomical region, nurses can appreciate the importance of their findings to patient care. For instance, immune function relies heavily on the lymphatic system, and dysfunction of the system can indicate serious health conditions. Evaluation of cervical lymph nodes is particularly pertinent to oncology since nodal involvement is one of the strongest prognosticators in conditions such as oral/oropharyngeal squamous cell carcinoma (OSCC). New techniques like sentinel node biopsy (SNB) have changed the way nurses and other health care workers assess lymphatic involvement, and an ongoing education and proficiency in these procedures are needed.

This practice change mirrors the significance of integrating new technology developments into nursing assessment to improve patient outcomes. The addition of an examination of the entire head, face, neck, and lymphatics to evaluation within nursing practice not only prepares nurses to detect immediate health concerns but allows them to note patterns that can suggest underlying systemic issues. Presented in the form of an address to a diverse audience comprised of practicing healthcare professionals as well as nursing students, this essay will look at the importance of assessment techniques and their effect on patient care. Through a consideration of current best practice, clinical practice, and the underpinning research evidence, this essay aims to raise awareness about holistic patient assessment. Apart from that, with the application of evidence-based best practices and recommendations, nursing practitioners can enhance their skillset to the maximum, thereby promoting improved quality care for the patient. This comprehensive introduction sets the stage for a critical examination of the head, face, neck, and lymphatics assessment methods, thus contributing to an enrichment of knowledge in the nursing profession (Figure 7.1).

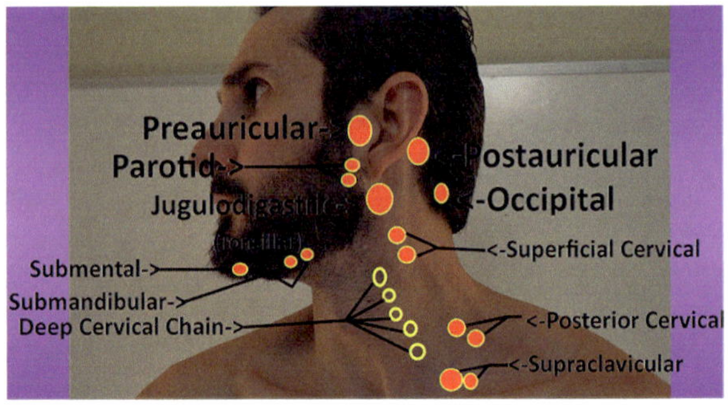

Figure 7.1. Head and neck assessment nursing.

Source: https://www.registerednursern.com/wp-content/uploads/2017/10/Health-Assessment-Lymph-Node-site.png.

Importance of Head, Face, Neck, and Lymphatics Assessment

Assessment of the head, face, neck, and lymphatics is a significant aspect in nursing practice due to its implications in the diagnosis of many medical complications. The head and neck have vital structures like the brain, sensory organs, and central vessels, making it necessary for nurses to perform thorough assessments. These assessments identify anomalies or abnormalities that can indicate underlying health complications. For instance, examination of the lymph system can identify infections or malignancies, and so there is a need for monitoring the health of lymph nodes as this suggests systemic disease. Additionally, localized examination plays a pivotal role in early identification of diseases, which results in improved patient outcomes and offers a chance for timely interventions. It is not merely routine to include a head and neck assessment; it is a fundamental nursing responsibility that is involved with disease prevention and health promotion. Nurses need to be competent in the identification of risk factors of head and neck complications, such as those palpable in older patients or cancer patients. The increase in the diagnosis of cancer, as highlighted in present studies, renders this assessment procedure an acute requirement. Cancer, being the leading cause of death globally, demands a keen consideration to identify symptoms early on (N/A, 2021). Lymphatic system assessment for this purpose is equally important because changes in lymph nodes might signal the advancement or recrudescence of malignancies, therefore placing emphasis on nurses' responsibility in monitoring patients' health beforehand. Further, the intricate relationship between head, face, neck, and systemic overall health is too involved to be overemphasized. For instance, lymphatic disease often appears in the forms of swelling or pain in the head and neck, which can lead to life-threatening consequences if unaddressed. Nurses are at the forefront of being caregivers who not only perform these assessments but also educate patients on what signs and symptoms to look out for and report on their own behalf. Awareness of possible danger and preventive measures plays a critical role in the management of chronic diseases, including cancer and cardiovascular disease. The ability to perform a comprehensive assessment of the head, face, neck, and lymphatics thus contributes to nursing practice and fosters an environment where anticipatory care can flourish, ultimately promoting patient well-being and quality of life (Petrashenko et al., 2017).

Overview of Nursing Roles in Patient Assessment

In head, face, neck, and lymphatics examination, nursing practice extends well beyond superficial data collection; it involves a general interaction with patients that allows for a holistic understanding of health. Nurses are first observers who are able to detect early abnormalities by observing and palpating. For example, when assessing the neck area, a nurse can check the range of motion, check for lymph nodes, and observe for swelling, each finding that could be indicative of underlying medical conditions. Nurses also help patients communicate with doctors so that patients can clearly report symptoms and worries. Such pre-emptive action is critical in recognizing conditions such as lymphedema, in which timely intervention makes a considerable difference to patients' experience, underlining the central function of nursing in patient-centered care and examination procedures. Instructional aspects integrated into nursing activities also make an important contribution to patient assessment. Patients are best instructed by nurses on what to expect from tests, which minimizes anxiety and maximizes compliance.

By explaining the significance of the head, face, neck, and lymphatic check-up, nurses empower patients to take an active role in their own wellness. Besides, constant education about diseases such as lymphedema is needed since improper control is mostly the result of ignorance. Research has indicated that the majority of healthcare professionals are poorly prepared to diagnose and treat lymphedema, which increases patient distress and makes recovery more difficult (Dreiling et al., 2022). Thus, nurses not only assess physical well-being but also provide patient awareness, fostering a culture in which patient education enables patients to control their statuses better. Lastly, the role of nurses in encouraging shared care cannot be overelaborated, particularly in treating complicated diseases like cancer. With approximately half of the men and one-third of the women eventually getting cancer in their lifetime, nursing's role in assessing not just physical symptoms but emotional and psychological well-being is paramount (N/A, 2021). During comprehensive assessment, nurses assess patient response, monitor treatment side effects, and recognize signs of distress, affirming medical and individual needs. By actively engaging with interprofessional groups, nurses help create individualized plans of care focused on addressing the immediate medical requirements as well as the overall psychosocial characteristics of health, thereby maximizing overall patient outcomes. Such an extended role is a demonstration of the central role played by nursing in patient assessment in fields such as oncology and others (Figure 7.2).

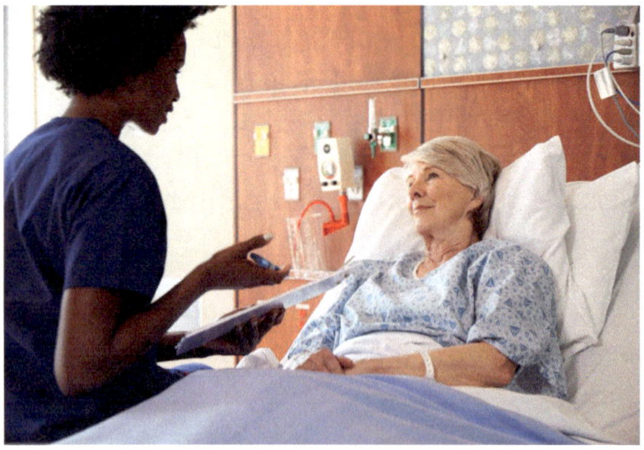

Figure 7.2. Nursing roles in patient assessment.

Source: https://wtcs.pressbooks.pub/app/uploads/sites/31/2020/08/361341143-huge-1024x683.jpg.

7.1. Anatomy of the Head and Neck

Learning Outcome

1. Key structures of the head;
2. Anatomy of the neck;
3. Lymphatic system overview.

The intricate anatomy of the head and neck offers a critical foundation for nursing assessments, particularly in terms of the vascular and muscular structures inherent to normal physiological function. The vascular anatomy in this region includes significant arteries like the common carotid and vertebral arteries, responsible for supplying blood to the brain and maintaining cerebral circulation. An understanding of these vascular pathways, along with any potential anatomical variations, is critical to nurses. For instance, trifurcation or quadfurcation terminations of the basilar artery, which have been demonstrated to occur in a high percentage of cases, can have critical ramifications in surgeries involving access to this region. Understanding these differences allows nurses to provide comprehensive care and anticipate patient management issues in intervening procedures (Jayapala et al., 2024). Apart from the vascular components, head and neck anatomy comprises various muscular components that facilitate movement and functioning. The neck itself comprises such essential muscles as the sternocleidomastoid and trapezius that assist in rotating, flexing, and stabilizing the head. Nurses must be proficient at assessing these muscles for dysfunction or tension, which is often an indicator of more critical health issues. Also, because this region has lymph structures, immunological defense becomes a component of this system as well. Lymph nodes are located strategically throughout the head and neck, and their inspection can give indications of infection or malignancy during assessments. The ability to palpate such nodes effectively is a nurse's competence that enhances with experience as nurses develop their skills, thus enhancing the opportunities for early diagnosis of potential health problems (Iddagoda et al., 2024). Lastly, head and neck assessment transcends basic anatomical education because it also entails screening of cranial nerves that perform sensory and motor functions. Each of the twelve cranial nerves has distinct functions, ranging from the olfactory nerves (CN I) for smells to the vagus nerve's (CN X) role in autonomic control of various body activities. Nurses must exercise additional care in examination of these nerves in physical assessments to ascertain patients' neurological function, especially those with symptoms like facial asymmetry or numbness. An extensive evaluation can reveal important health information and guide additional diagnostic tests if necessary. Knowledge of the anatomical and functional relationships within the head and neck supports a holistic practice of nursing, offering quality patient-centered care during the evaluation (Iddagoda et al., 2024) (Figure 7.3).

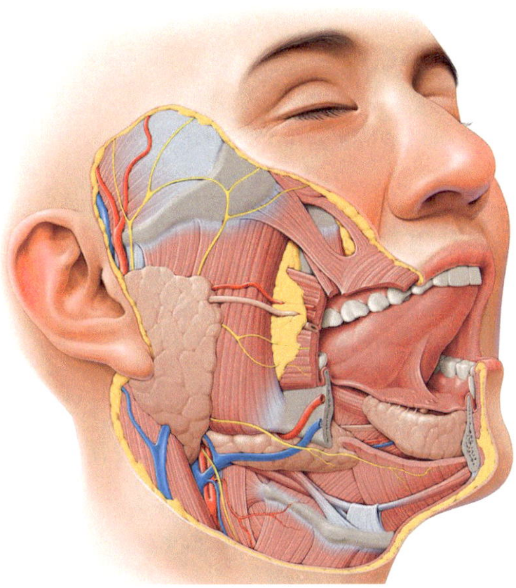

Figure 7.3. Head and neck anatomy.

Source: https://www.kenhub.com/thumbor/PD_d8HT-_hWCO2fqTDV0dcQpsj0=/fit-in/800x1600/filters:watermark(/images/logo_url.png,-10,-10,0):background_color(FFFFFF):format(jpeg)/images/article/head-and-neck-anatomy/uv0hJrE7NmPhrsFqOfj72A_Head_and_neck_anatomy.png.

7.1.1. Key Structures of the Head

The head is a complex structure consisting of numerous interconnected components that are of immense significance in the context of assessment in nursing. The skull is the covering for the brain, and the depiction of the frontal, parietal, temporal, and occipital bones highlights the importance of these bones. These bones enclose the central nervous system, which they safeguard against physical damage while offering attachment for facial movement and expression muscles. Assessment of these head structures is significant to nurses since head trauma has the potential to significantly affect neurological function. Profound understanding of cranial anatomy enables medical professionals to detect potential traumas or deformations that may need to be treated or assessed further. Overall, accurate assessment of head structures is an essential consideration when forming differential diagnoses in patient examinations across different healthcare settings. Other than the skull, the face holds numerous structures vital for a broad range of processes ranging from reception of sensory data to communication. Facial structure is mainly made up of the orbits, the nasal cavity, and the maxillary region, all of which have an important role to play in the sensory processes of seeing, smelling, and tasting. The facial muscles, which receive innervation from the facial nerve (cranial nerve VII) in great extent, not only contribute to expressions of emotion but also assist in functions such as chewing and speech. Thus, any deformities in these structures may suggest underlying neurological impairments or trauma and necessitate a strict policy during tests. For nurses at the practice level, understanding these relations enhances their ability to conduct comprehensive assessments and provide timely interventions in patients with facial injury or dysfunction-related symptoms, resulting in better patient outcomes. The lymphatic system of the head and neck plays an integral role in the immune response and homeostasis of body fluids. Key structures include the cervical lymph nodes, which are positioned to filter out harmful substances from lymph fluid and permit immune surveillance. In order to evaluate a patient's neck and head, nurses must palpate the nodes to search for such aberrations as swelling or tenderness, which may be indications of infections or cancers (Accettola et al., 2023). The information from the swollen lymph nodes is crucial regarding systemic disease or local pathology that can guide nursing interventions as well as consultations to other practitioners.

Secondly, understanding the function of lymphatic drainage in conjunction with the other head and neck structures assists nurses in providing holistic patient care such that all facets of a patient's life receive enough attention (Dobríková et al., 2017). By being cautious of these essentials, nursing assessments can prove successful in delivering thorough information regarding the patient's condition (Figure 7.4).

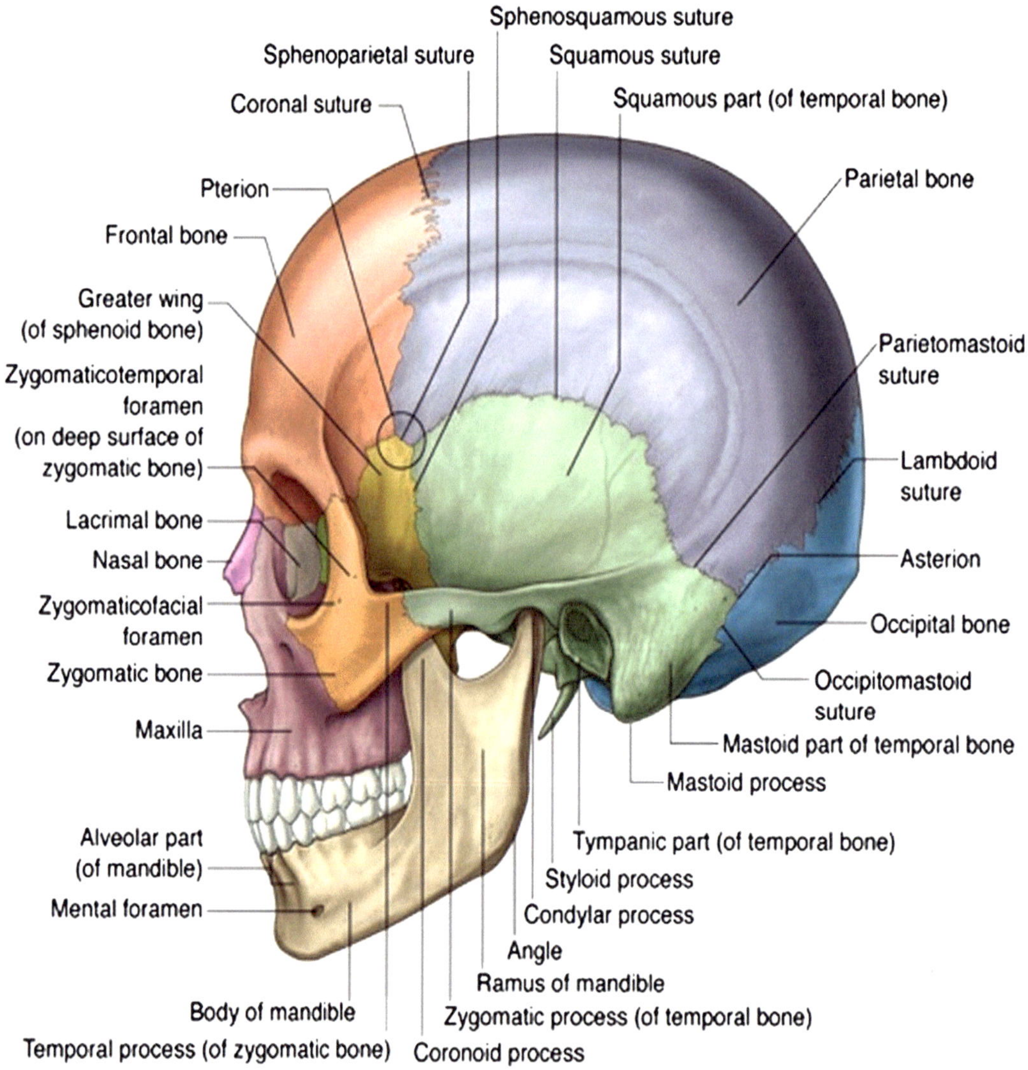

Figure 7.4. Key structures of the head.

Source: https://basicmedicalkey.com/wp-content/uploads/2016/06/B9780702051319000080_f008-019-9780702051319.jpg.

7.1.2. Anatomy of the Neck

The anatomy of the neck is a preeminently area of interest in nurse exams, especially because of its complex construction and the vital operations it supports. Composed of muscles, vessels, nerves, and lymphatic tissues, the neck serves as a conduit for anatomical and physiological functions central to human well-being. Cervical vertebrae provide structural support in guarding the spinal cord and serving as attachment points of head-moving muscles. The cervical region also houses the principal blood vessels, including carotid arteries and jugular veins, facilitating the flow of oxygenated blood to the brain and deoxygenated blood for reoxygenation. This intricate anatomy must be appreciated by nurses because any compromise of these structures can have a significant impact on the patient's overall well-being and mandate intervention. Neck lymphatic function is particularly important during patient assessment due to its role in fluid balance and immune status. The neck contains numerous lymph nodes that may be enlarged or tender secondary to infection or malignancy. This enlargement can be an indicator of localized or systemic disease, and therefore it is critical that medical practitioners perform proper evaluations of these lymphatic tissues. Moreover, because disorders like lymphedema can also happen following head and neck surgical procedures and radiation treatments, nurses must be vigilant in sensing manifestations of fluid accumulation (Schneider et al., 2000). In examinations, understanding the anatomical position of lymph nodes and their interactions with surrounding structures is able to enhance the diagnostic findings, ultimately resulting in effective interventions and treatments. Since lymphedema is a frequent sequela following head and neck cancer treatments, understanding the anatomy behind the condition can substantially be added to nursing practice (Arends et al., 2025). Lymphedema has to be distinguished from other possible complications in effective patient care. Nurses should be aware of measurement techniques used to assess and monitor lymphatic function, including provision for devices such as the revised Patterson scale, which offers sound measures for assessing lymphedema. In addition, incorporation of patient-reported outcomes regarding their experience of lymphedema captures the impact of lymphedema on quality of life. By incorporating both anatomical data and patient feedback, nurses are able to create inclusive care plans that address both the physical and emotional concerns that accompany illnesses of the neck, face, and lymphatics (Figure 7.5).

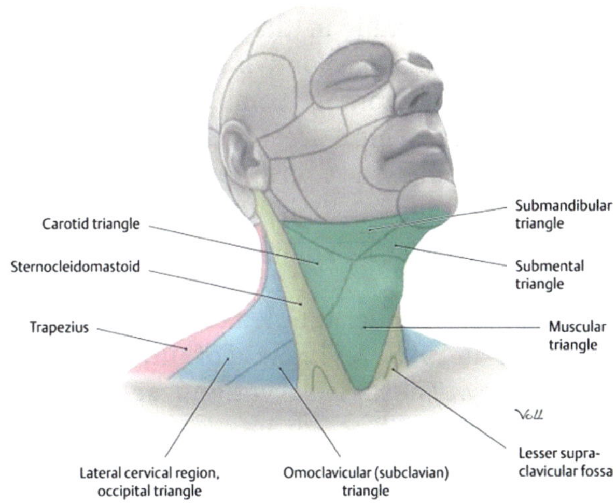

Figure 7.5. The anatomy and physiology of the neck.

Source: https://i0.wp.com/entokey.com/wp-content/uploads/2020/07/10-1055-b-002-74297_c001_f001.jpg?w=960.

7.1.3. Lymphatic System Overview

The lymphatic system is also critical in maintaining fluid balance within the body, and lymph is a clear, rich immune cell fluid perfused in the tissues by a network of lymph vessels. Fluid excess is drained efficiently by the system, thus preventing edema and homeostasis. The critical structures of the lymphatic system include the lymph vessels, lymph nodes, and lymphatic organs such as the spleen and thymus. Moreover, lymph vessels carry and bring this fluid back to the bloodstream where it plays a crucial role in eliminating wastes and cell detritus. This reciprocal relationship between immune system and fluid balance underscores the importance of the lymphatic system in overall health since any interruption could lead to compromised immunity or pathologic conditions, which nursing intake should keep in close observation in patient assessment, particularly head, face, neck, and regional lymphatics (Accettola et al., 2023). During clinical practice, especially in nursing, it is crucial to know about the anatomy and physiology of the lymphatic systems. This system is important in the immune process, serving as a passage for lymphocytes—white blood cells important for combating infections. Lymph nodes, which are strategically placed all over the body, act as filters that capture pathogens to inhibit their dissemination. In a head, face, neck, and lymphatics assessment, nurses also need to have the ability to palpate these nodes, for which they look for enlargement or tenderness as evidence of infection or malignancy. These observations are key to early detection of health issues, as literature in clinical practice suggests, further supporting the inclusion of nursing exams along with an in-depth understanding of the system's role of the lymphatic system in systemic processes of diseases and local infections (Franks et al., 2025). Moreover, the influence of the lymphatic system extends into other clinical conditions, particularly that of head and neck malignancies, where lymph node involvement is a critical prognostic determinant. Assessment of regional lymph nodes can yield useful information concerning the extent of the disease and metastatic potential. It is essential for nurses to understand the relationship between the lymphatic drainage pattern and tumor spread in developing effective care strategies and making appropriate referrals. Early identification of lymphatic obstruction or swelling, or lymphedema, during nurse assessments is also extremely critical, guiding interventions that will lead to symptom alleviation and quality of life enhancement in patients. Emphasizing the complexity of the lymphatic system in nursing programs will enhance clinical decision-making and guarantee equitable health outcomes since future nurses are in the process of addressing the complexity ushered in by future healthcare scenarios (Accettola et al., 2023) (Figure 7.6).

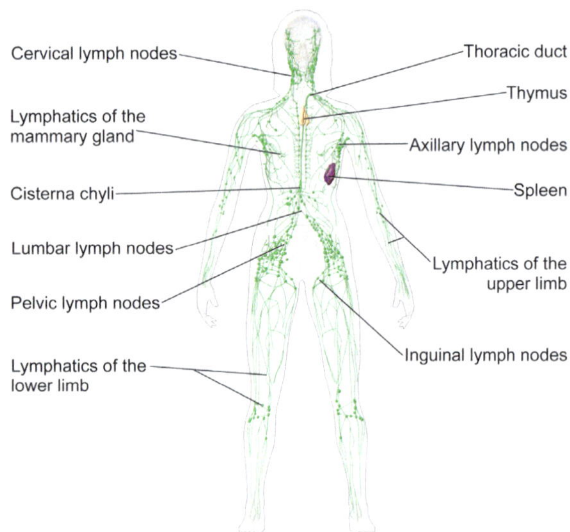

Figure 7.6. Lymphatic system overview.

Source: https://upload.wikimedia.org/wikipedia/commons/f/f4/Blausen_0623_LymphaticSystem_Female.png.

Test Your Knowledge

1. What are the major structures of the head and neck, and how do they relate to each other functionally?
2. How does understanding the anatomy of the head and neck assist in identifying abnormalities during assessment?

7.2. Assessment Techniques

Learning Outcome

1. Inspection methods;
2. Palpation techniques;
3. Auscultation in lymphatic assessment.

Assessment of the head, face, neck, and lymphatics is an essential aspect of nursing practice that entails a multidimensional approach to ensure comprehensive patient assessment. The assessment methods may vary widely but often involve systematic observation, palpation, and auscultation. During the visual inspection phase, nurses must make keen observations of any evident abnormalities on the neck and face, like lesions, asymmetry, or trauma. Palpation techniques are also important, allowing nurses to detect tenderness, swelling, or pathologic findings in lymph nodes and other tissues. Auscultation is employed to assess vascular sounds, particularly for patients with suspected vascular disease. These primary techniques provide a foundation which informs clinical judgment and assists in establishing conditions that may be in need of intervention or further examination. Furthermore, involvement of the cervical lymph nodes is a vital prognostic factor, particularly among patients with oral or oropharyngeal squamous cell carcinoma (OSCC). As is required under current guidelines, elective treatment of clinically negative necks remains a vital consideration in oncology care, including nursing. The employment of novel assessment technologies, such as Sentinel node biopsy (SNB), provides a new view. This minimally invasive surgical procedure is focused on increasing the accuracy of histologic staging and avoiding unnecessary tests on patients. Since SNB becomes defined in early OSCC, this also highlights the need for nurses to remain current with evolving practices that have an impact on patient care. Such assessment techniques require expertise, which is aligned with the delivery of evidence-based care that responds to the sophistication of oncological nursing. In addition to these established and emerging approaches to examination, general examination of the head, face, neck, and lymphatics also provides vital information regarding more systemic disease.

The examination may, for instance, reveal signs of systemic infection, autoimmune disease, or malignancy, and accordingly require regard for the patient's overall health from a holistic standpoint. Nurses are required to synthesize patient history and symptomatology with physical findings in order to build a general picture of the patient's condition. Such integration is critical not only for patient care in the here-and-now, but also in informing interdisciplinarity teamwork. Through the development and refinement of assessment skills in this area, nurses are empowered to take an active leadership role in the management of their patients. Continuing education and practice in these forms of assessment is needed so that nurses can maintain effectiveness as patient advocates in acute and chronic care settings (Figure 7.7).

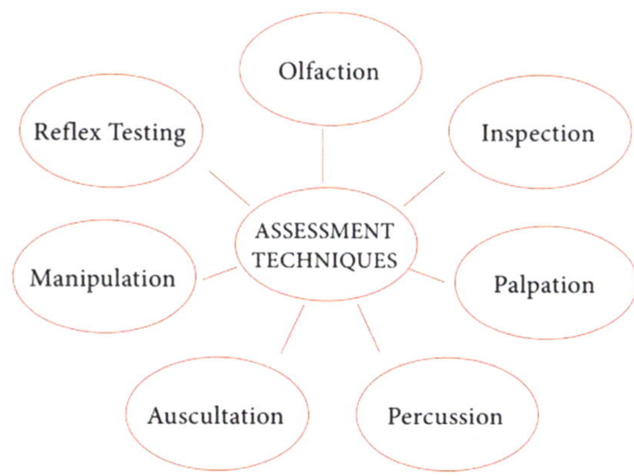

Figure 7.7. Assessment techniques.

Source: https://img.brainkart.com/imagebk36/In0FSuR.jpg.

7.2.1. Inspection Methods

The visual inspection methods employed during the assessment of the head, face, neck, and lymphatics are crucial in identifying normal anatomy and detecting deviations. Systematic visual assessment allows nurses to evaluate symmetry and variations in physical features that could indicate underlying illnesses. For instance, facial asymmetry could suggest neurological disease or trauma, while alterations in coloration or texture of the skin could suggest dermatological or systemic illness. Effective inspection requires not only keen observing skills but also recognition of the usual anatomical variations found in different populations, something nurses have to examine carefully during exams. Visual examination is a preliminary method employed in lymphatic tests to diagnose lymph node swelling or evidence of inflammatory response that may signify infection or neoplasm. Some special focus is placed in areas such as the cervical, submandibular, and supraclavicular zones, where the lymph nodes are readily palpable and visually examined. The combination of inspection methods with palpation helps to establish the tenderness and consistency of the lymph nodes and thus helps in proper diagnosis. For example, understanding the central role of cervical lymph nodes in the prognosis evaluation, particularly in diseases like oral/oropharyngeal squamous cell carcinoma, shows the ways in which inspection methods can inform clinical decision-making regarding elective therapy for clinically negative neck patients (Bilde et al., 2009). Furthermore, technological innovation such as imaging devices complements the traditional inspection methods and provides an even clearer picture of the patients lymphatic system. It is, however, necessary for nurses to remember that equipment in this regard is not a substitute for sharp observational skills acquired through practice and course work. The integration of these inspection techniques into routine examination fosters an overarching philosophy of patient care that embraces visual inspection and palpation in nursing. As emphasized in healthcare professional materials, strong foundation knowledge in anatomy and inspection procedures continues to be essential for clinicians engaged in head, face, neck, and lymphatic examination (Petrashenko et al., 2017).

7.2.2. Palpation Techniques

Palpation is one of the comprehensive assessments of the head, face, neck, and lymphatics in nursing. Palpation is the technique of feeling and evaluating the underlying anatomy and texture of these regions by using the hands, providing useful information regarding patient health. Efficient palpation skills enable nurses to identify abnormalities such as lymphadenopathy, tenderness, or masses that can reveal underlying pathology. Different palpation methods, including light, medium, and deep pressure, are used by clinicians to assess different types of tissues and locate structures effectively. By employing a systematic approach, healthcare providers can be able to perform complete exams, which ultimately can impact the diagnostic process as well as guide patient management plans. Anatomy knowledge and sensitivity to touch are required for familiarity with and mastery of palpation methods. For instance, during a lymphatic assessment, the nurses must palpate lymph nodes in the most critical anatomical sites, such as the cervical, submandibular, and supraclavicular regions, to assess their size, mobility, and consistency. This is particularly true in children, where lymphatic structures may be very different from adults. According to Petrashenko et al. (2017), comprehensive training in the nuances of such palpation skills enhances overall healthcare delivery, facilitating the early detection of potential health issues and allowing timely interventions. As they progress with clinical education, incorporating these skills in the learning process greatly assists in developing their clinical judgment and patient-centered care ideology. Furthermore, culturally sensitive approaches to palpation can have a profound impact on patient assessment and outcomes. Determining the ways in which problems such as race, gender, and body types contribute to physical examinations makes for a more diverse practice environment. Accettola et al. (2023) identifies the importance of integrating these aspects into nursing school so that new professionals can approach clinical assessments with a broad perspective. This question is a patient-warmer and trust-enhancing process that also promotes open communication about their health concerns. Finally, culturally competent advanced palpation skills are involved in enhanced clinical decision-making and patient safety to deliver thorough care to diverse multi-cultural patient populations to ensure nurses are well equipped (Figure 7.8).

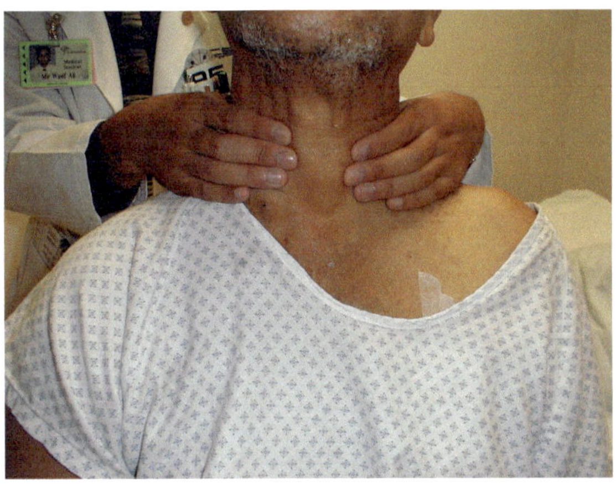

Figure 7.8. Palpation techniques.

Source: https://meded.ucsd.edu/clinicalmed/assets/img/head_thyroid_palpation.jpg.

7.2.3. Auscultation in Lymphatic Assessment

In clinical practice, auscultation is highly essential in lymphatic assessment, particularly in evaluating the lymphatic systems' function and identifying any pathology. Auscultation refers to the act of listening to some body sounds, and for the lymphatic system, it can identify abnormal results that require follow-up. This technique allows doctors to detect changes in lymphatic drainage or evidence of inflammation, which may be indicative of conditions such as lymphadenopathy or lymphoma. Discriminating between normal and abnormal sounds is vital to informed clinical decision-making. In addition, such auscultation techniques have the potential to further nurses' capacity for care planning and response to clinical signals, ultimately enhancing patient outcomes and safety in practice, also in alignment with goals promoted within pedagogical materials aimed at nursing professionals (Petrashenko et al., 2017). Beyond standard auscultatory technique, nurses must be instructed to incorporate culturally competent parameters in their assessments. The. connection between auscultation findings and culture is undeniable; certain populations will have certain health issues that will impact the health of the. lymphatics. For instance, illnesses like. lymphedema will manifest in patients in a different way based on the patients' ethnicity or other demographic affiliations. By implementing auscultation as part of an integrated assessment model incorporating cultural competence, not only are nurses receiving accurate clinical data but also providing holistic care. The integration facilitates creating stronger nurse-patient relationships as well as the ability to create patient-specific care plans according to a full assessment of the patient's history and health needs (Petrashenko et al., 2017). Auscultation in lymphatic assessment also bridges the overall goals of health promotion learned in nursing education. In the process of educating upcoming practitioners on the importance of auscultation, it is important that clinical judgment is integrated into the evaluation. The skill of recognizing abnormal sounds pertaining to lymphatic circulation educates the nurse's diagnostic skill and enhances their decision-making skill. Additionally, incorporating interactive clinical judgment practice in nursing education emphasizes the actual practice of auscultatory techniques in the clinical environment. Ultimately, the teaching approach aims to prepare nursing students to deal with the complexities of lymphatic examination confidently, prepared to identify clinical deterioration and intervene effectively on behalf of their patients in practice (Accettola et al., 2023) (Figure 7.9).

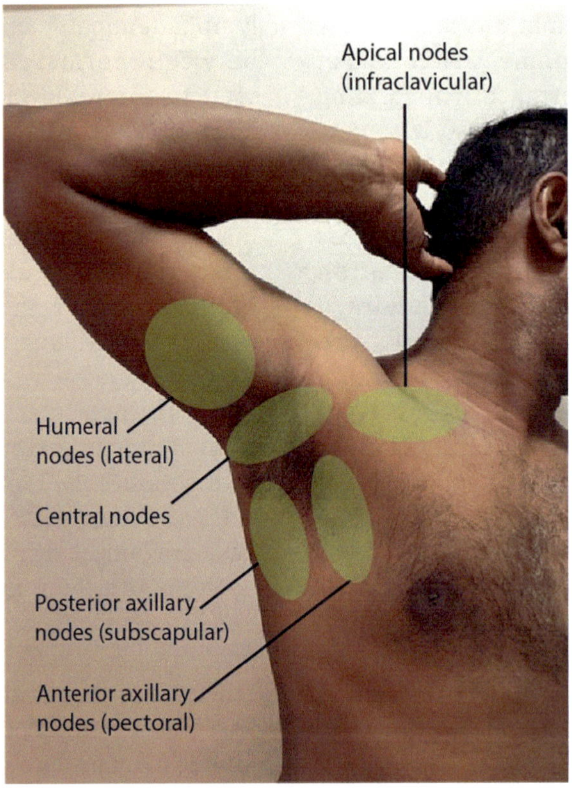

Figure 7.9. Inspection and palpation of the lymph nodes.

Source: https://pressbooks.library.torontomu.ca/assessmentnursingmain/wp-content/uploads/sites/421/2024/05/Axilla-labeled-1-225x300.jpg.

Test Your Knowledge

1. What techniques are used to examine the head and neck, including inspection, palpation, and auscultation?
2. How can a systematic approach to head and neck assessment improve accuracy and efficiency?

7.3. Common Conditions and Disorders

Learning Outcome

1. Headaches and their implications;
2. Neck pain and associated conditions;
3. Lymphadenopathy and its significance.

Referring to head, face, neck, and lymphatic examination in nursing, one of the normal conditions that need to be observed is lymphadenopathy. Lymphadenopathy typically precedes an underlying pathology, i.e., infection or malignancy. Lymph nodes are components of the lymphatic system and can become enlarged due to various factors, thus indicating regional or systemic pathologies at times. For instance, streptococcal pharyngitis and mononucleosis infection can result in palpable cervical lymph nodes. Assessment of lymphadenopathy involves proper palpation, noting the node characteristics, and attention to the presence of associated symptoms. Effective evaluation enables nurses to effectively inform the health team so that early intervention can be provided. The implications of unmanaged lymphadenopathy can be severe, with complications arising if the etiology is infectious or neoplastic in nature, thereby emphasizing the critical need for comprehensive evaluations in the nursing process. Another common condition in the region of head, face, neck, and lymphatic evaluation is temporomandibular joint (TMJ) dysfunction. The disorder entails disruption in articulation between the jaw and the skull, which most commonly results in pain and dysfunction in jaw movement. TMJ dysfunction can be caused by a variety of factors including misalignment, trauma, or stress. From a mild pain in the jaw, headaches, earaches, to clicking upon opening or closing the jaw, the signs and symptoms may vary. From a nursing practitioner's perspective, the full history considers the patient's history, a thorough physical examination, and knowing factors such as bruxism or stress resulting in the condition. Early diagnosis and effective management of TMJ dysfunction can improve quality of life in patients via relief of pain as well as enhanced jaw mobility. Nurses play a vital role in educating patients regarding lifestyle modification as well as potential treatment, thus integrating a holistic plan of care into their assessment. Lastly, allergies and sinusitis are prevalent in patients undergoing evaluation for the head and neck and contribute significantly to morbidity. Allergies may induce nasal passage irritation, which causes nasal discharge, sneezing, and congestion. Chronic sinusitis, often secondary to allergy, further contributes to these signs by causing facial pressure and pain that endure. In nursing practice, the identification of such conditions demands an extensive history of symptoms and allergies as well as facial tenderness and nasal obstruction. The nurses should also protect against the risk of complications that result from untreated sinuses, which can further lead to infections in the ears as well as breathing issues. Recommending treatment strategies for managing allergies and sinusitis, including pharmacological treatments and lifestyle modifications, is paramount in a nursing intervention. The holistic management of these conditions not only enhances patient outcomes but also highlights the importance of thorough assessments in nursing practice.

7.3.1. Headaches and Their Implications

The prevalence of headache as a primary complaint in clinical practice highlights the need for an adequate understanding of their importance in nursing assessment. Headaches show significant variability in etiology, classification, and severity, such as various forms like tension-type headache, migraine, and cluster headache. A greater depth of assessment is needed because they reflect such differences often of underlying conditions ranging from benign to life-threatening. The nurses' function in the evaluation of headache symptoms is beyond immediate alleviation; it encompasses understanding the patient history, identifying potential triggers, and identifying related symptoms that might indicate more serious health status. For instance, certain migraines have been connected with neurological dysfunction, and this points towards the need for a wholistic approach within the head, face, neck, and lymphatics assessment in nursing. Moreover, the impact of chronic headaches on a patient's quality of life cannot be overestimated. Chronic headache disorders usually lead to psychological effects, including depression and anxiety, further complicating patient management. The Red Cross's Therapeutic Care service, detailed in recent studies, stresses the importance of addressing not just physical but also emotional health of chronic headache and associated disease patients, like chronic pain and mental illness (Cavaye et al., 2009). In clinical practice, it is important to take measures not just to manage pain but also to enhance coping and overall wellness.

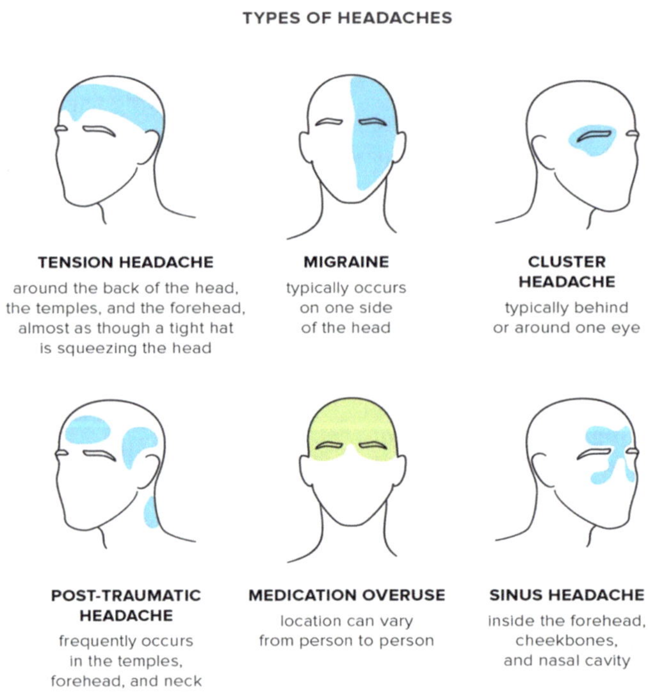

Figure 7.10. Headaches and their implications.

Source: https://i0.wp.com/post.medicalnewstoday.com/wp-content/uploads/sites/3/2021/07/headache-location-infographic-1296x1296-body-897x1024.jpg?w=1155&h=3110.

This collaborative care plan is essential in facilitating healing and improving patient outcomes, especially when the patients present incapacitating headache as part of other chronic conditions. Additionally, explanation of headache mechanisms can guide understanding of their implications within broader health contexts. Further research more recently mapped the intricacies of headache pathophysiology, revealing associations between neurological mechanisms and systemic disease (Brighina et al., 2017). For example, the relationship between peripheral chromatic and central visual impairment among migraine patients sheds light on how headaches can be an indicator of existing overarching neurological conditions. Therefore, nurses should be able to identify such correlations during an assessment, in consideration of the fact that a good assessment may initiate early interventions and referral. Through the incorporation of evidence obtained from existing research into clinic practices, nursing assessments can be guided and effective and, in the long term, enhance health outcomes among headache and other related condition patients (Figure 7.10).

7.3.2. Neck Pain and Associated Conditions

Neck pain is a widespread condition that has a direct impact on individuals quality of life and functionality, thus learning about its intricate nature is essential. Pathophysiology underlying neck pain may range from acute trauma, such as whiplash due to motor vehicle accidents to chronic illness, for instance, cervical spondylosis. Common symptoms of neck pain are restricted range of movement, stiffness, and radiation which can further go on to secondary areas such as the shoulders and arms. Notably, clinical assessment of neck pain frequently entails a careful assessment of the supporting anatomical structure, which can include musculoskeletal, neurological, or even vascular components. This in-depth analysis gives an impetus to create proper treatment plans with a goal to decrease pain and restore function, and also to facilitate health care providers to give importance to education and prevention strategies in patient management. In clinical practice, associated disorders of neck radiculopathy and myofascial pain syndrome are extremely prevalent along with neck pain.

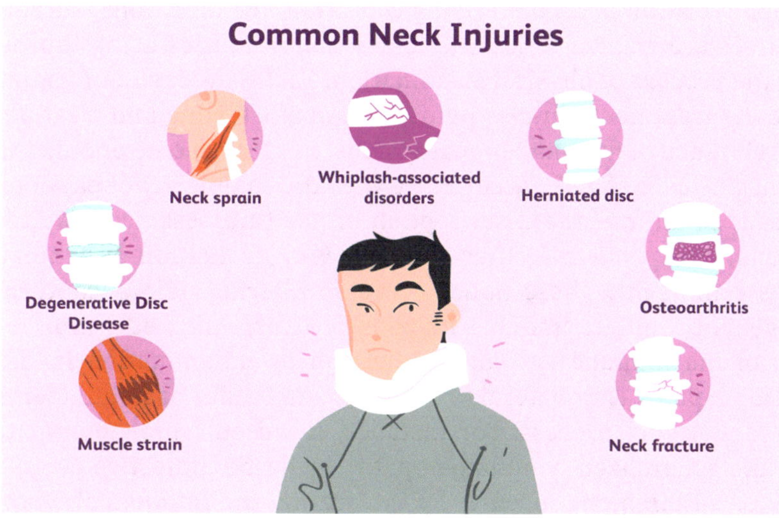

Figure 7.11. Neck pain and associated conditions.

Source: https://www.verywellhealth.com/thmb/jcr0ahb3BFeNNSlYaUJZ0UewpT8=/1500x0/filters:no_upscale():max_bytes(150000):strip_icc()/most-common-neck-injuries-described-296664_v4-HL-e923c5eb867744f89b62591a1dbd4dcf.png.

Cervical radiculopathy, most often caused by compression of the nerve roots by herniated discs or degenerative conditions, produces pain, numbness, and weakness of the upper limbs. Myofascial pain syndrome caused by trigger points in the muscles of the neck often causes pain localized to other areas. Knowledge of these associated conditions is vital for medical practitioners and nurses, as differential diagnosis ensures effective treatment as well as patient education. Additionally, the relationship between neck pain and psychosocial states, i.e., stress and anxiety, cannot be neglected. Understanding this relationship can direct an integrative care strategy that considers physical and psychological approaches to intervention, thereby enhancing patient outcomes. The scope of implications of neck pain extends to the assessment of lymphatic involvement, particularly in patients who have undergone head and neck cancer treatment. Evidence is present that neck pain could be an indicator of lymphatic dysfunction, including lymphedema, which affects the quality of life of patients (Arends et al., 2025). This necessitates comprehensive lymphatic assessment to become part of the diagnosis for neck pain to detect complications early. Because of the complicated presentation of neck pain, an evidence-based approach to nursing evaluations involves the application of standardized assessment tools to ensure accurate evaluation (Carl et al., 2025). Through the comprehensive knowledge of neck pain and related disorders, nurses can play an important part in the development of patient-directed care plans, fighting for adequate symptom management, and education of patients on lifestyle factors causing neck pain, thereby encouraging patient participation in self-care measures (Figure 7.11).

7.3.3. Lymphadenopathy and Its Significance

Lymphadenopathy examination is a key component of head, face, neck, and lymphatic system nursing examination. Lymphadenopathy or the swelling of lymph nodes in an abnormal manner is often a clinical manifestation of an underlying condition like infections, autoimmune conditions, and malignancy. Nurses are trained to identify these abnormalities using thorough palpation and observation during the process of physical examination. Lastly, detection of lymphadenopathy signs not only results in early treatment but also guides diagnostic testing and treatment planning. From understanding the relevance of lymphadenopathy, thus, nurses become enabled to optimize patient outcomes while managing care plans in accordance with the complexity of patients' clinical histories, which eventually leads to an integrated conception of health assessment. Multifunctional roles of lymph nodes in the immune system further highlight why evaluation of lymphadenopathy has to be considered in its complexity. These nodes serve as filtering points, capturing pathogens and possibly harmful agents to initiate immune responses. Thus, inflamed lymph nodes may indicate an active response of the immune system to infection or inflammation in the body. Moreover, whether the lymphadenopathy is unilateral or bilateral and tender or nontender may yield valuable information on the underlying process. For instance, localized lymphadenopathy would suggest a local infection, while generalized lymphadenopathy could be indicative of systemic pathologies, such as malignancy or autoimmune disease. By integrating the findings of lymphadenopathy into the broader context of patient assessments, nurses can appropriately set priorities for care and facilitate further diagnostic work that may lead to timely interventions (Accettola et al., 2023). In nursing practice, the dialogue surrounding lymphadenopathy is not just limited to clinical diagnosis but also encompasses patient education and support. Nurses play a key part in assisting patients in negotiating through the complexities of their diagnosis, reassuring them about implications of lymphadenopathy. Keeping an open dialogue about possible causes and treatment assists in establishing a care platform for patients. Furthermore, educating patients on self-examination and reporting changes has the ability to empower them as their own health care providers. Given the effect of lymphadenopathy on patient safety and well-being, incorporation of clinical judgment and empathetic communication are essential for nursing practice. This multi-pronged approach, as the precepts of culturally-responsive care illustrate, is essential in an effort to address patients' diverse needs and concerns and ensure that they receive equal evaluations and interventions based on their individual circumstances (Plotnikov et al., 2017) (Figure 7.12).

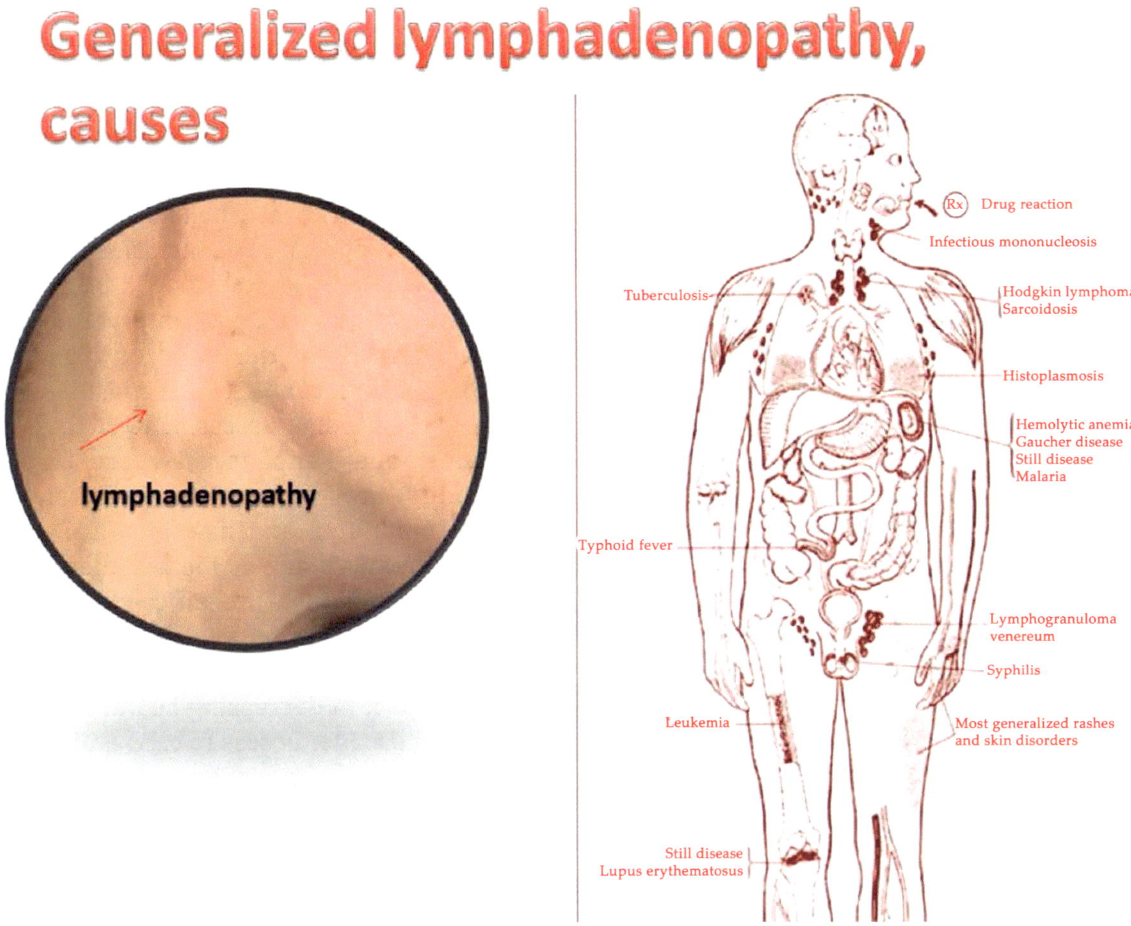

Figure 7.12. The generalized lymphadenopathies.

Source: https://www.gastroepato.it/en_lymphadenopathy-causes.webp.

Test Your Knowledge

1. What are some common conditions affecting the head and neck, and how are they identified during assessment?
2. How can early detection of disorders such as thyroid enlargement, lymphadenopathy, or cranial nerve deficits impact patient outcomes?

7.4. Cultural Considerations in Assessment

Learning Outcome

1. Variations in anatomy across different populations;
2. Cultural beliefs affecting health assessments;
3. Communication strategies for diverse populations.

Cultural elements occupy a significant position in the head, face, neck, and lymphatics assessment in nursing because they are responsible for the patients' values, beliefs, and conduct concerning illness. One should know a patient's culture to facilitate effective communication and trust. For instance, some cultures possess their own special beliefs over health practice and are not likely to embrace some medical interventions. Where patients are not congruent with dominant paradigms of health, nurses must undertake assessments from a culturally sensitive perspective. This involves recognizing and affirming the different views of health and illness, thus making the patients feel heard and appreciated in their treatment. By actively involving patients in conversation about their cultural beliefs, nurses can more effectively provide individualized and better care, encouraging a collaborative environment that fosters improved patient outcomes while addressing the individualized needs of patients. Cultural awareness also encompasses knowledge of the particular health disparities and issues of different groups. For instance, disease incidence and outcome disparities for such diseases as cancer highlight the importance of culturally competent care in assessments. As evident from the increased incidence of cancer, a proper understanding of cancer patients' cultural contexts is required. There is a stark difference in how different cultures perceive cancer and its treatment, and that affects how willing patients are to seek care and adhere to treatment recommendations. Knowledge of these cultural nuances not only allows for the evaluation process but also allows nurses to tailor interventions focusing on specific issues, for instance, stigma or myth surrounding the treatment of cancer. In doing this, an informed strategy can increase patient engagement and the effectiveness of health delivery to a great extent. Finally, culturally responsive evaluations involve an awareness of socio-economic factors that might overlap with health beliefs and practices. Most of the patients have histories that may influence whether they can or will be engaged in some health screening or intervention due to economic reasons, transport, or availability of access to health centers. Such considerations bear most in nursing assessment of the head, face, neck, and lymphatics, where physical accessibility may play an important role in a patient's emotional and psychological status. Nurses must make sure to include these socio-economic determinants in their calculations and considerations of care. In seeing and working through these barriers, nurses can become a dynamic aspect in decreasing health inequities and making broader access to care available for all, making their practice align with the inclusive and culturally framed approaches that current nursing demands (Accettola et al., 2023; N/A, 2021) (Figure 7.13).

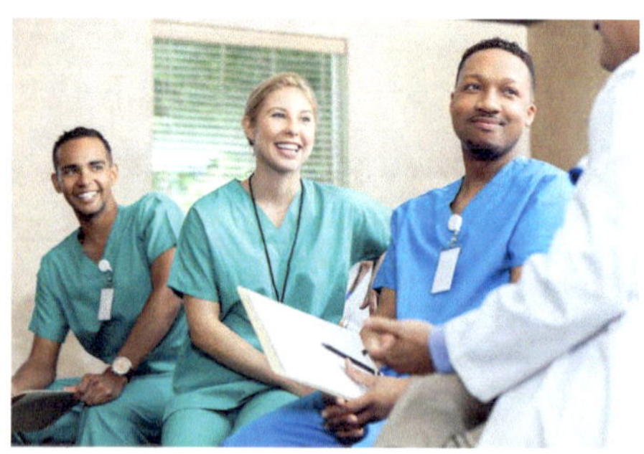

Figure 7.13. Cultural considerations in assessment in nursing.

Source: https://www.nurseregistry.com/wp-content/uploads/2016/09/diverse-group-nurses.jpg.

7.4.1. Variations in Anatomy Across Different Populations

The significance of knowledge regarding population anatomical differences is fundamental in the practice of nursing, particularly in the context of head, face, neck, and lymphatic assessment. Such differences will have significant implications for practice, ranging from physical assessment through surgery. For example, studies have revealed that certain vascular anatomical variants, such as those of the basilar artery, also exhibit enormous variations in prevalence across various populations, including trifurcation and quadfurcation incidences in more than 5% of cases in various groups of individuals (Jayapala et al., 2024). This diversity highlights the importance of nurses being adept at difference identification and accommodation of these differences, otherwise leading to misdiagnosis or inappropriate treatment. Enhancing cultural competence in nursing practice is required for the provision of care adapted to the variations in anatomy and physiology that occur in various ethnic groups. The use of inclusive approaches to health assessment, as highlighted in open learning resources, ensures that nursing students are adequately equipped with the knowledge required to perform culturally-sensitive assessments of anatomical variations (Accettola et al., 2023). For instance, recognition that facial morphology will differ significantly among individuals from diverse ethnic groups can inform the way in which a nurse will continue with assessment methods and physical examinations. These variations must be identified in order to plan interventions effectively, ensuring increased patient engagement and improved health outcomes. The anatomical variations also call for ongoing education and adaptability among nursing professionals so that they may provide quality care. With nursing education focusing more on the application of clinical judgment and critical thinking, educators must incorporate anatomical variation into curricula. This is intended to prepare the prospective nurse with interactions involving different patient populations where the traditional assessment techniques might not be completely applicable. By having a greater insight into population-specific anatomical features, nurses can facilitate increased sensitivity and adaptability in service, which are critical for proper implementation of safe and effective health interventions that are sensitive to the unique attributes of every patient (Accettola et al., 2023). This forward-thinking approach will help with improved health equity and patient safety in practice nursing.

7.4.2. Cultural Beliefs Affecting Health Assessments

In nursing, cultural beliefs are central in establishing health assessments, particularly of the head, face, neck, and lymphatics. This is extremely crucial for medical professionals to give culturally related care. Patients from various cultures will have varied perceptions about health and illness that influence their susceptibility to health assessments. For instance, certain symptoms can be attributed by some groups to supernatural or spiritual instead of physical causes, with the risk of postponing life-threatening condition diagnosis. It not only fosters patient and physician trust through acknowledging and respecting these beliefs but also enhances the effectiveness of health assessments. By embracing a holistic approach with cultural awareness, nurses can improve patient outcomes and make accurate and culturally responsive assessments that are attuned to diverse cultural contexts. The influence of cultural belief extends beyond the mere perception of health; it includes attitudes toward healthcare systems and expert recommendations. In some cultures, forms of healing that have been traditionally practiced have significant meaning, perhaps being counterintuitive to standard Western medicine intervention. Patients will, in certain cases, opt to visit traditional healers or undergo alternative therapy before undergoing formal medical assessments. Such inclinations bring about a communication disparity, resulting in inadequate health histories and compromised assessments (N/A, 2021). Nurses should understand these dynamics and incorporate appropriate culture-based practices into their assessments. This not only requires active listening but also the adaptation of measurement techniques to align with patient values, hence leading to more effective and inclusive treatment. Additionally, the concept of health literacy intersects with cultural belief in very profound ways, shaping how patients respond to health assessment. Other cultural patients might have other aspects of health literacy, significantly affecting their ability to understand medical terminology and procedures. For example, patients with lymphedema may not fully appreciate the implications of their condition due to cultural stigma or lack of information in their language or level of education (Dreiling et al., 2022).

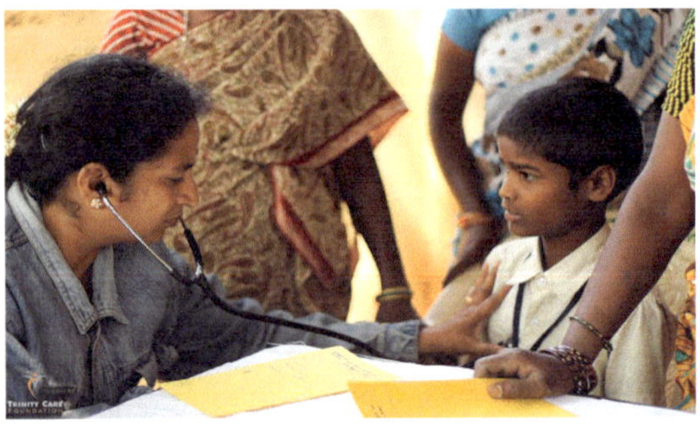

Figure 7.14. Cultural beliefs affecting health assessments.

Source: https://theindianpractitioner.com/wp-content/uploads/2022/03/November_Socio-cultural-dimensions-of-Public-Health.jpg.

This lack of health literacy has a bearing on adherence to recommended interventions, thus complicating nursing assessment and treatment planning. In order to alleviate such concerns, nurses have to employ culturally competent communication strategies that break down technical medical language into common parlance, enabling all patients to effectively participate in their health assessments. The act solidifies cultural competence as an integral part of the nursing practice, practically enhancing assessment accuracy and patient satisfaction (Figure 7.14).

7.4.3. Communication Strategies for Diverse Populations

Effective communication skills are crucial in nursing, particularly with head, face, neck, and lymphatic checks, because they often need to involve explaining complex information in sensitive circumstances. It is equally crucial to be aware of and respond to cultural variation as nurses must realize that both linguistic variation and differences in health beliefs may influence patient interactions. For instance, patients of diverse backgrounds can construct unique meaning of treatment outcomes or symptoms, necessitating a personalized communication strategy. Simple language usage, avoiding jargon, and utilization of instructional aids will enhance comprehension, which enhances nurse-patient relationship that is healing-friendly. This style of effective communication is not only helpful in accurate assessments but also ensures active patient involvement in their treatment process, thereby enhancing health outcomes to the fullest. In addition to language issues, non-verbal communication plays a critical role in rapport building with various populations in nurse assessments. Non-verbal behaviors such as body gestures, facial expressions, and physical contact can convey empathy and understanding, particularly where verbal communication is restricted by language or cultural barriers. For example, gentle touch can reassure and comfort patients, particularly when conducting sensitive head and neck area examinations. Empirical evidence highlights the importance of touch interventions in nursing practice, as revealed by studies indicating that deliberate and culturally appropriate touch enhances the therapeutic relationship between nurses and patients with backgrounds that vary (Kay et al., 1990). Through enhanced non-verbal communication, nurses can close gaps in their understanding and foster a trust climate conducive to enhanced assessment and interventions. In addition, the adoption of technology into plans of communication presents an opportunity to improve interactions across populations. Apps that translate and telemedicine services, for instance, have the ability to bridge linguistic gaps, enabling nurses to communicate more effectively with individuals who speak other languages. Also, these technologies can provide distant assessment of head, face, neck, and lymphatic issues, hence increasing access to such issues for the disadvantaged groups. However, the nurses should not forget that such technology has limitations and potential errors because it may fail to capture the cultural hues of communication. Overall, implementing an integrative framework that integrates verbal, non-verbal, and technological modes of communication ensures nurses are well-positioned to provide culturally competent care, ultimately leading to better quality assessments and patient outcomes for the diverse population (N/A, 2021).

Test Your Knowledge

1. How can cultural differences in facial features, hair, or neck structures affect assessment findings?
2. Why is it important to consider cultural norms when interpreting patient responses or presenting symptoms in head and neck assessment?

7.5. Documentation and Reporting

Learning Outcome

1. Importance of accurate documentation;
2. Standardized assessment tools;
3. Reporting findings to the healthcare team.

In nursing, accurate reporting and documentation of the assessment, particularly of the head, face, neck, and lymphatics, is imperative. All nursing assessments serve a twofold function: to first document basic clinical findings which will direct the care of the patient, and secondly, to facilitate communication between healthcare providers. This is a task to be approached with meticulousness so each finding is documented clearly and succinctly. Effective documentation not only forms a legal document of care but also increases care continuity for the patient because it guides subsequent healthcare decisions. The assessment information, when documented in an orderly format, forms a crucial factor employed to make judgments on patient conditions over time, thereby optimizing the effectiveness of intervention used in nursing practice. Furthermore, in reporting for some of these disorders such as oral/oropharyngeal squamous cell carcinoma (OSCC), precise reporting of lymphatic exams is critical. Familiarity with the impact of cervical lymph node metastasis directs therapy and prognostication. A case in point is the introduction of sentinel node biopsy (SNB) where findings of lymphatic staging can be more accurately reported by nurses with less invasion. Improved documentation practices in this discipline focus on the potential to minimize overtreatment, thus patient morbidity. Guidelines for SNB also highlight the importance of accurate and timely reporting, offering a standard by which nurses must acquaint themselves in order to conform to the best practices in handling patients. Such meticulous reporting not only aids in better individual patient outcomes but also towards the overall oncology nursing practice. The impact of quality documentation extends beyond patient care for the individual, into a culture of accountability and quality assurance among nursing personnel. As health care evolves, integration of technology into documentation processes has solidified the position of formalized types of reporting. Standardized assessment instruments, particularly for head and neck examination, assure that paramount data points are consistently obtained and transmitted. Furthermore, the documentation processes provide the background for multidisciplinary team discussion to enable well-informed decision-making that cuts across multiple clinical perspectives. Finally, effective nursing documentation and reporting greatly help to improve healthcare quality provided to patients, therefore bolstering the general goal of optimizing health outcomes among diverse patient populations (Figure 7.15).

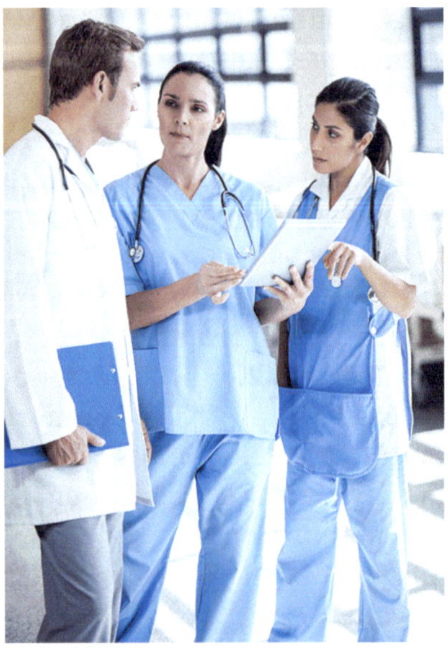

Figure 7.15. Documentation and reporting.

Source: https://medipharmsolutions.com/wp-content/uploads/2023/10/Program-Curriculum-5.png.

7.5.1. Importance of Accurate Documentation

Accurate documentation is the foundation of effective nursing practice, particularly in evaluating the head, face, neck, and lymphatics. The precision and clarity of recorded observations directly affect patient care because they enable healthcare practitioners to make informed decisions based on accurate data. Documentation maintains continuity of care by transferring important health information between various healthcare practitioners. This is especially the case in unstable clinical environments, where multiple practitioners may need to see a patient's background, evaluation data, and treatment protocols. Furthermore, detailed records are not only employed to support clinical decisions, but serve as legal protection for practitioners to avoid possible malpractice suits based on administrative error or miscommunication. Forgetting high documentation standards would result in severe lacunae in patient information, compromising both patient safety and care quality provided. Moreover, the significance of quality documentation is not only in direct clinical situations but also reaches to research and education as a nurse. Correct records also serve as an indispensable data source for gathering, enabling statistical computations with potential insights into trends in health and treatment effects. For instance, proper documentation of lymphatic exams can be interpretable in terms of better comprehension and control of diseases such as oral/oropharyngeal squamous cell carcinoma. With proper staging being the hallmark of treatment regimens, relevance of documentation is increased to an even greater extent; correct lymph node status reports direct vital prognostic factors and therapeutic planning. This aligns with best practice endorsed in the latest guidelines that advocate for newer documentations techniques that capture ongoing developments in clinical research and nursing education. The documentation process therefore has a dual role of not only satisfying immediate patient needs but also contributing to the broader pool of nursing knowledge. Embedding higher-order documentation techniques is vital in enhancing the quality and precision of healthcare service provision. Electronic recording systems, such as electronic health records (EHRs), have transformed the practice of documentation through tools that reduce data input and retrieval and lower the chances of human error. These systems can help clinicians perform thorough examinations of the head, face, neck, and lymphatics through an integration of a mixture of clinical tools and guidelines to provide a comprehensive method of patient assessment. Additionally, educating nursing students in proper documentation procedures can cultivate a culture of quality control and accountability. This is crucial for ensuring patient safety and compliance with relevant clinical standards. Together, these considerations highlight the significance of proper nursing documentation, not just individual patient care, but also the overall integrity and success of the profession.

7.5.2. Standardized Assessment Tools

Standardized assessment tools are an essential component of the nursing practice, particularly in the holistic assessment of head, face, neck, and lymphatics. Standardized tools ensure an equal process for evaluating patients, such that nurses can gather corresponding health information in a scientific way. Not only does the employment of standardized assessment enhance the reliability of findings but also facilitates better communication among medical professionals. Through the application of standardized measures of assessment, the nurses are in a position to compare outcomes for the various patients and environments, which ultimately leads to improved patient outcomes. Especially in the case of supervising symptoms for the various conditions, i.e., cancer in the lymphatic system, where it is crucial to recognize early signs so that treatment will be effective, as seen in N/A (2021). Standardized measures of assessment are thus key to guiding decision-making in clinical nursing assessment. Further, the incorporation of standardized test tools can refine the accuracy of post-concussion syndrome diagnosis, a crucial aspect of head and neck evaluations. Tools such as the Rivermead Post-Concussion Syndrome Questionnaire and the SCAT-5 battery enable clinicians to track cognitive and physical recovery in patients with great accuracy. These tests provide an objective index of symptom severity, which could influence future interventions and rehabilitation measures. In one such study specifically focused on teenagers, the efficiency of treatment interventions was evaluated using these standard measures, highlighting how systematic assessments assist in gaining insights into and improving patient health—particularly in cases involving concussions—as demonstrated by the findings of Gaudelli et al. (2020) related to VMLD therapy. The significance of these instruments cannot be overstated, as they direct best practice in nursing practice. In practice, standardized assessment instruments not only guide data collection but also allow nurses to deliver patient-focused care. By standardizing the assessment process, the nurses can attend to the unique problems of each patient, notably those patients with complex symptoms regarding head, face, neck, and lymphatics. The instruments can also be used to track the efficacy of interventions over time and determine that care plans are tailored to the patients evolving needs. This kind of flexibility is at the heart of treatment of diseases like cancer, whose control of symptoms can significantly enhance a patient's quality of life, as discussed in N/A (2021). Also, the addition of these standardized measures promotes accountability in nursing practice, allowing for constant professional growth and adherence to evidence-based criteria for patient care. Overall, benchmark assessment tools are indispensable in offering an organized, holistic philosophy to guide nursing assessments and ensure optimal patient safety and care quality (Figure 7.16).

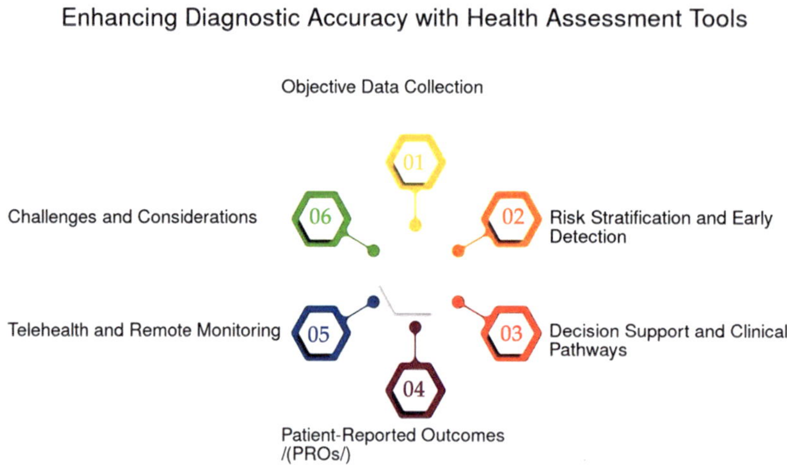

Figure 7.16. Understanding the role of health assessment tools in healthcare.

Source: https://fastercapital.co/i/Health-Assessment-Tool-Revolutionizing-Healthcare--How-Health-Assessment-Tools-Are-Disrupting-the-Industry--Enhancing-Diagnostic-Accuracy-with-Health-Assessment-Tools.webp.

7.5.3. Reporting Findings to the Healthcare Team

Clear communication of assessment findings to the healthcare team is critical to patient safety and care result maximization. In head, face, neck, and lymphatics assessment in nursing, clarity in report improves coordination among the health professionals, promoting an effective approach for patient management. This data should include relevant information such as reported lymphatic drainage deficiency, any infection, or observable masses, which play a significant role in the creation of an appropriate treatment plan. By meticulous documentation of such findings, nurses play a critical role in filling information gaps and facilitating timely interventions vital to patient recovery and safety. Use of standardized reporting tools, such as SBAR (Situation, Background, Assessment, Recommendation), still enhances the level of healthcare team communications. Use of the format ensures systematic reporting of head, facial, neck, and lymphatic findings to allow all key aspects of patient care to be addressed. For instance, the nurse may document enlarged cervical lymph nodes as results that indicate probable malignancy according to head and neck cancer surgery guidelines for managing head and neck cancer.

Proper application of such guidelines avoids unwarranted interventions while providing the team with details regarding matters of concern that could affect treatment decisions, justifying the place of nurses in the multidisciplinary setting (Bilde et al., 2009). Secondly, the function of ongoing education and training in the nursing practice supports the integration of clinical judgment into these reporting processes. Participation in professional development interventions allows nurses to hone their capacity for assessment, which immediately contributes to how results are relayed to the healthcare team. Inclusion of culturally-responsive approaches, such as those in nursing educational resources, ensures consideration of different patient perceptions during assessments and subsequent reporting (Accettura et al., 2023). Such transparent communication not only contributes to optimal patient safety but also facilitates an inclusive and equitable culture in healthcare settings, resulting in improved health outcomes among diverse populations.

Test Your Knowledge

1. How should abnormal findings in head and neck assessment be documented to ensure clear communication among healthcare providers?
2. What are the key elements to include when reporting assessment findings related to the head and neck?

7.6. Nursing Interventions

Learning Outcome

1. Patient education on self-assessment;
2. Referral processes for further evaluation;
3. Collaborative care approaches.

In Head, Face, Neck, and Lymphatics Assessment, nursing interventions play a critical role in providing holistic patient care. The interventions begin with effective communication that enables a trusting relationship between the patient and nurse, such that patients can openly discuss their concerns. For instance, evaluating lymphatic function, nurses must be competent to take a thorough health history, for instance, swelling or pain of the lymph nodes. This initial contact does not simply bring together pertinent data; it sets the stage for a holistic response, combining physical, emotional, and psychological elements. Education of the patient is essential at this juncture; nurses are able to provide some insight regarding the importance of reporting alterations in lymphatic function, maybe through early detection of difficulties. Systematic physical examination of the head, face, neck, and lymphatics is an important intervention. Applying conventional assessment techniques allows nurses to identify potential abnormalities, such as lymphadenopathy or masses. In the process, nurses must observe signs of malignancy or infection while bearing in mind the significance of their observation on follow-up for diagnosis. By integrating observational skills and palpation techniques, nurses can identify the mobility, size, and consistency of lymph nodes. Moreover, the assessment must further include determination of the range of motion of the neck since restriction may be indicative of associated conditions. Systematic approach will prevent anything from being overlooked, leading to increased patient safety and quality care in general. Finally, interventions by nurses extend beyond immediate assessment into planning care and referral. After assessment is conducted, nurses can integrate findings in a view of creating individualized care plans that meet identified needs. For example, in the event of a patient presenting with features suggestive of malignancy, it is essential to refer them urgently to a specialist so that timely intervention can be facilitated, particularly against the backdrop of rising cancer mortality rates. Cancer, currently the leading cause of death globally, should be closely monitored and aggressively nursed to minimize patient distress and optimize outcome (N/A, 2021). These endeavors can be from pain symptom control or emotional support, with the final aim of enhancing the patients quality of life and engagement during therapy. Therefore, a whole-person strategy characterized by proper assessment, individually tailored interventions, and collaboration with the healthcare team is necessary in nursing care of the head, face, neck, and lymphatics (Figure 7.17).

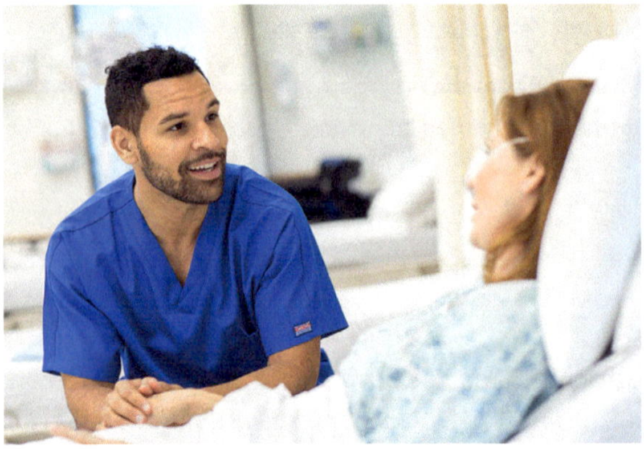

Figure 7.17. Nursing interventions.

Source: https://i0.wp.com/www.usa.edu/wp-content/uploads/2021/04/nurse-interventions-1.jpg?resize=1476%2C984&ssl=1.

7.6.1. Patient Education on Self-Assessment

Self-assessment of head, face, neck, and lymphatics by patients is important in nursing practice. Patient education regarding the importance of doing regular self-assessment enables earlier detection of abnormality. It also empowers patients through sensitizing them to their own health, allowing them to notice changes that require intervention by medical staff. Nurses may also educate patients on some ways of carrying out self-assessment, for instance, feeling the lymph nodes and assessing any distortion of the skin or underlying tissue. Apart from promoting patient participation, it also emphasizes the interprofessional aspect of health care, where patients are made participants in their own wellness process. Student-centered education for patient teaching on self-assessment enhances health outcome overall because it provides intervention at the correct time when things are not normal. Secondly, effective communication of self-assessment skills should be tailored to each patient's demographic features and health literacy. Different individuals may possess different levels of knowledge, which demands a systematic approach to instruction. For instance, the application of visual aids, demonstrations, and individual discussions will contribute significantly to better comprehension and retention. This personalized education approach is particularly relevant to populations with specific healthcare needs, like cancer patients who are more vulnerable to requiring ongoing surveillance of their conditions, as outlined in N/A (2021). By presenting self-assessment as a natural part of maintaining one's own health, patients come to learn about their bodies and feel at ease with them, thus ensuring improved detection of issues early on, which is highly significant in conditions that could otherwise go undetected. Finally, integration of self-assessment education into nursing school curricula is required for the future nursing workforce. With ongoing changes in health care, nurses must have both the technical skills required for assessments and the pedagogical skills required to teach patients effectively. This includes acquiring knowledge about cultural and individual determinants of a patient's acceptance with self-examination as well as the health care relationship, as indicated by Kay et al. (1990). By developing a culture of patient education of self-assessment, nursing education can prepare upcoming professionals to cope with these aspects. Eventually, such education creates more robust patient-nurse collaborations that enhance trust and responsiveness in the patient care relationship and support long-term health management.

7.6.2. Referral Processes for Further Evaluation

Referral procedures for follow-up assessment are significant in nursing assessment of the head, face, neck, and lymphatics. These procedures are part of ensuring that patients are provided with comprehensive care based on preliminary findings. Nurses conducting assessments may identify abnormalities, including lymphadenopathy or signs of infection, which may determine the presence of underlying issues that require further examination. Having a defined referral protocol in place can help in streamlining the response to such results to enable timely intervention. A patient, for example, can be referred by a nurse to a specialist in case there are indications of systemic disease observed during a lymphatic assessment. Proper communication and documentation between healthcare providers are fundamental because they establish a common concept of how patient care is to be handled so that all the practitioners involved are informed about the status of the patient and the reason for referral. Head, face, neck, and lymphatics assessment is rather complicated and requires a proper referral system in nursing practice. This is compounded by the demand for specialized diagnostic and treatment modalities that would be beyond the expertise of general nursing practice. For instance, patients with significant lymphedema or other lymphatic conditions may need to gain from the services of specialists such as oncologists or vascular surgeons. The development of programmatic guidelines to make referrals helps in minimizing diagnostic and treatment delays. Referral urgency is particularly applicable in the sense that illnesses like lymphedema can become chronic and lead to increasingly severe complications if not managed appropriately. The relatively recent development of e-learning materials on the topic of lymphedema management speaks to an increasing recognition of the need by nurses to aid their work in patient assessment and referrals (Lanning et al., 2020). Lastly, referral process not only enhances patient outcome but also adds to improved nursing practice via ongoing professional development. Exposure to referral indications also enables nurses to understand better how to educate patients on potential health issues regarding head, face, neck, and lymphatics assessment. Ongoing training on good referral procedures, as well as interprofessional practice, offers holistic care to the patient. Moreover, as noted in other medical fields, well-ordered referral systems ensure accountability among health professionals, in line with the better practices of patient management. Such emphasis on a systematic model of referrals not only ensures improved care efficiency but aligns with an integrated system of health, guaranteeing patient welfare through facilitating access to needed evaluation and interventions (Petrashenko et al., 2017).

7.6.3. Collaborative Care Approaches

The collaborative care models are increasingly essential in nursing, particularly in the evaluation of head, face, neck, and lymphatics. Collaborative care stresses interprofessional collaboration when working on intricate health issues, as in patients presenting with symptoms in these anatomical regions. Patients with cancer, for instance, are likely to experience intricate symptoms that require thorough assessment and intervention strategies. Since cancer is the most common cause of death globally, with significant effects on quality of life, the incorporation of collaborative approaches enables multifaceted assessments that treat not only clinical symptoms but also psychosocial factors like pain, depression, and dysfunction (N/A, 2021). The interaction of a number of healthcare professionals—ranging from doctors and nurses to social workers—enables a broader perspective on the patient's needs, hence providing a more efficient therapeutic space. In addition, the role of nurses in multidisciplinary models of care is significant since they often serve as the first point of contact for patients being evaluated for head, facial, neck, and lymphatic diseases.

Nurses possess unique abilities through which they can identify and rank patients' needs from their experiences and observations. Such an ability is complemented by education resources, including the one prepared for nursing staff with a focus on culturally competent health screenings (Accettola et al., 2023). Such preparation equips nurses with clinical expertise that allows them to identify early warning signs, which is essential in an interdisciplinary environment. Through coordination with other health professionals, nurses are in a position to plan on-time interventions that improve patient results, demonstrating the power of collaboration in the health care field. Furthermore, models of care involving interprofessional collaboration generally enhance the quality of the patient experience, particularly for those facing challenging diagnoses such as cancer. Shared responsibility facilitates effective communication between health care professionals, providing room for coordinated action in line with the specific needs of individual patients. For example, in cancer patient care, multidisciplinary forums can usher in innovative solutions to managing treatment side-effects. This teamwork not only addresses physical concerns, such as disfigurement and pain management, but also couples emotional factors with measures that promote well-being so that the well-being of the patient can be addressed in a more holistic manner (N/A, 2021). To achieve these results, curricula emphasize the significance of clinical decision-making and collaboration, which produce improved health equity and safety of patient care (Accettura et al., 2023). Overall, collaborative approaches improve not only nursing practice but also the quality of care given to patients to a large extent.

Test Your Knowledge

1. What nursing interventions can be implemented for patients with common head and neck conditions identified during assessment?
2. How can nurses educate patients on preventive measures and self-care for maintaining head and neck health?

SUMMARY

The culmination of a complete head, face, neck, and lymphatics assessment is important for nursing practice, particularly the detection and treatment of disorders that may occur in these regions. The assessments provide nursing professionals with important information on the general health of patients, enabling them to identify abnormalities or signs of diseases such as cancer. As observed, cancers in these areas are likely to have serious effects on patient health, given that they can cause complex physical and psychological complications past the point of first diagnosis (N/A, 2021). A good understanding of anatomy and function, then, alongside competent assessment skills, equips nurses with the ability to deliver quality care and support and guarantees positive results. Furthermore, the interaction between lymphatic function and cancer development attests to the value added by including lymphatics in routine assessments. Lymphatics play a central role in the metastasis of various forms of cancer and, by and large, influence treatment results and patient prognosis.

Chemotherapy, specifically, may be less effective in treating lymphatic disease due to poor drug penetration, as demonstrated by Cai et al. (2011). This limitation benefits the essential requirement for nurses to be attentive to lymphatic health changes as part of the assessments to optimize patient care, including the option of local drug delivery methods that may provide improved interventions for lymphatically metastatic cancer. Overall, head, face, neck, and lymphatics assessment is a must for nurses to excel at because it allows them to recognize early signs of systemic diseases and actively react. Adding comprehensive nursing assessments with an understanding of the pathophysiologic processes of the conditions affecting these areas enhances the degree of patient-centered care. Being knowledgeable about the significance of lymphatic involvement in disease will inform treatment strategies and aid in improved patient outcomes. Lastly, as the nature of healthcare keeps evolving, the role of nurses in carrying out holistic assessments will increasingly be essential in dealing with head and neck assessment-related issues, solidifying their importance in contemporary nursing practice.

Assessment of the head, face, neck, and lymphatics is a crucial nursing skill that serves as a foundation for health assessments. Structural defects and assessment of sites for lymphatic drainage are significant areas of assessment. Head assessment involves recognition of any defect such as facial asymmetry that may be a symptom of underlying health issues. Clinically, the nurses ought to examine the neck for the presence of any range of motion and swelling or tenderness, indicating cervical pathology issues. An extensive familiarity with these regions of anatomy allows nurses to catch potential complications early enough, thereby ensuring prompt intervention. A thorough process of assessment is generally part of the best outcomes for patients. In addition to observational skills, nursing practitioners need to engage patients in discussing their symptoms and medical history during the examination of the head, face, neck, and lymphatics. By creating a communicative environment, nurses can obtain important information regarding any discomfort or health alterations that patients may be unaware of. Besides, the interaction promotes trust, which plays an essential role in promoting compliance with follow-up tests and treatment protocols. Evaluation of lymph nodes, for example, involves the meaning of detecting swelling or tenderness that can reveal infections or cancers. Not just is extensive evaluation optimized in clinical findings, but it also supports nursing goals of whole-person patient care and education. Impacts of effective head, face, neck, and lymphatics assessment extend as far as patient education and advocacy. By knowing the significance of lymphatic exams and changes in facial anatomy, nurses are better able to inform patients about the significance of follow-up exams and observation of apparently slight symptoms. This aggressiveness is particularly suitable for these higher-risk groups for head and neck cancer. For instance, as noted, cancer is the leading cause of death worldwide, breaking out in populations of all kinds and necessitating the need for early detection measures (N/A, 2021). The incorporation of educational strategies in assessments enhances the possibilities of early diagnosis and intervention, thereby indicating the central position of nursing practice in promoting public health. By being engaged in their care through informed conversations, patients are really involved in the management of their health which is a core component of practice nursing.

KEY TERMS FROM THIS CHAPTER

- Skull
- Temporal Artery
- Sinuses
- Submandibular Gland
- Trachea
- Preauricular Nodes
- Submental Nodes
- Cervical Nodes
- Fontanelle
- Facial Symmetry
- Parotid Gland
- Thyroid Gland
- Lymph Nodes
- Postauricular Nodes
- Submandibular Nodes
- Supraclavicular Nodes

CRITICAL THINKING QUESTIONS

1. **Which cranial nerve is assessed when a nurse asks a patient to shrug their shoulders against resistance?**
   a. Cranial Nerve V (Trigeminal)
   b. Cranial Nerve VII (Facial)
   c. Cranial Nerve XI (Accessory)
   d. Cranial Nerve XII (Hypoglossal)
2. **A nurse palpates a firm, non-tender, enlarged lymph node in the neck. This finding is most likely:**
   a. Normal variation
   b. Acute infection
   c. Chronic inflammation or malignancy
   d. Trauma-related swelling
3. **During assessment of the thyroid gland, the nurse asks the patient to swallow. This maneuver helps the nurse:**
   a. Detect tracheal deviation
   b. Palpate the thyroid lobes for size and nodules
   c. Assess cervical lymph nodes
   d. Evaluate cranial nerve function
4. **A patient presents with facial asymmetry when smiling. Which cranial nerve is most likely affected?**
   a. Cranial Nerve V (Trigeminal)
   b. Cranial Nerve VII (Facial)
   c. Cranial Nerve IX (Glossopharyngeal)
   d. Cranial Nerve X (Vagus)
5. **Which of the following is a normal finding during lymph node assessment?**
   a. Nodes that are hard, fixed, and painless
   b. Nodes that are tender, mobile, and less than 1 cm
   c. Nodes that are matted together
   d. Rapidly enlarging, firm nodes

Short Answer Questions

1. What are the key structures assessed in a head, face, and neck examination?
2. How can a nurse assess the symmetry and movement of facial muscles?
3. What are the normal findings when palpating the temporal and occipital regions of the head?
4. Describe the technique for assessing the thyroid gland and what abnormalities might be detected.
5. How is lymph node assessment performed, and what characteristics indicate abnormal findings?

Answer to Critical Thinking Questions

1. (c) 2. (c) 3. (b) 4. (b) 5. (b)

REFERENCES

1. Accettola, E., Bogdan, A., Callahan, S., Chawda, A., et al. (2023). *Introduction to Health Assessment for the Nursing Professional: Part II*. https://core.ac.uk/download/622362029.pdf (accessed on 16th July 2025).
2. Arends, C. R. (2025). Lymphedema in head and neck cancer survivors: From diagnosis to daily life. https://core.ac.uk/download/631131520.pdf (accessed on 16th July 2025).
3. Bilde, A., Brobeil, A., Cheng, A., Khafif, A., Terada, A., Wagner, A., et al. (2009). Joint practice guidelines for radionuclide lymphoscintigraphy for sentinel node localization in oral/oropharyngeal squamous cell carcinoma. https://core.ac.uk/download/pdf/8339770.pdf (accessed on 16th July 2025).
4. Brighina, F., Catalano, E., Cillino, S., Cosentino, M., et al. (2017). 11th European Headache Federation Congress jointly with 31st Congress of the Italian Society for the Study of Headaches: Rome, Italy. 01–03 December 2017. https://core.ac.uk/download/286078050.pdf (accessed on 16th July 2025).
5. Cai, S. (2011). Development of lymphatic drug delivery platforms for the treatment of carcinomas. https://core.ac.uk/download/213394397.pdf (accessed on 16th July 2025).
6. Carl, J. G., & Furukawa, S. (2025). Skylab IMSS checklist application study for emergency medical care. https://core.ac.uk/download/pdf/42887448.pdf (accessed on 16th July 2025).
7. Cavaye, J. (2009). Service users' views of therapeutic care. https://core.ac.uk/download/3433.pdf (accessed on 16th July 2025).
8. Dobríková, P., Littlechild, B., Slaná, M., Stachurová, A., et al. (2017). The quality of life of hospitalized and outpatient oncological patients. https://core.ac.uk/download/159073173.pdf (accessed on 16th July 2025).
9. Dreiling, M. L. (2022). Promoting adherence to lymphedema management: A resource guide for OT practitioners in interprofessional teams. https://core.ac.uk/download/539325011.pdf (accessed on 16th July 2025).
10. Franks, P., Mercier, G., Moffatt, C. J., Murray, S., et al. (2025). The development and validation of the LIMPRINT methodology. https://core.ac.uk/download/96621180.pdf (accessed on 16th July 2025).
11. Gaudelli, M. (2020). Effectiveness of Vodder manual lymphatic drainage massage in adolescents with post-concussion symptoms. https://core.ac.uk/download/335015409.pdf (accessed on 16th July 2025).
12. Iddagoda, S., Mathangasinghe, Y., Singappuli, K., Weeraddana, D., et al. (2024). A rare presentation of infantile mediastinal mature cystic teratoma leading to progressive respiratory failure–A case series. https://core.ac.uk/download/642711584.pdf (accessed on 16th July 2025).
13. Jayapala, D., & Mathangasinghe, Y. (2024). The prevalence of termination variations of the basilar artery: A systematic review and meta-analysis. https://core.ac.uk/download/642711585.pdf (accessed on 16th July 2025).
14. Kay, S. C. (1990). Time series analysis of touch interventions: Case study of the therapeutic relationship of a hospice client and a nurse-massage therapist. https://core.ac.uk/

download/642338340.pdf (accessed on 16th July 2025).

15. Lanning, B. A. (2020). The development of an e-learning resource on lower limb lymphedema for continuing care nurses. https://core.ac.uk/download/395081014.pdf (accessed on 16th July 2025).
16. N/A. (2021). *Topics in Cancer Survivorship*. https://core.ac.uk/download/478140895.pdf (accessed on 16th July 2025).
17. Petrashenko, V. O., Redko, O. K., Tarasova, I. V., Zaitsev, S., et al. (2017). *Neonatology: Introduction*. https://core.ac.uk/download/141462979.pdf (accessed on 16th July 2025).
18. Plotnikov, P. V., & Zebentaev, A. A. (2017). *Urology*. https://core.ac.uk/download/80152221.pdf (accessed on 16th July 2025).
19. Schneider, L. (2000). The lymphatic system, lymphedema, and a discussion of methods for treatment: A review of the literature. https://core.ac.uk/download/235074037.pdf (accessed on 16th July 2025).

EYE ASSESSMENT IN NURSING

8

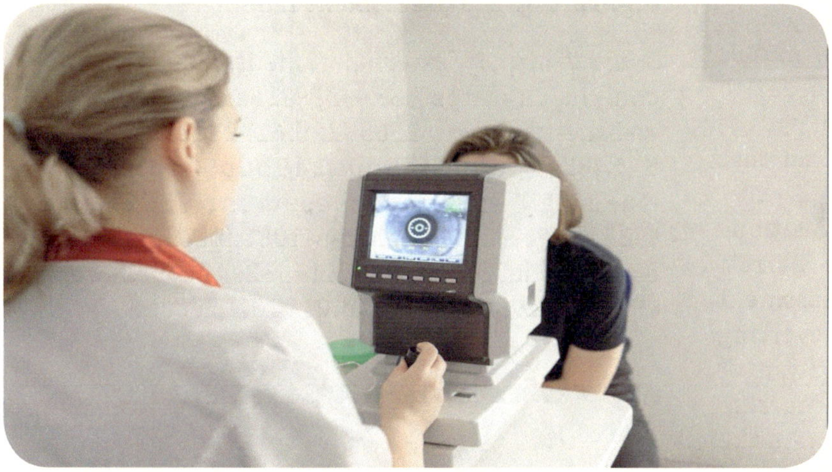

LEARNING OBJECTIVES

After studying this chapter, you will be able to:

1. Elaborate the anatomy of the eye;
2. List the techniques for eye assessment;
3. Identify the common eye disorders;
4. Discuss about patient history and eye assessment;
5. Explaore the documentation and reporting;
6. Define the role of technology in eye assessment.

Introduction

The importance of thorough eye exams in nursing cannot be overstated, given that the eyes are critical markers of overall health. Eye exams are within routine nursing practice, often acting as a window to systemic disease states like diabetes, hypertension, and neurological disease. Nurses have not just an observation role; they are tasked with interpreting visual data accurately in order to support diagnosis and ongoing patient management. In increasingly complex healthcare environments, with technology playing a central role, it is essential for nursing professionals to remain proficient at conducting detailed eye checks. This fundamental skill not only facilitates earlier detection of possible health issues but also underpins successful interdisciplinary communication on the healthcare team so that interventions can be provided in a timely manner. Eye examination is thus a bedrock of nursing expertise with an impact on patient outcomes and the quality of care. Furthermore, advances in telehealth and electronic communication are revolutionizing how eye examination is performed within nursing. Enhanced application of teleconsultation enables remote patient examination using video technology to undertake assessments previously unachievable. This new approach can improve access to care, particularly among individuals who are in underserved or rural populations. Teleconsultation in nursing, however, functions based on the practitioners' ability to maintain a nursing presence though physically remote. According to the findings of a recent study, the teleconsultation interactions need nurses to employ a number of strategies in order to overcome the inherent limitations of video-mediated communication. It is essential that nurses learn about these dynamics as they grapple with the issues of virtual examinations in trying to provide quality patient care (Barrett et al., 2017). Furthermore, eye care assessment practices are influenced not only by evolving technology but also by the incorporation of electronic health records (EHRs) into nursing practice. With EHRs increasingly present in the clinical setting, they introduce an additional factor to documentation and communication of patient information. Effective use of EHRs can easily enable streamlined patient assessment, reducing data collection into a more coordinated form, with easier follow-up. Having another third party—the EHR—engaged in the process of interacting with the patient does require nurses to effectively work on developing their communication skills in order to cover, if any, gaps in connectivity with their patients. Strategies that optimize collaborative practices among nurses and EHRs are vital to achieving optimal patient outcomes as well as high rates of provider and patient satisfaction (Leamon et al., 2016). The role of eye exams within nursing, thus, remains fluid, reflecting a nexus of technological advancement and clinical expertise (Figure 8.1).

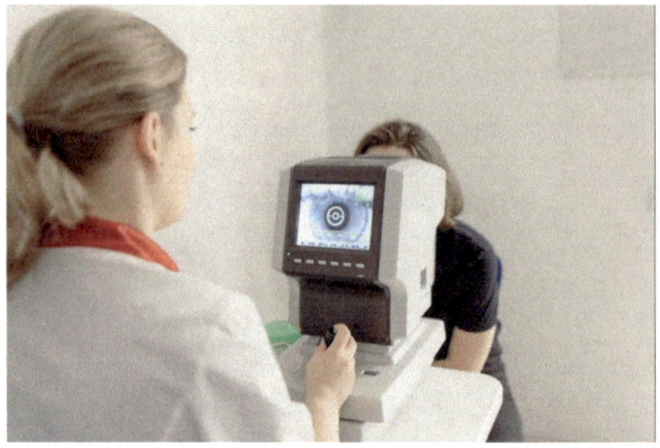

Figure 8.1. Eye assessment nursing.

Source: https://external-content.duckduckgo.com/iu/?u=https%3A%2F%2Fassets-global.website-files.com%2F6572fdb617211ce3d9d76878%2F 660cd48dbd249b6b977e2ddf_Nursing%2520 Assessment%2520of%2520Eye%25 20image-p-1080.jpg&f=1&nofb=1&ipt=ae73ebcbe62022f9b32e42e69a2406e975fb47c98032ec09dadf01976a65ee6f.

Importance of Eye Assessment in Nursing

Eye assessment in nursing is invaluable as it allows health workers to determine potential sight conditions and systemic illnesses at a preliminary stage. Eyes are a critical window to patients overall health because illnesses like diabetes and hypertension can first manifest through eye symptoms. With adequate eye assessment, nurses are able to find out abnormalities that require further evaluation or immediate intervention. This anticipatory practice not only enhances patient outcomes but also facilitates a preventive care culture within the clinical setting. Correct communication of results is paramount; thus, with eyesight assessment becoming more adept among nurses, they facilitate seamless incorporation of information into electronic medical records, encouraging coordination among healthcare providers (Leamon et al., 2016). These skills increase the quality of care and result in improved knowledge of patient health. Moreover, the addition of eye examinations to nursing practice increases patient education and involvement. Nurses are in a position to give good advice and information concerning the maintenance of eye health if they are well informed regarding their patients' eye health. Involving patients in discussions about their eye health and the requirement for regular assessment promotes adherence to recommendations. The information gathered from eye examinations educates nurses to initiate discussions about the risk factors for visual impairment, hence empowering patients to be responsible for their own care. This reinforces the new nursing role for teleconsultation, with video contact enhancing the delivery of health education for eye care, and establishing so-called nursing presence through technology as a vehicle for delivering important health messages (Barrett et al., 2017). Enhanced dexterity of the eyes also enables thorough patient assessment. Lastly, the effect of eye examinations extends beyond direct clinical practice, into broader public health programs as well. Nurses with eye assessment skills can be most useful to community eye health screening programs in early detection and control of visual impairment, ultimately reducing the global burden of eye disease. The programs serve a two-fold purpose: they improve individual patient care as well as augment public awareness in the significance of eye health. By integrating eye testing into their practice, nurses encourage preventive intervention that can counteract the onset of severe disease. In addition, such participation helps encourage interdisciplinary care, bringing together varied healthcare professionals to confront the intricate issues of eye health. Lastly, the broad role of nurses in eye testing emphasizes commitment to whole person care and reinforces the value of education and outreach in nursing practice.

Overview of Common Eye Conditions

Knowledge of common eye problems is important for nursing practitioners since it directly affects patient assessment and intervention. Of the common eye conditions, refractive errors such as myopia, hyperopia, and astigmatism are a major issue in eye health. Myopia, often referred to as nearsightedness, causes objects at a distance to be out of focus, whereas hyperopia or farsightedness causes objects nearby to be out of focus. Astigmatism results from an uneven curvature of the cornea or lens and causes blurred vision. They are generally easily correctable with the use of glasses or contact lenses but must be fully assessed by nurses for referral to ophthalmologists to continue the management and assessment in a timely manner. A second large category of eye disorders includes cataracts, glaucoma, and AMD. Cataracts lead to the clouding of the lens and tend to present as watery vision and glare. Cataracts have the capability of greatly impairing the quality of vision, and therefore nurses play a vital role in teaching patients on the routine eye checks to identify such conditions early enough. Glaucoma, which is a rise in intraocular pressure, may not present with visible signs until a lot of harm has been done, and thus screening is essential. AMD, which impacts central vision, is particularly prevalent in older adults. Early identification and management by nurses with comprehensive assessment can improve patient results and preserve quality of life. In addition to these conditions, ocular infections such as blepharitis and conjunctivitis frequently occur and must be addressed promptly. Conjunctivitis, also referred to as pink eye, can be caused by bacteria, viruses, or allergies and causes redness, discharge, and irritation. Nurses must be adept at recognizing these symptoms and providing adequate education on medication adherence and hygiene. Blepharitis, or inflammation of the edges of the eyelid, may result from seborrheic dermatitis or bacterial infection, necessitating proper management. With the ongoing evolution of the healthcare environment, including the integration of current best practices and patient education into eye exams, nurses' effectiveness in the treatment of these prevalent eye diseases will be optimized for maximum patient outcome and care (Figure 8.2).

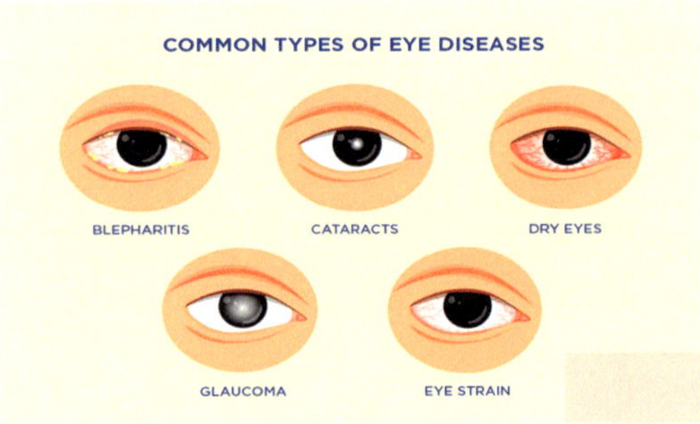

Figure 8.2. Common eye conditions.

Source: https://external-content.duckduckgo.com/iu/?u=https%3A%2F%2Fdj3im2gm3txew.cloudfront.net%2Fpub%2Fmedia%2Fwysiwyg%2Fimage-folder%2Fglasses%2Feye%2Fhealth%2F1-Common-Types-of-Eye-Diseases-900x600.jpg&f=1&nofb=1&ipt=22ae06762dfc5486ca691470568879a4177b28d6dc997cb7d66be9e38b9972a7.

8.1. Anatomy of the Eye

Learning Outcome

1. Structure of the eye;
2. Function of different eye components;
3. Common anatomical variations.

The anatomy of the eye is a complex arrangement of structures serving varying but essential functions in seeing. Light enters the eye through the cornea, which adds the majority of eyes refractive power. This transparent outer layer of the eye refracts forward-moving light rays and funnels them into the pupil, the adjustable opening regulated by the iris. Under the iris lies the lens, which focuses the light rays onto the retina in its sharp focus. Such a complicated structure allows light to be translated into neural impulses, something that is required for seeing. It is crucial to comprehend such complicated details while doing an eye checkup in nursing practice. A nurse should understand how structural abnormalities can impair sight and lead to various ocular diseases. Through comprehensive reviews that consider this anatomy, nurses can provide better care for the patients and assist with targeted treatment plans. The retina at the back of the eye possesses the vital task of changing light into electrical signals. Comprised of various layers, including photoreceptors rods and cones, the retina is responsible for image processing. Rods are sensitive to light and enable us to perceive vision during the night, while cones give us color vision and sharpness of vision. The optic nerve transfers all these electrical impulses obtained from the retina to the brain, where they are interpreted as visual images. In the realm of nursing assessment, examination of the retina is highly essential. With the use of tools such as the ophthalmoscope, nurses can identify signs of diabetic retinopathy, retinal detachment, or macular degeneration. Understanding the anatomy and physiology of the retina allows nursing specialists to provide holistic care and early intervention for patients suffering from vision-related complications, thus enhancing their lifestyle. In addition, other important elements of the eye, including the vitreous body and aqueous humor, enhance its function and integrity. The vitreous body, being a gel filling the area between the lens and retina, helps maintain the shape of the eyes and upholds their inner structures. The aqueous humor, on the other hand, which is secreted by the ciliary body, supplies nutrients to the cornea and lens and helps regulate intraocular pressure. Imbalance in the drainage or production of this fluid is what causes glaucoma, a condition that can potentially destroy vision. Nurses are tasked with intraocular pressure measurement and detection of signs that could indicate disorders during eye checks. This knowledge of anatomical functions and structures enables nurses to manage ocular health preemptively.

Through combining anatomical information with nursing assessments, clinicians can contribute to more effective patient care, in keeping with contemporary best practices for eye health care (Figure 8.3).

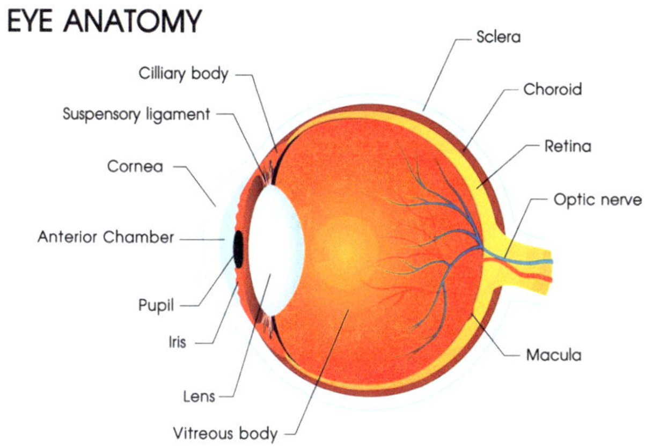

Figure 8.3. Anatomy of the eye.

Source: https://external-content.duckduckgo.com/iu/?u=https%3A%2F%2Fwww.specialtyeyeinstitute.com%2Fwp-content%2Fuploads%2F2021%2F09%2FEye-Anatomy-Image-Specialty-Eye-Institute.jpg&f=1&nofb=1&ipt=a65d3e755c175efb0fb34a78077fe0a8797658b804847f4a43672eb2ab28fb4e.

8.1.1. Structure of the Eye

The human eye is a highly developed organ that is the focal sensory interface for vision. It contains several central structures, and each plays a significant part in the process of sight. The cornea, which lies in front of the eye, is a transparent layer that deflects entering light into the eye and assists with overall focus. Aqueous humor in the anterior chamber, lying behind the cornea, not only nourishes neighboring structures but also controls intraocular pressure. The iris, the structure controlling color, controls the size of the pupil and, consequently, the entry of light into the eye. The lens, lying behind the iris, also refines the focus by changing its shape, a process known as accommodation. It is necessary for nursing practitioners to realize these basics so that they can conduct efficient eye checks to detect potential abnormalities. The uvea is the intermediate layer of the eye and includes the choroid, ciliary body, and iris. All of these are responsible for maintaining healthy vision. Choroid is vascular in nature, supplying oxygen and nutrients to vital tissues while protecting them from excessive light to prevent scatter.

Meanwhile, the ciliary body is equipped with muscles that change the lens to focus effectively on varying distances. The ability of this muscle to contract and relax adapts to dynamic focusing needs for activities ranging from reading to driving. In clinical practice as a nurse, understanding the anatomy of uveal tracts is critical when conducting assessments related to issues such as uveitis or other inflammatory processes that can affect a patient's vision and require appropriate medical treatment. The retina lies at the back part of the eye, and it is a laminated structure composed of light-sensitive photoreceptor cells that convert light into electrical stimuli, which are interpreted by the brain. The retina contains two primary photoreceptors: the light-sensitive rods, which allow for night vision, and the cones, which allow color vision and function best in bright light. The densely cone-populated macula serves to perform functions that involve acute vision, such as reading and recognition of faces. Any such assessment aimed at the eye must consider the integrity of these retinal structures because diseases like diabetic retinopathy or age-related macular degeneration can lead to significant impairment of vision. Therefore, awareness of the intricacy of the retinal structure is invaluable for nursing practitioners who are tasked with the monitoring and management of ocular health problems, as it informs assessment as well as potential interventions (Bianchi et al., 2012; Manigold et al., 2019) (Figure 8.4).

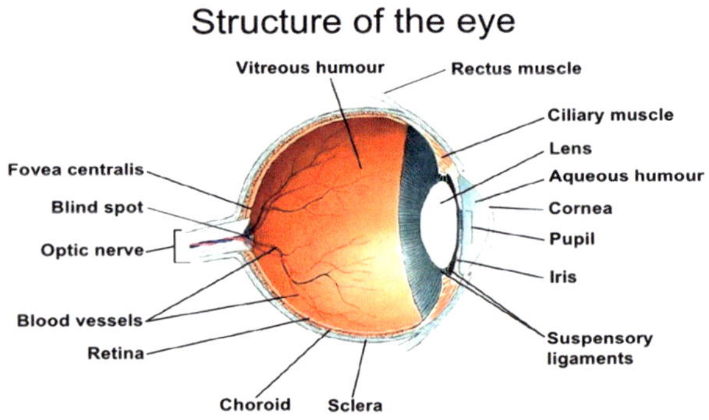

Figure 8.4. Structure of the eye.

Source: https://external-content.duckduckgo.com/iu/?u=https%3A%2F%2Fblog.stuidapp.com%2Fwp-content%2Fuploads%2F2022%2F10%2Feye-structure-1024x658.jpg&f=1&nofb=1&ipt=75a9fdecb51922d731449ec42a77d8447ba431c03da4bd21b86855cb9aa52076.

8.1.2. Function of Different Eye Components

The eye is a highly complex organ with numerous components that act in concert to facilitate vision detection. Preeminent among these components is the cornea, which serves as the chief light entry point. The cornea's curvature and transparency allow light rays to bend, a process known as refraction, which facilitates the convergence of images to the retina. Following the cornea, aqueous humor—formed in the anterior chamber—maintains intraocular pressure and delivers nutrients to the avascular cornea and lens. The iris also regulates light entry into the eye via the pupil. This dynamic interaction highlights the interdependence of these structures and the collective contribution of these structures to the eyes optical processes, which must be considered by nursing exams when evaluating eye function and health. Another extremely crucial component of the eye is the lens, a transparent tightly packed structure that varies in shape to accurately focus light. Accommodation is achieved by the variation in curvature of the lens to permit light rays to hit the retina directly, enabling clear vision at varying distances. The retina, covering the posterior of the eye, is made up of light-sensitive photoreceptor cells—rods and cones—that convert light into neural signals. Rods are responsible for vision in low light, while cones enable perception of color and detail in bright light. Nursing assessments of the eye should include tests for visual acuity and color perception because these are essential functions in identifying potential dysfunctions from various ocular diseases or systemic conditions.

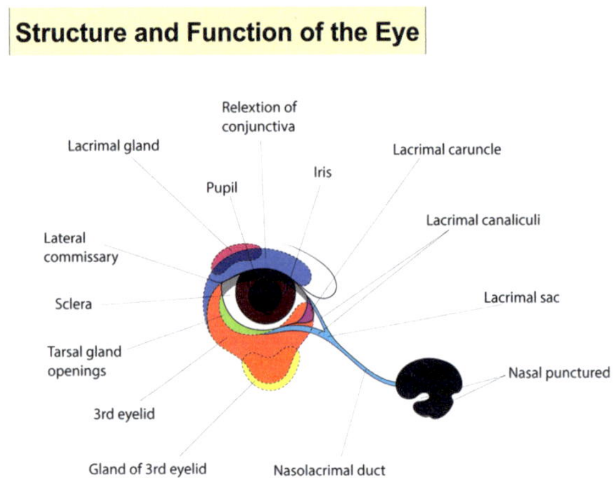

Figure 8.5. Function of different eye components.

Source: https://external-content.duckduckgo.com/iu/?u=https%3A%2F%2Fcdn2.vectorstock.com%2Fi%2F1000x1000%2F37%2F81%2Fstructure-and-functions-of-the-eye-main-parts-vector-48313781.jpg&f=1&nofb=1&ipt=13cfb9cfb197a6ce3a86e3bfb52e9293e0f9c96ace30642bc0eee59fa7c2a07e.

The optic nerve is also an essential part that carries visual information from the retina to the brain for interpretation. This visual pathway is crucial to vision, but it is also susceptible to a variety of conditions, such as glaucoma and diabetic neuropathy, which, if left untreated, result in permanent loss of vision. Comprehensive eye exams in the nursing environment must include not only assessments of the superficial structures of the eye, but also assessments of these deeper structures. Additionally, with advancing medical technology, inclusion of such assessments in electronic health records (EHRs) ensures that pertinent information is adequately recorded and easily accessible, allowing for informed clinical decision-making. By understanding the functions exerted by these different elements of the eye, nurses are able to provide meaningful care and timely interventions, ultimately optimizing patient outcomes in vision health (Leamon et al., 2016; Malek et al., 2025) (Figure 8.5).

8.1.3. Common Anatomical Variations

Understanding normal anatomical variations in the eye is essential for eye examination for nursing professionals. Variations may be present in different forms like anatomical differences of eyelids, corneal morphology, and optic nerve paths. The differences may be caused by genetic tendencies, congenital defects, or environmental factors, potentially influencing the function of vision. For instance, patients may exhibit ptosis, in which the eyelid falls because of muscular or neurological reasons, or variations in pupil size and form, with implications for reflex to light stimulus. Nurses are able to make adjustments in assessment accordingly by recognizing such variations, thus enabling thorough evaluation and adequate patient education regarding ocular health. Another feature of anatomical differences is the variation in positioning of structures within the eye, and such variations can influence diagnostic therapy. For example, the depth of the anterior chamber varies among individuals, and this impacts the susceptibility to developing diseases like glaucoma. Variations in lens shape and positioning can influence refractive defects and thus need specialized ocular examinations. Also, the angle of the anterior chamber comes into consideration when one thinks about the type of tonometry to be used after measuring pressure. Nurses who are aware of such differences are in a better position to screen for preventable eye diseases, and refer early to ophthalmologists when needed. Finally, the realization of variations in ocular anatomy is carried forward to understanding of neuroscientific factors determining the manner in which eye tests should be conducted. The connectivity of nerves such as the optic and oculomotor nerves is important in vision acuity as well as ocular movement. Changes in their paths may result in diplopia or visual field deficit. As prioritized in nursing teaching, effective pedagogy, including the use of miming and gesture, can aid in understanding such complexities to foster an even more interactive learning environment to support future practitioners (Dickson et al., 2015). By integrating anatomical knowledge with hands-on assessment skills, nursing practitioners are in a position to provide extended care and meet the diversified needs of patients to be assessed for eyes (Helmich et al., 2015).

Test Your Knowledge

1. What are the major anatomical structures of the eye, and what are their primary functions?
2. How does knowledge of eye anatomy assist in identifying abnormalities during assessment?

8.2. Techniques for Eye Assessment

Learning Outcome

1. Visual acuity testing;
2. Inspection and palpation methods;
3. Use of specialized equipment.

The eye assessment techniques of nursing are significant for identifying ocular health issues, especially in critical care. Thorough assessment is preceded by visual inspection, allowing nurses to observe the external ocular structures, such as eyelids, conjunctiva, and sclera. Visual inspection for redness, puffiness, or discharge may assist in the early identification of conditions such as conjunctivitis or keratitis. In addition, assessment for lid closure is crucial in mechanically ventilated patients who are at risk for exposure keratopathy. Knowledge of the anatomy of the eye and common conditions enables nurses to recognize abnormalities and institute appropriate interventions in a timely manner, significantly improving patient outcomes. Knowledge of these fundamental techniques is essential for both student and practicing nurses who wish to deliver quality eye care in different clinical environments, hence the necessity for specialized training in the practice area (Mahadevan et al., 2024). In addition to visual inspection, the use of particular devices such as the Snellen chart in determining visual acuity is required. This is the approach that allows the nurses to assess the vision of a patient at varying distances, which turns out to be an important factor influencing eye health. Proper pupillary response and extraocular movement examination is also necessary; any irregularity in these conditions can be an indicator of serious underlying neurological conditions. Techniques such as penlight use for the measurement of pupillary size and light response can be utilized to identify conditions such as afferent pupillary defect. Incorporating these assessments in routine tests enhances early identification of potentially vision-threatening conditions and underscores the essential role of nurses in whole patient evaluations in clinical settings. Inefficient examinations can critically prolong diagnoses, and thus ongoing training in eye examination is paramount (Mahadevan et al., 2024). Teleconsultation has been a groundbreaking technique which builds on traditional eye examination techniques, allowing nurses to access patients at a distance and provide on-time assessments. Teleconsultation has unique benefits, particularly in rural or resource-poor populations where specialist eye care is suboptimal. With video calls, nurses are able to administer initial eye exams, taking advantage of technology to perform visual screening and patient histories quickly.

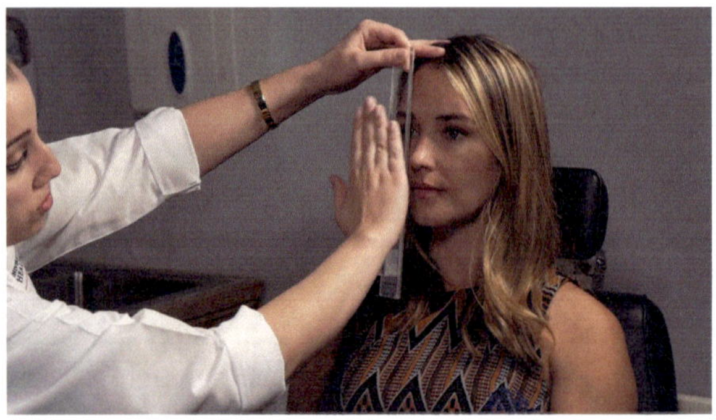

Figure 8.6. Techniques for eye assessment.

Source: https://external-content.duckduckgo.com/iu/?u=https%3A%2F%2Fi.ytimg.com%2Fvi%2FxW6B05a-LTw%2Fmaxresdefault.jpg&f=1&nofb=1&ipt=369c2a189a25c61cffd3594b12856cb792e74a0980047027d498d719eb8fb96c.

The ability to see patients visually from a distance has the potential to enhance the presence of nursing, since nurses compensate using mechanisms when physical assessment is not possible. Incorporating teleconsultation training into nursing programs has the potential to enable nurses to leverage technology to enhance reach without diminishing quality care. With integration of these modern techniques along with traditional measurements, ophthalmic nursing practice can be modified to meet the requirements of multi-diverse populations and enhance global patient outcomes (Figure 8.6).

8.2.1. Visual Acuity Testing

Visual acuity screening is a major instrument of eye examination in nursing, enabling practitioners to quantify the sharpness and clarity of a patient's eyesight. This quantification is especially important in patients with various visual needs, e.g., infants and space travelers who are engaging in long-duration spaceflight. The test of acuity can be done through numerous different techniques, including the Snellen chart and the Acuity Card Procedure, which is best suited for infants. For instance, a study with low-birth-weight neonates highlights the effective evaluation of visual acuity using the Acuity Card Procedure, with a 77.5% success rate in screening this high-risk group. These results highlight the need for proper assessment tools based on specific populations and highlight the need for nurses to be skilled in the use of such techniques for early detection of visual impairments (Arduini et al., 1992). Aside from determining levels of visual acuity, testing enables healthcare providers to track changes across time and assess the effects of any given conditions or environments on eye health. This aspect is particularly significant in unique environments, such as space travel, where there may be significant ocular adjustments due to extended periods of exposure to microgravity. For example, research on astronauts has reported refractive changes and other ocular anomalies following six-month missions on the International Space Station. Such findings not only confirm the necessity of routine visual acuity screening but also require ongoing study of mechanisms underlying such changes, possibly directing nursing practice in monitoring both spaceflight health and recovery at mission end (Cromwell et al., 2011). Thus, knowledge regarding implications of visual acuity testing goes beyond routine clinical environments and can find means to be translated in specialized contexts. Ultimately, the inclusion of visual acuity testing in eye examination processes within nursing involves ongoing education and acknowledgment of emerging methodologies and study findings. Nurses must be apprised of the most current practices and advances in ocular testing, capable of performing thorough assessments potentially resulting in timely interventions. Moreover, as increasing numbers of individuals with different needs require clinical care, from neonates to astronauts, nurses' role in assessing visual acuity will become increasingly valuable. Having a full comprehension of visual function not only maximizes patient outcomes but also reinforces the integrated role of eye exams in overall nursing practice. Offering such assessments promotes active identification of visual impairments, which leads ultimately to enhanced quality of life in populations of patients (Figure 8.7).

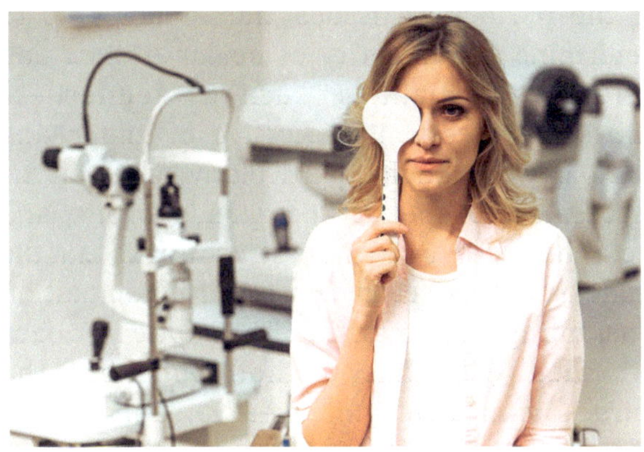

Figure 8.7. Visual acuity testing.

Source: https://external-content.duckduckgo.com/iu/?u=https%3A%2F%2Fmyvision.org%2Fwp-content%2Fuploads%2F2022%2F03%2Fvisual-acuity-testing.jpg&f=1&nofb=1&ipt=696d73f7ac80f780780dce52e948716372c041c9363ca19a52812831b31b54ab.

8.2.2. Inspection and Palpation Methods

During nursing practice, eye examination is a critical skill that begins with inspection and palpation methods. These processes allow nurses to evaluate the overall health of a patient's eyes and provide crucial data for diagnosing potential diseases of the eye. During inspection, visual observation grants the clinician the capacity to document abnormalities within the eyelids, lashes, and conjunctiva, and shape and hue of the iris. This initial assessment is important, as it can detect symptoms of systemic disease, infection, or allergic reaction. Additionally, routine and thorough assessments can lead to the early identification of diseases such as conjunctivitis or cataracts, with significant implications for patient outcomes. This foundational approach not only reminds us of the significance of ocular wellness but also emphasizes the role of the nurse in holistic patient care. Following examination, palpation is an ancillary method that helps in further assessment of ocular structures. By means of soft pressure applied to the periocular tissues, nurses are able to determine the integrity of ocular tissues and detect abnormalities, such as tenderness and swelling that is indicative of underlying pathology. Palpation is particularly helpful in the assessment of the lacrimal glands, orbits, and facial muscles around these structures so that the clinician can detect any masses or inflammation warranting further testing. The haptic feedback provided with this method enhances the nurse's clinical judgment—a valuable aspect in nursing education, as outlined in textbooks like "Introduction to Health Assessment for the Nursing Professional (Accettola et al., 2023)." Hence, the integration of palpation in the process of eye examination allows for detailed analysis encompassing both the visual and physical aspects. The integration of inspection and palpation techniques in eye examinations not only assists in identifying immediate visual problems but also helps accentuate the role of ongoing professional development in nursing practice. As such methods change, nurses' understanding of the underlying principles behind such an assessment change as well. The implementation of effective instructional models in nursing education can enhance the decision-making in eye health to further support students to develop clinical expertise (Edison et al., 2020). In this context, educational materials should provide interactive and practical means of learning that enable nurses to identify clinical signs and adopt culturally-responsive approaches in the context of ocular health. By giving priority to a complete and empathetic eye examination, nursing education can have a significant impact on maintaining improved patient outcomes as well as the quality of care delivered within clinical settings.

8.2.3. Use of Specialized Equipment

In the practice of eye examination in nursing, utilizing advanced equipment is integral to conducting thorough evaluations. Equipment such as the slit lamp and the indirect ophthalmoscope plays an essential role in visualizing intricate eye anatomy. The slit lamp, which is a microscope-high intensity light combination, allows nurses to view the anterior segment of the eye in detail and spot abnormality such as a cataract or abrasion of the cornea. The indirect ophthalmoscope also allows for a wider view of the retina and optic nerve and facilitates the spotting of abnormalities such as diabetic retinopathy or glaucoma. Such devices' precision enhances the nurse's ability for effective and comprehensive patient care, augmenting their diagnostic capabilities and offering early intervention designs when necessary. Moreover, technology use in eye examination with special equipment has guaranteed critical improvements in patient outcomes. The application of digital imaging technologies, for instance, allows one to make high-resolution images of the retina that can be used to monitor change over time. This capability not only allows for increased real-time visualization of eye disease but also aids in longitudinal studies of patient health. These technologies facilitate better communication among healthcare providers, as they can simply share images and findings during interdisciplinary conferences. Moreover, through the data analysis enabled by these sophisticated technology tools, nurses can practice evidence-based intervention enhancing the quality of care and response times for correcting vision issues, and ultimately support enhanced patient health outcomes. Finally, the applied use of advanced equipment in eye exams points to the significance of nurse training and competency. Proficient operation of such equipment as tonometers and vision charts requires more than technical skills; it requires a complete understanding of eye anatomy and pathophysiology. Education and hands-on experience are needed so that nursing practitioners can utilize such equipment with confidence and accurately interpret results. Continuous development of clinical practice guidelines utilizing these instruments is consonant with healthcare goals more generally outlined in quality measurement models. By cultivating a quality culture that encompasses the technical as well as people sides of care, nurses are in a better position to master the complexity of patient assessment and, in turn, affect the quality of care delivered in eye care (Figure 8.8).

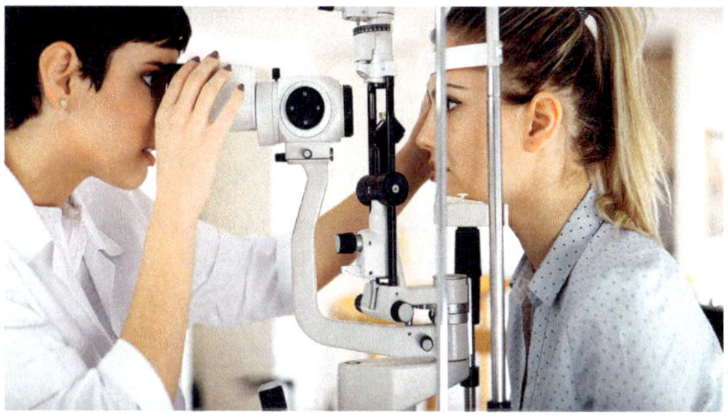

Figure 8.8. Use of specialized equipment of eye assessment.

Source: https://external-content.duckduckgo.com/iu/?u=https%3A%2F%2Fdepisteo.com%2Fwp-content%2Fuploads%2F2018%2F04%2Fadobestock_203369207.jpg&f=1&nofb=1&ipt=1361283495a2c44fa252dd8b542b734ba1f7385d8a057889391163209a7b00e8.

Test Your Knowledge

1. What are the key techniques used to assess visual acuity, pupillary response, and ocular movements?
2. How can inspection and the use of tools like an ophthalmoscope improve the accuracy of eye assessments?

8.3. Common Eye Disorders

Learning Outcome

1. Refractive errors (e.g., myopia, hyperopia);
2. Cataracts and their impact on vision;
3. Glaucoma and its assessment.

The prevalence of common eye conditions highlights the necessity of eye assessment in nursing. Myopia, hyperopia, and presbyopia are prevalent conditions and are frequently encountered in clinical practice. Myopia, or nearsightedness, occurs when the eye elongates and renders distant objects indistinct. Hyperopia, or farsightedness, is due to a reduced eyeball and makes close vision troublesome. Presbyopia is an old age-related condition where the lens of the eyes lose their elasticity, affecting the ability to focus on objects close to them. Not only are such refractive disorders prevalent, but they also have a significant impact on daily functioning, and therefore proper eye assessment by the nursing staff to enable early referral or corrective measures. In addition to refractive disorders, nurses should be vigilant in detecting other prevalent eye conditions such as cataracts and glaucoma. Cataracts, which are the opacification of the eyes lens, are typically expressed through manifestations such as blurred vision and sensitivity to glare. With the aging of the population, cataracts will increase in frequency, with a focus on early identification and intervention within nursing practice. Glaucoma is generally asymptomatic until there has been a significant loss of vision, and it is the routine eye examination that makes early detection possible. The disease is linked with high intraocular pressure, which, if left untreated, causes permanent damage to the optic nerve. Nurses play an important role in tracking patients vulnerable to such diseases and creating awareness in them for repeated eye examinations. Age-related macular degeneration (AMD) and diabetic retinopathy are also critical threats to vision health, particularly for the elderly and diabetics. AMD affects the macula, the region at the middle of the retina that allows for detailed vision, which leads to difficulty reading and recognizing faces. Detection at an early stage is essential since treatments can stop disease worsening and preserve vision. Diabetic retinopathy also needs close supervision due to slow development, with chronic high blood sugar levels damaging the blood vessels on the retina. The interconnectedness of such disorders with systemic illness necessitates a holistic approach to nursing assessment. Through educating patients on the risk factors and lifestyle change, the nursing practitioners have a catalytic role to play in preventing severe visual impairment from these common eye conditions (Figure 8.9).

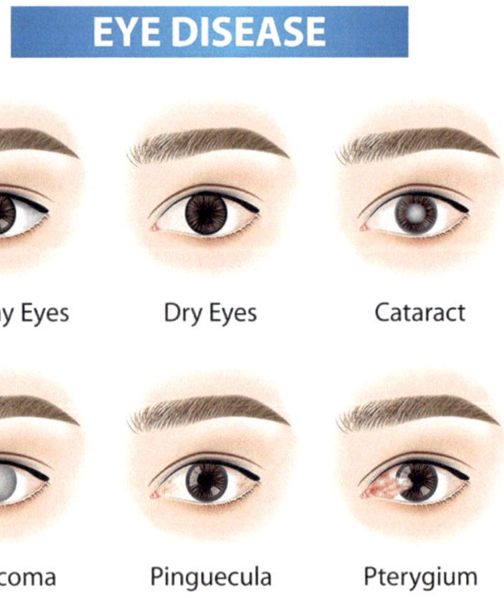

Figure 8.9. Common eye disorders.

Source: https://static.bangkokhospital.com/uploads/2021/07/shutterstock_1101541718.jpg.

8.3.1. Refractive Errors (e.g., Myopia, Hyperopia)

Refractive errors such as myopia and hyperopia occupy a prime position in the scenario of eye test, especially in nursing practice. Myopia, also known as nearsightedness, is a condition in which light rays passing through the eye converge in front of the retina, making it difficult to see things that are distant. In hyperopia, or farsightedness, light converges behind the retina, and it is difficult to view things close by. These conditions are likely to impact a patient's quality of life, so early detection and control are crucial. Proper eye evaluations carried out by nursing staff are critical in the identification of such refractive errors since untreated conditions can progress to other complications, with amblyopia being one of them, especially in children. The early diagnosis is therefore not merely a problem of visual acuity but of overall health care because uncorrected refractive errors may hinder general development progress in children. The methods of detection of refractive error have evolved, and composite ocular assessment in nursing has become vital. The use of automated visual testing machines can enhance the detection of refractive error more than the traditional method. The latest evidence indicates that devices like the PlusOptix™ S12 vision screener can detect more refractive problems in children through frequent screenings, which is significant for prompt intervention. Studies affirm that the integration of such automated screeners into well-child visits allows nurses to effectively manage visual impairment within the visit, ultimately leading to better patient outcomes. This kind of technological advancement fits with the shifting paradigm of nursing practice, which ever more strongly focuses on evidence-based approaches. These practices highlight the nurses' work in being at the forefront of using technology to enable more precise diagnosis, all culminating in quick referrals to ophthalmology whenever the case presents itself, and confirming the interprofessional aspect of managing a patient. In addition, an understanding of how refractive errors occur is crucial for nursing professionals. Visual impairments like amblyopia, which can occur due to undiagnosed refractive errors that go uncorrected, are a significant contributor to visual health among children (Slominski et al., 2018). Amblyopia is not only a condition of the eyes; it is an indication of neuroplastic adjustment of the growing brain which, if not addressed, can result in catastrophic visual deprivation (Slominski et al., 2018). An effective nursing interview should thus also determine the risk factors that may lead to refractive errors in various groups, for example, children. By recognizing the intricate dynamics of refractive anomalies and other conditions like amblyopia, nursing practitioners will be integral to preventive health. Not only will their interventions enhance visual wellness in their patients, but also overall well-being by fostering early detection and regular checks for vision acuity (Figure 8.10).

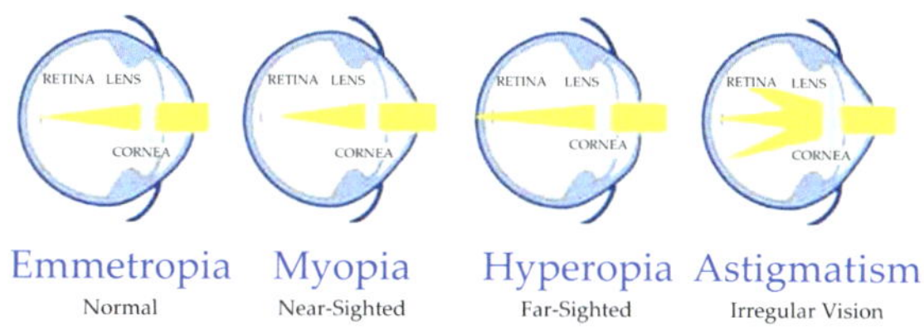

Figure 8.10. Refractive errors.

Source: https://insighteyeok.com/wp-content/uploads/2020/10/INS_Refarctive-Errors.jpg.

8.3.2. Cataracts and Their Impact on Vision

The formation of cataracts is a serious threat to the vision acuity, ultimately affecting the lifestyle of millions of individuals around the world. Characterized by the fogging of the eye lens, cataracts disrupt the transmission of light, producing symptoms such as blurred vision, halos around lights, and night vision impairment. As such signs become more pronounced, patients will find daily functioning increasingly impaired, highlighting the need for accurate assessment and intervention in nursing practice. Correct eye examination is the most important factor in establishing the presence of cataracts because nurses are most often on the ground in dealing with patients and are tasked with identifying early signs and appropriate referrals for further diagnosis. Lastly, understanding the impact of cataracts on vision allows nursing practitioners to provide important education and support, facilitating greater patient autonomy and safeguarding. Furthermore, the development of cataracts points to the importance of eye health education for nurses. Nurses are in a key position to encourage routine eye screening, particularly in groups at increased risk, for example, the elderly and individuals with co-morbid conditions such as diabetes. Patient education about lifestyle modifications can also be a significant factor in cataract development, as smoking, sun exposure over time, and dietary deficiencies have all been linked to cataract formation. By incorporating this information into ongoing nursing assessments and patient education, individuals can be facilitated to become proactive in their eye care. By establishing a feeling of awareness regarding these risk factors and the importance of early diagnosis, nurses reassert their position as not only caregivers but also educators in the eye care discipline. Finally, efficient prevention measures against cataracts must be highlighted in the nursing model to facilitate the maximum possible outcomes in patients. Surgical intervention is the treatment of choice in the case of established cataracts, but pre-operative assessment and postoperative care fall under the ambit of nursing. Comprehensive eye testing has an important part to play in determining the suitability of patients for surgery, thus highlighting the importance of proficiency in assessing visual skills. Postoperative care is all about monitoring complications, teaching patients about visual rehabilitation, and assessing functional vision following surgery. Working in a multidisciplinary team, nurses play a pivotal role in delivering whole-patient care, which helps individuals regain their vision and enhances the quality of life. Because cataracts have a significant impact on visual function, eye examination and management are given prominence in nursing practice to provide effective patient-centered care (Figure 8.11).

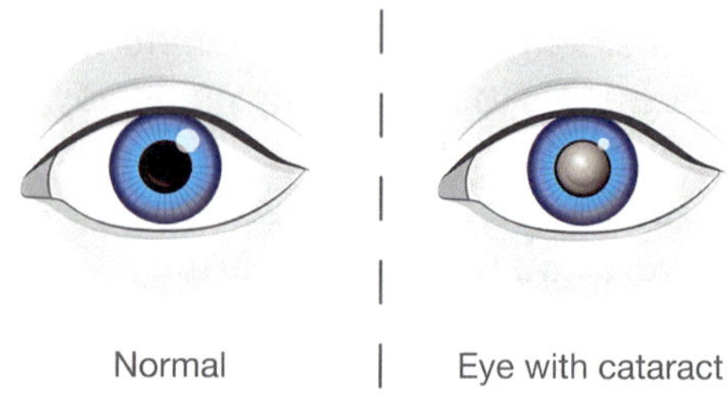

Figure 8.11. Cataracts and their impact on vision.

Source: https://www.aoa.org/AOA/Images/Patients/Eye%20Conditions/Eye-Cataract.jpg.

8.3.3. Glaucoma and Its Assessment

Assessment of glaucoma is an important aspect of comprehensive eye exams among nurses, particularly since the illness has an insidious onset. Glaucoma will progress without overt symptoms, so most patients are unaware that they are losing their eyesight progressively until it is worse. Regular screening using intraocular pressure measurement, visual field testing, and optic nerve assessment must be initiated in order to facilitate early detection. The nurse practitioners play the central role since they can elicit awareness among the patients about the importance of having such assessments and adherence to therapy. When the medical professionals identify barriers to compliance, including lack of pain or visible symptoms, they can improve their approaches to communication so as to improve patient outcomes, in this case, the management of their glaucoma (Cox et al., 2012). Patient compliance with glaucoma drug treatment is a complex issue, with intricate environmental and psychological determinants. The seriousness of the eye drops they have been prescribed is not always realized by patients, and it is not until they have lost their sight severely that patients understand the gravity of their condition. This does reflect a discrepancy between patient awareness and reality in terms of the progression of their illness, founded in the stealthy manner of the disease's progression. Nursing assessments should therefore consider the patient's cognitive states, such as dementia, which complicates medication management (Harper et al., 2018). Effective communication and patient- and caregiver-provider relationship establishment between providers, patients, and caregivers can allow for compliance. In specific, patient-specific information on home circumstances and recall memory capabilities enables nurses to undertake tailored approaches to eliciting compliance with treatment strategies. Moreover, the inclusion of supportive interventions in combination with glaucoma assessment is important for optimal patient outcomes. Nurses must also be equipped to recognize social determinants that influence a patient's capacity to remain on treatment regimens. For instance, presence of concerned family members will aid in monitoring medication adherence, a valuable service for patients with cognitive impairment (Harper et al., 2018). Family-based strategies can serve to bring external support to patients, closing gaps created by non-adherence secondary to dementia or comorbidities. As such, educational interventions clarifying the relationship between adherence and long-term visual function can empower patients throughout their treatment. Through promoting understanding and support, nursing practitioners can greatly improve the management of glaucoma and counteract its deleterious effects on vision (Figure 8.12).

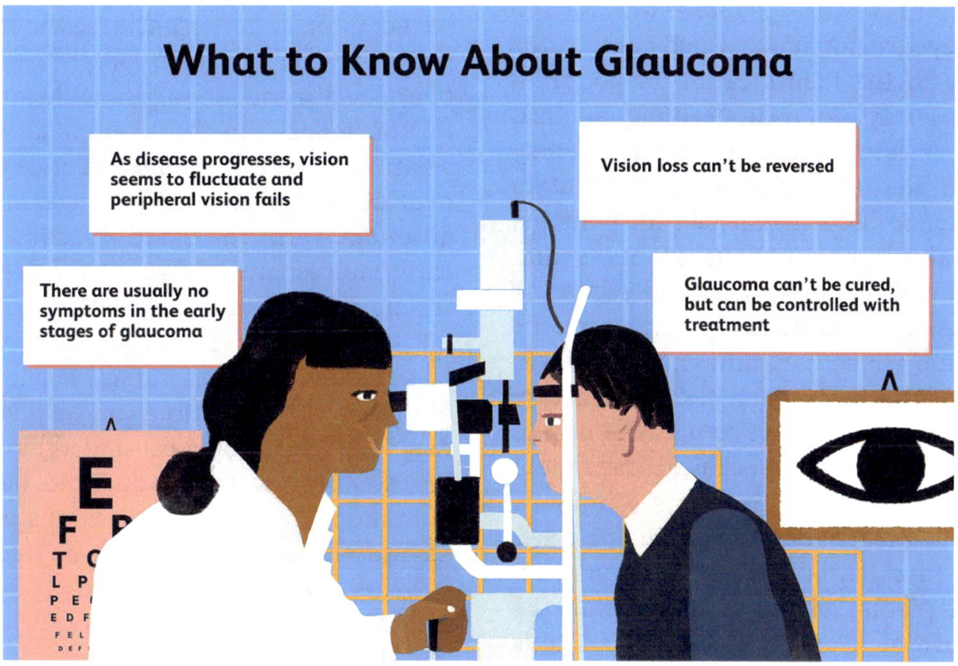

Figure 8.12. Glaucoma and its assessment.

Source: https://www.verywellhealth.com/thmb/CXci8IKARjfe4Lu5ahpaTD-xtio=/1500x0/filters:no_upscale():max_bytes(150000):strip_icc()/Glaucoma-overview-3421722_final-6a69af8338584e2ab11102d00ca1ad11.jpg.

Test Your Knowledge

1. What are some common eye disorders, and what assessment findings are typically associated with each?
2. How can early detection of conditions like glaucoma, cataracts, or conjunctivitis affect patient outcomes?

8.4. Patient History and Eye Assessment

Learning Outcome

1. Importance of patient history in eye care;
2. Key questions to ask during assessment;
3. Identifying risk factors for eye diseases.

Taking patient history is essential in the practice of eye examination, which contributes significantly to the identification of potential ocular diseases as well as underlining medical conditions. A comprehensive patient history should entail not only prior ocular complaints but also systemic diseases that have the potential to impact the eyes, such as diabetes and hypertension. Family history inquiry regarding ocular disease can also identify potential genetic predisposition which may influence diagnosis. This wide-ranging exploration of patient history is the core of nursing practice because nurses are often on the frontlines of clinical assessment within clinical practice environments. By optimal collection and interpretation of patient histories, nurses are in a better position to construct an accurate picture of the causes behind the patient's current eye health status, and thus enhance their ability to intervene and facilitate optimal patient care. An important aspect of eye assessment is the interfacing of assessment techniques and devices that support the obtained patient history. Nurses should possess the expertise to operate instruments such as the ophthalmoscope to allow direct viewing of the retina and ocular abnormalities. Visual acuity testing, pupil reaction, and confrontational visual fields are other tests that cumulatively allow for complete examination of the ocular system. Moreover, patients' symptom clarification, i.e., vision disturbance, pain, or discomfort, can lead to significant streamlining of the assessment process. It is critical for nurses to observe and monitor the subtle signs during such examinations, which can be indicating pointers for wider health complications. Through the integration of patient history and evidence-based information from assessment, nursing personnel can develop a comprehensive picture of eye health and identify suitable interventions. Furthermore, the moral implications of eye examination in nursing practice cannot be overlooked, particularly concerning patient autonomy and informed consent. As health care choices grow increasingly dependent on technology and advanced techniques, the onus for learning these innovations with dignity and wisdom rests on nurses. For instance, eye examination procedures can involve advanced diagnostic technologies, and thus nurses are responsible for presenting the benefits and limitations of these interventions clearly. This data supports a co-production approach, gaining patients trust and enabling informed decision-making regarding their care. Furthermore, the integration of ethics of technology design can ensure that eye testing innovations are such that patient dignity and wellbeing are preserved, as emphasized by care-focused strategies that place central importance on the voice of patients throughout their healthcare journey (Wynsberghe et al., 2012). The integration of ethical consideration into eye tests ultimately yields a dignified and empowering patient experience (Gottlieb et al., 1979) (Figure 8.13).

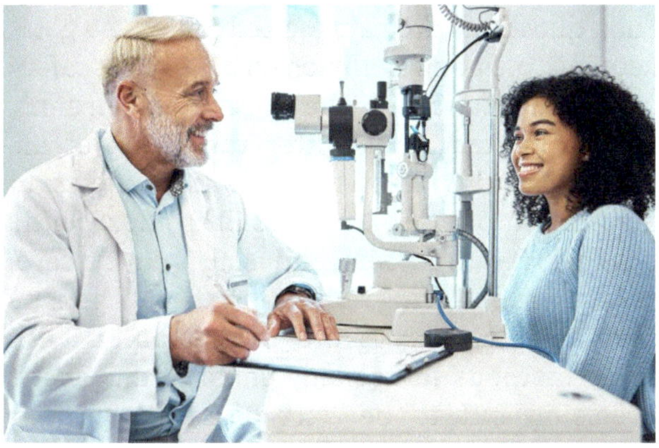

Figure 8.13. Patient history and eye assessment.

Source: https://greathillseyecare.com/wp-content/uploads/2024/06/comprehensive-eye-exam-hero-1-1024x672.jpg.

8.4.1. Importance of Patient History in Eye Care

During conducting eye examinations, taking of thorough patient history is most crucial in establishing potential ocular as well as systemic diseases. An excellent history does not just show the primary reasons for a patient's consultation but also insight one into the underlying conditions of well-being that can influence ocular health. For example, patients with autoimmune illnesses, for instance, those associated with HLA-B27 positivity, can have eye-associated symptoms that are an expression of systemic disease. Nurses thus have to work assiduously to evaluate medical histories in an effort to identify any relationship between systemic diseases and ocular manifestations. This first step is significant since it will allow health care providers to formulate individualized assessment plans and interventions guided by the patient's own health terrain, thereby enhancing the quality of care delivered in ophthalmic centers. Besides accommodating medical history, a patient's medication profile needs to be comprehended by the eye examiner. Certain drugs have also been discovered to induce ocular side effects that complicate diagnosis when not accurately documented. For instance, patients using corticosteroids may develop elevated intraocular pressure leading to glaucoma. Inclusion of medication history alongside general health information allows nurses to recognize potential interactions and foretell complications during the administration of these medications. Moreover, taking a holistic patient history supports a collaborating environment in which patients are motivated to provide relevant information. This interview ultimately benefits the promotion of a more comprehensive understanding of ocular health, which allows for alignment of treatment plans with the unique patient needs and enhances nursing effectiveness in eye care assessment. Finally, the intersection of clinical observation and patient history provides the unique benefit for nurses to formulate evidence-based, informed interventions tailored to specific cases. The integration of detailed patient history and clinical examination can significantly influence the diagnosis of such illnesses as uveitis, which is also related to systemic illness such as Crohn's disease and ankylosing spondylitis. The nurse's most crucial role to play in this image cannot be overstated; they are directly responsible for assessing not only the ocular manifestations but also the broader implications of any systemic disorder that may be inferred from the patient's presentation. Using data from evidence-based studies, nurses are better placed to navigate the complexities of patient care so as to address immediate and long-term ocular requirements. Consequently, patient history is a bedrock of eye care nursing practice, which reinforces the need for careful and close attention during patient examination.

8.4.2. Key Questions to Ask During Assessment

Effective eye assessment in nursing is mostly based on the strategic formulation of key questions that guide practitioners to elicit relevant information. To begin, the patient's ocular history must be queried. Examples include "Have you noticed any alterations to your vision recently?" or "Do you have a history of eye disease in your family? "Can provide important information regarding the patient's current vision health as well as any genetic problems. This initial question provides a baseline of the patient's visual acuity and highlights the appropriate areas that need to be questioned in greater detail. By open discussion, nurses promote an atmosphere that is conducive to correct assessments, allowing for a complete appreciation of the patient's vision." This rapport is vital in that, besides facilitating data collection, it also ensures enhanced patient comfort and co-operation in divulging significant information regarding their eye condition. Aside from visual history, it is also vital to assess the impact of lifestyle and environmental factors on the patient's eye condition. Areas in daily life discussed through queries include, for example, "How many hours a day do you spend in front of screens? " or "What kind of lighting do you usually work in?" enable nurses to identify potential harms from long-term exposure to noxious stimuli. Secondly, being aware of a patient's occupation can disclose some hazards that would affect vision, which in turn can guide relevant preventive measures or intervention. For instance, health care providers can prescribe protective glasses for patients engaged in high-risk occupations. Integrating these questions into eye exams not only contributes to the nurses' awareness of potential risk factors, but also educates patients on optimal practices for ocular health, ultimately resulting in proactive participation in their own care. Lastly, it is crucial that nursing exams cover questions related to patients' overall health and medication use because these have heavy implications on ocular issues. The types of questions such as "Are you currently taking any medications at all, including over-the-counter drugs?" or "Do you have any chronic illnesses such as diabetes or hypertension?" aid in the revelation of systemic problems that can lead to ocular manifestations(undefined). Such questions are categorized under the gate-keeping role of nurses in ensuring patient safety and competence in eye care interventions, as highlighted in the literature (Cox et al., 2013). Besides, knowledge of side effects of medication on vision can result in therapeutic changes required for rendering quality care, yet again solidifying the importance of holistic assessments. Nurses are thus enabled with these methods to not only enhance diagnostic precision but to be part of better patient outcomes through a deeper appreciation of the intricate eye-wellness connection (Figure 8.14).

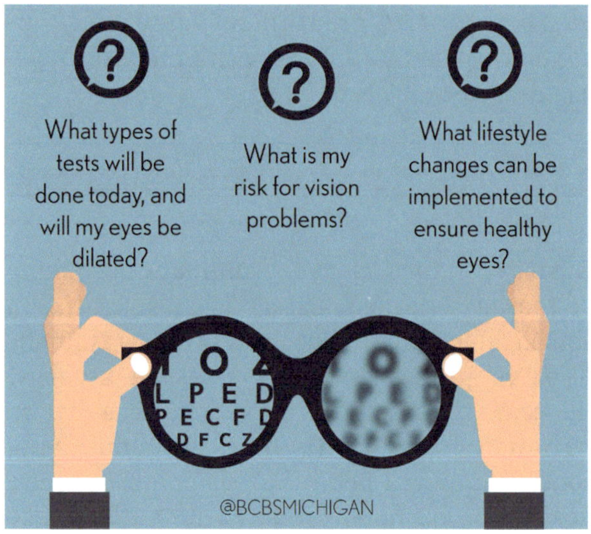

Figure 8.14. Key questions to ask during assessment.

Source: https://www.ahealthiermichigan.org/wp-content/uploads/2022/08/Questions-to-Ask-an-Optometrist-01-1.jpg.

8.4.3. Identifying Risk Factors for Eye Diseases

Risk factor identification for ocular disease forms an essential part of the role of nursing, particularly in the context of general patient assessment. Nurses play a central role in evaluating ocular status in patients, particularly those with predisposing conditions such as diabetes and hypertension. Such chronic conditions are most commonly associated with complications such as diabetic retinopathy and hypertensive retinopathy, whose resultant vision loss can be devastating if not properly monitored. Also, factors such as family background, ethnicity, and age predispose individuals to most of the eye conditions. For instance, older adults have a greater incidence of conditions including age-related macular degeneration and cataracts, thus making nurses need to be vigilant to identify such risk factors within their patient population (Mahadevan et al., 2024). Eye assessment nursing practice is not simply observing; it is a proactive practice that prevents and minimizes the impact of eye disease. In critical care settings, nurses discover that a large number of patients are at risk for ocular issues as a result of prolonged immobility or mechanical ventilation. For example, exposure keratopathy can result from poor eyelid closure in mechanically ventilated patients, and therefore intervention becomes imperative. Nurses must remain vigilant to the acute ocular risks of critical illness, as well as to the long-term outcomes of undiagnosed eye disease. Thoughtfully constructed protocols for eye care—with emphasis placed on patient identification at risk—can enhance patient outcomes by allowing early intervention and treatment of visual impairment (Andrew et al., 2017). Lastly, the interconnectedness of vision impairment and international health cannot be underestimated, particularly in elderly individuals. Research has indicated that older individuals with self-reported eye disease also experience reduced mobility and increased fear of falling, contributing to health complications inherent in visual impairment. These findings suggest that nurses must incorporate comprehensive assessments of eye health as a component of fall risk assessment, dealing with the complex problems surrounding vision and mobility. Nurses can be more effective at meeting their patients' needs if they apply tools such as the Fear of Falling Avoidance Behavior Questionnaire (FFABQ) when screening for patients exhibiting avoidance behavior based on their vision status. By incorporating these items into their assessments, nursing professionals can more effectively encourage an integrative model in the management of their patients' care, ultimately leading to improved quality of life for those at risk of eye disease (Andrew et al., 2017).

Test Your Knowledge

1. What questions should be included in a patient's eye health history to identify risk factors or previous ocular problems?
2. How can a thorough patient history complement physical eye assessment findings?

8.5. Documentation and Reporting

Learning Outcome

1. Importance of accurate documentation;
2. Standardized reporting formats;
3. Legal implications of documentation errors.

Accurate documentation and reporting are important aspects of the nursing practice, particularly in conducting eye exams. Accurate documentation not only serves as a tool of patient data documentation but also as a critical tool that aids in continuity of care. When nurses document thoroughly after an eye exam, they create a complete picture of the patient's ocular status that can inform follow-up interventions and assessments. This systematic documentation facilitates clinical decision-making and communication between multidisciplinary teams. Furthermore, by adhering to established guidelines for documentation, nurses are able to avoid the danger of miscommunication due to incomplete or ambiguous records. Under this, electronic health records (EHRs) have transformed the world of documentation, thereby enhancing the efficiency as well as effectiveness of reporting processes in nursing settings (Leamon et al., 2016). In clinical practice of nursing, documentation of eye assessment findings is a fundamental determinant of quality care and safety of patients. Sharing of information on outcomes of assessments, either abnormal or within the limits, is crucial in ensuring timely intervention. Documentation provides a history that can be useful in follow-up assessment or in situations where patients condition changes. By situating data collected through eye exams within context, nurses can narrate a story that represents the overall health state of the patient and thereby influence treatment. Furthermore, systematic reporting frameworks like SBAR (Situation, Background, Assessment, Recommendation) allow nurses to convey findings in clear and effective terms and thus facilitate improved coordination between other healthcare practitioners. This practice not only helps in patient care on an individual basis but also aids in fulfilling the expectations of nursing documentation within healthcare systems (Patty et al., 2014). Finally, the worth of thorough documentation and reporting isn't only viewed in current patient care but also in influencing bigger picture healthcare quality initiatives. Since healthcare is more and more emphasizing safety and effectiveness, the ability to track and analyze documented eye exams becomes paramount to quality improvement efforts. Analysis of trends and patterns of eye health information can be employed to identify likely risk areas and inform institutional policy to maximize patient outcomes. Along with ongoing research and development in technology, documented practices enable evaluation of the impact of interventions along with possible areas for nursing staff education and training. This integrative practice of documenting and reporting not only reinforces individual practice as a nurse but also aligns with organizational goals in delivering quality care to patients in the dynamic healthcare industry (Leamon et al., 2016) (Figure 8.15).

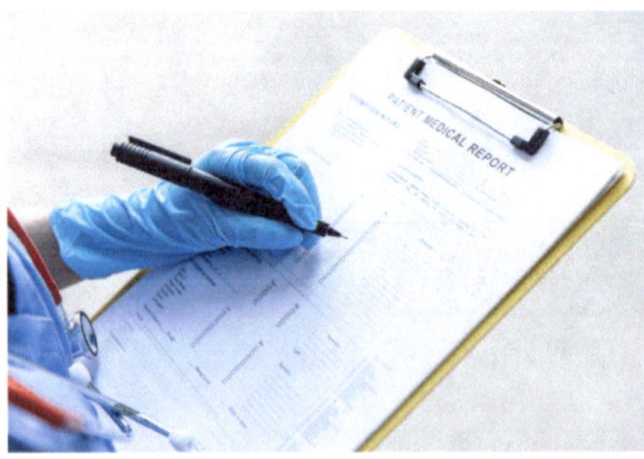

Figure 8.15. Documentation and reporting.

Source: https://wf-labs.s3.amazonaws.com/public/courses/249/images/cover/observation%2C_reporting%2C_and_documentation_1710744462947.jpg.

8.5.1. Importance of Accurate Documentation

Proper documentation of nursing practice, particularly in performing eye examinations, is a building block of patient safety and quality care. Proper and timely recording of observations regarding visual acuity, range of motion, and ocular conditions allows for the creation of comprehensive patient histories, which in turn inform informed clinical decisions. Not only does it reveal the possibility of ocular complications but also assists in tracking the trend of treatments over time. In the arena of electronic health records (EHRs), accurate documentation enhances the communication among the health providers, enhancing a care continuum essential to address the needs of the patients. Possession of the ability to refer to an organized record creates a foundation for ongoing monitoring, thereby enhancing the nursing process with rich information that guides patient outcomes (Leamon et al., 2016). The effects of inadequate documentation are far-reaching, causing misinterpretation and potential injury to patients. During eye examination, defective records can cause failure to note crucial changes in a patient's status, adversely prejudicing treatment. Furthermore, inconsistency in recording encourages dilapidation of communication among interdisciplinary teams and leads to piece-meal care. For instance, if the recorded results of the patients are incomplete or misleading, future clinicians will lack vital information, and this can lead to inaccurate diagnoses or incorrect treatment options. Emphasizing strict documentation practice can bring about a great improvement in the quality of care and patient well-being (Armstrong et al., 2012). Besides, investing in education and training on correct documentation is essential for nursing practitioners. As more healthcare organizations implement EHR systems, nurses must learn effective skills in communications and documentation to practice appropriately. Documentation improvement programs improve not only confidence in technology use but also significantly impact overall patient experience and satisfaction. As demonstrated across a range of clinical environments, incorporation of best practice documentation techniques gives nurses the power to describe their observations and choices concisely, minimizing the chance of errors. By adopting good habits of documentation, nurses are a part of a safety culture and an environment of accountability that will ultimately promote improved care for the patient (Leamon et al., 2016).

8.5.2. Standardized Reporting Formats

Standardized reporting templates are crucial in nursing, particularly when taking an eye examination, because they facilitate the uniform presentation of patient observations and assessments. Employment of standardized reporting templates guarantees that healthcare professionals effectively convey critical information, thereby enhancing inter-professional communication and ultimately patient outcomes. Employment of standardized reporting avoids ambiguity and inconsistencies that may arise as a result of variation in individual documentation methods. Clinicians may refer to specific criteria and measures in a systematic way, and this helps the reliability as well as the transparency of the results in the test. Standardized formats help in adherence to evidence-based nursing practices and help transfer critical information effectively. Standardization in eye tests enables nurses to identify significant changes in patients' eye health more effectively. For instance, in reporting outcomes from visual acuity tests, standardized guidelines can be employed by nurses that require necessary parameters such as measurement procedures and scoring. It is not only necessary for proper assessment but also for creating appropriate care plans. The standardized formats can also serve as educational tools for nurses, helping new recruits become properly familiar with required assessment methods and reporting protocols. Furthermore, by having consistency throughout paperwork, health centers can easily examine data trends over time, which allows for ongoing quality improvement programs (John, 2007). Furthermore, the effectiveness of standardized reporting forms extends to their ability to enhance patient safety and continuity of care. Effective communication during handovers is especially essential where eye tests are conducted, e.g., hospitals or outpatients clinics. Research proves that poor standardized communication procedures may compromise the safety of patients because critical information regarding test results may be omitted or miscommunicated (Tasseri et al., 2013). The incorporation of standardized reporting procedures into the nursing protocol can significantly reduce such errors in institutions. Not only do these structures standardize information delivery, but also build nurses' confidence in making the same as well as in taking action following results from assessment, so that patients' care stays at the heart of nursing practice (Figure 8.16).

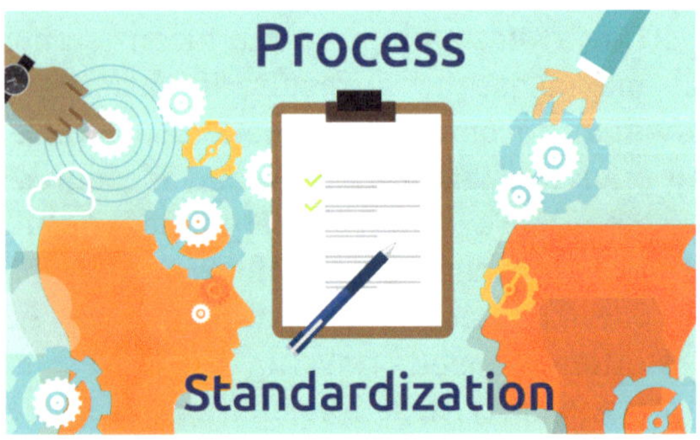

Figure 8.16. Standardized reporting formats in nursing.

Source: https://external-content.duckduckgo.com/iu/?u=https%3A%2F%2Fcheckflow.io%2Fimg%2Fbanner-process-standardization.png&f=1&nofb=1&ipt=8f8630d09d6fd9bf8188732384afc2b0ed4a557f202d11920f2cea3b91ec8e48.

8.5.3. Legal Implications of Documentation Errors

When conducting eye examinations in nursing, the level of accuracy in documentation is paramount since inaccuracy may carry heavy legal implications for health practitioners. Nurses need to maintain accurate patient examination records, including findings during the process of examination. Incomplete or inaccurate documentation may not only jeopardize patient safety but also hold nurses accountable in the event of a malpractice claim. If a patient undergoes harmful effects from a failure to record important results, such as changes in vision or potential signs of eye ailments, the legal implications are severe. Courts are prone to base judgments on documentation as a key determiner of whether proper standards of care were met, as record quality is essential within nursing practice, particularly in situations such as eye evaluation for health (Campbell et al., 2019). Furthermore, the legal ramifications of documentation errors extend beyond individual liability to include institutional penalties. Health facilities may be legally harassed if a pattern of poor documentation is established among their staff. Compliance with nursing procedures by regulatory bodies is monitored, and failure to comply with documentation standards can result in loss of accreditation, legal penalties, and increased insurance premiums for facilities. Proper documentation in eye examinations is given importance by the need for open communication among health professionals. This is especially important at handoff times when crucial patient information is being transferred from one caregiver to another. The threat of miscommunication is higher if documentation is incomplete or missed at such transfers, hence impacting patient care and possibly exposing both individuals and healthcare organizations to increased legal risk (Baker et al., 2014). Moreover, to reduce the legal implication of documentation errors, nursing education must include training for correct documentation procedures. The emphasis on proper record-keeping must be integrated into the curriculum of nurses to equip future practitioners with the skills and knowledge necessary to avoid legal problems. Simulation-based education, as mentioned in the context of clinical handoffs, can bring to the fore the significance of written communication in nursing. The application of systematic, evidence-based documentation systems in documentation processes fosters a culture of accountability and promotes compliance with the law. By recognizing the critical role documentation plays in upholding legal and ethical healthcare standards, nurses can better cope with the intricacies of patient care and safeguard against documentation errors that can lead to the consequences of eye tests (Campbell et al., 2019).

Test Your Knowledge

1. How should normal and abnormal eye assessment findings be documented to support continuity of care?
2. What details are essential when reporting eye assessment results to other healthcare providers?

8.6. Role of Technology in Eye Assessment

Learning Outcome

1. Advancements in diagnostic tools;
2. Telehealth and remote eye assessments;
3. Future trends in eye assessment technology.

The introduction of technology in eye examination has essentially changed the way nursing is practiced, with greater efficiency and precision in patient evaluation. The use of high-tech diagnostic equipment helps medical practitioners conduct extensive examinations with higher accuracy, and thus they are able to identify and treat ocular ailments earlier. For example, tools like optical coherence tomography (OCT) offer detailed imaging of the retina, allowing for easier identification of conditions like macular degeneration and diabetic retinopathy. Besides, the integration of artificial intelligence (AI) tools in ophthalmology comes with real-time image analysis, which reduces human error potential and offers nurses a uniform method of determining patients' needs. This technology underscores the necessity for ongoing education for nursing professionals to adopt such innovations and thereby effectively implement such equipment in practice. Another significant feature of technology in eye examination is the enabling of communication among healthcare teams and patients. Electronic health records (EHRs) streamline patient documentation and data sharing, enabling nurses to easily access detailed information while conducting eye examinations. As shown in existing findings, interoperability characteristics and hand-held qualities are crucial for nurses to allow them to see patient data without being interrupted and provide care continuity (N/A, 2010). In addition, telehealth services have proven to be a valuable asset that allows remote eye examination and follow-ups, which prove useful in patients who may find it difficult to present themselves to healthcare centers. With the integration of these technologies, nursing professionals can prepare themselves with evidence-based data that favors decision-making and leads to improved patient outcomes. Through cooperation between the various stakeholders in the technology arena, solutions are found for developing innovative solutions to the dynamic issues encountered in eye examination. Such programs as those sponsored under DAAD in Germany and CRUP in Portugal are aimed at developing methodologies of technology appraisal, particularly those for robotics and autonomous systems applicable in healthcare settings (António B Moniz). Identifying how the trends of knowledge production and control of technology are shifting will allow nurses to easily integrate new technologies into practice while shaping policies that make it easy to utilize cutting-edge innovations. This multi-pronged technology strategy goes not only beyond the capability of nurses to perform eye examinations but also toward a complete system centered on patient safety and quality of care in the rapidly changing area of eye care (Figure 8.17).

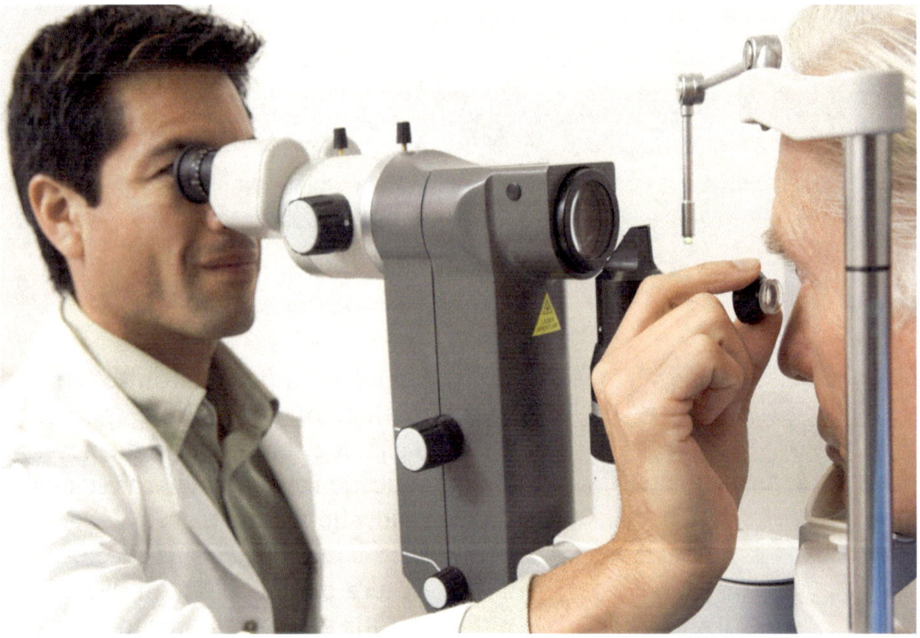

Figure 8.17. Role of technology in eye assessment.

Source: https://external-content.duckduckgo.com/iu/?u=https%3A%2F%2Fwww.infinityvisiondallas.com%2Fwp-content%2Fuploads%2F2019%2F04%2FiStock-179323312.jpg&f=1&nofb=1&ipt=d18885946388552 98fa10cba9ca84a953d47a3c20c1f99f1b2c1bdeccdac56af.

8.6.1. Advancements in Diagnostic Tools

Nursing eye testing has long been revolutionized by technological advancements in diagnostic devices, enhancing ocular checks to be more precise and time-saving. The development of OCT and fundus cameras has revolutionized the way healthcare professionals are now able to examine the retina and other internal structures of the eye. Both take high-quality images, allowing for early detection of conditions such as diabetic retinopathy and glaucoma. The ability to detect subtle changes in eye tissues enables nurses to contribute positively to patient care, and better results are obtained through facilitating interventions at the right time. Furthermore, with such technologies becoming more accessible, they can become integrated into routine assessment, hence proving the worth of proper eye examination in comprehensive patient care (N/A, 1988). In addition to imaging technologies, technological innovations in artificial intelligence (AI) are changing eye assessments in nursing. Machine programs are able to analyze ocular images with unprecedented precision, identifying abnormalities that may elude the naked eye. Not only do this smart diagnosis systems guide healthcare practitioners in making informed choices, but they also conserve time in assessments. As AI technology continues to advance, the collaboration of nurses with technology will increasingly enhance diagnostic capabilities and optimize clinical processes. The integration of artificial intelligence-based technology into nursing practice serves as one indication of a bigger shift toward data-driven health, eventually leading to better patient outcomes through earlier detection and treatment of eye disease (Tirrell et al., 2016). The development of portable diagnostic equipment also has the potential to deliver improved eye exams in a range of settings, from underserved to remote areas. Portable technology, such as hand-held fundus cameras and smartphone retinal imaging devices, allows nurses to perform significant checks without having to deal with clunky machines. Portability brings access to eye care service to include screenings and testing in a variety of settings, from clinics to community outreach. As a result, such developments affirm the pivotal role of nursing in the development of ocular health in populations, including vulnerable populations who can be confronted by challenges to traditional eye care. By embracing such innovations, nursing professionals have the ability to enhance practice and adequately address healthcare disparities in eye examinations (N/A, 1988).

8.6.2. Telehealth and Remote Eye Assessments

Adding telehealth into eye exams is a huge step forward towards enhancing healthcare accessibility, particularly for people who reside in rural areas. The majority of Australians have severe barriers to accessing healthcare, such as being far away from healthcare centers and experiencing shortages of healthcare providers in rural communities. Consequently, patients end up enduring either the ordeal of being on long-distance travels or the negative consequences of not receiving requisite care at all. Telehealth is a contemporary reaction that employs telecommunications and information technology to promote the delivery of healthcare services without the need for physical presence. By remote consulting, healthcare workers can perform eye examination via video conferencing and computer tools, hence overcoming barriers and attaining timely intervention for conditions which otherwise would have catastrophic outcomes if left unchecked. Telehealth technology for eye testing in rural locations not only increases access but promotes an interdisciplinary approach to patient care. As experiences in North Dakota, where medical care has been adapted to regional requirements, indicate, telehealth may strengthen primary care through a system of coordination that allows for patient management by various types of healthcare providers. These systems foster the idea of a "medical home," in which patients are given holistic and continuous care specifically tailored for them regardless of whether they are distant from the typical healthcare site. The use of technology in such instances not only makes interactions between patients and providers easier but also promotes specialized screenings and follow-ups crucial to conditions such as diabetic retinopathy or glaucoma. By incorporating eye care screenings into wider telehealth systems, practitioners can ensure that rural communities are given quality treatment. With nursing landscape still evolving, the viability of telehealth as a method to conduct remote eye exams grows increasingly relevant. The capacity of the nurse to learn how to function on virtual platforms not only broadens their skill set but also extends access to eye care services without diminishing the level of quality.

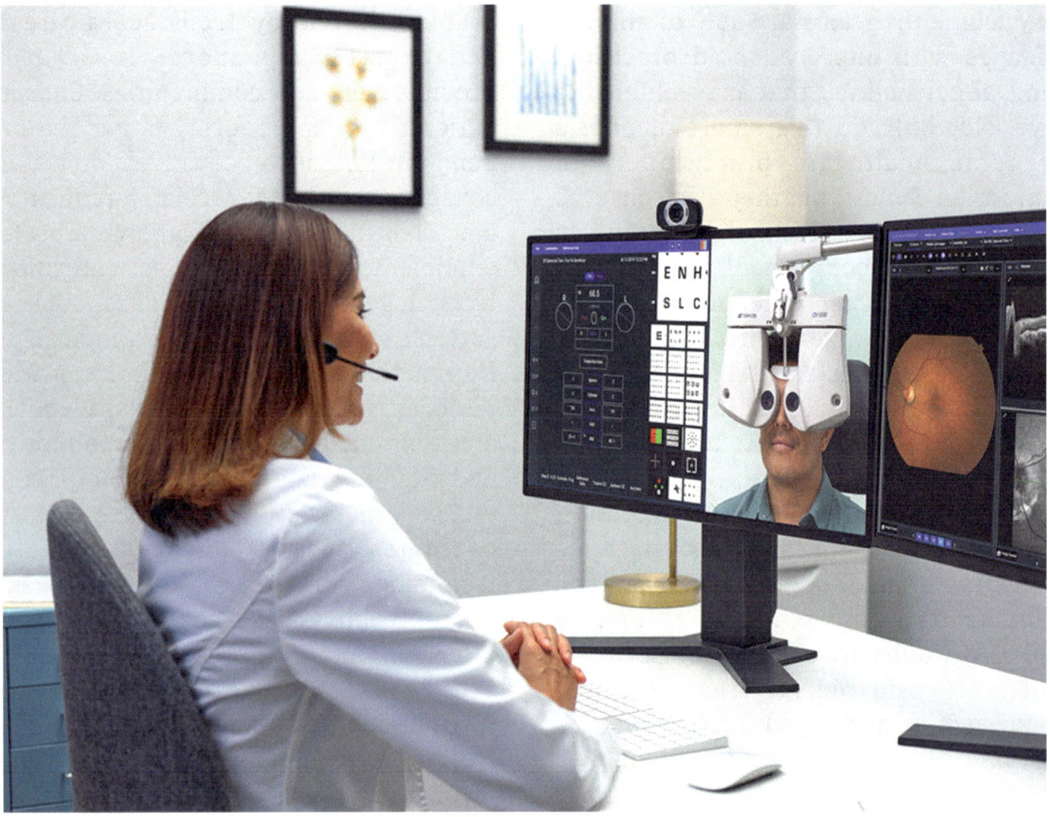

Figure 8.18. Telehealth and remote eye assessments.

Source: https://external-content.duckduckgo.com/iu/?u=https%3A%2F%2Ftopconhealthcare.com%2Fwp-content%2Fuploads%2F2020%2F12%2FRDx_from_TopconHealthcare.jpeg&f=1&nofb=1&ipt=a69c8c2f089779af0277c3ae8f797d18659e01b03ece99fc0b29bd16f308836d.

Training nurses in the application of digital aids and telecommunication methods equips them to assist patients' self-examination or relay critical information to eye specialists. Moreover, integrating telehealth into nursing practice offers a convenient forum for inter-professional collaboration, with nurses engaging jointly with ophthalmologists and other medical professionals to deliver an integrated care. Through telehealth channels, nursing is inextricably involved in revamping eye assessment, that everyone, free from geographical constraints, receives personalized, quality care appropriate to their unique needs (Figure 8.18).

8.6.3. Future Trends in Eye Assessment Technology

Eye testing technology seems to be on the verge of revolutionary change, largely due to advancements in telemedicine and artificial intelligence. As more nurses use teleconsultation, they are now in a position to conduct eye tests over distant locations to enhance patient convenience and accessibility. The technology enables real-time communication between patients and health care providers for timely diagnosis and intervention. The effectiveness of teleconsultation is established on aspects like nurses' presence, which identifies how much nurses can transmit clinical information and also aid in patient care through video-mediated communication (Barrett et al., 2017). Integration of telemedicine in eye examination means nursing practice would not only enhance the outcomes of patients but also make healthcare delivery systems more efficient. Additionally, the integration of artificial intelligence (AI) into eye examination technology is transforming the diagnostic model. AI programs are capable of reading retinal images and other visual data with remarkable precision, allowing for early detection of disease such as diabetic retinopathy and glaucoma. Use of AI along with normal examination protocols can assist nurses by providing improved decision-making tools and simplifying the intellectual demands of complex assessments. The recent study demonstrates how professionals enhance increased confidence and improved knowledge application when employing AI-based tools for practice in clinical settings (Perea et al., 2020). The innovation indicates a promising future where technology not only increases the efficiency of nursing professionals but also leads to improved accuracy in eye tests. Furthermore, the employment of mobile and smartphone-based diagnostic instruments signifies the democratization of eye care. These innovative technologies allow nurses to perform initial eye exams in a wide range of settings, from rural health centers to home visits, thus broadening the scope of complete vision care. The simplicity of use and scalability of these devices can significantly alleviate barriers to access, especially for marginalized populations. As eyesight assessment technology advances, education on these new technologies needs to be included in nursing education so that the practitioners can use them with proficiency. So, the future of eye assessment within nursing is not merely a function of technological advance but also of nursing curriculum adapting to advance competence in using them.

Test Your Knowledge

1. How can technology, such as visual field analyzers or retinal imaging, enhance the accuracy of eye assessments?
2. What are the advantages and limitations of using teleophthalmology for remote eye examinations?

SUMMARY

The process of eye examination in nursing is a vital aspect of comprehensive patient care. With its capacity to yield important information regarding systemic illnesses, the eyes are said to be windows to vision as well as health. Nurses have a crucial role in the early detection and care of eye conditions, allowing for early referral to specialists when indicated. This forward-thinking practice of eye testing leads to improved patient outcomes and an enhanced quality of care. By the incorporation of comprehensive exams and encouraging patient education regarding eye health, nurses are able to take a significant role in reducing the incidence of visual impairments and their corresponding complications. The incorporation of evidence-based practices also strengthens the practice of nursing by guaranteeing examinations are conducted uniformly and reliably. Besides, eye examination is not a task alone; it is a nurses commitment to patient care. Knowledge of how a patient's overall health is affected by eye health underscores the importance of thorough examinations in facilities of all kinds. Acquiring skills such as vision testing and inspection of ocular structures enables nurses to detect abnormalities that indicate serious underlying illness. The need for regular training and exposure to emerging technologies further underpins the imperative of continuous professional development among nursing practitioners. Thus, eye examination becomes not only a norm but also an avenue of expression for nurses to battle for the health and wellness of their patients. Finally, the future of eye examination in nursing remains promising, with emerging technologies bringing about enhanced diagnostic capacity. With telemedicine gaining ground, nurses can utilize virtual examinations to provide treatment to patients in remote areas, further enhancing access to essential eye care. Artificial intelligence and machine learning will become increasingly integrated into diagnostic testing, increasing accuracy and speed. All of this must be complemented by a solid emphasis on ethical consequences and patient privacy. Moving forward, nursing education must also adapt by incorporating training in digital tools, data privacy, and the ethical use of technology in clinical settings.

In the nursing profession, vision testing is a key component of giving holistic care to patients. Not only is the health of the eyes indicative of the overall health of an individual, but it is also a critical surveillance for several systemic diseases, including diabetes and high blood pressure. Nurses must be skillful in conducting visual acuities, testing the ocular surface, and measuring pupils because the tests can lead to the detection of early indications of potential complications. By following systematic guidelines and using standardized procedures can enhance the validity of these assessments as well as consistency in reporting and outcomes. Having a basic understanding of common eye disease can cause nursing practitioners to identify signs that need further medical evaluation and become a fundamental part of health promotion and disease prevention in practice (Matthew et al., 2021). Moreover, the integration of eye examinations within routine nursing assessments is consistent with the general aims of universal health coverage. Although there are many patients with avoidable eye conditions, the necessity for regular eye examinations is frequently overlooked, leading to a disparity of eye health between groups. There has been evidence to demonstrate that there are specific inequities in the delivery of eye treatment, particularly amongst vulnerable communities and in poorer countries. A successful eye examination protocol for nursing can overcome such division, referring patients to needed resources and interventions. Nurses are able to bargain for comprehensive eye health services that attend to ocular care as integral to general health by working with multidisciplinary teams, hence strengthening broader public health initiatives (Matthew et al., 2021). Last but not least, the need for special training in eye examination for nurses cannot be overstated. With the population changing, as an aging population is more likely to experience increased vision impairment, nurse education must adapt to address these issues in equipping practitioners with them. This adaptation includes remaining up to date with technological advances in eye care interventions and eye treatment, which can help to produce improved patient outcomes.

KEY TERMS FROM THIS CHAPTER

- Pupil
- Sclera
- Lens
- Optic Disc
- Extraocular Muscles
- Pupillary Light Reflex
- Consensual Response
- Snellen Chart
- Iris
- Cornea
- Retina
- Conjunctiva
- Visual Acuity
- Accommodation
- Ophthalmoscope
- Peripheral Vision

CRITICAL THINKING QUESTIONS

1. **The nurse uses the Snellen chart to assess:**
   a. Visual field
   b. Color vision
   c. Visual acuity
   d. Pupillary light reflex
2. **Pupils that are equal, round, and react to light and accommodation are documented as:**
   a. PERRLA
   b. 20/20 vision
   c. Mydriasis
   d. Anisocoria
3. **Which cranial nerves are involved in extraocular movements?**
   a. II, III, IV
   b. III, IV, VI
   c. III, V, VII
   d. II, V, VII
4. **The nurse observes yellowing of the sclera. This is indicative of:**
   a. Anemia
   b. Jaundice
   c. Conjunctivitis
   d. Glaucoma
5. **When using an ophthalmoscope, the nurse can assess:**
   a. Corneal reflex
   b. Optic disc and retina
   c. Lens opacity only
   d. Extraocular muscles

Short Answer Questions

1. What are the main structures of the eye that should be assessed during a physical examination?
2. Describe the steps of the visual acuity test and explain its significance.
3. How is the pupillary light reflex tested, and what does it indicate about neurological function?
4. What is the difference between direct and consensual pupillary response?
5. Explain how to assess extraocular movements and why this is important.

Answer to Critical Thinking Questions

1. (c) 2. (a) 3. (b) 4. (b) 5. (b)

REFERENCES

1. Abrams, A., Barer, B., Brittain, K., Brittain, K., Brittain, K., et al. (2008). Treatment of urinary incontinence after stroke in adults. https://core.ac.uk/download/339635.pdf (accessed on 16th July 2025).
2. Abrouk, M., Bhutani, T., DaLovisio, R., Farahnik, B., et al. (2016). The patient's guide to psoriasis treatment. Part 2: PUVA phototherapy. https://core.ac.uk/download/323063370.pdf (accessed on 16th July 2025).
3. Accettola, E., Bogdan, A., Callahan, S., Chawda, A., et al. (2023). *Introduction to Health Assessment for the Nursing Professional: Part II*. https://core.ac.uk/download/622362029.pdf (accessed on 16th July 2025).
4. Adams, D., & Christopher, O. (2011). The expression and assessment of emotions and internal states in individuals with severe or profound intellectual disabilities. https://core.ac.uk/download/pdf/18498841.pdf (accessed on 16th July 2025).
5. Andrew, L., Davis, T., & Johnson, C. (2017). The impact of visual impairments on mobility performance in community-dwelling older adults. https://digitalscholarship.unlv.edu/cgi/viewcontent.cgi?article=3923&context=thesesdissertations (accessed on 16th July 2025).
6. Arduini, R., Atkinson, H., Baraldi, M., Bekedam, H., Birch, R., Brown, T., et al. (1992). Visual acuity in low birth weight (1500–2500 g) neonates. https://core.ac.uk/download/43318297.pdf (accessed on 16th July 2025).
7. Armstrong, S., Avery, A. A., Barber, N., Crowe, S., et al. (2012). Investigating the prevalence and causes of prescribing errors in general practice: The PRACtICe study. https://core.ac.uk/download/29841235.pdf (accessed on 16th July 2025).
8. Baker, P., Bates, D., Darbyshire, D., Gordon, M., et al. (2014). Physicians' practice of dispensing medicines: A qualitative study. https://core.ac.uk/download/42138091.pdf (accessed on 16th July 2025).
9. Barrett, D. (2017). Rethinking presence: A grounded theory of nurses and teleconsultation. https://core.ac.uk/download/151161610.pdf (accessed on 16th July 2025).
10. Bayley, K. D. (2016). The applications of sub-Tenon's anesthesia for canine ophthalmic surgery: A thesis presented in fulfilment of the requirements for the degree of Master of Veterinary Science (MVSc) at Massey University, Manawatu, New Zealand. https://core.ac.uk/download/148644296.pdf (accessed on 16th July 2025).
11. Bianchi, J., Cook, L., Fumarola, S., Ousey, K., et al. (2012). The missing link: The key to improved wound assessment. https://core.ac.uk/download/9555354.pdf (accessed on 16th July 2025).
12. Burton, M. J., Ramke, J., Marques, A. P., Bourne, R., Congdon, N., Jones, I., Ah Tong, B. A. M., et al. (2021). The Lancet Global Health Commission on global eye health: Vision beyond 2020. *The Lancet Global Health, 9*, e489–e551. https://doi.org/10.1016/s2214-109x(20)30488-5 (accessed on 16th July 2025).
13. Bywood, P. T. M. (2013). Allied health video consultation services. https://core.ac.uk/download/43335675.pdf (accessed on 16th July 2025).
14. Campbell, L. (2019). Textual mediation in simulated nursing handoffs: Examining how student writing coordinates action. https://core.ac.uk/download/223025148.pdf (accessed on 16th July 2025).

15. Chan, C. L. W., Chi, I., & Wang, C. (2014). Overview of quality-of-life research in older people with visual impairment. https://core.ac.uk/download/38046267.pdf (accessed on 16th July 2025).

16. Charles, N. (2011). A brief guide to carrying out research about adult social care services for visually impaired people. https://core.ac.uk/download/223324.pdf (accessed on 16th July 2025).

17. Colmers, J. M. (2007). Public reporting and transparency. https://core.ac.uk/download/71354121.pdf (accessed on 16th July 2025).

18. Cox, C. L. (2012). Adherence, compliance, persistence and concordance in the management of glaucoma, Part I. https://core.ac.uk/download/9983106.pdf (accessed on 16th July 2025).

19. Cox, C. L., Evans, P., Gibbons, H., Titmus, A., et al. (2011). HLA-B27 positivity: Associated health implications. https://core.ac.uk/download/9983108.pdf (accessed on 16th July 2025).

20. Cox, C. L., Jones, M., & Rutkowski, K. (2013). On being a mentor. https://core.ac.uk/download/9983102.pdf (accessed on 16th July 2025).

21. Cromwell, R. L. (2011). Surveillance of ocular parameters and visual function in bed rest subjects. https://core.ac.uk/download/pdf/10559124.pdf (accessed on 16th July 2025).

22. Dickson, K., & Stephens, B. W. (2015). It's all in the mime: Actions speak louder than words when teaching the cranial nerves. https://core.ac.uk/download/33476062.pdf (accessed on 16th July 2025).

23. Edison, C. C. (2020). The design and application of a decision-making process for identification of critical curricular variables which affect optimal application of CAI in a baccalaureate school of nursing. https://core.ac.uk/download/344444036.pdf (accessed on 16th July 2025).

24. Finnegan, A., Hernandez, D., Hynes, C., Kip, K., et al. (2015). Accelerated resolution therapy: An innovative mental health intervention to treat post-traumatic stress disorder. https://core.ac.uk/download/42155395.pdf (accessed on 16th July 2025).

25. Gohman, N. (2018). The relationship between community dwelling older adult's fall risk and beliefs of risk for falling in Northwest Arkansas and Bolgatanga, Ghana. https://core.ac.uk/download/159417149.pdf (accessed on 16th July 2025).

26. Gottlieb, M. L., & Moore, C. B. (1979). Activities of nurse practitioners as identified by medical directors of university student health services. https://core.ac.uk/download/215482198.pdf (accessed on 16th July 2025).

27. Harper, R., Morgan, J., Read, S., Spencer, C., et al. (2018). Glaucoma, dementia and the 'precipice of care': Transitions between states of medication adherence. https://core.ac.uk/download/159767753.pdf (accessed on 16th July 2025).

28. Helmich, I., Holle, H., Lausberg, H., Rein, R., et al. (2015). Brain oxygenation patterns during the execution of tool use demonstration, tool use pantomime, and body-part-as-object tool use. https://core.ac.uk/download/151156569.pdf (accessed on 16th July 2025).

29. Leamon, A. E. (2016). *The Electronic Health Record Scorecard: A Measure of Utilization and Communication Skills.* https://core.ac.uk/download/79664897.pdf (accessed on 16th July 2025).

30. Mahadevan, K., Raghavan, R., & Thomas, R. A. (2024). Knowledge, attitude and practice pattern among intensive care nursing staff on eyecare practices in ICU patients. https://core.ac.uk/download/613230160.pdf (accessed on 16th July 2025).

31. Malek, I., Ramani, K. V., & Trivedi, P. (2025). *IIMA in Healthcare Management: Abstract of Publications (2000–2010)*. https://core.ac.uk/download/pdf/6815495.pdf (accessed on 16th July 2025).
32. Manigold, R. (2019). *ACR Accreditation for Utah Valley Hospital's Radiation Oncology Center*. https://digitalscholarship.unlv.edu/cgi/viewcontent.cgi?article=4649&context=thesesdissertations (accessed on 16th July 2025).
33. McCarthy, D., Wrenn, J., Wakefield, M., Nuzum, R., & Mika, S. (2008). The North Dakota experience: Achieving high-performance health care through rural innovation and cooperation. https://core.ac.uk/download/71353481.pdf (accessed on 16th July 2025).
34. Moniz, A. B. (2025). Synthesis about a collaborative project on "Technology Assessment of Autonomous Systems." https://core.ac.uk/download/pdf/6815454.pdf (accessed on 16th July 2025).
35. N/A. (1967). *Barnes Hospital Bulletin*. https://core.ac.uk/download/70380906.pdf (accessed on 16th July 2025).
36. N/A. (2010). *Technology Target Studies: Technology Solutions to Make Patient Care Safer and More Efficient*. https://core.ac.uk/download/71355358.pdf (accessed on 16th July 2025).
37. Page, M. J., Moher, D., Bossuyt, P. M., Boutron, I., Hoffmann, T., Mulrow, C. D., Shamseer, L., et al. (2021). PRISMA 2020 explanation and elaboration: Updated guidance and exemplars for reporting systematic reviews. *BMJ*. https://doi.org/10.1136/bmj.n160 (accessed on 16th July 2025).
38. Patty, C. M. (2014). A novel method for assessing medication-related adverse outcomes in a community hospital. https://core.ac.uk/download/70419796.pdf (accessed on 16th July 2025).
39. Perea, J. D., & Sit, W. (2020). Comparing learning platform impact on low vision education for occupational therapists. https://core.ac.uk/download/286641353.pdf (accessed on 16th July 2025).
40. Slominski, R. D. (2018). Screening amblyopic risk factors in a pediatric population using an automated vision screener. https://core.ac.uk/download/216808975.pdf (accessed on 16th July 2025).
41. Slominski, R. D. (2018). Screening amblyopic risk factors in a pediatric population using an automated vision screener. https://core.ac.uk/download/303863909.pdf (accessed on 16th July 2025).
42. Stichler, J. F., & Weiss, M. E. (2000). Through the eye of the beholder: Multiple perspectives on quality in women's health care. https://core.ac.uk/download/213077269.pdf (accessed on 16th July 2025).
43. Tasseri, A., Malekzadeh, J., Mazluom, S. R., & Etezadi, T. (2013). A standardized shift handover protocol: Improving nurses' safe practice in intensive care units. https://core.ac.uk/download/pdf/26788131.pdf (accessed on 16th July 2025).
44. Tirrell, G. (2016). The emergency department evaluation and outcomes of elderly fallers. https://open.bu.edu/bitstream/2144/15371/1/Tirrell_bu_0017N_10816.pdf (accessed on 16th July 2025).
45. Wynsberghe, A. van. (2012). Designing robots for care: Care centered value-sensitive design. https://core.ac.uk/download/pdf/11487391.pdf (accessed on 16th July 2025).

9

EAR, NOSE, MOUTH, AND THROAT (ENT) ASSESSMENT IN NURSING

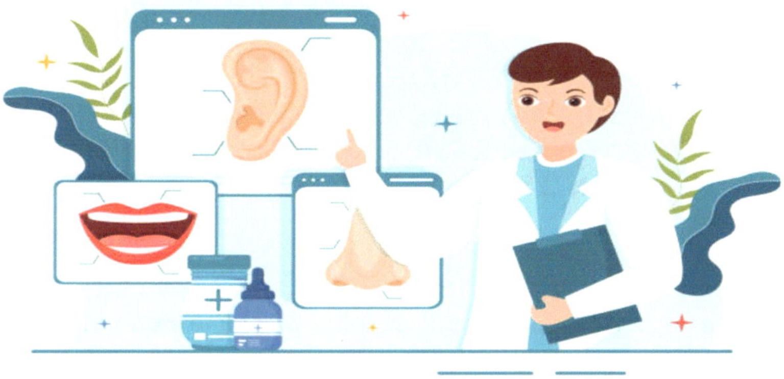

LEARNING OBJECTIVES

After studying this chapter, you will be able to:

1. Illustrate the anatomy of the ear, nose, mouth, and throat;
2. List the common ENT disorders;
3. Explain the assessment techniques in ENT;
4. Define patient history and symptoms;
5. Explore the diagnostic tests and procedures;
6. Identify the nursing interventions and care plans.

Introduction

The need for effective assessment in the Ear, Nose, Mouth, and Throat (ENT) region in nursing cannot be overstated, as it forms the foundation of patient management as a whole. Effective assessment is critical to the diagnosis of many conditions, ranging from common colds to severe sinusitis, to facilitate timely interventions and management. Nurses who have in-depth ENT anatomy and physiology knowledge are better positioned to record subtle changes in patient status and make the appropriate interventions. Such emphasis on ENT examination is also amplified by the complexities of contemporary healthcare environments, where understanding and integrating the application of advanced health information technologies is crucial in the delivery of high-quality care. As emphasized in recent literature, successful assessment is dependent upon the integration of intellectual and technological skills, which affirms the value of nurses continuously enhancing their knowledge in these areas (Cachata et al., 2025). In addition to important anatomical and physiologic knowledge, the adaptation of health information technology into practice has been a major factor in enhancing the effectiveness of ENT evaluations. As healthcare becomes increasingly digital, nurses must cross many technology instruments facilitating clinical decision and patient care. The ongoing creation of such technologies presents challenges requiring nursing professionals to possess certain skills, not only the mastery of the applications of clinical tools but also an understanding of their ethical dimensions and use in patient-centered care. By gaining a firm understanding of technological competency, nurses can advance their assessment abilities significantly, aligning their practices with the latest standards of care. This demand for additional training and education, particularly in ENT assessment contexts, is increasingly being established as a necessary component of nursing school curricula (Liu et al., 2024). Also, the study skills in nursing schools are changing to introduce diversified evaluation practices that improve both knowledge and moral aspects of practice. The change is most critical in equipping nursing students for handling patients' needs holistically and effectively. For instance, research that investigates different assessment systems indicates the inclusion of ideological and political instruction principles can result in dramatic enhancement of students' learning results and overall satisfaction with their education. By advocating an incorporated environment of learning that involves both traditional and non-traditional assessment processes, prospective nurses can achieve a balance between technical skill acquisition and ethical decision-making necessary for high-quality ENT assessments. This interprofessional approach ensures that the graduate nurses are not only skilled in conducting clinical examination but also adequately equipped to deal with the intricacies of modern healthcare (Liu et al., 2024) (Figure 9.1).

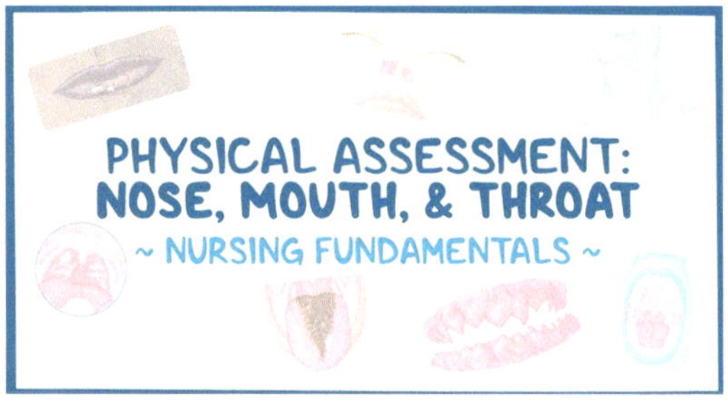

Figure 9.1. Ear, nose, mouth, and throat (ENT) assessment.

Source: https://external-content.duckduckgo.com/iu/?u=https%3A%2F%2Fosmose-it.s3.amazonaws.com%2FETQX8CCRRYqzlcrCqLkXsCC_R5WSBC0Y%2F_.jpg&f=1&nofb=1&ipt=042f73bcd7c3b64d853f0dea8f02774486744f775efcb403cf7735b8edb67c7d.

Definition of ENT Assessment

ENT assessment is one of the fundamental nursing practices addressing various issues of a wide scope affecting these interrelated areas. ENT assessment refers to the systematic process of examination employed to identify any abnormalities or illnesses that may influence a patient's auditory, olfactory, and oral functions. ENT assessment is crucially performed by visual inspection, palpation, and auscultation, and history and symptom questioning. The relevance of a proper ENT examination lies in its capacity to disclose infections, allergies, or anatomical abnormalities that could interfere with daily living and health. Nurses play a crucial role in ensuring that these examinations are performed competently so that early detection and management of various ENT conditions with possible consequences for the overall health and well-being of a patient are realized. In actuality, the components of an ENT examination are a combination of clinical techniques and patient presentation. A full examination involves visual assessment of the external ears, nasal passages, and mouth, frequently augmented by digital palpation of tissues directly adjacent to them in order to assess for any signs of tenderness or irregularity. In such a case, nurses may employ devices such as otoscopes in the performance of ear exams and tongue depressors to view the oral cavity and throat effectively. Additionally, they must be trained to observe clinical signs that may indicate pathologies like pharyngitis or otitis media. Involving patients through detailed questioning about their symptoms, medical histories, and life patterns is empathetically linked to the determination of their complaint causes, management of the subsequent procedure, and ensuring continuity of care. The development of evidence-based practice truly enhances the efficacy of ENT examinations among nurses.

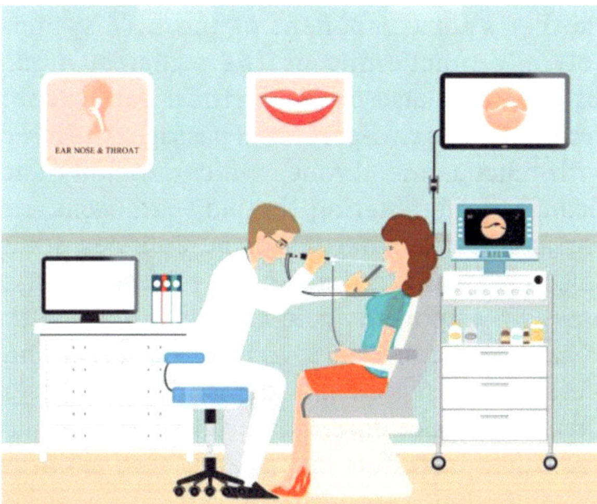

Figure 9.2. ENT assessment.

Source: https://www.westsidehn.com/wp-content/uploads/2020/11/fshlakjdfhaksjdhf-1.jpg.

Incorporation of the latest evidence and research-based guidelines in clinical practices ensures that nurses practice the best evidence-based treatments and diagnoses of ENT diseases. For instance, standardized assessment instruments and guidelines can facilitate the evaluation process, making it more effective in its diagnostic potential. Furthermore, evidence-based theories improve the nursing observation techniques that are a must in an ENT evaluation. As noted by new dysphagia assessment challenges guidelines, keen observation of the risks involved in various procedures informs enhanced patient care practice (Bolton et al., 2020; Brian et al., 2023). Thus, properly done ENT assessment empowers nurses to deliver holistic, patient-focused healthcare provision and perform specific needs arising from ears, nose, mouths, and throats (Figure 9.2).

Importance of ENT Assessment in Nursing

The role of thorough ENT tests in nursing practice cannot be overstated, as such examinations are most critical for the diagnosis and management of many diseases of the ear, nose, mouth, and throat. Nurses are frontline practitioners who are likely to identify signs of diseases that require early treatment. Through proper assessments, nurses facilitate early diagnosis of conditions such as ear infection, sinusitis, and throat infections, which could prevent complications and improve patient outcomes. The authority to diagnose and treat ENT-related health concerns allows nurses to provide holistic care, tailoring interventions based on individual patients' needs. Moreover, proactive testing can enhance patient education, giving people information about their conditions and treatment processes, thus encouraging greater participation in their care process and further emphasizing the importance of ENT testing in nursing. Moreover, ENT testing is a key in influencing nursing interventions and care planning. ENT testing enables nurses to capture valuable information that can be used in influencing the management of a patient's health in general. For instance, identifying a patient's respiratory history, either chronic sinus infection or sleep apnea, allows nurses to effectively take preventive measures or recommend specialty treatment if needed. Such evidence-based nursing practice adheres to standards emphasizing the importance of accurate assessments and ongoing management plans. The integration of ENT tests within normal nursing practice enhances the quality of care, as well as ensures patient safety and well-being through avoiding risks of incurable ENT complications. Hence, the role of nurses in carrying out the tests is central to bringing about the optimal health outcomes in patients across various environments. Finally, continuous education and training in ENT tests for nursing professionals is of the highest priority. It is essential to keep up with new research and clinical practice guidelines, as evidenced by recent updates of clinical practice guidelines in areas such as the management of complex conditions that can impact ENT health. The continuous evolution of medical knowledge and practices necessitates that nurses should be capable of performing related assessments competently. According to the recent guidelines, best practice needs to be updated following a critical review of literature and the most current evidence to enhance the quality of nursing care provided to patients with ENT pathology (Brian et al., 2023; Speiser et al., 2018). By giving priority to professional growth, nurses can make sure they are competent in performing thorough ENT examinations, ultimately resulting in better patient care and reinforced health results in the community.

9.1. Anatomy of the Ear, Nose, Mouth, and Throat

Learning Outcome

1. Structure and function of the ear;
2. Anatomy of the nasal passages;
3. Overview of the oral cavity and throat.

Ear anatomy is essential to understanding its various functions and their bearing on overall well-being. The ear consists of three main parts: the outer ear, middle ear, and inner ear, each playing a different role in the hearing process. The outer ear collects sound waves and channels them into the auditory canal and onto the tympanic membrane, or eardrum. It vibrates when it is struck by a sound, transferring its vibration to the ossicles of the middle ear, i.e., the malleus, incus, and stapes. These bones subsequently amplify the sound waves before they reach the inner ear, where sensory cells in the cochlea convert these vibrations into electrical impulses for the brain. Understanding these anatomical structures is relevant to ENT evaluation by nurses because dysfunction in this complex system can lead to hearing loss and other health conditions that need to be thoroughly examined and treated. The nose is another vital component of the ENT system, not only functioning as the principal organ for smell but also being a critical pathway for breathing. The two-part nasal passage is covered with mucous membranes which humidify and cleanse the air entering, trapping pathogens and particulates. Furthermore, the complex sinus structure, which drains into the nasal passage, plays an important role in breathing health. Nasal dysfunction can lead to mouth breathing, which, as research has demonstrated, has a negative impact on craniofacial growth. It has been demonstrated in research that children with habitual mouth breathing exhibit varying dental and skeletal changes due to the lack of nasal airflow, and intervention at an early stage in pediatric assessment is important to prevent such potential complications (Chowdhary et al., 2024). Proper knowledge of nasal anatomy enables nurses to conduct effective assessment and plan appropriate treatment regimens for patients. The mouth is an organ with multiple functions that play a significant role in digestion, navigation of speech, and organization of respiratory procedures through its association with the throat. The mouth consists of the lips, cheeks, gums, tongue, and palate and plays a significant role in the first process of digestion, in which mechanical and enzymatic food digestion occurs. Moreover, the function of adenoids and tonsils in the region of the throat as a line of defense for children against infection cannot be overstressed. Nevertheless, infections such as adenoid hypertrophy are able to initiate habitual mouth breathing, which can make it more probable to develop periodontal diseases and dental caries as an outcome of changes in oral flora and pH (Farahzadi et al., 2024). Thus, critical assessment of the mouth, throat, and adjacent structures by nurses was important not only for acute care but also for long-term health outcomes, illustrating the unity of ENT anatomy in clinical practice.

9.1.1. Structure and Function of the Ear

The ear is a complexly developed organ, with intricate design to enable hearing and balance functions. It is anatomically divided into three major areas—the outer ear, the middle ear, and the inner ear—each playing a vital role in hearing. The outer ear, which houses the pinna and the auditory canal, is a projecting funnel and directs sound waves into the tympanic membrane. This membrane vibrates when it is stimulated by sound, transferring the vibrations to the ossicles in the middle ear. The ossicles are the malleus, incus, and stapes. This mechanical amplification is vital to the transmission of sound, ultimately allowing for sound waves to reach the fluid-filled inner ear in an effective way. The physical layout of such parts is intrinsic to their function, as each must be treated sequentially in order for optimal auditory processing to occur in the context of ENT scans (Dai et al., 2025). The ear has a role not just in hearing, but also in equilibrium, which is regulated primarily by the vestibular apparatus in the inner ear. This organ contains semicircular canals and otolithic organs that are respectively responsible for sensing rotations and linear head movements. Coordination between the sensory input from the vestibular apparatus, together with vision and proprioception, is essential to ensure equilibrium. Dysfunction of vestibular function can lead to dizziness or vertigo, conditions that frequently present in ENT practice. Hence, nurses must be well aware of the structures involved in balance to conduct good evaluations and utilize beneficial interventions. Evaluating vestibular function through caloric testing or vestibular evoked myogenic potentials (VEMP) tests can provide information regarding underlying pathologies that may be causing balance deficits (Dai et al., 2025).

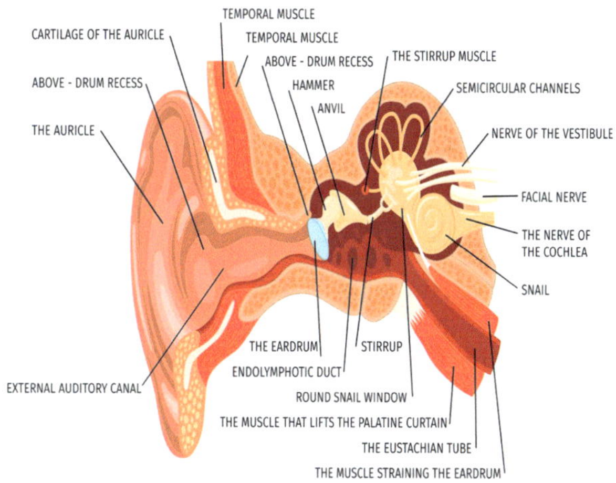

Figure 9.3. Structure and function of the ear.

Source: https://www.vedantu.com/seo/content-images/9d7924d2-ba18-4c14-9f0f-269f72a51397_1.png.

The integrity of the ears structure is not only an anatomical concern, but it is also very significant to auditory and vestibular health. Assessment of the ears structure using advanced imaging techniques, such as 3D-Flair MRI, can be very informative regarding probable pathologies, such as infection or structural abnormalities affecting the hearing outcomes. For instance, research has determined that abnormal MRI outcomes are correlated with reduced hearing recovery rates in patients presenting with sudden sensorineural hearing loss. Therefore, the inclusion of imaging assessment in routine evaluations enables nurses to formulate holistic care plans that integrate both the structure and function of hearing health. The relationship between structural deformities and the resulting functional effects is a central area of reflection in the realm of nursing practice due to its optimization of the delivery of comprehensive ENT assessments (Li, 2024) (Figure 9.3).

9.1.2. Anatomy of the Nasal Passages

The anatomy of the nasal passages is crucial in understanding their function in the upper respiratory tract. The nasal passages, or more precisely the nasal cavity, possess a well-developed structure for filtering, warming, and humidifying air during inspiration before its delivery to the lungs. The nasal septum divides the nasal cavity into two halves and contains various structures, such as turbinates—bony projections that increase the surface area for filtration and olfactory reception. The anatomy of this structure is extremely significant to respiratory health since any type of blockage or deviation in these passages can result in problems like sinusitis or insufficient ventilation. In addition, the relationship between the paranasal sinuses and nasal passages is essential to normal mucosal function and drainage, highlighting the importance of thorough evaluation of these structures in nursing care. The complete picture of the nasal passages encompasses their role within the overall context of ENT examinations. Symmetry, patency, and mucosal health of the nasal passages are essential parameters during nursing evaluations. The medical providers will need to employ techniques such as inspection and palpation in order to diagnose for nasal blockage, inflammation, or discharge since these symptoms are suggestive of pathology. Anomalies of the nasal passage are more likely to be indicative of systemic processes and thus demand a multidisciplinary management plan for further evaluation. For example, nasal airflow and turbulence measurement can be indicative of acquired velopharyngeal dysfunction since nasal airflow physics is linked to oropharyngeal function. As such, these anatomical considerations should not be omitted during ENT assessment in nursing.

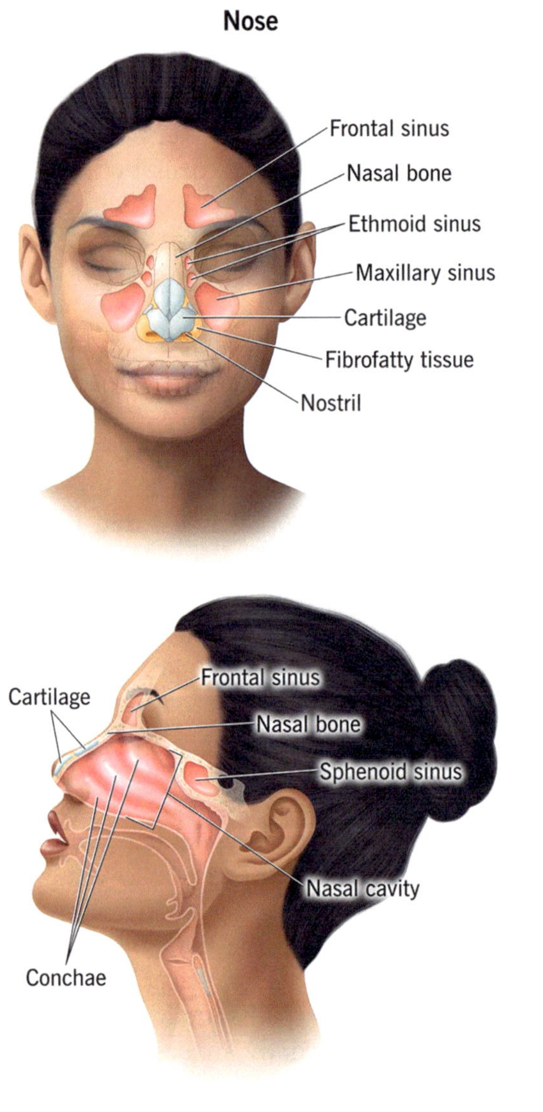

Figure 9.4. Anatomy of the nasal passages.

Source: https://my.clevelandclinic.org/-/scassets/Images/org/health/articles/21778-nose.

The anatomical complexity of nasal passage is even further heightened by the interactions with other structures around it, such as paranasal sinuses and oral cavity. Nasal passages are connected to sinuses, air spaces that are utilized to increase voice resonance and decrease the weight of skulls. If this system is not functioning or if there is an obstruction, the symptoms may be severe, ranging from nasal blockage to potential speech impairments, especially in patients with oropharyngeal dysphagia. Furthermore, nasal passage diseases may affect the overall assessment procedures in nursing. For instance, the failure to agree on clinical guidelines in the management of velopharyngeal disorder-related conditions is a clear indication that there is a necessity for stronger frameworks. Thus, an in-depth understanding of nasal anatomy does not just improve clinical assessments but also proves the interactive relationship of ENT structures towards the theory that significant nursing practice should be accompanied by holistic assessment (Doris-Denk et al., 2022; Kelsey et al., 2018) (Figure 9.4).

9.1.3. Overview of the Oral Cavity and Throat

Mouth and throat are significant components of the upper respiratory and gastrointestinal tracts and are focal points both for physiology and communication. The mouth, which is the oral cavity, consists of the lips, cheeks, palate, tongue, and teeth and is tasked with numerous functions including mastication, phonation, and swallowing. Within this multidimensional framework, the tongue is a primary food manipulator and a significant sensory organ with taste buds involved in flavor detection. Moreover, the oral cavity also harbors salivary glands that secrete saliva, which is of immense importance in digestion and oral health. Understanding the anatomy and functions of the oral cavity is essential to nursing assessments because it provides significant clues to potential health issues that may arise in this region. Continuing beyond the oral cavity, the throat or pharynx is an air and foodway between the oral cavity and the larynx and esophagus. The pharynx consists of three segments: the nasopharynx, oropharynx, and laryngopharynx, each with a distinct function that is crucial for normal physiological process. For instance, the oropharynx plays a critical role in swallowing, while the nasopharynx participates in respiratory processes. Assessment of the throat can detect various pathologies, including infection, obstruction, and neoplasms. Some conditions, such as tonsillitis and epiglottitis, can have serious complications if they are not detected immediately and treated accordingly. Nurses should conduct throat assessment using palpation of lymph nodes and visual observation to identify deviations at the initial stage of the clinical process since this emphasizes the inter-relationships among these anatomical components. Empirical evidence shows that oral health assessment integration in nursing education may enhance nurse practitioners' confidence and competency in practice significantly. Educational institutions have incorporated interprofessional educational (IPE) exercises where dental educators get nursing students to engage in practical work concerning whole-mouth examination and identification of pathologies specific to the oral cavity. Survey of participants indicates that students feel more comfortable and confident once they have undergone such training sessions, which goes to prove the importance of having a multidisciplinary strategy in healthcare education (Krista et al., 2018). Secondly, recognizing the importance of oral health in the overall status of patients—such as its connection to systemic diseases—increases the need for generalized nursing assessment that involves the oral cavity and pharynx as integral components of the comprehensive Ear, Nose, Mouth, and Throat (ENT) assessment process (Roland et al., 1995) (Figure 9.5).

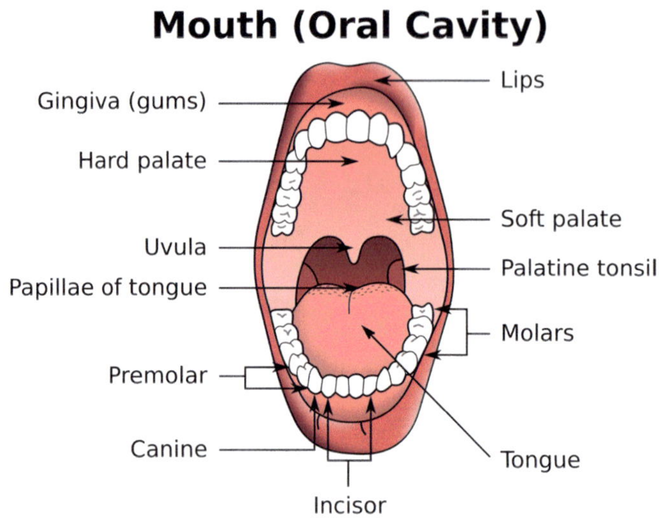

Figure 9.5. Overview of the oral cavity and throat.

Source: https://study.com/cimages/multimages/16/mouth3674724355892505108.png.

Test Your Knowledge

1. What are the major anatomical structures of the ear, nose, mouth, and throat, and how do they function together in respiration, digestion, and hearing?
2. How does understanding ENT anatomy assist nurses in identifying abnormalities during assessment?

9.2. Common ENT Disorders

Learning Outcome

1. Ear disorders: otitis media and hearing loss;
2. Nasal disorders: sinusitis and allergies;
3. Throat disorders: pharyngitis and tonsillitis.

The spectrum of ear, nose, and throat (ENT) disorders encompasses a variety of prevalent disorders with significant impacts on patient health and quality of life. Among these, otitis media is one of the most prevalent disorders, particularly in childhood. It is characterized by inflammation or infection of the middle ear and symptoms of ear pain, irritability, and hearing loss. In children, chronic otitis media can lead to impairment of hearing, potentially undermining the development of speech and learning. Good nursing assessment is vital for early diagnosis and appropriate care, which could include pain relief strategies and antibiotic therapy if required. To nurses, as well as in educating parents about the condition and treatment, understanding the nuances of otitis media and its management is vital. Other common ENT condition is allergic rhinitis, which affects a significant portion of the population and generates a range of symptoms, including sneezing, nasal congestion, and watery eyes. Allergic rhinitis is often elicited by environmental allergens such as pollen, dust mites, and pet dander. For patients, allergic rhinitis can have a profound effect on activities of daily living as well as global quality of life. Nurses play a central part in assessing the impact of allergic rhinitis on a patient's well-being, educating the patient on prevention strategies, and administering pharmacological interventions such as antihistamines or topical corticosteroids for symptom relief. Having a holistic management strategy including educating the patient on potential exposure to allergens can empower the patient to better control their condition and improve their long-term outcomes. Other than allergic rhinitis and otitis media, pharyngitis is another prevalent ENT illness. The illness, normally characterized by pharyngeal inflammation, can either result from viral or bacterial infection. Nurses must be capable of distinguishing between the two properly since bacterial pharyngitis requires antibiotic treatment in order to prevent such complications as rheumatic fever. Symptoms typically manifest in the form of sore throat, throat swelling, and fever. A critical aspect of nursing assessment is the assessment of the severity and the persistence of the symptoms, as well as recent exposure to infectious agents. Patient education on symptom management and when to return for further medical evaluation will be important in effective pharyngitis management. With these nursing interventions, relief not just from acute symptomatology but also reduced frequency of recurrent infections can be felt by the patients, underscoring the role of comprehensive ENT examinations in nursing practice.

9.2.1. Ear Disorders: Otitis Media and Hearing Loss

Otitis media is a prevalent ear disorder characterized by inflammation of the middle ear, and in most cases, it leads to severe health conditions, including hearing loss. The incidence of otitis media is highest in children, where physicality of the eustachian tube exposes them to infection. There are multiple factors that cause otitis media to occur, including environmental, genetic, and allergen exposure. Recurrent or chronic incidence of otitis media causes chronic otitis media (COM), with persistent discharge from the ear through a perforated tympanic membrane. Otitis media needs to be treated to prevent permanent effects, particularly hearing loss, which affects language development and socialization in children. Early nursing assessment and interventions are essential in the treatment of otitis media, in the aim to remit symptoms and reduce the risk of further complications. Otitis media-induced hearing loss is either conductive or sensorineural type, with conductive hearing loss more probable in middle ear infection. In chronic cases, there is possibility of damage to the ossicular chain, leading to additional hearing impairment. Nursing duty for the screening of hearing loss due to otitis media involves meticulous assessment of auditory function and identification of any associated symptoms, such as pain or discharge in the ear. For instance, Kujur et al. (2024) identifies the importance of preoperative assessment using high-resolution computed tomography (HRCT) to diagnose ossicular chain erosion in patients with chronic suppurative otitis media (CSOM), which can decide on surgery. Nurses must be proficient in reading the implications of these assessments in order to discuss the patient's treatment plan with other medical practitioners. Surgical treatment of otitis media, particularly through surgeries such as tympanoplasty, has been proven to reverse hearing with significant improvement. Studies indicate that type-1 tympanoplasty patients exhibit dramatic hearing improvement, especially those with small perforations (Safi et al., 2025). Appreciation of the interrelationship of otitis media and hearing loss is vital in order to give comprehensive care. Evaluation after surgery is important to assess the effectiveness of surgical procedures since documented gains in hearing can significantly improve the quality of life for the patients. As the role of nursing continues to progress, maintaining through ENT evaluations will be central to better patient outcomes, especially for those afflicted with the ill effects of otitis media and resultant hearing loss (Figure 9.6).

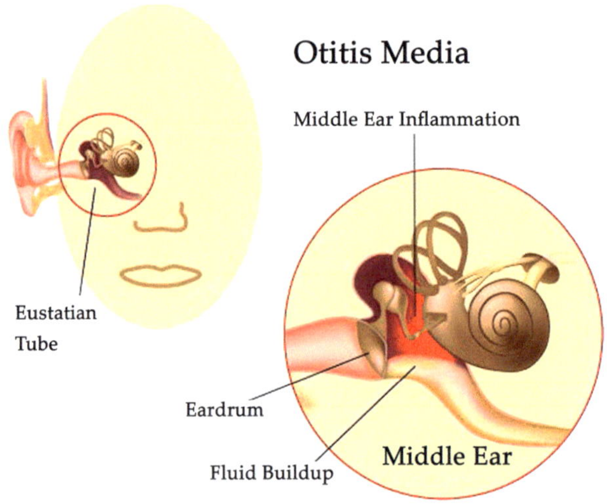

Figure 9.6. Ear disorders: Otitis media and hearing loss.

Source: https://sp-ao.shortpixel.ai/client/to_webp,q_glossy,ret_img,w_500,h_405/https://www.nyogmd.com/wp-content/uploads/Otitis-media-Diagram.jpg.

9.2.2. Nasal Disorders: Sinusitis and Allergies

Nose disorders, particularly sinusitis and allergies, are serious conditions that need detailed assessment in nursing practice. Sinusitis, an inflammation of the sinuses' linings, can be acute or chronic, and it may result from infections or blockages of the nose. The symptoms often include facial pain, nasal congestion, and purulent drainage, which can significantly impact a patient's quality of life. During nursing assessment, viral and bacterial sinusitis should be differentiated since the modes of treatment are quite distinct. The awareness of the nuances of sinusitis allows nurses to apply targeted education and interventions that can minimize symptoms and recurrences. General assessment can involve the determination of other potential factors such as environmental allergens or causative anatomic differences so a holistic approach is made in clinical practice. Allergic rhinitis is another extremely prevalent nasal condition, in which an intensified immune response to external allergens like pollen, dust, or mold occurs. It is typically accompanied by sneezing, itching, congestion, and rhinorrhea, causing significant distress and disruption of daily functioning. Nursing assessment in such patients is of prime importance; the symptom severity should not only be assessed by nurses but also the patient's history taken in detail to determine the particular provoking agents and the measures to be recommended for lifestyle changes. Effective management of allergic rhinitis depends greatly on implementing measures to teach patients avoidance methods and pharmacotherapy like antihistamines and corticosteroids. Moreover, understanding the impact of allergies on mental health and overall well-being is important to nursing professionals as they seek to take patients through complex symptom management. The increased rates of allergic disorders and the complexity of the conditions further necessitate an integrated approach within healthcare systems. An up-to-date report labeled the suffering of patients with allergies as such, highlighting their inappropriate clinical services and management inconsistency within the healthcare systems, particularly in the UK (N/A, 2024). The discomfort these diseases impose on patients will result in drastic reductions in their quality of life, justifying the necessity for specialist nursing assessment incorporating a multi-disciplinary approach. As nursing experts become educated about these disorders, they have a core role to ensure enhanced clinical services and patient care approaches that address unmet needs in managing sinusitis and allergy. Emphasizing the importance of patient-centered care helps for better interventions that enhance health outcomes in practice (Seylanova et al., 2024) (Figure 9.7).

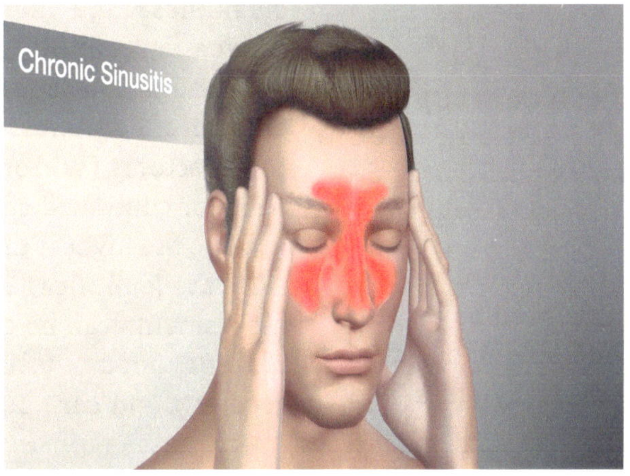

Figure 9.7. Nasal disorders: Sinusitis and allergies.

Source: https://allergysc.com/wp-content/uploads/2020/07/sinus-allegeries.jpg.

9.2.3. Throat Disorders: Pharyngitis and Tonsillitis

Pharyngitis and tonsillitis are prevalent throat infections normally evaluated during ENT visits during nursing. Pharyngitis, which is pharyngitis inflammation, may be due to viral or bacterial causes, and the differentiation is necessary to effectively manage the conditions. Dysphagia, sore throat, and fever are common symptoms that impair the quality of life of a patient. On the other hand, tonsillitis is inflammation of the tonsils and may also produce similar symptoms, but with accompanying swollen lymph nodes and white patches on the tonsils. The nursing assessment process calls for careful throat examination by visual inspection and palpation of local lymph nodes to differentiate between them and determine the course of action. When faced with recurrent attacks of tonsillitis, the process of treatment decision-making—particularly the balancing of tonsillectomy—comes into play. It has been established that tonsillectomy helps in reducing the number of sore throat days suffered by the patient more than conservative management, as indicated by recent studies (Wilson et al., 2023). For nurses, having an understanding of the significance of such intervention is essential. It not only involves assessing the patients' previous medical history and how the disorder is impacting daily life but also talking about surgery-related risks, such as potential complications like post-operative hemorrhage.

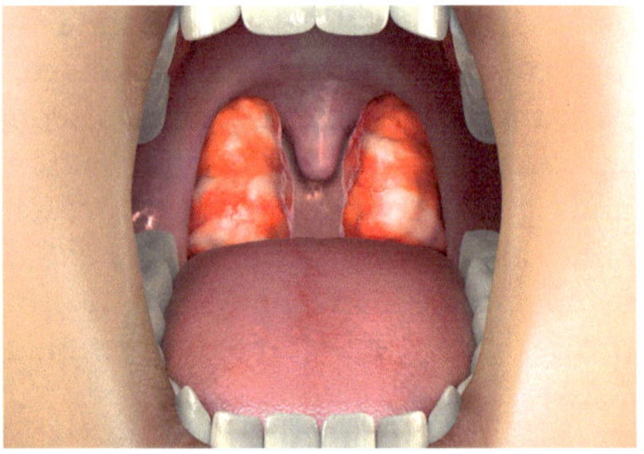

Figure 9.8. Pharyngitis.

Source: https://images.squarespace-cdn.com/content/v1/5d26b16e3c8b190001ab4906/1569462538075-4TTXHH242MH32B4ZJFP9/image-asset.jpeg.

Therefore, detailed patient education and shared decision-making become a part of the nursing assessment. Beyond acute care, overall assessment of pharyngitis and tonsillitis patients globally also needs to take into account long-term outcomes and overall health consequences. Chronic throat illness sufferers usually experience recurring episodes, leading to absence from school or work, further contributing to social and psychological stressors. By applying evidence-based practice principles, patients can be guided to explore preventive strategies, such as good personal cleanliness and lifestyle changes that might reduce susceptibility to such infections. The new studies into the cost-effectiveness and clinical effectiveness of interventions such as tonsillectomy (Wilson et al., 2023) highlight the need for continued education and assessment to achieve the highest therapy of throat conditions. With the identification of these factors, nursing assessments can be tailored to meet individual patient needs, ultimately enhancing their recovery and care outcomes (Figure 9.8).

Test Your Knowledge

1. What are some common disorders affecting the ear, nose, mouth, and throat, and what are the typical clinical signs for each?
2. How can early recognition of ENT disorders, such as sinusitis, otitis media, or pharyngitis, impact patient outcomes?

9.3. Assessment Techniques in ENT

Learning Outcome

1. Inspection methods for the ear, nose, and throat;
2. Palpation and percussion techniques;
3. Use of specialized tools: otoscope and laryngoscope.

In nursing practice, there is a need for proper assessment of patients in the ear, nose, mouth, and throat (ENT) region to identify underlying conditions. ENT assessment skills follow a holistic approach which integrates observational skills and physical examination skills. The nurses initially must conduct a comprehensive history-taking process, collecting information on symptoms, duration, and history in relation to past medical conditions. This first step lays the foundation for subsequent assessment techniques, including inspection of the external ear, nose, and mouth. For instance, observation for any visible deviation can indicate probable underlying conditions such as infection or malignancies. Application of a structured approach assists nurses in building up their ability to detect crucial changes in the patients' health status, which can lead to timely intervention and referral to specialists where necessary. Thus, the robustness of the assessment process is critical to offering the best patient care in nursing practice. There is a complete series of assessment tools that can be applied when evaluating ENT-related complaints. In the ears, nurses have the option of using otoscopic examination to view the tympanic membrane and evaluate for infection or fluid behind the tympanic membrane as part of the diagnosis of otitis media. Similarly, nasal examinations involve assessment of nasal passages for swelling, discharge, or other deviation that may be a sign of infection or allergies. Depending on proper technique, such assessments require experience and expertise, hence the importance of ongoing education and mentorship among nursing practitioners. As shown, professional development and mentorship opportunities significantly influence nursing specialization choices, suggesting a need for formal mentorship programs in nursing education (Onyenwenyi et al., 2025). These programs are essential to build the skills and confidence of nurses in their diagnostic abilities, which are crucial to effective ENT care. Oral cavity examination in ENT is also vital and involves checking the tongue, gums, and overall oral hygiene. Techniques may include looking for lesions, odor of the breath, and palpation for abnormal growths within the oral cavity. These tests can bring out underlying conditions such as dental caries, periodontal disease, or systemic illness, reflecting the diverse function of oral health in the overall health of patients. The relationship between clinical competency and nursing professional education continues to be at the center of focus in nursing literature, with findings to support correlations between educator competency and student performance results (Youssif et al., 2024). Through clinical competency development through extensive training programs, nurses will be capable of conducting detailed ENT evaluations, thereby improving patient care quality. In summary, effective testing techniques in ENT not only enhance patient outcomes but also contribute to ongoing development in nursing practice (Figure 9.9).

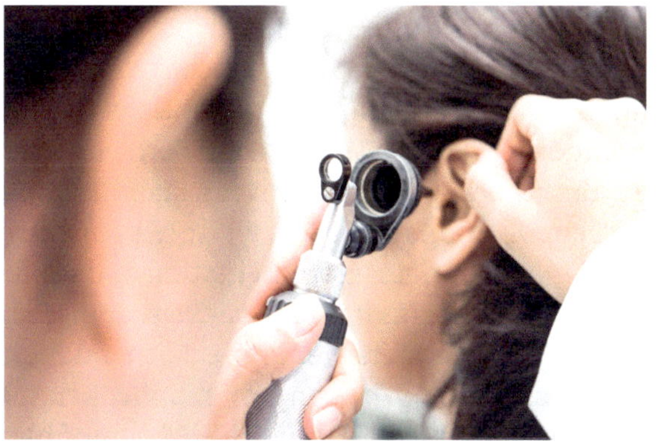

Figure 9.9. Assessment techniques in ENT.

Source: https://www.bluemedicalcenter.com/wordpress/wp-content/uploads/2017/09/shutterstock_667507708.jpg.

9.3.1. Inspection Methods for the Ear, Nose, and Throat

Evaluation of the ear, nose, and throat (ENT) is an essential component of nursing practice, highlighting the significance of specialized examination techniques. Otoscopy, an essential ear examination technique, entails the use of an otoscope to observe the tympanic membrane and external auditory canal. The technique enables one to detect conditions like otitis media, perforation, or cerumen impaction, which can compromise auditory function. In addition, the necessity of the use of otoscopic equipment should not be exaggerated; losses can lead to late diagnosis and adverse patient outcomes, as underscored by recent studies that focus on the economic burden and treatment delays brought about by shortages in equipment (Bass et al., 2025). Thus, with proper training and resource management, nurses can enhance their proficiency in performing effective ear examination, ultimately improving patient care quality. In addition to otoscopy, assessment of the nasal passages often involves flexible nasendoscopy—a low-risk procedure that allows direct visualization of the nasal cavity and sinuses. The technique is particularly valuable in the diagnosis of many conditions, e.g., chronic rhinosinusitis or nasal polyps, which can be characterized by significant symptoms impairing quality of life. Not only does flexible nasendoscopy increase diagnostic effectiveness but also therapeutic maneuvers such as nasal cautery or biopsy. However, the procedure requires appropriate instrumentation and skilled individuals, and thus it is imperative that medical facilities are adequately equipped. The financial burden created by missing or inappropriately stored devices, as the surveyed ENT clinics have reported, demands anticipatory measures such as the implementation of tracking technology, which can reduce loss of equipment and enhance clinical efficacy (Bass et al., 2025). Lastly, throat examination often includes techniques that quantify tonsil and oropharyngeal wellness. In inpatient and outpatient settings, peritonsillar abscess drainage might be necessary in the case of severe tonsillitis. Nursing process in such procedures stands as an absolute priority since it encompasses pre-procedure education and post-procedure observation. Charting what the literature currently says regarding ENT processes for children, as proposed in recent scoping reviews, would enhance nurses' education on nursing diagnosis and intervention in ENT care. This knowledge pool helps not just in complication management but also in evidence-based clinical decision-making, thus leading to better health outcomes in patients undergoing ENT evaluations and interventions.

9.3.2. Palpation and Percussion Techniques

Effective palpation and percussion skills are an integral part of the Ear, Nose, Mouth, and Throat (ENT) assessment in nursing practice. Palpation refers to the application of tactile pressure to various regions of the body in order to enable the nurse to assess for tenderness, swelling, or structural abnormalities. During ENT assessments, palpation can detect minute details that the nurse can use to infer underlying conditions. With the assistance of palpation over the neck and the throat regions, clinicians can identify lymphadenopathy or masses that are indicative of malignancies or infections. Palpation is thus a simple skill enhancing the reliability of ENT examinations as well as assisting in the development of proper care plans. Percussion, on the other hand, is utilized when assessing the air-filled or fluid-filled structures within the ENT region. This technique, involving tapping to generate sound and vibration at known locations, aids the clinician in the evaluation of the presence of effusion or amount of abnormal air in the middle ear or sinuses. Percussion may also aid in differential diagnosis of ENT disease such as otitis media or sinusitis by detecting variability of sounds obtained over normal and diseased tissue. In clinical practice, percussion technique is often used after preliminary palpation for gathering further information regarding potential health conditions to assist nurses in clinical judgment during examination. The practice of both palpation and percussion as part of routine ENT examinations facilitates the thorough assessment of patients. Research has established that when these techniques are mastered by nursing professionals, patient outcomes improve significantly, particularly in terms of detection and management of conditions like postoperative gastrointestinal dysfunction, where percussion enables timely complication diagnosis (Siby et al., 2024). Similarly, clinical assessment such as the therapeutic ultrasound test and percussion method have documented high specificity in identifying certain conditions, emphasizing the importance of proficiency in these skills within nursing practice (Rosenthal et al., 2022). Ultimately, proficiency in palpation and percussion skills not only refines a nurse's assessment tool but also anchors their important position in patient-centered care, allowing for integrative and effective evaluations within ENT healthcare settings (Figure 9.10).

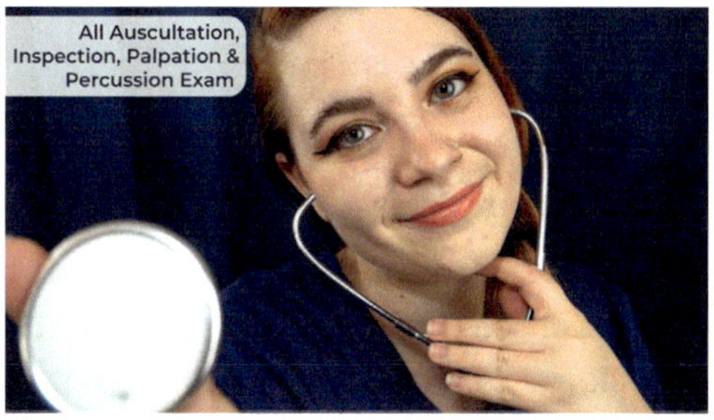

Figure 9.10. Palpation and percussion techniques in ENT.

Source: https://external-content.duckduckgo.com/iu/?u=https%3A%2F%2Fi.ytimg.com%2Fvi%2Fn2FxdTkl5Sk%2Fmaxresdefault.jpg&f=1&nofb=1&ipt=9c7026ef37d6b59c05e408f685e21dd5ea0035fc2e18a3ebedeb72b1d99e5bce.

9.3.3. Use of Specialized Tools: Otoscope and Laryngoscope

In ENT examination, unique devices such as the otoscope and the laryngoscope are core within nursing practice. The otoscope is primarily utilized to examine the external ear canal and tympanic membrane, providing critical information on hearing status. The examination is quite crucial, particularly in children where ailments such as acute secretory otitis media (SOM) are prevalent. With the use of an otoscope, nurses are able to identify signs of infection or fluid retention that, if not addressed, can lead to hearing deficits. Findings from research emphasize that SOM among school children may lead to permanent auditory impairments, so having regular exams using certain instruments like the otoscope in nursing care is necessary (Siyad et al., 2021). The laryngoscope, another crucial ENT examination instrument, is responsible for visualizing the larynx and the upper airway. The device provides the means to perform procedures such as intubation and direct visualization of laryngeal anatomy, thereby facilitating the nurses to explore voice and respiration-related conditions. Through a laryngoscope, healthcare professionals can identify problems like swelling, lesions, or blockages that may complicate airway management.

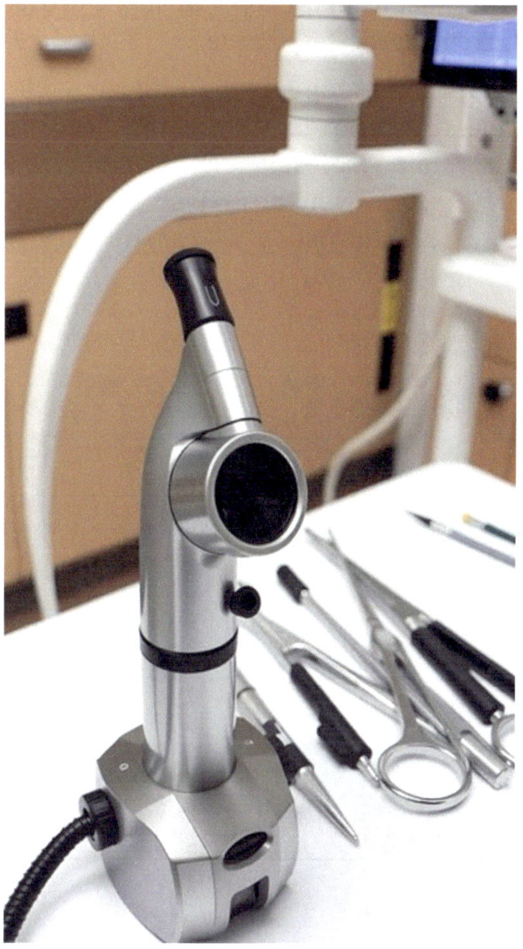

Figure 9.11. Modern laryngoscope with otoscope.

Source: https://external-content.duckduckgo.com/iu/?u=https%3A%2F%2Fimg.freepik.com%2Fpremium-photo%2Fmodern-laryngoscope-with-otoscope-medical-instruments_1264082-261700.jpg&f=1&nofb=1&ipt=da4eab3c8d4e0e822d1ed9554273c45b27794eeb0658a0301e7725350094ba57.

The application of technology to nursing, particularly in laryngoscope use, makes the assessment precision higher so that interventions are accomplished promptly through findings observed. This kind of assessment is convenient in emergency rooms or even in routine visits to patients with known respiratory disorders, ensuring that nursing interventions are proactive and client needs-responsive.

Both otoscopes and laryngoscopes complement the quality of care that is provided by nursing professionals, demonstrating their worth in general ENT screening. Their role transcends purely diagnostic use; they are also tools for education through patient sensitivity and involvement. Through visual display of conditions observed on a patient's ear or throat, nurses can better communicate health concerns, promoting an environment of teamwork in patient care. Also, the statistical foundation of such analyses, as highlighted by the research work on otolaryngologic measuring devices, supports the significance of introducing such specialist equipment into general nursing practice. Such inclusion finally enhances the ENT-associated disorder evaluation and benefits the patient outcome, cementing the significance of specialist devices in the contemporary age of nursing (Chakrabartty, 2023) (Figure 9.11).

Test Your Knowledge

1. What assessment techniques are used to evaluate hearing, nasal patency, oral health, and throat condition?
2. How can inspection, palpation, and use of specialized tools like an otoscope or tongue depressor improve ENT assessment accuracy?

9.4. Patient History and Symptoms

Learning Outcome

1. Importance of a thorough patient history;
2. Common symptoms to inquire about;
3. Cultural considerations in patient communication.

The taking of patient history and symptoms is a signature aspect in the ear, nose, throat (ENT) examination procedure. Comprehensive patient questioning allows healthcare professionals to obtain contextual details necessary for informed decision-making, which often reveals rich information about their condition that would not be revealed through physical examination. Patients' histories regarding their symptoms provide valuable information on the duration, severity, and changeability of their experiences, thus facilitating accurate diagnoses. Second, knowledge of medical and social histories—like previous illness, allergy, or familial tendencies—is also essential to constructing an integrated picture of the patients' health. This is particularly pertinent in an ENT environment, where lifestyle or environmental exposure can most powerfully predispose a patient to particular pathologies, and therefore inform nursing interventions aimed at maximizing patient outcomes and satisfaction. Another critical element of optimal patient history collection is the integration of validated assessment tools. Instruments such as the Charlson Comorbidity Index allow for the assessment of patients' global disease burden to enable practitioners to identify individuals at greater risk for complications or adverse effects. For instance, in one research on the measurement of fluid volume among patients who were undergoing dialysis, the investigators presented a positive correlation between rising comorbidity scores and intradialytic hypotension rates as well as related events, thereby affirming the necessity for individualized approaches to patient care (Choo et al., 2025). These approaches confirm the significance of the systematic process of patient history taking, since they not only aid in risk stratification but also enable nurses to formulate individualized care plans for specific health issues. Moreover, the influence of traumatic events, such as those encountered by healthcare professionals in health emergencies, cannot be ignored while analyzing patient history and symptoms. Evidence has shown that traumatic grief can significantly affect the psychological well-being of nurses and, therefore, the quality of care provided to them (Gilart et al., 2025). Along with the rising amount of stress that comes with such experiences, nursing assessments must take into consideration not only the patient's physical condition but the emotional state of the caregiver, as a result of which clinical interactions may be affected. The inclusion of wellness protocols that encompass mental health as well as physical testing can result in improved patient outcomes and an empathetic health care culture, the interconnectedness of nursing practice and the wholeness of patient care in ENT settings.

9.4.1. Importance of a Thorough Patient History

The history taking of an all-encompassing patient is a core component of the ENT assessment in nursing, giving clinicians the power to effectively address both presenting symptoms and underlying etiology. The comprehensive history assists nurses in observing patterns, which may then herald definite diagnoses, particularly in the complicated realm of ear, nose, mouth, and throat pathology. For instance, a patient's diagnosis, as seen in a case report, of acute onset fever and confusion is improved through understanding their present illness history, prior medical issues such as cancer or past ENT history. Such levels of information may influence test selection and treatment plans, all in all contributing to better patient outcomes. As can be seen from this case, detailed histories not only aid in diagnosis but also help in predicting likely complications based on an individual's medical history, affirming the importance of comprehensive medical histories in practice (Ilyès et al., 2024). Moreover, obtaining a complete social and functional history is equally important when performing ENT examinations, particularly in elderly patients. Nurses who assess patients 65 and older, as they do at St John's Hospital, find that social determinants of health like housing, mental status, and support systems play a significant role in treatment. Accurate documentation of the above goes hand-in-hand with better patient-centered care because an environment of the patient can influence compliance and recovery after ENT surgeries. Such as identifying mobility or activity of daily living that is restricted, the ability for nurses to quantify frailty and adapt care plans accordingly. As illustrated by one study in which interventions improved the accuracy of social history documentation, having a systematic process of obtaining this information changes how multifaceted patients are treated (McGinlay et al., 2022). In ENT nursing, patient history becomes more important with the possibility of peculiar presentations of common conditions. Nurses encounter different cases that may seemingly look straightforward but are found to be complex after detailed scrutiny of the patient's history. The following example of CNS infection due to *Gemella* species illustrates this point forcefully, as understanding the patient's previous ENT history and history of cancer treatment was essential to guiding the diagnosis and subsequent treatment interventions. This example illustrates idealized patient history's ability to enable more than simply contemporaneous clinical assessment; it creates an integrative mindset that guides medical decision-making and interprofessional practice. Lastly, the practice of taking an active comprehensive patient history contributes to a better understanding of the individual's special health narrative and hence the overall quality of care offered within ENT nursing (Figure 9.12).

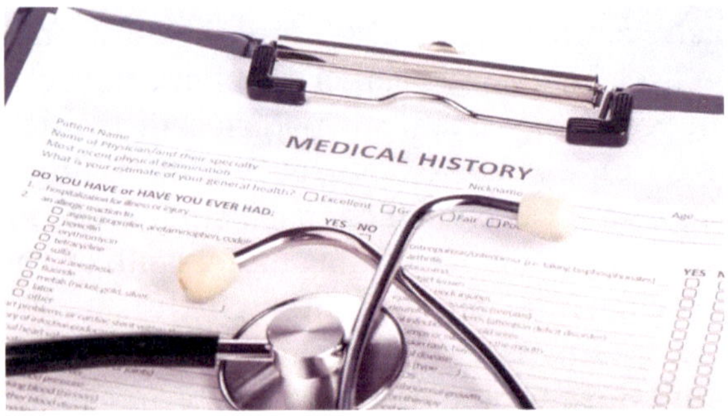

Figure 9.12. Importance of a thorough patient history.

Source: https://denpedia.com/wp-content/uploads/2024/01/medical-history-724x398.webp.

9.4.2. Common Symptoms to Inquire About

In ENT examinations of nursing, asking for fundamental symptoms is essential to condition diagnosis and management. The nurses must conduct rigorous interviews with patients, highlighting symptoms such as pain or discomfort in the ear, nose, and throat. Symptoms of the ears might be depicted as otalgia, which can indicate otitis media or impairment of the eustachian tube. Questions regarding the presence and severity of symptoms are most important because they contribute to a differential diagnosis. In addition, nasal congestion, discharge, or epistaxis must be considered because they may signal underlying infections or systemic disease that must be evaluated and treated. In addition, throat symptoms like dysphagia (swallowing difficulty) and odynophagia (painful swallowing) must be explored during ENT visits. These findings can be caused by a variety of possible reasons, ranging from infection like pharyngitis to structural abnormalities like tumors. In assessing these findings, nurses would assess concomitant factors such as change in voice or persistent cough that can give them a suspicion about the issue.

Also, inquiry regarding concomitant systemic signs like fever or tiredness can provide further clues regarding the patient's condition overall. This integrated approach allows for the nurses to provide focused care and make appropriate referrals as and when needed, thereby enhancing patient outcomes. Even the assessment of the general symptoms is extended to cover identification of otologic findings such as tinnitus and vertigo. Tinnitus, or the perception of ringing or noise in the ears, can greatly compromise a patient's quality of life and is associated with a number of conditions such as hearing loss, exposure to noise, or ototoxic drugs. Similarly, inquiry into vertigo—best explained by patients as a spinning sensation or a feeling of falling—is indicative of vestibular disorder or neurological illness. By recognizing these symptoms, nurses can treat them early on using evidence-based practice recommendations to manage discomfort or refer patients for additional treatment, especially in more complex cases. Most importantly, a well-developed knowledge of these common symptoms enables ENT nurses to offer comprehensive and patient-centered care that facilitates optimal health outcomes in their practice.

9.4.3. Cultural Considerations in Patient Communication

Cultural sensitivity in communication with patients is central to the delivery of effective care, particularly in specialized practice such as Ear, Nose, Mouth, and Throat (ENT) nursing. Understanding the diverse sociocultural backgrounds of patients assists medical professionals in modifying communication strategies to respond to individual needs. Cultural competency involves understanding language issues, health beliefs, and cultural practices which may influence a patients perception of their condition. For instance, there are cultures that have specific beliefs regarding health, illness, and healing which may affect how patients will accept ENT assessments and treatments. Through open communication and respect for one another, nurses are able to build trust and facilitate enhanced patient outcomes, all of which are congruent with goals of successful nursing collaboration as outlined in research (Bakht et al., 2024). Also, culturally competent practice is required in effective communication during ENT examinations. This might involve the use of interpreters or technology to bridge language differences so that essential information is relayed accurately. Cultural competence enables nurses to navigate successfully potentially sensitive topics regarding health, such as dietary restrictions, religious observance, or beliefs about traditional healing that may overlap with medical advice. For example, a patient who is from a culture that has a strong affinity towards home remedies might be skeptical about the use of pharmaceutical treatments. Thus, shared decision-making and patient education in their cultural heritage enhances adherence to the treatment and enhances patient satisfaction. The patient-centered approach, as highlighted by various studies, highlights the essence of cultural sensitivity in establishing effective nurse-patient relationships in ENT facilities (Saif et al., 2023). Ultimately, the consideration of cultural factors in patient communication in ENT nursing highlights the essence of comprehensive care. By recognizing that communication is greater than information exchange, yet an interactive process influenced by cultural perception, health professionals can improve patient experiences and outcomes. This is particularly significant in the assessment of patients who may have possibly unique anatomical or auditory challenges that require tailored approaches. Incorporating culturally responsive communication into practice encourages a caring environment where patients feel valued and understood. Thus, this shift to cultural competence enhances not only the quality of nursing care but also aligns with the broader agenda of health care to improve equity and promote health literacy across communities, thereby warranting the necessity for teamwork in achieving these objectives as presented in the literature (Bakht et al., 2024).

Test Your Knowledge

1. What key questions should be asked to obtain a thorough patient history for ENT assessment?
2. How can patient-reported symptoms, such as hearing loss, sore throat, or nasal congestion, guide further examination?

9.5. Diagnostic Tests and Procedures

Learning Outcome

1. Audiometry and hearing tests;
2. Nasal endoscopy and throat cultures;
3. Imaging studies: X-rays and CT scans.

Diagnostic procedures and tests in the case of Ear, Nose, Mouth, and Throat (ENT) assessment play a crucial role in drawing valid conclusions and guiding treatment plans. Essential tools are endoscopic assessments, audiometry testing, and imaging tests, all of which are employed to finalize the assessment of patients. Endoscopy, for example, enables practitioners to observe within the nasal tract and throat, so detection of tumors or polyps can occur. Audiometric testing, also crucial to the assessment of hearing ability, helps to diagnose conductive or sensorineural hearing loss, a vital element of ENT assessments. By incorporating a combination of these diagnostic modalities, clinicians can develop a composite image of a patient's condition and thereby lead to more effective and tailored treatment protocols. Blood work and allergy testing are also very important components of ENT diagnostic workups. Blood tests can reveal underlying infections, autoimmune conditions, or inflammatory processes involving the ear, nose, or throat, while allergy testing identifies specific allergens causing chronic sinusitis or other ENT disorders. Allergy testing through skin prick tests or serum immunoglobulin tests helps providers tailor treatments to help minimize symptoms effectively and can significantly enhance patient outcomes. The integration of such tests not only directs the immediate clinical treatment but also establishes the foundation for long-term patient care plans. Knowledge and use of these diagnostic tests, therefore, contextualize the individual's clinical presentation and allow a more comprehensive management of ENT care. In addition, they must be interpreted by considering a deeper understanding of their practice implications. For example, abnormal results of imaging studies can lead to further diagnostic testing, such as biopsies or referral for surgery. Also, the results of audiometric testing may portend referral to specialist services for rehabilitation support, such as hearing aids or cochlear implant. The importance of having a methodical approach in the identification of potential complications cannot be overstated, as misinterpretation could lead to delays in diagnosis and treatment. Therefore, healthcare workers and nurses must take care to stay up to date with current guidelines and evidence-based practices in ENT examination, as exemplified in the regular review of treatment for conditions such as aneurysmal subarachnoid hemorrhage (Brian et al., 2023) and urticaria (Zuberbier et al., 2021). Overall, well-established diagnosis procedures pave the way for effective nursing interventions and improved patient results in dynamic ENT practice.

9.5.1. Audiometry and Hearing Tests

Assessment of hearing function is a critical component within the framework of Ear, Nose, Mouth, and Throat (ENT) examination within nursing practice. Utilization of audiometry as a primary diagnostic tool enables clinicians to evaluate a patient's hearing ability and, in turn, ascertain the presence or absence of any hearing impairment, or compromised ear function. Conducting hearing testing, particularly through automated and manual techniques of audiometry, enables clinicians to identify the quality and degree of hearing impairment. In existing studies, application of non-specialist health workers to perform the tests has been seen to yield high sensitivities and specificities, which demonstrate their effectiveness in correctly diagnosing bilateral hearing loss. This ease of application has critically significant implications for poor-resource settings, where specialized ENT specialists are not always easily accessible, hence ensuring maximum community health participation in hearing testing (Bright et al., 2019). Besides, the utilization of technology in audiometric assessment has transformed traditional processes into more convenient and quicker ones. That mobile-based audiometers exist is a relief in the hearing test arena since there can be instant results that can facilitate expedited clinical decision-making. Audiometric testing may be conducted successfully by trained nurses and non-specialist health workers, further bridging patient needs and specialist involvement. It is important that nursing education includes thorough training in audiometry, both for the optimization of hearing examination effectiveness and for empowering nurses as active participants in preventive care. This empowerment can have immediate effects on the outcomes of patients since identification of auditory complications at an early stage usually leads to timely intervention (Bright et al., 2019).

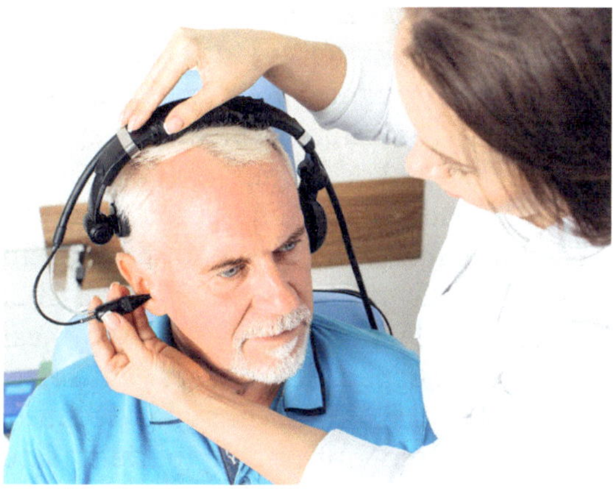

Figure 9.13. Audiometry hearing test.

Source: https://www.mediright.co.uk/wp-content/uploads/2021/03/audiometry.jpg.

In the management of tinnitus, audiometric testing is also important. Tinnitus, as a general rule, is secondary to hearing loss and therefore requires thorough audiological assessment to rule out associated conditions and guide treatment accordingly. Current clinical guidelines in various nations emphasize the value of audiometric testing, along with physical examination and filling out standardized questionnaires. The identical recommendations for the incorporation of audiometry in tinnitus evaluations reflect an overall consensus of its significance in addressing auditory discomfort. Furthermore, having uniform guidelines available for the treatment of tinnitus potentially has the ability to enhance the quality of care for tinnitus patients, in that nurses and other professionals are adequately trained to address both the auditory and psychological components of tinnitus management (Figure 9.13).

9.5.2. Nasal Endoscopy and Throat Cultures

Nasal endoscopy is an important advance in the field of otolaryngology, particularly in the diagnosis of chronic rhinosinusitis (CRS). It's considered the gold standard for the identification and measurement of nasal disease severity. With this minimally invasive procedure, physicians can visualize the nasal passages, identifying obstructions, swelling, and anatomical abnormalities not discernable by physical examination.

Evidence has shown that symptoms such as nasal congestion are closely linked to findings on nasoendoscopy, as demonstrated in clinical research where CRS patients displayed strong correlations between the severity of nasal congestion and the Lund-Kennedy score—highlighting the significance of endoscopy in understanding the pathophysiology of nasal symptoms (Chandra et al., 2024). This method not only enhances diagnostic accuracy but also guides the treatment interventions such that patients receive particular care based on their individual conditions. Throat cultures are another key component of ENT assessment, particularly for the detection of etiologic pathogens responsible for pharyngitis, tonsillitis, and other throat pathologies. By obtaining a sample from the throat, health professionals are then able to test for the exact pathogens responsible for causing the patient's symptoms, whether bacterial, viral, or fungal. This is significant because it determines the management plan, such as whether to prescribe antibiotics for a bacterial infection or schedule supportive therapy for a viral condition. In addition, throat cultures are able to uncover atypical presentations, i.e., abscesses or malignancies, explaining why thorough evaluations in patients presenting with a mass in their throat or chronic symptoms are crucial (Tanthry et al., 2021).

Thus, including throat cultures in routine evaluations helps ensure that physicians can respond promptly and effectively, preventing complications from misdiagnosis or delayed intervention. The integration of nasal endoscopy and throat cultures in the ENT assessment system highlights the importance of proper assessment in nursing practice. Both modalities perform different functions that complement an overall picture of a patient's status.

Endoscopy provides an excellent visualization of the nasal anatomy and disease, whereas throat cultures provide biochemical data regarding infective etiologies. Both are demanding in terms of skilled clinical administration and interpretation, and there is a focus on the importance of continuous training and education in practice nursing. Furthermore, their combination allows for improved patient outcomes through evidence-based interventions that are targeted at the individual. In brief, strategic use of nasal endoscopy and throat cultures highlights the crucial role played by thorough ENT examinations in nursing practice, providing diagnostic accuracy and patient care in addition to mitigating potential health risks caused by undiagnosed or inappropriately treated conditions (Figure 9.14).

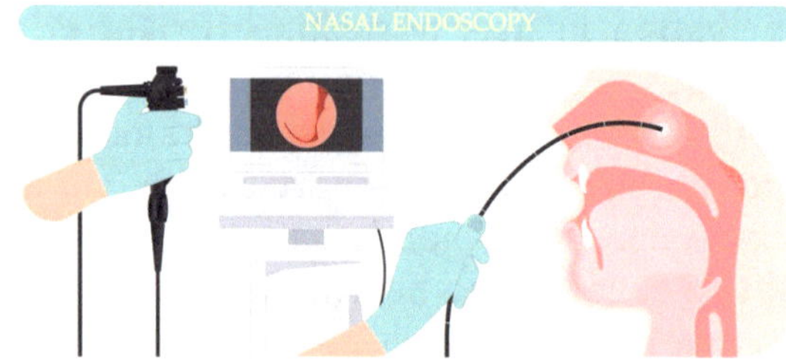

Figure 9.14. Nasal endoscopy.

Source: https://www.aglow-ent.sg/wp-content/uploads/2024/03/Naso-endoscopy.jpeg.

9.5.3. Imaging Studies: X-Rays and CT Scans

Imaging examinations, such as X-rays and computed tomography (CT) scans, play an important part in the diagnosis of ear, nose, mouth, and throat (ENT) diseases. X-rays are, in fact, a convenient and efficient means of visualizing anatomical structures, particularly in conditions such as sinusitis or nasal cavity foreign bodies. However, overutilization of X-ray imaging has brought about concerns about unnecessary radiation exposure, especially among children. For instance, a pediatrician review of head trauma suggested that while most children underwent imaging, few required it for accurate diagnosis (Gharaibeh et al., 2025). This is an appeal for more engagement by health practitioners, especially nurses, in serious scrutiny of whether an imaging technique is needed, hence optimizing patient safety and resource allocation. CT scans also offer more details and understanding compared to conventional X-rays, and hence are particularly valuable in complex ENT cases. They are essential in diagnosing conditions that would not be appropriately imaged through the use of X-rays, such as sinusitis, tumors, or structural abnormalities. CT scans may also create cross-sectional images of the neck and head that may be utilized for surgical planning or intervention. The incorporation of newer technologies, such as artificial intelligence, can help further enhance diagnostic accuracy and efficiency (Syed et al., 2024). By integrating AI technology with CT scans, health care professionals have access to more precise risk assessments and improved imaging protocols, which can ultimately lead to better patient outcomes. In ENT nursing, understanding the results of imaging tests is relevant to patient-centered care. Nurses often are the first point of contact for patients who require an ENT workup, and their knowledge of when to refer or order X-rays and CT scans affects immediate clinical decision-making. Outside of technology, nurses must also be able to communicate with patients effectively in order to answer their questions about the necessity and safety of these imaging studies. By establishing a cooperative environment where there is much discussion about potential harms and benefits, nurses are able to allow patients to make informed choices about their health. As technology improves, current education about new imaging technologies and applications will be necessary to help promote quality ENT exams and the highest quality of care.

Test Your Knowledge

1. What common diagnostic tests are used to assess ENT disorders, and what information does each provide?
2. How can results from audiometry, throat swabs, or nasal endoscopy influence nursing care and treatment planning?

9.6. Nursing Interventions and Care Plans

Learning Outcome

1. Developing individualized care plans;
2. Patient education on ENT health;
3. Collaboration with interdisciplinary teams.

Effective nursing interventions and care plans are a central feature of patient care for ENT evaluation. These care plans are intended to identify discrete patient needs, establish realistic objectives, and ensure nursing actions are adequately coordinated and evidence-based. For example, effective ENT symptom evaluations are not only physical exams but also the utilization of patients' histories as guides to care maneuvers. By addressing issues like otitis media or pharyngitis, follow-up patient education on medication compliance, symptom management, and follow-up can be included in nursing interventions. Such particular care plans not only improve patient outcomes but also provide assistance to a healing nurse-patient relationship crucial for compliance and communication in the health care setting. Moreover, incorporation of evidence-based guidelines in nursing care plans enhances the quality of ENT assessment and treatment. With the ongoing development of medical research, especially on disorders such as aneurysmal subarachnoid hemorrhage, nurses must keep up with new recommendations. The *2023*

Guideline for the Management of Patients with Aneurysmal Subarachnoid Hemorrhage (Brian et al., 2023) emphasizes a comprehensive, global approach to diagnosis and management. These standards also prescribe not only the on-the-spot actions of care but also the longer-term follow-up measures necessary for optimal patient outcomes. By using these best practices, nurses can rest assured that they are providing care that is based on the most current scientific evidence and thereby minimizing complications and maximizing prospects for recovery in patients with ENT-related complaints.

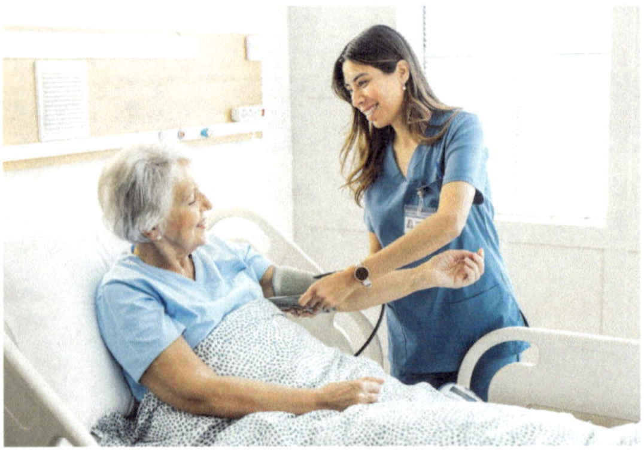

Figure 9.15. Nursing interventions and care plans.

Source: https://cdn.prod.website-files.com/5babc11099f97ea5dbcf24d5/653ad10165a9716ee31bd67d_64de3ec56db3d89c7d78cab0_med-surg-nurse.jpeg.

In the last couple of years, the use of telehealth services in nursing practice has also been an efficient mechanism in managing ENT assessments. Telehealth not only provides greater access to care but also makes it easy to track patients at home. As outlined in recent reviews, the potential for telehealth to expand health care delivery across much of the country is huge (Dorsey et al., 2016). For ENT assessment, this might mean virtual consultations, distant symptom monitoring, and remote access to preventive care and management tips information. By incorporating these innovative technologies into nursing interventions, nurses can enhance patients' degree of engagement, adhere to care plans more comprehensively, and act quickly in response to patients' changing needs, thus improving the overall quality of care in the ENT sector (Figure 9.15).

9.6.1. Developing Individualized Care Plans

Individualized care planning forms the core of practice in Ear, Nose, Mouth, and Throat (ENT) nursing in advancing patient outcomes and promoting effective care. Each patient presents a unique combination of presenting symptoms, medical history, and personal preferences that need to be addressed by tailored interventions. For instance, patients' specific ENT problems, such as recurrent sinusitis or tonsillitis, enable nurses to tailor-assessment strategies and treatment options to address individualized needs. Further, patient participation in the care plan fosters collaboration, giving them ownership of their own care. With data gathered by nurses through comprehensive assessments, they can create care plans that include not just medical interventions but also lifestyle modifications and psychosocial interventions, thus facilitating holistic care responsive to the individual complexities of every patient's case. Moreover, the use of evidence-based practice in creating care plans that are individualized per patient is most important in ENT nursing. With the use of the latest clinical guidelines and evidence-based literature, nurses can ensure that care plans are aligned with the latest information and best practices within the profession. An example is the ongoing revision of guidelines such as the "2023 Guideline for the Management of Patients with Aneurysmal Subarachnoid Hemorrhage"—patient-centered care—that demonstrates the ongoing need to make changes in clinical practice (Brian et al., 2023). Such evidence-based interventions not only enhance the quality of care provided but also contribute to the overall patient satisfaction by ensuring congruence with determined standards and evidence-based interventions. Therefore, this commitment to evidence-based individualized care planning serves to advance the level of practice in the ENT specialty. Additionally, the application of artificial intelligence (AI) to health care presents promising opportunities for enhancing the process of individualized care planning in ENT nursing. As found by the NAIL team's collaborative efforts, integrating AI can help in the development of advanced care plans by helping nurses to analyze clinical data more effectively and detect patterns to guide patient-specific intervention (Ronquillo et al., 2021). By empowering nurses to better understand the connection between the information they collect and the AI tools they have at their disposal, more accurate and nuanced care plans can be constructed. Furthermore, involving nursing professionals in the development of AI ensures that created tools are functional and practical within practice settings, ultimately delivering more effective care for patients with diverse ENT needs. Embracing this technological revolution is not only essential for the further progress of nursing practice but for enhancing the overall quality of care within the ENT field as well.

9.6.2. Patient Education on ENT Health

Appropriate patient education on ear, nose, and throat (ENT) health is an essential predictor of enhanced patient outcomes and forms a basic aspect of nursing practice. By sharing reliable information on the health status of patients, nurses can empower patients to take on active roles in managing their healthcare. The key domains of concern in ENT education are identification of symptoms, information on treatment, and recognition of the need to seek additional medical assistance. Lack of readiness among junior doctors and medical students towards ENT practice has been proven to create a gap in healthcare provision, and thus incorporation of specialized educational modules in nursing curriculum becomes critical to bridge these gaps (Gary et al., 2016). These enhancements in education methodologies could potentially extend to more effective patient interactions, establishing an environment where patients become informed and engaged in their own treatment procedures. Focused interventions that are directed towards treating individual conditions of the ENT can also improve compliance and satisfaction among patients. For instance, informing patients about the need for compliance with therapies in cases of allergies, sinusitis, or hearing impairments can extend far in improving patient outcomes. Furthermore, multimodal interventions such as the employment of visual aids or digital health tools can enhance patient understanding and retention of information. Evidence shows that patients waiting for long periods for elective ENT surgeries are likely to develop frustration and stress, which can exacerbate their conditions (Ballini et al., 2015). Nurses play a pivotal role in addressing such issues through educating patients about the reason behind delays and potential alternatives, hence improving the patient experience as well as strengthening the healthcare system's trust. Additionally, patient education must evolve with advancements in the science of medicine and shifts in healthcare delivery. As advancing technologies and treatments in ENT become available, nurses need to make sure that patients receive current information that is relevant to their own conditions. This continuous education not only promotes a trusting patient-nurse relationship but also makes patients aware of new therapies that may help them. Including education on lifestyle changes, including quitting smoking and the avoidance of allergens, further promotes global health management. By ensuring active patient participation in their ENT healthcare through health education, nurses help promote better health outcomes, reduce preventable complications, and ultimately promote a culture of well-being in society.

9.6.3. Collaboration with Interdisciplinary Teams

The health care setting is increasingly characterized by the requirement for interprofessional team working, particularly in such procedures as Ear, Nose, Mouth, and Throat (ENT) examination in nursing. These interprofessional teams bring together professionals of diverse backgrounds including nursing, audiology, speech-language pathology, and otolaryngology, each with specialist expertise. By facilitating an environment where a team's members share their skill and knowledge, health care providers are able to enhance patient outcomes and results. In this setting, the collaborative model facilitates end-to-end assessment that is essential in diagnosis and treatment of ENT disorders. The blending of various perspectives, besides improving the quality of care provided, fosters a learning and improvement culture among providers, which leads to enhanced clinical decision-making during the assessment and treatment process. Multidisciplinary team working demands awareness of roles and relationships between team members. Communication is essential to facilitate exchange of information and aid collective problem-solving. In ENT nursing clinical assessments, team members will need to deal with such variables as disparity in clinical practice and terminology, which call for respect for each other and open communication. In addition, the procedure includes conflict resolution and rapport-building skills, which are very important in maintaining a harmonious working environment. The fusion of expertise from numerous disciplines not only enhances the teams capabilities to tackle intricate problems in patient care but also evokes innovative ideas in the concept development and acceptance phase of patient assessments, according to research focusing on interdisciplinary collaboration in intricate clinical settings (Merty, 2025). Aside from that, interdisciplinarity promotes the effectiveness of curricula aimed at improving competencies in ENT examinations. Research in project-based learning emphasizes collaboration and independent learning in the constantly evolving healthcare environment (Kirilova, 2024). With collaborative approaches such as workshops and debates through case studies, nursing experts will better grasp many ENT conditions and best practices for assessment. This pedagogy fosters experiential learning while presenting the participants with the chance to assess their peers, hence cementing learning outcomes. Eventually, interdisciplinary collaboration not only improves the nurses' skill set but also fosters a learning setup that is productive for the practitioners and the patients they handle, leading to enriched clinical practice and greater patient satisfaction.

Test Your Knowledge

1. What nursing interventions can be implemented for patients with ENT disorders to relieve symptoms and prevent complications?
2. How should nurses develop and document care plans for patients with chronic or acute ENT conditions?

SUMMARY

The importance of thorough Ear, Nose, Mouth, and Throat (ENT) screenings within nursing cannot be overstated. ENT screenings are essential for diagnosing a wide array of illnesses, ranging from mild infections to serious systemic issues. The multifaceted nature of ENT screenings allows nursing staff not only to identify existing issues but also to identify potential underlying health conditions. This interprofessional process not only enhances patient care but also promotes early intervention actions, which further improve patient outcomes. With new guidelines coming in, as directed by the Endocrine Society with regard to safety and quality of life in clinical care (Speiser et al., 2018), the nurse must stay updated in order to deliver the optimal level of care in its evaluation. A complete ENT assessment also plays a critical part in the interdisciplinary health model. Interdisciplinary working between healthcare professionals like physicians, specialists, and pharmacists enhances the quality of care offered to patients. Through effective ENT assessments, nurses can support referrals and communicate important findings well, contributing to enhanced interdisciplinary decision-making processes. As shown by the correlations of recent research, for example, between lower cerebral perfusion and cognitive impairment (Frank et al., 2017), an ENT assessment offered by a nurse can yield significant information that influences the general health management interventions. The collaboration not only optimizes resources but also maintains patient-centered care throughout. Finally, considering the evolving face of medicine, continuous education and training in ENT examinations are essential to nurses. Combining evidence-based practice into routine examination allows nurses to identify and treat serious ENT complications. Continuous professional development ensures nursing practice remains at par with advances in medicine and that a culture of patient safety and quality is enhanced. As research continues to reveal connections between ENT health and general health, nurses must be firmly grounded in these assessments. Therefore, there is a necessity to campaign for training centers that continue to prepare nurses in their crucial role of providing comprehensive ENT care to patients.

The full assessment of the ear, nose, mouth, and throat (ENT) is a fundamental component of nursing practice that needs to be supported by sound anatomy knowledge and common pathologies. A logical sequence begins with an adequate patient history that includes inquiry into presenting symptoms such as pain, discharge, or alterations in hearing and swallowing. Such information not only helps in the identification of acute and chronic diseases but also allows for proper understanding of individual needs of all patients. The inclusion of an orderly physical examination adds to the process of evaluation as it involves visual observation, palpation, and, if needed, some specific maneuvers like otoscopy or laryngoscopy. As the healthcare systems continue to develop, nursing professionals must be proficient in these fundamental approaches to render skilled and evidence-based care. Technology application for ENT examinations significantly enhances diagnostic accuracy and patient outcomes. Advances, for instance, with telehealth consultations, have significantly revolutionized the manner in which assessments are conducted from traditional methods, with remote tests and follow-ups that can be facilitated by patient mobility issues and time factors. Further, imaging technology and software using Artificial Intelligence improve the ability to evaluate complex cases and detect abnormalities that would have otherwise remained unnoticed. Such developments are particularly handy in the instance of ENT consultations, where diverse presentations of ailments render them challenging to identify. As has been evidenced through the continued medical research in numerous fields, the advent of new technologies presents with it opportunities and challenges that doctors need to stay aware of and adapt, eventually positioning them to deliver cutting-edge care which addresses patients' needs in a holistic manner. Finally, awareness of the psychosocial effects of ENT conditions is crucial during the nursing assessment. EAR, NOSE, and THROAT conditions are likely to have significant effects on the patients' quality of life, impacting on their social interaction, emotional status, and overall well-being. Nurses play an important role in providing not only clinical interventions but also psychologic support, counseling patients on the challenges that come with their diseases. This underscores the importance of communication skills and cultural competence in delivering empathetic care. Furthermore, responsiveness to social determinants of health can maximize the potential of interventions to respect patients' histories and contexts. As evidence underscores the importance of patient-centered care, nurses must continue to focus on these psychosocial factors in routine assessments to deliver complete care that respects both the physical and emotional dimensions of health.

KEY TERMS FROM THIS CHAPTER

Auricle
External Auditory Canal
Otoscope
Weber Test
Nasal Septum
Sinuses
Lips
Hard Palate
Uvula
Pharynx
Tympanic Membrane
Eustachian Tube
Hearing Acuity
Rinne Test
Turbinates
Nasal Mucosa
Tongue
Soft Palate
Tonsils
Gag Reflex

CRITICAL THINKING QUESTIONS

1. **Which cranial nerve is primarily assessed when testing the gag reflex?**
   a. Cranial Nerve V (Trigeminal)
   b. Cranial Nerve VII (Facial)
   c. Cranial Nerve IX (Glossopharyngeal)
   d. Cranial Nerve XII (Hypoglossal)
2. **A nurse is assessing a patient's hearing. Which test evaluates the ability to hear high- and low-frequency sounds?**
   a. Rinne test
   b. Weber test
   c. Audiometry
   d. Romberg test
3. **During nasal assessment, the nurse notes pale, bluish, boggy turbinates. This is most consistent with:**
   a. Allergic rhinitis
   b. Bacterial sinusitis
   c. Nasal polyp
   d. Deviated septum
4. **The nurse inspects the oral cavity and notices white patches on the tongue that cannot be scraped off. This is indicative of:**
   a. Oral candidiasis
   b. Leukoplakia
   c. Geographic tongue
   d. Oral herpes
5. **Which technique is correct when using an otoscope to inspect the adult ear canal?**
   a. Pull the pinna downward and backward
   b. Pull the pinna upward and backward
   c. Pull the pinna straight back
   d. Pull the pinna forward and upward

Short Answer Questions

1. What are the key structures assessed in the ear, and what is their primary function?
2. Describe the technique for assessing hearing and balance in a patient.
3. What abnormalities in the external ear and tympanic membrane might indicate infection or trauma?
4. How is the nose assessed for patency, symmetry, and signs of infection?
5. What should a nurse observe when inspecting the oral cavity, including the teeth, gums, and tongue?

Answer to Critical Thinking Questions

1. (c) 2. (c) 3. (a) 4. (b) 5. (b)

REFERENCES

1. Abreu, C., Esteves, I. M., Pires, R., Santos, M. P., & Santos, M. (2024). Nursing knowledge of school-age children undergoing ear, nose and throat surgery and their families–A scoping review protocol. *Research, Society and Development.* https://www.semanticscholar.org/paper/fc1d71f7b565e30f4e3b0d04f1e482c1777c396e (accessed on 16th July 2025).

2. AL Saif, N. A., Alharthi, M. S., Alshammari, A. M., Altamimi, A. M., Azw alanazi, M., Hawbani, R. F., Alanazi, N. W., et al. (2023). Pediatric nursing in primary care: Strategies for holistic child and family support. *Journal of Survey in Fisheries Sciences.* https://www.semanticscholar.org/paper/66cd2719c7021270041502377f9e3cc86db7de40 (accessed on 16th July 2025).

3. Bakht, K., Mir, S., & Shah, S. A. (2024). Nursing teamwork: An in-depth concept analysis with Walker & Avant's framework. *Journal of Health and Rehabilitation Research.* https://www.semanticscholar.org/paper/f685c9967b1d3c995717584ee62228ae82667f64 (accessed on 16th July 2025).

4. Ballini, L., Negro, A., Maltoni, S., Vignatelli, L., Flodgren, G., Simera, I., Holmes, J., et al. (2015). Interventions to reduce waiting times for elective procedures. *The Cochrane Database of Systematic Reviews, 2,* CD005610. https://www.semanticscholar.org/paper/33df9f526d11f0f524d1a2a87d0d7fb839b04d2a (accessed on 16th July 2025).

5. Bass, J., Patel, M., & Kapoor, K. (2025). Utilizing tracking technology to reduce the financial and patient care impact of lost ear, nose and throat equipment. *Annals of the Royal College of Surgeons of England.* https://www.semanticscholar.org/paper/98d802616777eb8a84cd5a1c951d81b39419a65d (accessed on 16th July 2025).

6. Benhalima, I., Jacquemont, L., Milière, L., Tone, A., Ettahar, N., Dewulf, G., & Mazars, E. (2024). Meningitis due to *Gemella* sp. in a patient with severe ENT conditions: Case report and review of the literature. *Annals of Clinical Microbiology and Antimicrobials, 23.* https://www.semanticscholar.org/paper/69f1507c05b94f77981b2462ecb53e55a4d59bb6 (accessed on 16th July 2025).

7. Bolton, L., Mills, C., Wallace, S., & Brady, M. (2020). Aerosol generating procedures, dysphagia assessment and COVID-19: A rapid review. *International Journal of Language & Communication Disorders, 55,* 629–636. https://doi.org/10.1111/1460-6984.12544 (accessed on 16th July 2025).

8. Bright, T., Mulwafu, W., Phiri, M., Ensink, R. J. H., Smith, A., Yip, J., Mactaggart, I., et al. (2019). Diagnostic accuracy of non-specialist versus specialist health workers in diagnosing hearing loss and ear disease in Malawi. *Tropical Medicine & International Health, 24,* 817–828. https://doi.org/10.1111/tmi.13238 (accessed on 16th July 2025).

9. Cachata, D., Costa, M., Magalhães, T., Lucas, P., & Gaspar, F. (2025). Information technology in nursing practice: A scoping review of assessment tools for evaluating nurses' competencies. *Journal of Healthcare Leadership, 17,* 211–223. https://www.semanticscholar.org/paper/7f5b85669787635db7c68e958b87fd93e7c417df (accessed on 16th July 2025).

10. Caffrey, M. K. (2022). Value-based care will "continue to evolve" even if OCM expires. *The American Journal of Managed Care, 28,* SP208–SP209. https://doi.org/10.37765/ajmc.2022.89177 (accessed on 16th July 2025).

11. Chakrabartty, S. N. (2023). Assessment tools in rhinology and otology and quality of life: Methodological issues. *International Journal of Medical and All Body Health Research, 04*(1), 17–23. https://www.allmedicaljournal.com/uploads/archives_upload/20230503170255_A-23-08.1.pdf (accessed on 16th July 2025).
12. Chandra, C. M., Kristyono, I., Soegiarto, G., & Nugroho, P. S. (2024). Nasal symptoms of chronic rhinosinusitis were related to its nasoendoscopic findings: A retrospective cohort study at Dr. Soetomo General Academic Hospital, Surabaya. *JUXTA: Jurnal Ilmiah Mahasiswa Kedokteran Universitas Airlangga*. https://www.semanticscholar.org/paper/35c0a1dde58bd61f69e27f8d09d7595025a70b58 (accessed on 16th July 2025).
13. Chowdhary, K., Yadav, G., Rai, A., Saha, S., Dhinsa, K., & Sharma, A. (2024). Mouth breathing habit and their effects on dentofacial growth in children in the age range of 6–14 years: A cephalometric study. *International Journal of Clinical Pediatric Dentistry, 17*, 545–551. https://www.semanticscholar.org/paper/9570673d2e659b518d275403efdd623c71541d02 (accessed on 16th July 2025).
14. Dai, Q., Xiong, W., Wang, Y. J., Hu, N., Sun, X., Fan, Z. M., Wang, H. B., et al. (2025). [Application of 3D-Flair MRI and vestibular function assessment in profound sudden sensorineural hearing loss patients]. *Zhonghua Er Bi Yan Hou Tou Jing Wai Ke Za Zhi (Chinese Journal of Otorhinolaryngology Head and Neck Surgery), 60*(1), 2–9. https://www.semanticscholar.org/paper/c3324a8726defa36174113df3d38e0ae0f05490f (accessed on 16th July 2025).
15. Denk-Linnert, D.-M., Farneti, D., Nawka, T., am Zehnhoff-Dinnesen, A., Moerman, M., Zorowka, P., Farahat, M. F., et al. (2022). Position statement of the Union of European Phoniatricians (UEP): Fees and phoniatricians' role in multidisciplinary and multiprofessional dysphagia management team. *Dysphagia, 38*, 711–718. https://doi.org/10.1007/s00455-022-10502-9 (accessed on 16th July 2025).
16. Dorsey, E. R., & Topol, E. J. (2016). State of telehealth. *New England Journal of Medicine, 375*, 154–161. https://doi.org/10.1056/nejmra1601705 (accessed on 16th July 2025).
17. Elmetwaly, R. M., Ali, A. S., Abd Elsalam, S. N., & Sherif, D. E. M., & Elsayed, S. M. (2024). Nursing guidelines on safety measures awareness among patients with thyroid disorders undergoing radioactive iodine therapy. *Egyptian Journal of Health Care*. https://www.semanticscholar.org/paper/fc93c694117b148e71611221c27b3c4a927a08a2 (accessed on 16th July 2025).
18. Estes, K. R., Callanan, D., Rai, N., Plunkett, K., Brunson, D. K., & Tiwari, T. (2018). Evaluation of an interprofessional oral health assessment activity in advanced practice nursing education. *Journal of Dental Education, 82*(10), 1084–1090. https://www.semanticscholar.org/paper/715d1fad1b8ad9a0aa23d7a1db274371c460e1cd (accessed on 16th July 2025).
19. Farahzadi, Z., Khodadadi, E., Abesi, F., & Gholinia, H. (2024). Assessment of the relationship between oral health and adenoid hypertrophy in children aged 8 to 15 years. *Journal of Oral Health and Oral Epidemiology*. https://www.semanticscholar.org/paper/690c18bf594fa54bd277fa8e4fa7e93355cb2ccf (accessed on 16th July 2025).
20. Ferguson, G. R., Bacila, I. A., & Swamy, M. (2016). Does current provision of undergraduate education prepare UK medical students in ENT? A systematic literature review. *BMJ Open, 6*. https://www.semanticscholar.org/paper/f09df91ed1a07d0aef310aee96270effda57f3b6 (accessed on 16th July 2025).

21. Fuller, T., Haider, H. F., Kikidis, D., Lapira, A., Mazurek, B., Noreña, A., Rabau, S., et al. (2017). Different teams, same conclusions? A systematic review of existing clinical guidelines for the assessment and treatment of tinnitus in adults. *Frontiers in Psychology, 8*. https://doi.org/10.3389/fpsyg.2017.00206 (accessed on 16th July 2025).

22. Gharaibeh, A., Lackova, A., Gharaibeh, M. M., Alwadiya, A., Čellár, R., Mitró, I., Filip, V., et al. (2025). Overuse of ionizing radiation imaging by skull X-ray scans for minor pediatric head trauma. *European Journal of Clinical and Experimental Medicine*. https://www.semanticscholar.org/paper/5cd1b5cd98f2aa51ef4b8b02eaed2cc74e0a117a (accessed on 16th July 2025).

23. Gilart, E., Bocchino, A., Lepiani, I., Gilart, P., Cantizano Nuñez, M. J., & Dueñas, M. (2025). Psychometric properties and validity of inventory of symptoms of professional traumatic grief among nursing professionals. *BMC Nursing, 24*. https://www.semanticscholar.org/paper/ba9f65917597c2c5bd58519a2e651cfe53c7df9e (accessed on 16th July 2025).

24. Groen, J., Gordon, M., Chogle, A., Benninga, M. A., Borlack, R. E., Borrelli, O., Darbari, A., et al. (2025). ESPGHAN/NASPGHAN guidelines for treatment of irritable bowel syndrome and functional abdominal pain-not otherwise specified in children aged 4–18 years. *Journal of Pediatric Gastroenterology and Nutrition*. https://www.semanticscholar.org/paper/4bb46422605368da297d44d8175df14ab1d72f63 (accessed on 16th July 2025).

25. Guyton, K. B., Sandage, M. J., Bailey, D. J., Haak, N. J., Molt, L. F., & Plumb, A. M. (2018). Acquired velopharyngeal dysfunction: Survey, literature review, and clinical recommendations. *American Journal of Speech-Language Pathology, 27*, 1572–1597. https://doi.org/10.1044/2018_ajslp-17-0222 (accessed on 16th July 2025).

26. Hanson, S., Bruyere, S., Forber-Pratt, A. J., Reesman, J., & Sung, C. (2023). Guidelines for assessment and intervention with persons with disabilities: An executive summary. *The American Psychologist*. https://www.semanticscholar.org/paper/d3a1e4c332d60d9f3da674a049416520e2a7da67 (accessed on 16th July 2025).

27. Hoh, B. L., Ko, N., Amin-Hanjani, S., Chou, S., Cruz-Flores, S., Dangayach, N., Derdeyn, C. P., et al. (2023). 2023 guideline for the management of patients with aneurysmal subarachnoid hemorrhage: A guideline from the American Heart Association/American Stroke Association. *Stroke, 54*. https://doi.org/10.1161/str.0000000000000436 (accessed on 16th July 2025).

28. Kirilova, B. (2024). Addressing challenges in enhancing team collaboration and evaluating interdisciplinary projects. *Pedagogika-Pedagogy*. https://www.semanticscholar.org/paper/4641526988b66997898300be762cabe5a718d9fc (accessed on 16th July 2025).

29. Kobkam, K., Aree-Ue, S., & Roopsawang, I. (2024). Prevalence of lower urinary tract symptoms and their associations with health outcomes among older nursing home residents: A cross-sectional study. *Pacific Rim International Journal of Nursing Research*. https://www.semanticscholar.org/paper/3165838304475c7f8d0c130d756bf584f4aecc03 (accessed on 16th July 2025).

30. Kujur, N. A., Sinha, B. K., Murmu, I. M., Karmbir, Tudu, M., & Ranjan, R. K. (2024). A comparative study between preoperative computed tomography and intraoperative ossicular chain status in patients of chronic suppurative otitis media at RIMS, Ranchi. *Journal of Pharmacy & Bioallied Sciences, 16*, S3853–S3855. https://www.semanticscholar.org/paper/295ad1d0574d44ae894f65d6fc65ca2eeeef8cde (accessed on 16th July 2025).

31. Li, Z. (2024). Research on computer intelligent nursing home service quality assessment factor scoring feedback system. *2024 IEEE 3rd International Conference on Electrical Engineering, Big Data and Algorithms (EEBDA)*. https://www.semanticscholar.org/paper/1b390fa08953927de46dd4a7ccf06729ce870d83 (accessed on 16th July 2025).

32. Liu, S., Lu, X. X., & Wang, Y. (2024). Construction and practice of diversified curriculum assessment system in the course of introduction to nursing theory under the ideological and political background. *2024 14th International Conference on Information Technology in Medicine and Education (ITME)*. https://www.semanticscholar.org/paper/32c1273ffbd6797b8cb6338797ed84b1431b6ee1 (accessed on 16th July 2025).

33. McGinlay, A., & Munang, L. (2022). 794 Standardized social history documentation in medical clerking improves identification of frailty. *Age and Ageing*. https://www.semanticscholar.org/paper/2ce9400c11570f39b373148d862d92a9573b7bde (accessed on 16th July 2025).

34. Mertyürek, S. (2025). Interdisciplinary collaboration and teamwork in design issues: Assessment of team performance conditioned by professional backgrounds. *Online Journal of Art and Design*. https://www.semanticscholar.org/paper/6d14d98d4dd550d384ac5ed631ec98bc686b57b6 (accessed on 16th July 2025).

35. Mohammed Siyad, A., Venkataramanan, R., & Latheef, M. N. (2021). Secretory otitis media–A clinical prospective study and its management. *World Wide Journal of Multidisciplinary Research and Development, 7*(5), 107–110. www.wwjmrd.com (accessed on 16th July 2025).

36. Ng, L. C., Lim, C., Tan, S. B., Tan, H. K., & Turner, B. S. (2025). Fluid volume assessment in acute hemodialysis by dialysis nurses using clinical signs, symptoms and bio-electrical impedance–A pilot implementation study. *Journal of Advanced Nursing*. https://www.semanticscholar.org/paper/1879c86ce4408586e3821034fdf230cb8a31e808 (accessed on 16th July 2025).

37. Onyenwenyi, A. O. C., Abosede, E. C., Ojei, T. I., Okechukwu, I., Jolayemi, K., Anene, J. A., et al. (2025). Assessment of determinants of limited specialization in nursing practice among student nurses at Adeleke University, Ede, Osun State. *World Journal of Advanced Research and Reviews*. https://www.semanticscholar.org/paper/4ebc19e3d260e86cc44abc104898974fd6fc386e (accessed on 16th July 2025).

38. Prasetya, A., Santosa, A., & Suroso, J. (2024). Nursing intervention: Kinesio taping to reduce restless legs syndrome symptoms in patients undergoing hemodialysis. *Ukrainian Journal of Nephrology and Dialysis*. https://www.semanticscholar.org/paper/cec90163a95b91e725bd996cf8f52d3c866752de (accessed on 16th July 2025).

39. Roland, N., McRae, R. D., & McCombe, A. (1995). *Key Topics in Otolaryngology and Head and Neck Surgery*. https://www.semanticscholar.org/paper/f2d12d15ed5624d2665fa94f5d8a8c34a12f97cd (accessed on 16th July 2025).

40. Ronquillo, C., Peltonen, L., Pruinelli, L., Chu, C. H., Bakken, S., Beduschi, A., Cato, K., et al. (2021). Artificial intelligence in nursing: Priorities and opportunities from an international invitational think-tank of the Nursing and Artificial Intelligence Leadership Collaborative. *Journal of Advanced Nursing, 77*, 3707–3717. https://doi.org/10.1111/jan.14855 (accessed on 16th July 2025).

41. Rosenthal, M., Rauh, M., & Cowan, J. E. (2022). Prospective assessment of clinical tests used to evaluate tibial stress fracture. *Orthopedic Journal of Sports Medicine, 10*. https://www.semanticscholar.org/paper/08e4dfcdd1c0f8f877889ec7bdf4797d44505135 (accessed on 16th July 2025).

42. Safi, M. A., Karim, M. A., & Islam, M. A. (2025). Hearing improvement after Type-1 tympanoplasty in chronic otitis media. *Bangladesh Armed Forces Medical Journal*. https://www.semanticscholar.org/paper/175f7b23364e470db5c6a435e3f8a86a79965621 (accessed on 16th July 2025).

43. Seylanova, N., Chernyavskaya, A. S., Degtyareva, N., Mursalova, A., Ajam, A., Xiao, L., Aktulaeva, K., et al. (2024). Core outcome measurement set for research and clinical practice in post-COVID-19 condition (long COVID) in children and young people: An international Delphi consensus study "PC-COS Children." *European Respiratory Journal, 63*, 2301761. https://doi.org/10.1183/13993003.01761-2023 (accessed on 16th July 2025).

44. Siby, T., Shajimon, A., Mullen, D., Gillani, S., Ong, J. R., Dinkins, N. E., Kruse, B. C., et al. (2024). Leveraging nursing assessment for early identification of post operative gastrointestinal dysfunction (POGD) in patients undergoing colorectal surgery. *Current Oncology, 31*, 3752–3757. https://www.semanticscholar.org/paper/c398a416ff0bba4d8d4d57ee125ff9d908702a16 (accessed on 16th July 2025).

45. Speiser, P., Arlt, W., Auchus, R. J., Baskin, L. S., Conway, G. S., Merke, D. P., Meyer-Bahlburg, H. F. L., et al. (2018). Congenital adrenal hyperplasia due to steroid 21-hydroxylase deficiency: An Endocrine Society* clinical practice guideline. *The Journal of Clinical Endocrinology & Metabolism, 103*, 4043–4088. https://doi.org/10.1210/jc.2018-01865 (accessed on 16th July 2025).

46. Syed, S., Ahmed, R., Iqbal, A., Ahmad, N., & Alshara, M. (2024). MediScan: A framework of U-health and prognostic AI assessment on medical imaging. *Journal of Imaging, 10*. https://www.semanticscholar.org/paper/f50ffc3440b091e4e6050d7adcca89a49cfdf3f6 (accessed on 16th July 2025).

47. Tanthry, D., Perdoor, P. S., Santhraya, M., Pannen, D. P., Bhandary, R., & Pai, V. K. (2021). Rare cases of nasal mass with bleeding: Case series. *International Journal of Otorhinolaryngology and Head and Neck Surgery*. https://www.semanticscholar.org/paper/d9d030a350aba7d59f5151ec6bc7866a6b2aa1ff (accessed on 16th July 2025).

48. The Pharmaceutical Journal. (2024). Changing the culture of fluoroquinolone prescribing. *The Pharmaceutical Journal*. https://doi.org/10.1211/pj.2024.1.228064 (accessed on 16th July 2025).

49. Tombesi, P., Cutini, A., Di Vece, F., Grasso, V., Politti, U., Capatti, E., & Sartori, S. (2025). Surgery or percutaneous ablation for liver tumors? The key points are: When, where, and how large. *Cancers, 17*. https://www.semanticscholar.org/paper/214bb196b3569fd963a995208a2652d9b2a83b41 (accessed on 16th July 2025).

50. Wilson, J. A., Fouweather, T., Stocken, D., Homer, T., Haighton, C., Rousseau, N., O'Hara, J., et al. (2023). Tonsillectomy compared with conservative management in patients over 16 years with recurrent sore throat: The NATTINA RCT and economic evaluation. *Health Technology Assessment*. https://doi.org/10.3310/ykur3660 (accessed on 16th July 2025).

51. Wolters, F. J., Zonneveld, H. I., Hofman, A., van der Lugt, A., Koudstaal, P. J., Vernooij, M. W., & Ikram, M. A. (2017). Cerebral perfusion and the risk of dementia. *Circulation, 136*, 719–728. https://doi.org/10.1161/circulationaha.117.027448 (accessed on 16th July 2025).

THORAX AND LUNGS ASSESSMENT IN NURSING

10

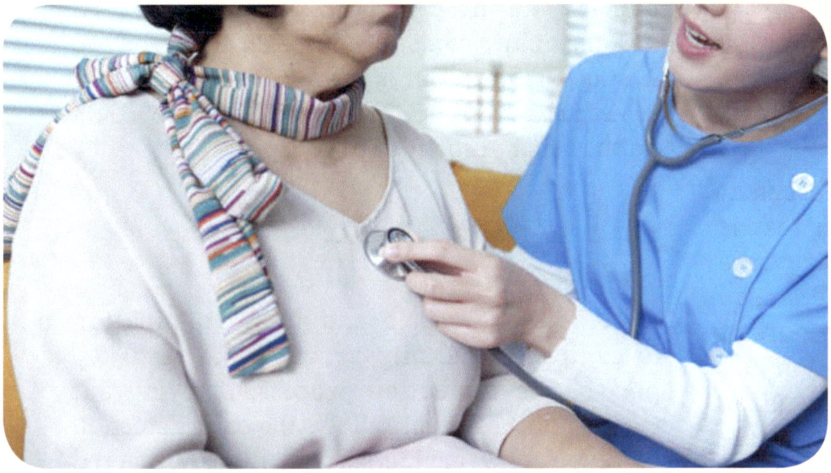

LEARNING OBJECTIVES

After studying this chapter, you will be able to:

1. Understand the anatomy of the thorax;
2. Describe the physiology of breathing;
3. Discuss the assessment techniques;
4. Identify the common thoracic and pulmonary conditions;
5. Explore the nursing interventions;
6. Focus on the challenges in thorax and lung assessment.

Introduction

Examination of the thorax and lungs is a fundamental aspect of nursing practice that is essential to maintaining respiratory health. Familiarity with the subtleties of thoracic anatomy and lung physiology makes it possible for nurses to identify potential respiratory issues early, allowing effective intervention. The thoracic cavity harbors life-supporting organs such as the lungs, heart, and great vessels, and it is therefore important for nurses to be competent in evaluating any abnormality in this region. Besides, the nature of the respiratory systems demands whole assessment techniques using observation, palpation, percussion, and auscultation to properly examine a patient's respiratory condition. As the healthcare environment continues to evolve, knowledge of these techniques becomes increasingly important, as nurses are often on the front lines for treating and monitoring patients with respiratory illness. The utility of a complete thorax and lung examination extends beyond the immediate clinical evaluation. Chronic disease, such as chronic obstructive pulmonary disease or asthma, must be continuously evaluated to measure the progression of disease and to evaluate treatment efficacy. To this end, nurses are most important facilitators between the healthcare system and patients, working in the patient's interest by advocating appropriate treatments according to their assessments. The risks of respiratory disease, including non-tuberculous mycobacterial disease, underscore the need for an ordered process of lung assessment as established by current evidence-based guidance. As highlighted in contemporary literature, there is a need to possess an advanced understanding of such factors so that patient outcomes can be optimized and holistic care delivered, hence the need for the integration of effective assessment measures into the nursing curriculum that is necessary for the future of respiratory care (Haworth et al., 2017). In addition, effective thorax and lung assessment relies on nurses' competence in clinical data interpretation and integrating their observation into individualized care plans. Nurses not only have to be aware of abnormal sounds in the lungs or changes in the pattern of breathing but also put these observations into patients greater health profiles, including comorbidities and lifestyle. Identifying body composition, for instance, can significantly impact the assessment process because variability in fat and lean mass can influence respiratory function and general health (Clifton et al., 2021). With growing numbers of healthcare practitioners adopting comprehensive paradigms of patient care, the function of respiratory assessment becomes all the more paramount for bridging the gap between acute clinical evaluation and chronic health care. By improving their thorax and lung assessment competencies, nurses become integral to an integrated paradigm of patients' respiratory needs, ultimately producing better health outcomes in diverse groups of patients (Figure 10.1).

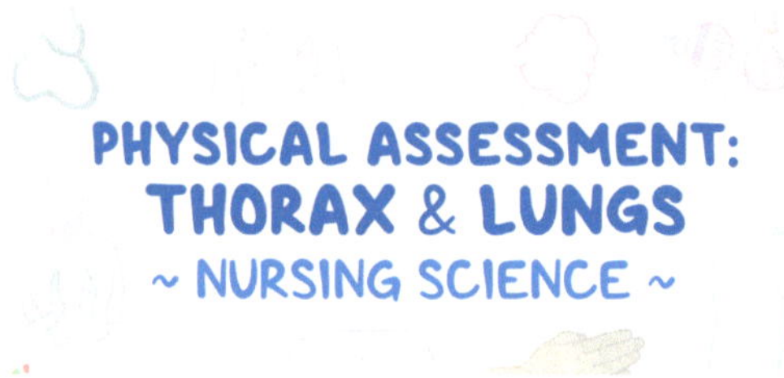

Figure 10.1. Thorax and lungs assessment in nursing.

Source: https://external-content.duckduckgo.com/iu/?u=https%3A%2F%2Fosmose-it.s3.amazonaws.com%2FeTmJxcPIQFqwWbx04CAf3CqQTTi9nRij%2F_.jpg&f=1&nofb=1&ipt=08cc42a53a2e62a2962756b0806b752500987831d8b21dcaf71aba2008b705be.

Importance of Thorax and Lung Assessment in Nursing

A complete thoracic and lung examination is central to nursing practice and is a key part of the evaluation process. Carrying out extensive assessments allows the early detection of respiratory problems, which can be acted upon in a timely manner. Early intervention is particularly important for patients with underlying chronic respiratory diseases or for those presenting in the acute care environment, where subclinical deterioration may result in serious complications. These results during these tests – such as breath sounds, oxygen saturation level, and respiratory rate – are crucial in developing personalized care plans such that each patient can be administered intervention as required based on his/her own unique clinical presentation. Becoming skilled in thorax and lung examination skills is important for improved patient outcomes and optimizing the quality of care provided by nursing professionals. In the past decades, the importance of thorax and lung assessment has been highlighted by worldwide respiratory infection health concerns, mainly experienced throughout the COVID-19 pandemic. The pandemic has revealed that proper and timely assessment of respiratory function can significantly influence decisions concerning patient isolation, treatment, and resource allocation. For instance, an abnormal breath sound or oxygen saturation level can prompt healthcare workers to suspect a COVID-19 infection, and the clinician may order diagnostic tests and control measures in a timely manner. Furthermore, the identification of unusual results from sputum or feces samples has raised questions about the disease transmission potential of respiratory illnesses and the need for rigorous testing protocols. Thus, the growth of assessment skills not only consolidates nurses' practice but also consolidates their important roles in public health programs during emergencies like epidemics and pandemics (Chen et al., 2020; Shadmi et al., 2020). Thorax and lung assessment continuing education and professional development are critical for nursing professionals. With continued evolution of healthcare via new technology and modes of treatment, the nurse must stay up to date with best practice for lung examination techniques. Incorporation of newer devices such as handheld ultrasonography or digital spirometry into routine exams can complement normal listening abilities with a more comprehensive understanding of a patient's respiratory status. Ongoing education courses focusing on these developments ensure nurses can provide state-of-the-art care individually suited to the patient. Emphasizing proficient assessment of thoracic and pulmonary function enhances not only clinical proficiency but also nurses' confidence, ultimately affecting patient health by diagnosing respiratory issues early and intervening accordingly.

Overview of Assessment Techniques

Relevant assessment techniques are the foundation of nursing practice, particularly in thoracic and lung health assessments. A systemic approach to assessment typically includes inspection, palpation, percussion, and auscultation. The initial step is through visual examination of the thorax for abnormality or asymmetry, respiratory distress, or abnormal chest wall movement. Following inspection, palpation entails use of the sense of touch by the nurse to identify areas of tenderness, mass, or irregular vibration on respiration. Such kinesthetic information may give significant hints about underlying pulmonary pathology, allowing for more targeted nursing intervention. All of these initial steps lead the clinician to perform more precise evaluation and are essential in enabling patient-oriented care in thoracic exam. The percussion comes afterwards after the initial visual and palpation in order to check the density of underlying tissues, particularly identifying hyper-resonance or hyper-fluidity areas. As the nurse percuss rhythmically over the thoracic wall, the resulting sounds may direct towards conditions such as pneumothorax or pleural effusion. Additionally, the technique also aids in observing diaphragmatic movement, a significant factor in lung inflation. Auscultation is generally performed after percussion and allows for assessment of airflow as well as any lung sound abnormality. It is important to differentiate between vesicular and bronchial, which are both normal breath sounds, and wheezes or crackles, which are abnormal breath sounds, during the process of developing a differential diagnosis. Using the incorporation of these techniques, nursing assessments become comprehensive, allowing for better clinical outcomes in the patient with various respiratory illnesses. Last, the culmination of these assessment techniques is developing an informed nursing care plan. Nurses must not just rely on such diagnostic methods but also consider patient histories to place findings more meaningfully. The nursing process extends beyond the initial assessment to include monitoring and modifying interventions as patient status changes. In high-volume environments such as intensive care units, where risks for illness like ventilator-associated pneumonia are highest, standardized protocols become important. As an example, studies have shown that multimodality chest physiotherapy is able to sharply lower pneumonia rates among mechanically ventilated patients, evidencing the significance of incorporating clinical evidence into practice (Younes et al., 2022). Therefore, marrying different assessment methods with current evidence is critical in enhancing patient outcomes in thoracic and lung health evaluation (Haworth et al., 2017) (Figure 10.2).

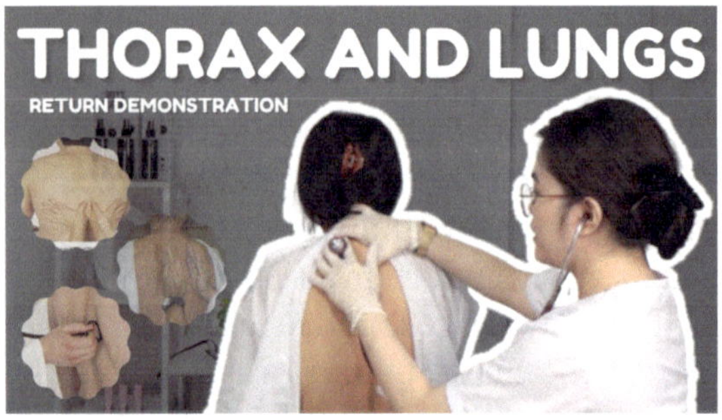

Figure 10.2. Thorax and lungs assessment techniques in nursing.

Source: https://external-content.duckduckgo.com/iu/?u=https%3A%2F%2Fi.ytimg.com%2Fvi%2Frtk07UkOETY%2Fmaxresdefault.jpg&f=1&nofb=1&ipt=f6d7061bb97f596ed31f824704c8e8b16a93f1bc7d9ffe9191929dacd7364094.

10.1. Anatomy of the Thorax

Learning Outcome

1. Structure of the Thoracic Cavity
2. Major Organs Within the Thorax
3. Role of the Thorax in Respiratory Function

Thorax, as a critical component of the body, is not just a protective covering of the lungs and heart but also has an active function in respiration and hemodynamics. The thorax is made up of the sternum, rib cage, and thoracic vertebrae and contains the lungs, mediastinum, and supporting structures within. It is necessary for nurses to know its anatomy while conducting comprehensive assessments since alterations in thoracic structures can have a direct impact on the function of the respiratory system. The thoracic cavity is also divided into pleural spaces that encase the lungs; nurses are aided by comprehensive knowledge of the spaces in recognizing manifestations of conditions such as pneumothorax or pleural effusions. A knowledge of how these anatomical features work in combination can optimize nursing interventions, particularly when physical exams are being conducted during which nurses use procedures such as auscultation and palpation to detect abnormalities in thoracic form and function. The significance of accurate anatomical information in nursing examination of the thorax extends beyond observation. In particular, the auscultation and percussion techniques are essential in identifying respiratory disorders. According to current studies, nursing students all too often lack proper application of these skills in clinical rotations, and therefore more effective training and guidance would be needed here (Egilsdottir et al., 2019). As nursing students progress, reinforcement of essential physical assessment skills (B-PAS) is necessary. Nurse educators are obligated to train students to perform techniques proficiently, aware that preceptors play a key role in utilizing learned skills practically in the field. Finally, reinforcing education strategies can ensure nursing graduates to confidently apply their knowledge of thoracic anatomy in combination with assessment skills when treating patients. Lastly, proper assessment of thoracic and lung function is the pathway to improved patient outcomes. Monitoring of respiratory rate, for instance, is a nursing practice core of essential critical care skills. Despite its importance, noted variations in how nurses take and chart respiratory rates can potentially lead to misconceptions in the clinical setting (Rolfe, 2019). As medical care professionals, nurses ought to be aware of noticing as they build their evaluating processes to understand the impact of thoracic anatomy on respiration. Emphasizing the relationship between anatomical structure and physiological function can guide nursing evaluations towards more accurate diagnosis and treatment. By promoting an in-depth understanding of thoracic anatomy, nursing education can equip practitioners to provide quality care and actively prevent potential respiratory disorders (Figure 10.3).

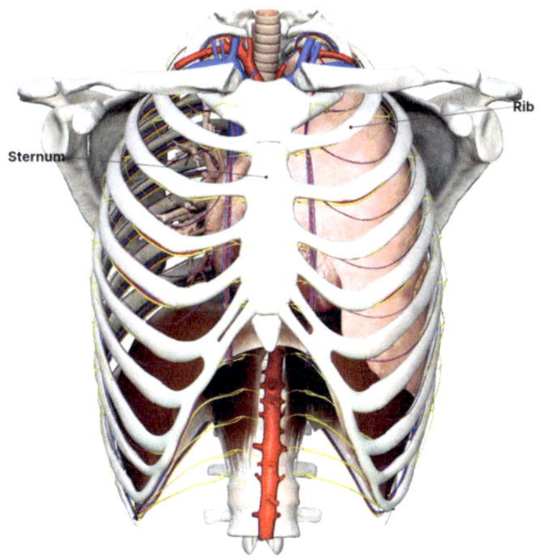

Figure 10.3. Anatomy of the thorax.

Source: https://anatomy.app/Media/slides/thorax-overview-3-9785_medium.jpg.

10.1.1. Structure of the Thoracic Cavity

The thoracic cavity is a fundamental body anatomical region that harbors vital organs such as the heart and lungs and houses major respiratory processes. Lateral walls are supported by the ribs, and inferior support is offered by the diaphragm. The thoracic cavity is then divided into three cavities: mediastinum, two pleural cavities, and pericardial cavity. The mediastinum is in the central position and houses the heart, trachea, esophagus, and large blood vessels and is crucial for achieving stability and regulation of thoracic pressure. Pleural cavities, divided by the mediastinum, surround the lungs and create a friction-free environment for breathing movements. Thus, it is crucial for clinicians, specifically nurses, to be well aware of the thoracic cavity's anatomical setup to direct clinical assessments and the management of pulmonary and thoracic wellness. Nursing assessment of the thoracic cavity must be geared towards an exhaustive understanding of its anatomy and physiology to effectively identify abnormal states. The thoracic cavity anatomy allows for expansion and contraction of the lungs during respiration; thus, nurses must observe any sign of respiratory distress or pathological abnormality. Some diseases, such as pneumothorax or pleural effusion, can compromise the integrity and function of this cavity with resultant serious clinical implications. For example, a buildup of excess fluid in the pleural cavity can hinder lung expansion, while air accumulation causes lung collapse. Understanding these dynamics is essential to assessing a patient's respiratory condition, guiding diagnosis, and determining the most appropriate therapeutic measures, such as any procedures outlined for managing pleural pathology (Asciak et al., 2023) or spontaneous pneumothorax (Schnell et al., 2018). In evaluating the structure of the thoracic cavity, the nurses should also learn about its significance for many clinical interventions. Significant interventions like thoracentesis or chest tube placement are in turn established by the cavity's anatomical structures. Smooth transit through the thoracic cavity spaces requires knowledge of its boundaries, e.g., the rib cage and diaphragm, to prevent complications related to the intervention. Apart from that, adherence to given guidelines, for instance, those issued for spontaneous pneumothorax management, is also vital in helping bring about patient safety and enhanced outcomes. The S3 guidelines, for instance, require practice on an individual basis in regard to the unique situation of the patient, both the anatomical structure of the thoracic cavity and the unique health needs of the patient (Schnell et al., 2018). Therefore, comprehension of the structural dynamics of the thoracic cavity not only directs assessment but enhances the effectiveness of nursing interventions in respiratory therapy (Figure 10.4).

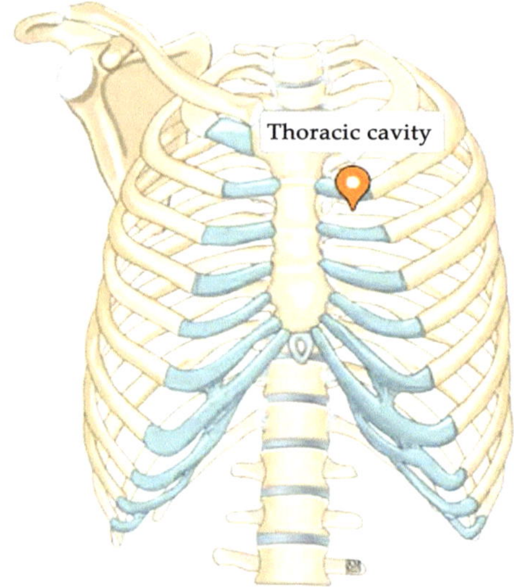

Figure 10.4. Structure of the thoracic cavity.

Source: https://cdn1.imaios.com/i/imaios-images/web/images/eanatomy/modules/paroi-thorax-sein-illustrations/images/v3/0e8a0d69da5cacfc02cdfcc2550b60e9ea1ed4016f834a247b53b9532 9122e6f?ar=640:670&bg=FFFFFF&fit=crop&p64=NzU2LDQ4NA&t=VGhvcmFjaWMgY2F2aXR5&tx =756&ty=484&w=350&wk=1&s=9c17bacfcc5e396a794b56a459ab49a0.

10.1.2. Major Organs Within the Thorax

The thorax, a critical anatomical chamber in the human body, holds some of the significant organs involved in respiration as well as circulation. The lungs, which are tasked with the process of gas exchange, are very likely the most visible organs located within the chamber. They are divided into lobes; the right lung holds three lobes, and the left lung, in order to fit the location of the heart, holds only two. Surrounding the lungs, the pleura create a fluid-filled space through which expansion and contraction of the lungs are made easy during breathing. Such intricate balance is very important, with slight damage able to compromise the respiratory system and overall health. Understanding the lung structure and function as well as its interaction with surrounding organs is important in nursing assessments to detect pulmonary disease early and inform the management. In addition to the lungs, the thoracic cavity accommodates the heart, a muscular structure responsible for circulating blood throughout the body. Located in the center and left, the intricate structure of the heart has four chambers: the left atrium and the right atrium and the left ventricle and the right ventricle. Each chamber plays a critical role in the circulatory process, accepting and pumping the blood harmoniously. The pericardium, or two-layered sac that encloses the heart, serves to protect it and hold it in position within the thoracic cavity. Nurses' heart evaluation includes the recording of vital signs, auscultation for heart sounds, and observation for manifestations of cardiovascular distress. Knowledge of the anatomy and physiology of the hearts will provide nurses with a complete understanding of how disease processes affecting this organ may influence respiratory status and general patient health. The thorax also harbors important structures such as the trachea and esophagus. The trachea is the primary airway, branching into the bronchi that extend to each lung. The airway must be open to allow for breathing; therefore, any obstruction can be life-threatening immediately. The esophagus, situated posterior to the trachea, is responsible for transporting food from the mouth to the stomach. The proximity of these structures establishes the intricate interrelation between gastrointestinal and respiratory functions. For the nurses, understanding these anatomical relationships is significant during assessment since it can direct decisions with regard to intervention for patients with respiratory impairment or swallowing difficulties. Anomalies in any of these thoracic organs may significantly influence general well-being, which highlights the importance of comprehensive thoracic assessments in nursing practice (Ferdinand et al., 2021; Rohrig et al., 2020).

10.1.3. Role of the Thorax in Respiratory Function

The thorax provides a significant structural support that keeps the respiratory system in place to enable effective lung functioning. Its anatomical features, including the ribs, sternum, and thoracic vertebrae, create a shielding covering over the lungs while enabling their expansion and contraction process during the process of breathing. The diaphragm, the central muscle of the thoracic base, is a significant muscle in ventilatory mechanics that contracts to increase intrathoracic volume so that air will flow into the lungs.

The intercostal muscles connect neighboring ribs and assist rib cages to move during inspiration and expiration. In addition to supporting efficient gas exchange, this process maintains intrathoracic pressure influencing blood flow and lymphatic drainage. Understanding the anatomy of the thorax is basic to nursing assessments because it gives insight about potential complications that may be caused by respiratory disorders. In nursing assessments, the significance of the thorax is recognized beyond its mere structural function. The impact of other pathophysiologic conditions, such as pneumonia or chronic obstructive pulmonary disease (COPD), has the ability to alter the thoracic dynamics, which in turn significantly impacts respiratory function.

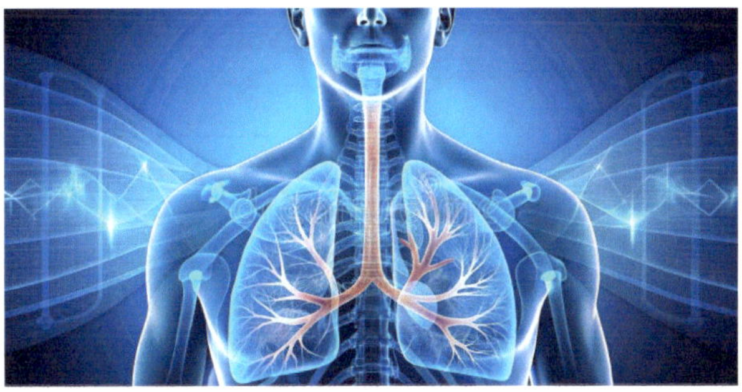

Figure 10.5. Role of the thorax in respiratory function.

Source: https://thumbs.dreamstime.com/b/anatomical-structure-respiratory-system-detailed-visual-representation-lungs-trachea-human-thorax-stunning-388622395.jpg.

For instance, infections like viral pneumonia associated with COVID-19 have imaging characteristics of thoracic abnormalities that need to be sensitively evaluated and monitored (Peter et al., 2020). Expansion of the thorax during respiration can be restricted by factors like inflammation or fluid in the pleural space, leading to ineffective gas exchange. Thus, a good inspection, palpation, and auscultation of the thorax is called for to be able to identify abnormal results and facilitate proper interventions, particularly among at-risk groups prone to respiratory complications. The role of the thorax in breathing also calls for an integrated approach to post-acute care, particularly for patients with serious respiratory conditions such as SARS-CoV-2 infections. Many survivors of COVID-19 continue to experience symptoms, one of which is breathlessness, weeks after recovery from the acute illness (Arnold et al., 2020). This highlights the need for follow-up care that is not only physiological but also psychosocial. Nurses must be equipped to develop rehabilitation plans that are holistic, focusing not just on the recovery of lung function but on overall quality of life as well. With healthcare systems changing to accommodate the increasing demand for respiratory follow-up, understanding the thorax's role in respiratory function can be essential to the delivery of outstanding, patient-centered care capable of addressing the complexity provided by long-term complication (Figure 10.5).

Test Your Knowledge

1. What are the major structures of the thorax, including bones, muscles, and organs, and how do they support respiratory function?
2. How does knowledge of thoracic anatomy assist in identifying abnormal findings during assessment?

10.2. Physiology of Breathing

Learning Outcome

1. Mechanisms of Ventilation
2. Gas Exchange Process
3. Factors Affecting Respiratory Function

Breathing physiology is complex cooperation of several anatomical and physiological mechanisms that facilitate gas exchange in the lungs. The secret to this mechanism is the thoracic cavity and the diaphragm, both working together to generate negative pressure to facilitate air being drawn into the lungs. When contracting, the diaphragm lowers, increasing the volume of the thoracic cavity. This expansion lowers intrathoracic pressure, which opens the trachea to allow air to pass through and into the bronchial tree. It is thus crucial that nursing professionals are well aware of these mechanisms, in order to assess respiratory function effectively and identify any deviation from normal physiology which could indicate pathology or impairment of gas exchange. In critical or perioperative care, accurate assessment of pulmonary function is the issue with particular importance in the context of viral infections such as COVID-19 that result in respiratory illnesses. Physiological effects of compromised respiratory function can possess severe clinical presentations in the forms of hypoxemia and respiratory distress. Increased monitoring using innovative technologies has gained momentum, supporting the need for nurses not just to implement traditional assessment practices but also to leverage innovations such as telehealth and wearable tech. These devices provide real-time feedback regarding a patient's pulmonary status, and it enables nurses to make informed evidence-based choices on interventions and changes in care models for the betterment of patient outcomes. This is consistent with current best practice for the management of oxygen therapy in acute care environments where prompt, evidence-based intervention is paramount (O'Driscoll et al., 2017).

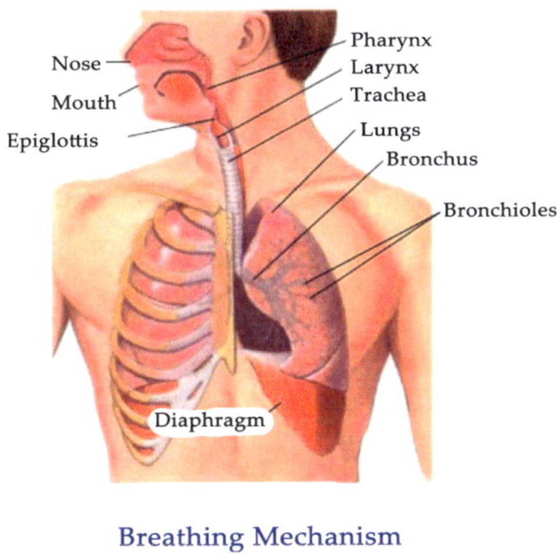

Figure 10.6. Physiology of breathing.

Source: https://meditationiseasy.com/subdir/wp-content/uploads/2015/06/mechanism-of-breathing2.jpg.

Knowledge of respiratory physiology also requires an understanding of common pathophysiologies that compromise respiratory efficiency. They also trigger considerable alterations in the normal mechanics of breathing, leading to workload on breathing and gas exchange efficiency that becomes abnormal. Nurses must be capable of recognizing signs of respiratory distress and utilize assessment tools to critically review lung function. Auscultation of lung sounds and monitoring respiratory rate are just a few methods through which underlying conditions can be discovered early enough for timely interventions. Moreover, with the emergence of new issues like infectious disease-related ones, patient education and self-management of respiratory status training by nurses is vital in enabling patients to participate in their own care and perhaps enhance their respiratory health outcomes (Ding et al., 2020) (Figure 10.6).

10.2.1. Mechanisms of Ventilation

Ventilation mechanisms are essential knowledge for thoracic and pulmonary nursing assessment because the processes underlie normal ventilation. Ventilation is the cyclical movement of air in and out of the lungs driven by pressure gradients created by the movement of diaphragm and intercostal muscles. On inhalation, the diaphragm relaxes and flattens, increasing the thoracic cavity and creating a negative pressure gradient into which air can pass into the lungs. On exhalation, the diaphragm moves back to its original position and the elastic recoil of lung tissues and thoracic wall helps to force out air. Regulation of these processes is essential in nursing care since derangement of the process causes ineffective gas exchange and respiratory insufficiency, which needs immediate management. The assessment of the mechanisms of ventilation also encompasses understanding the role of neural control and the influence of other factors such as age, body position, and the presence of respiratory disease. The rhythm and depth of breathing are controlled by the brainstem, primarily the medulla oblongata and pons, through intricate feedback mechanisms with the help of carbon dioxide- and oxygen-sensitive chemoreceptors. In individuals afflicted with diseases like COPD or ARDS, these mechanisms are compromised, leading to ineffective ventilation. Such disruptions can be reflected in the manifestation of abnormal breath sounds, altered respiratory rate, and accessory muscle utilization with breathing. Nurses' recognition of these signs is paramount in creating effective care plans and interventions that address the restoration of effective ventilation and resultant improvement in patient outcomes. Aside from the physiological mechanisms, the nursing assessments must also consider the impact of environmental factors on ventilation. Environmental condition, for instance, high altitude or polluted air, significantly affects lung function and, consequently, respiratory mechanics. Also, acute infections, such as those caused by SARS-CoV-2 during the COVID-19 pandemic, pose unique challenges to ventilatory mechanics, typically causing hypercapnia and hypoxemia due to compromised lung function (Katerina et al., 2022). The present evaluation of long COVID-affected patients highlights the importance of identifying the nuances of ventilation mechanisms as long-lasting respiratory symptoms can arise even after full recovery from acute disease (Ding et al., 2020). The observations highlight the importance of regular training and education of nursing staff to properly identify and manage ventilation issues so that the patients who get respiratory conditions get proper care (Figure 10.7).

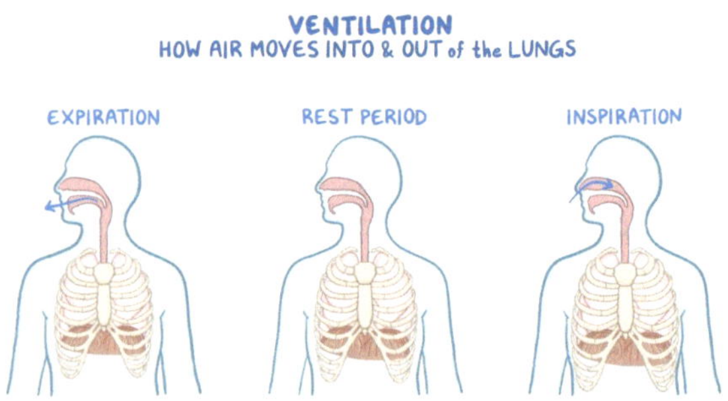

Figure 10.7. Mechanisms of ventilation of breathing.

Source: https://www.osmosis.org/_next/image?url=https%3A%2F%2Fd16qt3wv6xm098.cloudfront.net%2FEJB5u8QTTemEMAIUu4BvHdAURMKKbgYB%2F_.jpg&w=3840&q=75.

10.2.2. Gas Exchange Process

The gas exchange process is at the core of respiratory function in that it facilitates the uptake of oxygen into the bloodstream as well as the excretion of carbon dioxide. The intricate procedure is primarily executed in the alveoli, tiny air sacs of the lungs, where the thin alveolar membrane enables gases to diffuse based on concentration gradients. Oxygen in breathed air penetrates this membrane and is transported bound to hemoglobin in red blood cells, facilitating efficient transport of oxygen to tissues all over the body. On the other hand, carbon dioxide, which is a byproduct of cellular respiration, moves from the blood and into the alveoli to be removed by exhalation. Efficient operation of this gas exchange mechanism points to the significance of thoracic and pulmonary assessment in nursing, which provides the image of patients' respiratory effectiveness and general health. During the assessment of patients in nursing, measuring the efficiency of gas exchange, particularly in patients suffering from respiratory illness or infections, is significant. Diseases such as COPD and pneumonia may severely impair gas exchange by inflammation, accumulation of fluid, or changes in the pulmonary structure. Roles of nurses in respiratory function assessment include observation of vital signs, lung sounds, and reading of imaging tests, e.g., chest X-ray or CT scan in the event of suspected pulmonary pathology. Techniques such as lung ultrasound may be beneficial in emergent care to evaluate pleural effusions or consolidations that affect gas exchange, particularly in the setting of COVID-19, where imaging of the lung is paramount to evaluation. Together, these evaluations give clinicians the necessary information to make appropriate decisions regarding treatment protocols and follow-up. Furthermore, more recent literature underscores the necessity of ongoing care and monitoring of patients with respiratory sequelae caused by infection such as COVID-19, particularly long-term sequela concerning impaired gas exchange. Patient studies have revealed that patients may exhibit protracted pulmonary symptoms and compromised quality of life after infection, therefore necessitating individualized intervention and follow-up strategies. Measurements may include comprehensive evaluations of lung function, imaging studies, and patient-reported outcomes to determine the symptom burden and functional capacity of these patients. According to definitions that exist, nursing personnel should detect impairments in gas exchange on an early note and act accordingly, where feasible by way of treatment and rehabilitation of the respiratory type intended to enhance recovery outcomes and general respiratory function (Katerina et al., 2022; Vetrugno et al., 2020) (Figure 10.8).

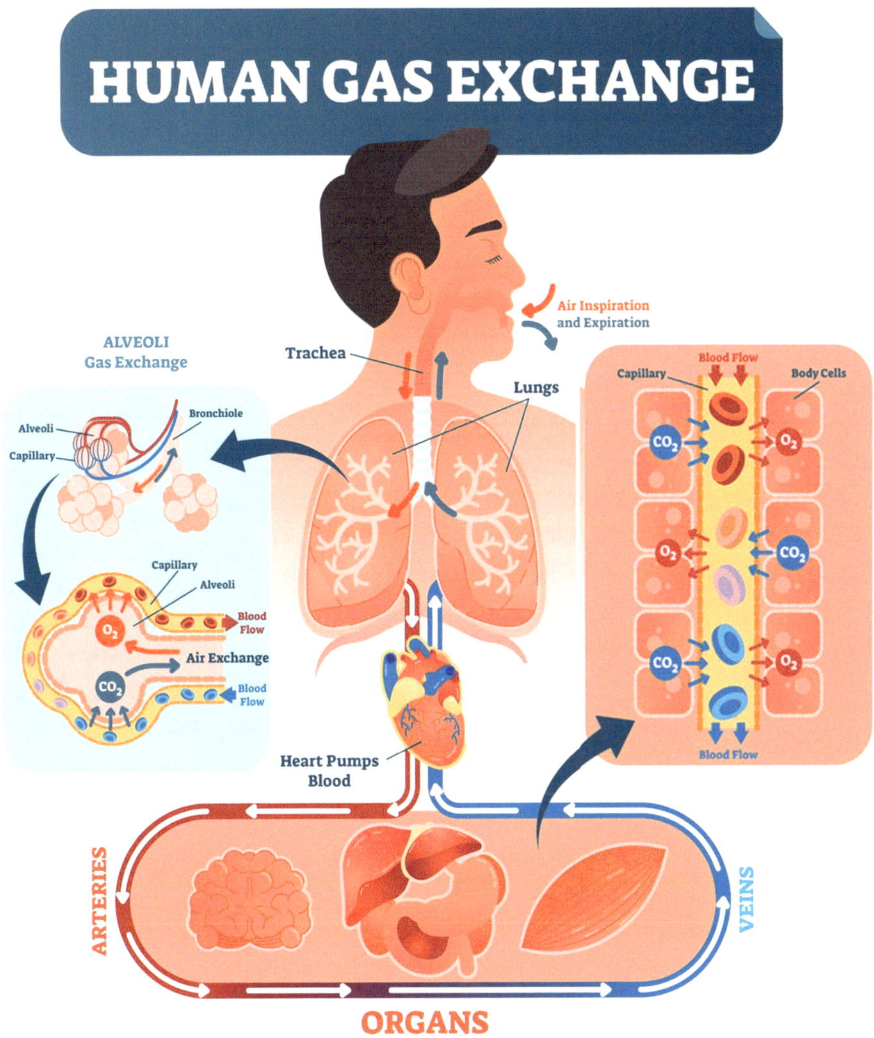

Figure 10.8. Gas exchange process.

Source: https://s3.us-east-2.amazonaws.com/medictests/app/public/ckeditor_assets/pictures/524/content_Human-gas-exchange-system-vector-illustration.-Oxygen-travel-from-lungs-to-heart_-to-all-body-cells-and-back-to-lungs-as-CO2.-948356058_962x1094_%281%29.jpeg.

10.2.3. Factors Affecting Respiratory Function

Respiratory function testing in the clinical setting is significantly affected by a number of intrinsic and extrinsic factors, which can compromise normal pulmonary function. Among the key determinants is the anatomical and physiological condition of the subject, including age, sex, and genetic predispositions. For instance, alterations with age, such as diminished lung elasticity and muscle strength, can contribute to compromised respiratory efficiency. Moreover, obesity plays an important role in reducing lung capacities and increasing the workload for respiratory muscles, hence complicating respiratory examinations. Furthermore, the presence of chronic conditions such as asthma or chronic obstructive pulmonary disease (COPD) may play a major role in affecting airflow as well as gas exchange and is therefore important to assess comprehensively during nursing examinations. Identifying these factors is crucial to the provision of effective care in a responsive way to the individual requirements of every patient, enabling nursing interventions that are relevant and effective in the facilitation of respiratory outcomes. Environmental conditions are also critical to respiratory function, and must be properly considered in assessment. Exposure to allergens, irritants, and pollutants can lead to acute or chronic respiratory disease, and it is vital for healthcare providers to address this. For example, individuals living in city environs will be subjected more to air pollution—well-documented to exacerbate pre-existing conditions such as asthma or precipitate new respiratory symptoms. Further, occupational hazards such as being exposed to toxic chemicals or dust can lead to pneumoconiosis, among other determinants to respiratory health. Further still, smoking remains a socio-environmental factor that profoundly impairs lung function and leads to respiratory disease. Nurse practitioners must integrate knowledge of these environmental risk factors into assessments in order to develop comprehensive care plans that address these influences and promote optimal respiratory function in complex populations. Where such complex conditions as long COVID and child bronchiectasis exist, specialist care is indicated to comprehend how these complex factors affect respiratory function. Long COVID presents specific difficulties in that it can manifest with a range of long-lasting respiratory symptoms that significantly affect quality of life (QoL) following initial infection (Katerina et al., 2022). Similarly, in pediatric populations, bronchiectasis is recognized as a chronic condition which leads to recurrent exacerbations and severely affects the children and their families, demonstrating the need for individualized management strategies (Anne et al., 2021). In taking on a multimodal strategy that includes careful evaluation of respiratory health determinants—whether anatomical, environmental, or chronic condition-type—nurses are best placed to intervene and optimize respiratory assessment and care strategies in acute and chronic settings. Interweaving these determinants is essential in bringing nursing practices for thorax and lung examinations to the next level and overall impacting patient outcomes in a positive manner.

Test Your Knowledge

1. How do the processes of ventilation, diffusion, and perfusion work together to maintain effective gas exchange?
2. What physiological changes occur in the respiratory system during exercise, disease, or aging?

10.3. Assessment Techniques

Learning Outcome

1. Inspection Methods
2. Palpation and Percussion
3. Auscultation of Lung Sounds

Methods of assessment of the thorax and lungs are important in nursing practice since they enable health care professionals to identify and monitor potential respiratory disorders effectively. A good assessment begins with inspection, which involves observation of the patient's respiratory rate, rhythm, and effort. Nurses must also assess for chest symmetry, shape, and visible deformity. Following examination, palpation is performed to evaluate tactile fremitus, searching for any abnormality like enhanced or diminished vibrations across the lung fields. These simple maneuvers provide insightful information about the patients respiratory condition and guide further tests, impacting clinical decision-making and interventions for improved patient management. As emphasized by studies, a specific assessment not only identifies current conditions but also forecasts complications, such as Ventilator-Associated Pneumonia (VAP), in order to facilitate immediate management measures (Younes et al., 2022). Auscultation is an essential assessment technique of respiratory nursing that allows practitioners to auscultate normal and abnormal lung sounds. Nurses employ the use of a stethoscope to listen to sounds such as wheezes, crackles, and rhonchi, which can be indicative of intrinsic pathologies such as pneumonia or bronchitis. Ongoing observation and comparison of lung sounds with repeated assessment over time enhance the clinicians' detection of changes in the patient's status. This is particularly crucial for high-risk patients for illnesses such as pneumonia, early detection of which can make a tremendous difference in treatment modalities. Integration of a multimodal approach that unites auscultation with other methods of assessment like chest physiotherapy can also prevent mechanical ventilation complications and the onset of VAP, demonstrating the integration of treatment and assessment techniques (Younes et al., 2022). Recognition of the patient's history and risk factors is also important in assessing thoracic and lung health. Nursing assessments must consider complete patient histories, including prior respiratory illness, smoking status, and environmental pollutant exposure. These could predispose patients to diseases such as non-tuberculous mycobacterial pulmonary disease. Directed interventions based on these assessments can be critical to the optimization of respiratory care. Nursing staff must also take special care to review and document changes in patient status and educate regarding decompensation symptoms. Pneumonia and other lung disease management guidelines emphasize the necessity of interprofessional collaboration to provide individuals with comprehensive care tailored to their unique needs, as evidenced by strategic recommendations for condition management, such as those for NTM (Figure 10.9).

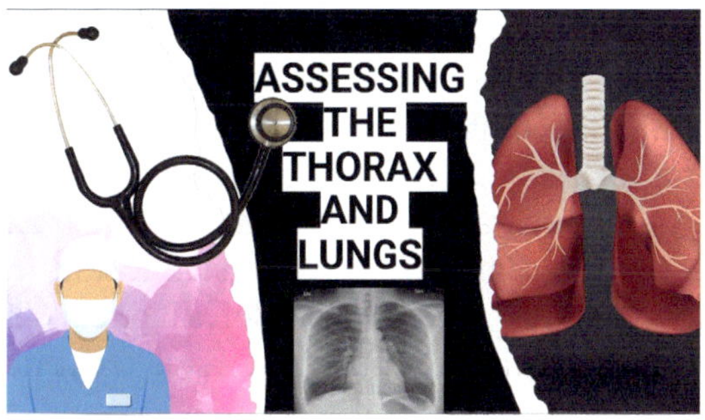

Figure 10.9. Assessing the thorax and lungs.

Source: https://i.ytimg.com/vi/3aRjaMRGkDo/maxresdefault.jpg.

10.3.1. Inspection Methods

Techniques of inspection form a crucial part of the thorax and lungs assessment process in nursing practice, providing useful information about a patient's respiratory health. During the inspection process, nurses observe the thoracic symmetry of a patient visually, noting any deviation such as deformity, uneven expansion, or signs of difficulty in breathing. This initial observation is helpful to detect illnesses like COPD or infection, which may have to be investigated further. An accurate investigation includes observing the respiratory rhythm, rate, and patterns to detect any deviation from normal physiological conditions, which may be associated with underlying pathologies. The merging of visual observation with the employment of other investigation devices has enhanced the clinician's effectiveness in allocating patient needs and addressing accumulating respiratory issues in due time, which makes it a constituent of effective nursing examination in respiratory health. Also, the incorporation of high-tech imaging modalities, such as ultrasonography, has transformed traditional inspection procedures in lung examinations. The method allows one to detect alterations in the lung tissue, which may be imperceptible during physical examination. Studies have established that a combination of ultrasonography with traditional inspection procedures improves substantially the diagnostic accuracy of respiratory diseases. For instance, when accompanied by clinical scoring instruments, ultrasonography is highly sensitive and specific, thereby enabling early disease diagnosis such as pneumonitis or emphysema. This multi-dimension lung evaluation not only facilitates the process of diagnosis but also aids in the administration of treatment regimens, quite efficiently curbing unnecessary antibiotic therapy in various settings, as seen in veterinary settings (Hoffelner et al., 2023). There is a growing need for the utilization of lab findings in combination with physical inspection processes for better diagnostic outcomes in respiratory health testing. Techniques such as analysis of blood eosinophil tests and computed tomography (CT) scans provide valuable information that is a supplement to findings based on inspection. For example, such methodologies can explain differential microbial compositions relevant to diseases like COPD, directing targeted interventions for the underlying disease processes (Rotevatn et al., 2025). Integrating inspection, imaging, and lab data allows nurses to build an integrated picture of a patient's respiratory status. This combined methodology ultimately generates evidence-based clinical decision-making that optimizes patient benefits from early interventions and responsive treatment strategies taking into consideration the complexity of lung disease (Figure 10.10).

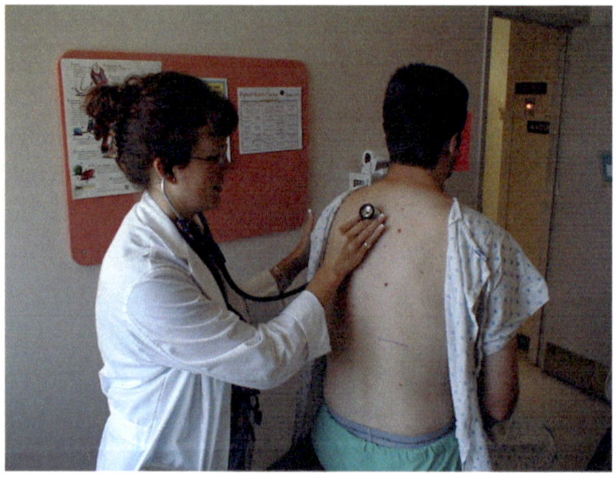

Figure 10.10. Inspection methods for the thorax and lungs.

Source: https://meded.ucsd.edu/clinicalmed/assets/img/lungs_auscutation.jpg.

10.3.2. Palpation and Percussion

In lung and thoracic examination, percussion and palpation are important techniques that enhance a nurse's ability to gain full information regarding a patient's respiratory function. Palpation is done methodically by exploring with the hands the thoracic area to assess for abnormality in texture, temperature, and tenderness, finally aiming to identify potential respiratory pathology. This physical examination allows nurses to detect asymmetry of thoracic structures that may indicate underlying pathologies such as pneumothorax or pleural effusion. Also, this check-by-touch encourages better understanding and acquaintance between the patient and the nurse, engendering trust and facilitating communication about symptoms that the patient may be experiencing. By the use of palpation in an efficient manner, nurses will be in a better position to build a complete picture of breathing health. Besides palpation, percussion is also another important evaluation technique utilized during thoracic assessment. Percussion involves hitting the chest wall using the fingers to produce sound waves that can pick up useful information about the lung tissue under it. The sounds that are elicited in percussion can differentiate between the normal lung resonance and areas of dullness which may represent fluid accumulation or consolidation. Percussion, therefore, is not only a diagnostic tool but also an additive to nurses' clinical judgment. Research has determined that nursing students enhance their test skills more effectively in environments in which systematic reflection on methods such as palpation and percussion is encouraged; this suggests that practical test practice plays a significant role in their ability to apply clinical knowledge to practice (Kirsten et al., 2022). Palpation and percussion interaction is central to the evolution of a more holistic and person-centered respiratory assessment methodology in nursing. Practice-oriented clinical education enables students to witness for themselves the nuances of these approaches, which are essential to the establishment of good clinical judgment. For instance, actively engaged students yield to checklist approaches in place of a customized assessment based on the unique context and requirement of every patient. This action is a step in the broader direction of nursing education, supporting the inclusion of practice reflection as well as the utilization of physical assessment skills when completing clinical rotations (Kirsten et al., 2020). In the end, as nurse students learn palpation and percussion, they can gain confidence, provide patient safety, and provide a higher quality of care given to those with respiratory distress.

10.3.3. Auscultation of Lung Sounds

Lung auscultation is a crucial component of the thorax and lungs assessment model utilized in nursing. By the proper utilization of a stethoscope, nurses can identify numerous normal as well as abnormal breath sounds, which are crucial markers of healthy pulmonary function. For instance, normal breath sounds such as vesicular, bronchial, and bronchovesicular sounds reveal good lung function and air passage. However, the presence of adventitious sounds like wheezes, crackles, or rhonchi can signal underlying conditions such as asthma or pneumonia. As research notes, observation and measurement of respiratory parameters like lung sounds have a considerable influence on the treatment and outcome of patients, particularly those with respiratory illnesses (El-Deeb et al., 2024). Therefore, effective auscultation skills are absolutely essential for nurses, not only to identify existing clinical issues but also to guide future diagnostic and therapeutic interventions. To strive towards quality patient care, placing auscultation results into clinical perspective is elementary. As noted by Ramsingh et al., while techniques such as point-of-care ultrasound have emerged as alternatives, they cannot replace the urgency of the normal auscultation (Priebe, 2016). For instance, in a patient presenting with respiratory distress, the fine examination of lung sounds can immediately signal the status of the patient, such as the need for oxygen supplementation or other interventions. In addition, the historic practice of auscultating lungs as a routine part of examination continues to be beneficial in picking up on change. Thus, the inclusion of auscultation within comprehensive nursing assessments guarantees that clinicians are able to respond optimally and promptly to evolving respiratory issues, thereby maximizing outcomes for patients. Lastly, technical abilities employed within auscultation, including technique and stethoscope positioning, impact finding accuracy. For optimal results, the clinician must have a good hand at applying proper auscultation technique, for instance, locating the diaphragm of the stethoscope on various lung regions to effectively capture airflow. Patient position and extraneous noise pose hazards to the quality of sounds perceived. Perhaps surprisingly, it has been observed that some maneuvers—such as getting patients to breathe deeply—can enhance clarity in breath sounds (El-Deeb et al., 2024). Thus, nurses must acquire both technical skill and contextual understanding of lung sounds. Acquisition of these skills not only enhances the thoroughness of respiratory histories but also secures the nurse's role as a primary caregiver in managing respiratory illness (Figure 10.11).

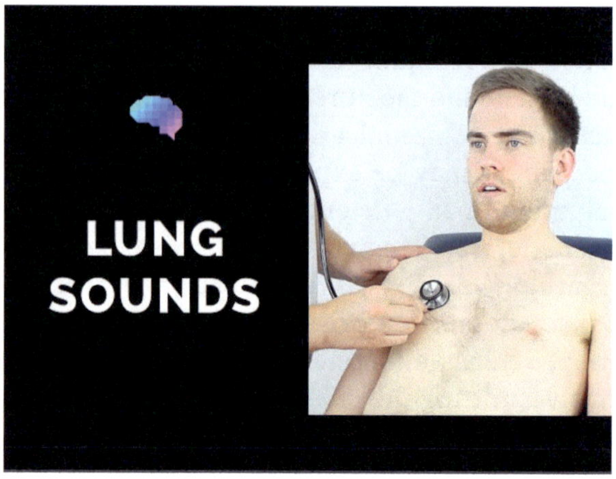

Figure 10.11. Auscultation of lung sounds.

Source: https://i.ytimg.com/vi/2NvBk61ngDY/sddefault.jpg.

Test Your Knowledge

1. What techniques are used to assess the thorax and lungs, including inspection, palpation, percussion, and auscultation?
2. How can nurses systematically evaluate respiratory rate, rhythm, and breath sounds for accurate assessment?

10.4. Common Thoracic and Pulmonary Conditions

Learning Outcome

1. Asthma and Its Assessment
2. Chronic Obstructive Pulmonary Disease (COPD)
3. Pneumonia and Its Implications

In-depth knowledge of common thoracic and pulmonary disorders is beneficial for nursing professionals who have the responsibility of assessing and managing patients suffering from respiratory diseases. Pneumonia, an often occurring yet dangerous lung infection, has significant morbidity and mortality implications, particularly for vulnerable subjects such as elderly individuals and those with chronic medical illnesses. Effective nursing assessment processes center on the detection of clinical signs, like cough, fever, and dyspnea, which are crucial for early intervention. Inasmuch as severe pneumonia involves implications beyond direct respiratory compromise, including extrapulmonary complications, strict compliance with standardized guidelines is vital. Empirical evidence indicates that early intervention with effective antimicrobial treatment significantly improves survival in critically ill patients, and therefore, highlighting the importance of nurses maintaining vigilance in monitoring and understanding pneumonia risk factors and treatment guidelines (Cill et al., 2021). Bronchiectasis is still another chronic lung disease that demands careful nursing assessment and management. Characterized by disease related and irreversible widening of the airways, bronchiectasis may lead to a perpetual cycle of chronic infection, inflammation, and worsening lung damage. Nursing assessments must search for the patients history of chronic respiratory infection, coughing, and sputum that is purulent, all of which are indicative of this disease. In addition, since bronchiectasis compromises the quality of life for its afflicted children and adolescents, as well as their families, education and counseling represent crucial roles that nurses play. By instituting evidence-based management strategies, as advocated by numerous guidelines, nurses can significantly enhance clinical outcomes for the patients (Anne et al., 2021). These plans entail personalized treatment schedules such as airway clearance techniques, chronic control of the exacerbations, and follow-up on underlying issues that may precipitate the progression of the disease. Asthma, in most instances characterized as a normal thoracic disorder, also requires some degree of subtlety when nursing diagnosis is being performed. The chronic inflammatory disease is characterized by reversible airway obstruction, wheezing, and shortness of breath. Good practice in nursing includes explicit patient education about the precipitating factors of asthma and the requirement for strict compliance with prescribed inhaled corticosteroids and bronchodilators. Assessment should include a review of frequency and severity of symptoms, and the patient's level of capability to manage acute exacerbations. Nurses have an important role to play in assisting in the development of action plans that help the patient recognize deteriorating symptoms and summon early intervention. By emphasizing self-management techniques and follow-up, nursing clinicians can be at the forefront of reducing asthma morbidity as well as overall patient outcomes. Understanding their pivotal role in evaluating and caring for these common thoracic and pulmonary disorders makes nurses become the leading promoters of respiratory health (Figure 10.12).

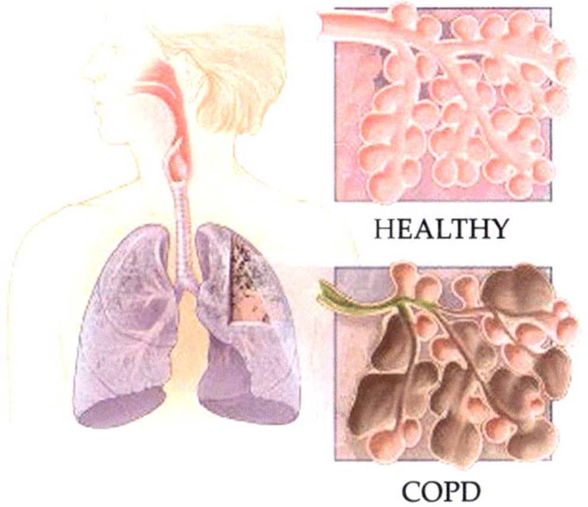

Figure 10.12. Common thoracic and pulmonary conditions.

Source: https://upload.wikimedia.org/wikipedia/commons/5/59/Copd_versus_healthy_lung.jpg.

10.4.1. Asthma and Its Assessment

The assessment of asthma is an essential component of nursing practice involving a condition found in millions worldwide. The extensive evaluation begins with a comprehensive patient history that covers the frequency and severity of asthma symptoms, triggers, and family or personal history of allergy. Utilization of standardized measures such as the Asthma Control Test (ACT) helps quantify the frequency of symptoms and their effect on daily living. Besides, physical assessment highlights the thorax and breath sounds, wherein wheezing and lengthened expiration may show bronchospasm. Implementing such procedures into nursing care necessitates not just knowledge of asthma's clinical presentations but also its pathophysiology. Such a two-way process informs nurses regarding appropriate interventions and care measures tailored to patient health profiles, thereby advancing patient outcomes. Other than clinical assessment, objective assessment is important in asthma evaluation using spirometry, among others. Quantification of lung function is done by spirometry through measurement of FEV1 and FVC, providing very significant information about airway obstruction. Abnormal results from spirometry tests can help decide on the severity of asthma and guide the treatment as per relevant guidelines. Most importantly, the monitoring of peak expiratory flow (PEF) gives patients an easy way to check their lung function, which encourages self-management and the early recognition of exacerbations. The role of advanced diagnostics, such as fractional exhaled nitric oxide (FeNO) tests, is also increasingly acknowledged in assessing airway inflammation. A close understanding of such measurements allows nurses to apply responsive pharmacological and non-pharmacological interventions, facilitating enhanced disease control and patient satisfaction. In addition, asthma care calls for a strategy that extends beyond transient clinical assessment. Part of educating patients is the skill to empower them to recognize early warning signs of increasing attacks and stick to treatment regimens. Nurses have to explain the importance of sticking to medication properly, including inhalers and preventive therapy, in an effort to establish optimal asthma control. It involves patients in action plans directed at their own requirements, which increases self-efficacy and participation in their own care. Psychosocial problems such as stress and anxiety need also to be addressed since these can actually increase symptoms. In the evolving management of asthma, evidence-based practice needs to be updated, as indicated in current guidelines, to ensure that nursing assessment is current and effective in maximizing patient care outcomes in asthma patients. Through the use of continuous education and advocacy, nurses can influence asthmatic patients' quality of life (Anne et al., 2021; Hardinge et al., 2015) (Figure 10.13).

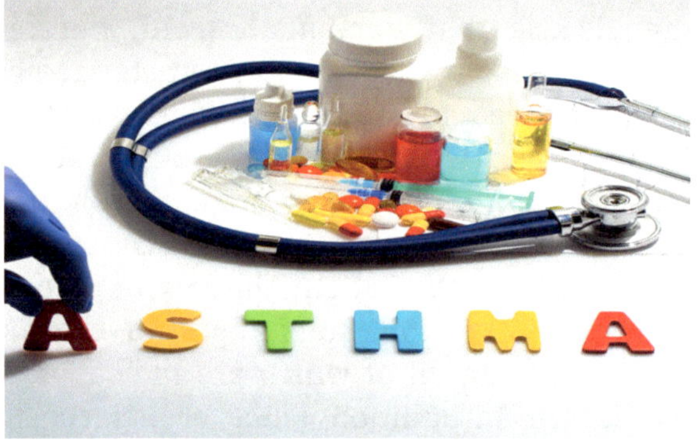

Figure 10.13. Asthma and its assessment.

Source: https://external-content.duckduckgo.com/iu/?u=https%3A%2F%2Flocalquoter.net%2Fwp-content%2Fuploads%2F2023%2F04%2FAsthma-Diagnosis-Involves-Multiple-Tests-and-Assessments.png&f=1&nofb=1&ipt=1f8398b209241b2793307d4c71852e5d0376d86c64cbccb5a201bac2ffdd55ed.

10.4.2. Chronic Obstructive Pulmonary Disease (COPD)

Chronic obstructive pulmonary disease or COPD is a serious health issue with chronic respiratory signs and airway limitation caused primarily by exposure to noxious gases or particles, typically cigarette smoke. During nursing assessments, care should be taken to understand the complexity of COPD because the condition typically leads to compromised pulmonary function as well as overall health status. The patients typically present with a chronic cough, production of sputum, and dyspnea that increase over a period. Systematic assessment, including patient history and physical examination, can ascertain the degree of airway obstruction, assess any comorbidity, and identify the patient's baseline function and quality of life. Early and extensive assessment can enable customized interventions, thereby facilitating better patient outcomes and management of this disabling chronic illness. Furthermore, the role of nursing in the daily management of COPD cannot be overstated. Effective nursing assessment facilitates preventive practice, such as the development of individualized care plans focused on symptom management and patient education. The incorporation of pulmonary rehabilitation programs, such as exercise training and smoking cessation literature, has been helpful in enhancing lung function and quality of life for patients with COPD. Also crucial is the regular tracking of exacerbations and identification of the triggers for these events, as it is the most important way to avoid complications and hospitalizations. For these reasons, ongoing patient education about early identification of the signs of exacerbation and inhaled drugs and nebulizer use is critical in the case of COPD, thus illustrating the nursing profession's influence on patient outcomes. In as much as the health environment adapts to meet new challenges, diagnosis of chronic respiratory diseases like COPD has significantly been impacted by recent global health situations. The intersection of COPD and COVID-19 presents the most critical issues of patient management, with those who have experienced a history of respiratory disease potentially experiencing increased risks and longer recovery times following viral illnesses. The literature identifies that COPD patients developing COVID-19 may have an increased symptom burden and require specialized follow-up care to improve quality of life (Katerina et al., 2022). The delivery of care for such patients encompasses an understanding of appropriate use of oxygen in the clinical setting, as explained under the amended guidelines of best practice orientation (Ronan et al., 2017). Therefore, patient management for patients with COPD must remain constantly responsive and adaptable to altering health concerns in order to supply the best possible management regimens (Figure 10.14).

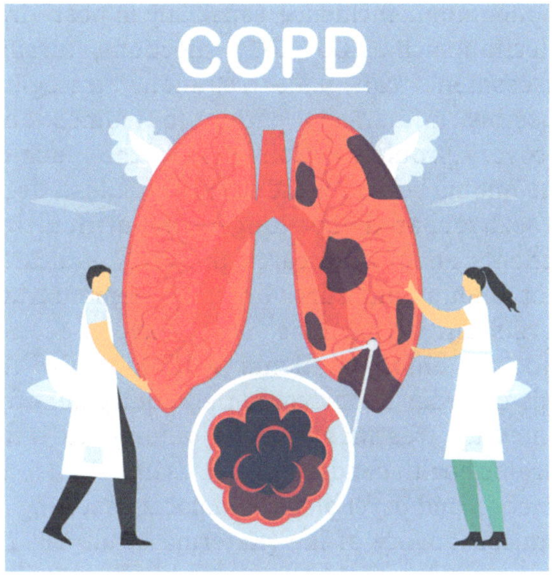

Figure 10.14. Chronic obstructive pulmonary disease.

Source: https://external-content.duckduckgo.com/iu/?u=https%3A%2F%2Fcdn.vectorstock.com%2Fi%2F1000v%2F38%2F44%2Fchronic-obstructive-pulmonary-disease-or-copd-vector-31783844.jpg&f=1&nofb=1&ipt=aab48ff870c793a3a0ae0418e5b8f063b7ca56b90563c8587d004015bfeb8b43.

10.4.3. Pneumonia and Its Implications

The diagnosis of pneumonia requires precautions in nursing practice because of the severity associated with the disease. Pneumonia is an infection and inflammation of the air sacs within the lungs or one of them that can lead to severe complications, particularly among the vulnerable population such as the elderly and those with existing diseases. They need to be effective because they guide the clinical symptoms of pneumonia diagnosis such as cough, fever, and abnormal lung sounds on auscultation. Also, understanding the patients' history, either recent infection or travel, can provide nursing professionals with context clues that are imperative for diagnosis. With a rise in pneumonia incidence, especially in post-viral infection such as COVID-19 infections, nursing assessments can guide treatment strategies, possibly influencing patient outcomes and recovery profiles. Prolongation of the reach of pneumonia beyond acute clinical manifestations is exacerbated by long-term difficulties patients endure. Research presently indicates that pneumonia survivors may demonstrate persistent symptoms that have become endemic among patients with long COVID. This disorder underscores the requirement for follow-up treatment that is tailored to treat chronic health conditions such as impaired lung function and psychological impacts, resulting in reduced quality of life (Katerina et al., 2022). Nursing assessments play a crucial role in the identification of these chronic complications through vigilant monitoring. Nurses do not only perform physical examinations but also educate families and patients about the risk of late sequelae, thus being in the center of comprehensive patient care and care giving. Pneumonia may also be further complicated by conditions such as bronchiectasis, in which chronic airway inflammation results in recurrent respiratory infections and exacerbations (Anne et al., 2021). This prolonged pulmonary illness vastly increases both the clinical and economic strain on healthcare systems and families because of its severity as well as the need for constant management measures. With respect to assessing patients who have pneumonia, nursing visits should further include screening for the potential development of such chronic illnesses so that early intervention and treatment can occur. With a comprehensive understanding of pneumonias repercussions, which include its progression to chronic lung disease, nursing professionals can effectively best champion relevant treatment avenues, hence ensuring patient care is not just reactive, but proactive to improve long-term health outcomes (Figure 10.15).

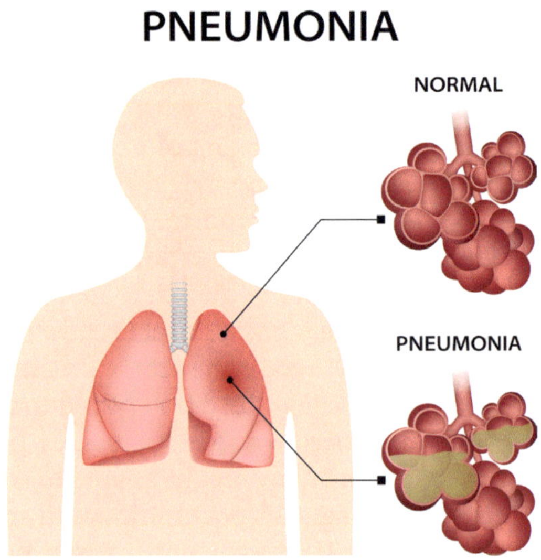

Figure 10.15. Pneumonia.

Source: https://external-content.duckduckgo.com/iu/?u=https%3A%2F%2Fwww.respiratorylondon.co.uk%2Fwp-content%2Fuploads%2FPneumonia-picture-amit-patel-scaled.jpeg&f=1&nofb=1&ipt=adcb781cd30c98bb88923b8eef5ae2920b33ab95bae4ea74bddf93d46d07006a.

Test Your Knowledge

1. What are some common thoracic and pulmonary conditions, and what assessment findings are associated with each?
2. How can early recognition of conditions such as asthma, pneumonia, or COPD improve patient outcomes?

10.5. Nursing Interventions

Learning Outcome

1. Patient Education on Respiratory Health
2. Techniques for Effective Breathing Exercises
3. Importance of Monitoring and Documentation

For optimal patient outcomes during thorax and lung assessment, nursing intervention is essential to facilitate proper assessment and prompt treatment. A prime intervention for that purpose is continuous monitoring of respiratory rate and pattern. Nurses must assess for manifestations of respiratory distress like abnormal breath sounds or changes in oxygen saturation levels, and those are indicative of latent pathologies such as pneumonia or chronic obstructive pulmonary disease. Through proper documentation of these findings, nurses will be able to clearly communicate with the healthcare team to expedite decision making regarding treatment. Further, interventions like instructing patients on breathing exercises will enhance lung capacity and overall respiratory function, hence nurses' role in ongoing patient education is paramount. Other than monitoring, proper infection control practices must be employed in patient safety while being subjected to thorax and lungs examination. With higher risk of transmission of respiratory diseases, especially in the context of infectious diseases like COVID-19, strict adherence to hygiene practices cannot be avoided. This includes the donning of personal protective equipment (PPE), adherence to hand hygiene, and appropriate environmental cleanliness. Effective decontamination of equipment that has been used during the period of assessment, including stethoscopes and peak flow meters, is necessary to prevent cross-contamination. Moreover, nursing interventions should address patient education on respiratory hygiene to empower them to take an active role in their health care and limit the spread of infection, as highlighted in corresponding guidelines (Chen et al., 2020). When managing specific respiratory conditions, tailor-made nursing interventions are essential for optimal care. For instance, individuals suffering from chronic disease such as asthma require multimodal treatment not only including regular assessment but also an individualized action plan. The medication use, like the use of bronchodilators or corticosteroids, along with patient education on the use of inhalers and symptom control, must be included in the plan. Furthermore, frequent reassessment and adjustment of care plans based on the reaction of the patient are crucial so that optimal therapy interventions are achieved. Such targeted interventions allow nurses to provide holistic care in managing chronic lung disease and its implications for patients' quality of life, consistent with informing clinical recommendations (Haworth et al., 2017).

10.5.1. Patient Education on Respiratory Health

Efficient patient education for respiratory health is key to enhancing self-management and general outcome among patients with chronic respiratory illnesses. Nurses' role in imparting empowering information to enable patients to understand their diseases, treatment regimens, and adjustment skills is paramount. Of prime concern to education are pathophysiology of respiratory illness, the need for medication compliance, and early warning signs of worsening. By establishing an environment in which patients can freely state their symptoms and concerns, nurses can encourage health-seeking behavior, ultimately leading to reduced hospitalization and improved quality of life. Educational interventions should be planned to cater to the diverse needs of patients, considering factors of health literacy and culture, so that all individuals receive proper and understandable information with regards to their respiratory health. In addition to general education on respiratory health, there are some measures that need to be taken to address the needs of vulnerable populations disproportionately affected by respiratory disease. The COVID-19 pandemic has made us focus more on the disproportionate health resource utilization and higher chronic respiratory disease burden among poor communities and highlighted the urgency of targeted educational interventions. Educational interventions must emphasize promotion of respiratory health, promotion of vaccination, and prevention to decrease risk of exposure to respiratory pathogens. Joint efforts between healthcare providers, community-based organizations, and public health agencies can expand the access of these educational messages to populations that otherwise might not have exposure in clinical settings. Placing importance on patient education with these populations allows nurses to reduce some of the inequalities that are being perpetuated through systemic injustices, as evidenced through the recurring problems observed during the pandemic (Shadmi et al., 2020). Additionally, the application of technology in patient education about respiratory health has changed how information is shared and received. Telehealth websites and mobile health applications offer new avenues for education, facilitating real-time communication between health care providers and patients. The technologies not only increase access to educational material, but also enable nurses to monitor patient outcomes, adjust treatment regimens, and provide timely support. But it is imperative that patients be empowered to engage fully with these technology platforms, possibly through additional training and assistance to build digital literacy. Also, identification of the psychosocial dimensions of respiratory health is of utmost importance; programming in education needs to incorporate stress and anxiety control with chronic lung disease. Comprehensive education programs that enhance clinical, as well as affective, patient needs can significantly enhance compliance with treatment and overall quality of life (Taplitz et al., 2018) (Figure 10.16).

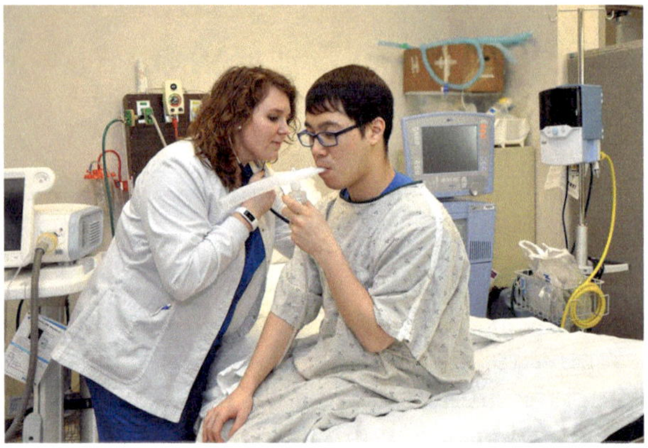

Figure 10.16. Patient education on respiratory health.

Source: https://external-content.duckduckgo.com/iu/?u=https%3A%2F%2Fwww.swic.edu%2Fwp-content%2Fuploads%2F2017%2F05%2FHealth-Sciences-Respiratory-Care-DSC-0091-1024x683.jpg&f=1&nofb=1&ipt=5028048aba9c588161e495bd4f4dd1344709fef6ad2bc7938f1d0b5cb95bcd40.

10.5.2. Techniques for Effective Breathing Exercises

Efficient respiratory exercises are an important aspect of assessing and enhancing pulmonary function in practice nursing. Diaphragmatic breathing, pursed-lip breathing, and rib-stretching exercises are the methods which allow patients to maximize ventilation and minimize respiratory effort. Diaphragmatic breathing encourages the use of the diaphragm and not accessory muscles for more effective and deeper breathing. This method can be particularly useful in individuals with chronic obstructive pulmonary disease (COPD), in whom shallowness of the breathing pattern is common. The application of these exercises, not just increases gas exchange but also patient overall respiratory muscle strength, as needed when assessing thoracic and lung status within the nursing setting, in agreement with research evidence that respiratory muscle training significantly impacted pulmonary function among a variety of patient groups (Ramli et al., 2023). In addition to diaphragm-focused approaches, pursed-lip breathing offers another valuable means of increasing patient outcomes. This approach involves inhaling through the nose and slow exhalation through pursed lips, helping to keep airways patent and alveoli from collapsing during expiration. Developing low resistance during the expiratory phase can help patients gain control over their breathlessness, especially during exertion or periods of increased dyspnea. Adding rib-stretching exercises can enhance thoracic mobility so additional lung expansion is achievable. These exercises, when implemented in nursing assessments, have the potential to give useful information regarding lung capacity and respiratory efficiency, ultimately leading to more specific and effective patients' care plans for those potentially suffering from limitations in lung function due to other certain underlying conditions (Patel et al., 2022). Nurses must assess personal patient needs and provide immediate feedback on how well the exercises are performed in order to gain most from these breathing exercises. In-depth evaluation with the use of respiratory pressure measurement and vital capacity measurement can yield information regarding weaknesses or limitations. Integration of technology with standard assessment, such as spirometry or electromyography, can give more comprehensive information regarding respiratory status. Systematic integration of these modes of assessment into clinical settings enhances clinicians' ability to diagnose respiratory dysfunction and utilize corresponding breathing exercises, leading to better patient outcome. Thus, such exercises serve not only to contribute to clinical goals but also enable the patient through giving them the ability to manage their breathing properly, highlighting the central role of nursing assessment in respiratory care (Ramli et al., 2023) (Figure 10.17).

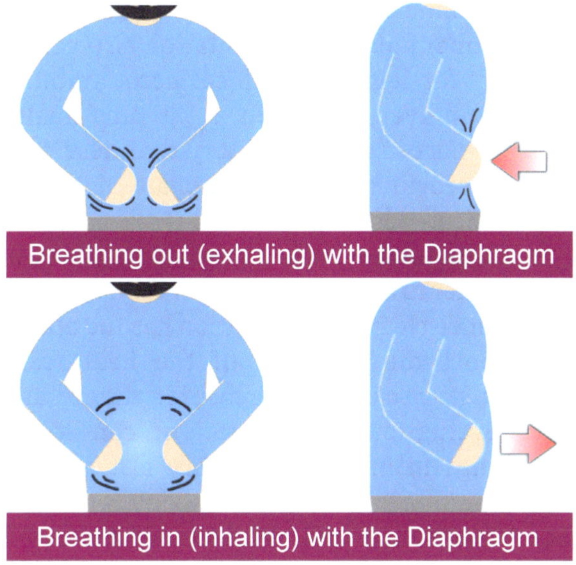

Figure 10.17. Techniques for effective breathing exercises.

Source: https://www.torbayandsouthdevon.nhs.uk/uploads/pain-service-breathing.jpg.

10.5.3. Importance of Monitoring and Documentation

Good monitoring and documentation are essential roles in thorax and lungs assessment within nursing practice. These procedures help ensure that healthcare practitioners adhere to set standardized procedures that facilitate adequate evaluation and timely intervention. Systematic monitoring assists in early detection of respiratory distress or abnormality, thereby preventing complications and improving patient outcomes. For instance, detailed documentation of a patient's respirations, oxygen saturation, and lung sounds findings provides invaluable baseline data. These are invaluable in determining trends and patterns in the patient's condition over time, and enabling nurses to adjust care plans accordingly on the basis of the evolving patient needs. Besides, precise documentation is a valuable communication instrument among members of multidisciplinary teams so that all members of the patients care team are presented with clear information about their clinical status and treatment plan. Documentation also comes in handy for legal and ethical accountability in nursing. Every entry on a patient's health record is part of an entire story that describes the care provided and the rationale that went into clinical decision making. This assumes a lot of importance when resolving possible disagreements and differences in the provision of care since clear documentation has the ability to support the accuracy of the healthcare provider's actions. In the case of thorax and lungs evaluation, where patient conditions can change in minute ways very fast, precise documentation guarantees that all interventions, observations, and patient reactions are noted clearly and accurately. This observance to evidence-based practice supported by guidelines like those of the European Respiratory Society excerpted by Anne et al. (2021) is reflective of monitoring and documentation roles in maintaining best patient care results and supporting overall quality improvement initiatives among healthcare systems. Additionally, having a successful monitoring and documentation function empowers nurses to play active roles in educating patients and in self-management. By maintaining detailed histories of patient assessments and responses to interventions, nurses are in a better position to educate patients and families regarding the patient's respiratory condition. These histories are educational tools that highlight the need for compliance with treatment, the significance of lifestyle modification, and tangible steps toward controlling conditions, such as bronchiectasis by Anne et al. (2021). Further, ongoing documentation offers a foundation for team care in order that nurses may identify learning gaps and support teaching at junctures along a patient's trajectory. Educating well-informed patients and families facilitates their empowerment to assume more responsibility for care, ultimately leading to more successful adherence and improved health outcomes. Therefore, good monitoring and documentation are essential parts of nursing care that enhance patient care through improved communication, accountability, and education.

Test Your Knowledge

1. What nursing interventions can support patients with respiratory conditions to improve oxygenation and airway clearance?
2. How can nurses educate patients on preventive measures such as smoking cessation and pulmonary hygiene?

10.6. Challenges in Thorax and Lung Assessment

Learning Outcome

1. Variability in Patient Presentations
2. Limitations of Assessment Tools
3. Cultural Considerations in Assessment

The assessment of thoracic and lung disease also creates numerous challenges that have a direct effect on the clinical outcome. Nurses often find themselves with an initial assessment role, being requested to identify impairments of the respiratory system that are not always easy to identify. Perhaps the greatest challenge is variation in patient presentation, which can be affected by numerous factors such as age, pre-existing illness, and the presence of comorbid illnesses. For instance, the patients with COVID-19 who recover show a wide range of persistent symptoms that complicate the assessment process. These symptoms, for instance, like fatigue and shortness of breath, might not necessarily be accompanied by objective imaging or pulmonary function test findings, leading to likely misinterpretation of the patient's status.

Here, understanding the subtle nature of respiratory disease becomes important in effective nursing practice and achieving the best patient outcomes. No less demanding in thorax and lung assessment is the weight of social determinants of health, which have a tendency to expand disparities in care. Impacted populations, such as marginalized or chronic health sufferers, may face multi-layered barriers to managing pulmonary disease. Particularly during the COVID-19 pandemic, disparities in access to healthcare were stark, with disadvantaged patients being adversely affected in disproportionate numbers due to lack of support structures and resources. The disproportionate prevalence of respiratory conditions among these groups has the possibility of generating inequalities in assessment and follow-up treatment, making it challenging to create effective nursing interventions. Correcting these disparities is crucial not only to better health outcomes but also to making sure all patients have access to the integrated care they need.

The barriers must be recognized by nurses and efforts must be made to promote fair healthcare access when performing thoracic evaluations. Finally, the changing nature of respiratory diseases must be considered, especially with respect to post-infection syndromes such as long COVID, and this adds an additional level of complexity to lung evaluation. There is ongoing investigation into the most useful follow-up care interventions, with evidence to indicate that a high symptom burden in most patients persists many weeks beyond initial recovery.

This chronic symptomatology—through persistent respiratory illness, functional impairment, and decreased quality of life—causes challenges for nurses in the area of diagnosis. With fresh evidence indicating a relationship between the severity of acute infection and the development of chronic symptoms, there exists a need for an efficient follow-up protocol.

However, existing research highlights a paucity of research in the topic, further limiting the scope of lung examination to nursing practice (Katerina et al., 2022). With these challenges, nurses must remain cautious and employ a patient-centered strategy in order to effectively adapt assessments within the context of evolving medical knowledge (Shadmi et al., 2020).

10.6.1. Variability in Patient Presentations

Heterogeneity in patient presentation is one of the greatest challenges in thorax and lung assessment by nurses, as the clinical presentation of respiratory illnesses may differ among patients. Role of age, comorbidities, and environmental factors is responsible for such differences. Older adults, for instance, may present with atypical presentations of respiratory illnesses with symptoms of other illnesses bearing the comorbid disease rather than the typical respiratory distress. In addition, certain conditions, including interstitial lung disease (ILD), manifest a range of symptoms largely influenced by individual patient histories and comorbidities. It is this heterogeneity that complicates the assessment and diagnostic process, requiring nurses to be very clinically suspicious and reactive to unique patient situations (Gupta et al., 2023). Such diversity is necessary in order to create individualized care models aimed at maximizing patient outcomes in the course of respiratory examinations. Recognition and interpretation of subtle respiratory findings are included in the care of diverse patient presentations. For instance, children with bronchiectasis will present with chronic cough and recurrent infection and have their symptoms falsely attributed to normal asthma symptoms and thereby at risk for misdiagnosis. Nurses must, therefore, apply extended assessment techniques, including thorough patient histories and physical examinations, in order to differentiate from similar respiratory conditions. Standardized recommendations can provide us with illumination, yet the absence of consensus in guidelines complicates the management approach to pediatric cases. The European Respiratory Society supports a multidisciplinary approach to addressing bronchiectasis, highlighting the importance of special care in the process of narrowing focus to unique presentation and treatment options (Anne et al., 2021). This highlights nurses' functions in tailoring assessments to become more patient profile-based. Management of variability in patient presentation involves ongoing education and adjustment of nursing practice to enhance clinical competence and the efficacy of assessments. Ongoing professional development helps nurses revise their methods as they realize how cultural perceptions, socioeconomic issues, and previous histories of health influence patient reports. Additionally, employing improved diagnostic technologies and instruments can further clarify respiratory illness, allowing for greater accuracy of assessments. As the nurses become more adept at detecting subtle presentations, they help to enhance care and patient satisfaction. In the long term, being tolerant of differences in respiratory examinations leads to a deeper perception of the needs of patients and increases successful intervention, which is very essential for the realization of successful nursing practice in thorax and lung examinations (Anne et al., 2021; Gupta et al., 2023).

10.6.2. Limitations of Assessment Tools

Evaluation tools are valuable in ensuring the proper assessment of pulmonary and thoracic health in nursing practice; however, they carry inherent limitations that cannot be overlooked. One of these limitations is the aspect of subjective interpretation of outcomes, which can lead to inconsistency among the practitioners. As an illustration, results of auscultation, while vital in establishing abnormal lung sounds, can significantly depend on the experience and ability of the clinician. Additionally, some of the tools lack a complete scope of respiratory issues, such that vital aspects of a patient's case may be omitted. The limitations of these assessment methods could thus result in poor patient care or misdiagnosis, further affirming the necessity for continuous training and standardization of assessment practices in nursing. Another significant limitation is that of specificity and sensitivity across various assessment tools. The ability to correctly identify specific lung conditions is apt to be undermined by interspersed symptoms and patient variability. For example, respiratory rate and pattern determination can be influenced by anxiety or fever, which are not necessarily linked to lung pathology. Additionally, while pulse oximetry is a very good way of measuring oxygen saturation, it gives incorrect results in patients who have compromised peripheral perfusion or reduced skin pigmentation. This has made the importance of supplemental assessing devices and an overall clinical assessment because sole dependence on a single approach would weaken the overall knowledge of a patients respiratory status. Also, the emergence of respiratory disease over a longer term, particularly with respect to new and emerging diseases, makes it challenging to restrict the diagnostic limitations. In the case of long COVID, for example, limited evidence remains regarding optimal follow-up management of patients dealing with symptom burdens beyond the acute phase of infection. According to recent data, even though overall lung assessment tests can provide an early warning, they may not be capable of meeting the subtle complications with post-acute sequelae of SARS-CoV-2 infection such as thromboembolic disorders and changes in long-term pulmonary function (Katerina et al., 2022). Consequently, nursing professionals must take these limitations into account when using assessment tools and look for an integrated strategy that combines comprehensive evaluations and patient-centered care in a bid to enhance quality of life and recovery outcomes. In addition, as highlighted in the body composition measurement case, the traditional markers like BMI do not take into account specific risk factors involving respiratory disease, hence the need for holistic evaluation methods (Clifton et al., 2021).

10.6.3. Cultural Considerations in Assessment

In terms of thorax and lung evaluation in nursing, cultural factors need to be considered in offering fair and efficient care. Cultural beliefs will shape perceptions of health, illness, and healthcare interaction and, consequently, may determine patient reactions to assessment. For instance, patients from different cultures may have differing understandings of a symptom or concern for a specific intervention, such as auscultation or percussion. A nurse must be sensitive to such cultural nuances in order to develop rapport and trust, particularly when discussing potentially sensitive topics like respiratory distress or chronic lung disease. By introducing cultural understanding into the nursing assessment, health care providers can give assurance that evaluations are not only medically correct but also culturally sensitive and therefore result in beneficial patient outcomes and an improved overall experience of care. Moreover, patients' cultural backgrounds influence their health literacy and communication style, which is a further aspect of complexity in thorax and lung examination. Non-verbal communication or reluctance to discuss respiratory issues directly may be significant in certain cultures, whereas other cultures may be frank. Such differences necessitate a tailored approach to taking patient history and conducting assessments, enabling nurses to identify symptoms and vital information more effectively. Use of culturally responsive assessment tools can earn better patient compliance and a better understanding of their health status. Incorporation of common-sense thinking, giving precedence to experiential knowing and everyday decision-making within the evaluation contexts, can also bridge communication gaps and result in more accurate diagnoses and treatment planning (Daved et al., 2021). Finally, a crucial part of cultural factors in thorax and lung assessment is to value the social determinants of health impacting respiratory well-being. Such factors involve socioeconomic status, environmental exposure to risk factors, and availability of health resources, which strongly interact with cultural settings. For example, individuals belonging to marginalized groups may experience increased rates of asthma or chronic obstructive pulmonary disease due to environmental and structural factors. Harnessing these factors within the evaluation process allows nurses to provide care that not only addresses immediate health concerns but also underlying causes. By realizing how culture, health behaviors, and social determinants influence each other, nurses can be able to advocate for focused interventions that resonate with cultural needs of patients and improve overall quality of care provided for thoracic and pulmonary diseases (Preusser et al., 2021).

Test Your Knowledge

1. What factors, such as obesity, patient cooperation, or underlying conditions, can complicate thoracic and lung assessment?
2. How can nurses address these challenges to ensure accurate and effective respiratory evaluations?

SUMMARY

An extensive thorax and lungs examination in nursing not only summarily reports the outcome of the evaluation but also highlights the dynamic role of continuous appraisal and intervention planning. Effective assessment techniques mold the nursing practice through the presentation of abnormalities of respiratory function and guiding effective interventions. Due to the fact that lung physiology is so intricate, multimodality assessments combined have a significant impact on patient outcome. As a case in point, studies have found that the application of interventions such as manual hyperinflation and chest physiotherapy can reduce the occurrence of complications like ventilator-associated pneumonia (VAP) among mechanically ventilated patients, highlighting the close connection between rigorous assessment and patient care quality (Younes et al., 2022). The nurses' predictive role in respecting respiratory needs is also fundamental to maximizing pulmonary disease patients' optimal care. Of equal importance is identifying body composition and its relationship with respiratory health and how it needs to be incorporated into the overall assessment plan. As body composition affects the overall health status, advanced practice nurses must evaluate how changes in lean mass and fat distribution could affect respiratory function and recovery outcomes. For instance, being able to recognize the increased risk for reduced skeletal muscle mass can enable nurses to take steps that facilitate and support muscle health, which is important for effective mechanics of breathing. This multifaceted understanding reinforces the argument for holistic assessments that extend beyond normal respiratory surveillance and permit clinicians to tailor interventions that address both short-term and long-term health concerns (Clifton et al., 2021). Ultimately, ongoing development of assessment techniques within the thorax and lungs specialty proves the adaptive nature of nursing practice. By implementing a unifying model combining both respiratory assessment and consideration of body composition, nurses can significantly enhance patient care. The application of evidence-based practice, such as multimodality chest physiotherapy, illustrates an obvious model of how best to improve clinical outcomes and reduce harmful effects like VAP among vulnerable populations. The nursing practice must then continue to promote advanced assessments to get a proactive management of the respiratory health, thus bringing nursing practices into line with the best possible evidence. This, in addition to enhancing better health outcomes, also reiterates the significance of nursing in delivering patient-centered care in the ever-evolving healthcare arena.

In thorax and lungs evaluation in nursing, an understanding of the complexities of pulmonary disease is relevant to optimal patient care. One area of interest is bronchiectasis, a chronic pulmonary disease that has a long-lasting impact on the quality of life for affected children and adolescents. The disease is marked by recurrent pneumonias and flare-ups and should be addressed through a multidisciplinary team to optimize management programs. The European Respiratory Society has issued evidence-based recommendations on numerous aspects of treatment and diagnosis, including long-term antibiotic treatment and airway clearance. Adherence to these guidelines will allow clinicians to offer improved clinical outcomes for the patient with bronchiectasis, as well as fulfill the greater need for comprehensive management plans in nursing practice (Anne et al., 2021). Similarly, assessment of sarcoidosis, another serious pulmonary illness, necessitates identification of its often-subtle clinical presentation. Respiratory exams will commonly be normal and therefore further disguise estimation of disease severity and morbidity. Due to this lack of certainty, pulmonary function tests cannot always reliably quantify disease activity or symptom burden of patients. Therefore, it is of utmost importance for nurses to perform thorough baseline screenings that include complete blood counts, biochemical examinations, and extra-thoracic disease screening. These measures not only provide pertinent information regarding controlling the condition, but they also accentuate the importance of meticulous assessment in clinical practice nursing. Engaging patients in conversations about overall health can encourage enhanced symptom perception of fatigue and mood changes, encouraging a more holistic approach (Thillai et al., 2020). Finally, a good understanding of both bronchiectasis and sarcoidosis adds significantly to thorax and lung nursing evaluation. The absence of clear diagnostic signs in illnesses like sarcoidosis compels nurses to rely on advanced imaging modalities and a multidisciplinary diagnosis to identify potential cardiac involvement that may be overlooked in general respiratory examination. On top of this, ongoing education with regard to new evidence-based practice guidelines is essential in order for nurses to continue to practice on optimal care for chronic pulmonary conditions. By achieving an all-around understanding of the intricacies, nursing practitioners can contribute immensely towards better clinical outcomes. Continual assessment and adjustment within nursing assessment, as supported through management of sarcoidosis and bronchiectasis, shows the essence of incorporating emerging evidence into daily practice (Anne et al., 2021; Thillai et al., 2020).

KEY TERMS FROM THIS CHAPTER

Thoracic Cage	Intercostal Spaces
Respiratory Rate	Chest Expansion
Breath Sounds	Vesicular Sounds
Bronchial Sounds	Bronchovesicular Sounds
Adventitious Sounds	Crackles
Wheezes	Rhonchi
Pleural Friction Rub	Tactile Fremitus
Percussion Note	Resonance
Hyperresonance	Dyspnea
Cyanosis	Barrel Chest

CRITICAL THINKING QUESTIONS

1. **Which of the following is a normal finding when auscultating the lungs?**
   a. Wheezes over all lung fields
   b. Vesicular breath sounds over the peripheral lung fields
   c. Crackles in the bases of the lungs only during deep inspiration
   d. Stridor during quiet breathing
2. **The nurse percusses over the lungs and hears a dull sound. This finding may indicate:**
   a. Normal lung tissue
   b. Pneumothorax
   c. Consolidation or pleural effusion
   d. Hyperinflated lungs
3. **During thoracic assessment, the nurse observes unequal chest expansion. This may indicate:**
   a. Normal variation
   b. Pneumothorax, atelectasis, or pleural effusion
   c. Hyperventilation
   d. Bronchitis
4. **Which of the following indicates effective diaphragmatic movement during breathing?**
   a. Use of accessory muscles
   b. Symmetric abdominal rise and fall
   c. Intercostal retractions
   d. Paradoxical chest movement
5. **A high-pitched continuous sound heard during expiration is called:**
   a. Crackles
   b. Rhonchi
   c. Wheezes
   d. Stridor

Short Answer Questions

1. What are the anatomical landmarks used in thoracic and lung assessment?
2. Describe the steps of a systematic respiratory assessment, including inspection, palpation, percussion, and auscultation.
3. What normal breath sounds are expected, and where are they typically auscultated?
4. Identify common adventitious lung sounds and their clinical significance (e.g., crackles, wheezes, rhonchi).
5. How can respiratory rate, rhythm, and depth provide information about a patient's respiratory status?

Answer to Critical Thinking Questions

1. (b) 2. (c) 3. (b) 4. (b) 5. (c)

REFERENCES

1. Antoniou, K. M., Vasarmidi, E., Russell, A. M., Andréjak, C., Crestani, B., Delcroix, M., Dinh-Xuan, A. T., et al. (2022). European Respiratory Society statement on long COVID follow-up. *European Respiratory Journal, 60*, 2102174–2102174. https://doi.org/10.1183/13993003.02174-2021 (accessed on 16th July 2025).
2. Arnold, D., Hamilton, F., Milne, A., Morley, A. J., Viner, J., Attwood, M., Noel, A., et al. (2020). Patient outcomes after hospitalization with COVID-19 and implications for follow-up: Results from a prospective UK cohort. *Thorax, 76*, 399–401. https://doi.org/10.1136/thoraxjnl-2020-216086 (accessed on 16th July 2025).
3. Asciak, R., Bedawi, E. O., Bhatnagar, R., Clive, A., Hassan, M., Lloyd, H., Reddy, R., et al. (2023). British Thoracic Society clinical statement on pleural procedures. *Thorax, 78*, s43–s68. https://doi.org/10.1136/thorax-2022-219371 (accessed on 16th July 2025).
4. Byermoen, K. R., Brembo, E. A., Egilsdottir, H. Ö., Heyn, L. G., Moen, A., & Eide, H. (2020). Reflection on actions: Identifying facilitators of and barriers to using physical assessment in clinical practice. *Nurse Education in Practice, 50*, 102913–102913. https://doi.org/10.1016/j.nepr.2020.102913 (accessed on 16th July 2025).
5. Byermoen, K. R., Eide, T., Egilsdottir, H. Ö., Eide, H., Heyn, L. G., Moen, A., & Brembo, E. A. (2022). Nursing students' development of using physical assessment in clinical rotation—a stimulated recall study. *BMC Nursing, 21*. https://doi.org/10.1186/s12912-022-00879-1 (accessed on 16th July 2025).
6. Chang, A. B., Fortescue, R., Grimwood, K., Alexopoulou, E., Bell, L., Boyd, J., Bush, A., et al. (2021). European Respiratory Society guidelines for the management of children and adolescents with bronchiectasis. *European Respiratory Journal, 58*, 2002990–2002990. https://doi.org/10.1183/13993003.02990-2020 (accessed on 16th July 2025).
7. Chen, C., Gao, G., Xu, Y., Pu, L., Wang, Q., Wang, L., Wang, W., et al. (2020). SARS-CoV-2–positive sputum and feces after conversion of pharyngeal samples in patients with COVID-19. *Annals of Internal Medicine, 172*, 832–834. https://doi.org/10.7326/m20-0991 (accessed on 16th July 2025).
8. Cillóniz, C., Torres, A., & Niederman, M. S. (2021). Management of pneumonia in critically ill patients. *BMJ*. https://doi.org/10.1136/bmj-2021-065871 (accessed on 16th July 2025).
9. Ding, X., Clifton, D. A., Ji, N., Lovell, N. H., Bonato, P., Chen, W., Yu, X., et al. (2020). Wearable sensing and telehealth technology with potential applications in the coronavirus pandemic. *IEEE Reviews in Biomedical Engineering, 14*, 48–70. https://doi.org/10.1109/rbme.2020.2992838 (accessed on 16th July 2025).
10. Egilsdottir, H. Ö., Byermoen, K. R., Moen, A., & Eide, H. (2019). Revitalizing physical assessment in undergraduate nursing education–what skills are important to learn, and how are these skills applied during clinical rotation? A cohort study. *BMC Nursing, 18*. https://doi.org/10.1186/s12912-019-0364-9 (accessed on 16th July 2025).
11. El-Deeb, H. A. A. E. M., Abd El Hafeez, N. A. A., Rashwan, M., El-Sayed, M., Khedr, M. A., & Dawood, R. F. A. (2024). Effect of self-proning on respiratory functions, pneumonia severity, and mortality risk among patients diagnosed with community-acquired pneumonia: A nursing-based quasi-experimental study. *Clinical Nursing Research, 34*, 47–57. https://

www.semanticscholar.org/paper/acba006a721ea845c7d173050ec952b7a0ce4fdc (accessed on 16th July 2025).

12. Ferdinand, J., Morrison, M., Andreasson, A., Charlton, C., Chhatwal, A., Scott, W., Borthwick, L., et al. (2021). Transcriptional analysis identifies potential novel biomarkers associated with successful *ex-vivo* perfusion of human donor lungs. *Clinical Transplantation, 36*. https://www.semanticscholar.org/paper/91848ad3d4010f63d8bef98b7c2519eafbf56931 (accessed on 16th July 2025).

13. Garbe, C., Amaral, T., Peris, K., Hauschild, A., Arenberger, P., Basset-Séguin, N., Bastholt, L., et al. (2022). European consensus-based interdisciplinary guideline for melanoma. Part 1: Diagnostics: Update 2022. *European Journal of Cancer, 170*, 236–255. https://doi.org/10.1016/j.ejca.2022.03.008 (accessed on 16th July 2025).

14. George, P. M., Barratt, S., Condliffe, R., Desai, S. R., Devaraj, A., Forrest, I., Gibbons, M., et al. (2020). Respiratory follow-up of patients with COVID-19 pneumonia. *Thorax, 75*, 1009–1016. https://doi.org/10.1136/thoraxjnl-2020-215314 (accessed on 16th July 2025).

15. Gupta, R., Koteci, A., Morgan, A., George, P. M., & Quint, J. K. (2023). Incidence and prevalence of interstitial lung diseases worldwide: A systematic literature review. *BMJ Open Respiratory Research, 10*, e001291–e001291. https://doi.org/10.1136/bmjresp-2022-001291 (accessed on 16th July 2025).

16. Hardinge, M., Annandale, J., Bourne, S., Cooper, B., Evans, A., Freeman, D., Green, A., et al. (2015). British Thoracic Society guidelines for home oxygen use in adults: Accredited by NICE. *Thorax, 70*, i1–i43. https://doi.org/10.1136/thoraxjnl-2015-206865 (accessed on 16th July 2025).

17. Haworth, C., Banks, J., Capstick, T., Fisher, A. J., Gorsuch, T., Laurenson, I. F., Leitch, A., et al. (2017). British Thoracic Society guidelines for the management of non-tuberculous mycobacterial pulmonary disease (NTM-PD). *Thorax, 72*, ii1–ii64. https://doi.org/10.1136/thoraxjnl-2017-210927 (accessed on 16th July 2025).

18. Hoffelner, J., Peinhopf-Petz, W., & Wittek, T. (2023). Diagnostic and prognostic value of clinical scoring and lung ultrasonography to assess pulmonary lesions in veal calves. *Animals: An Open Access Journal from MDPI, 13*. https://www.semanticscholar.org/paper/6f734555173ff3cbc57eb5b4b0825c906931f005 (accessed on 16th July 2025).

19. Holmes, C. J., & Racette, S. B. (2021). The utility of body composition assessment in nutrition and clinical practice: An overview of current methodology. *Nutrients, 13*, 2493–2493. https://doi.org/10.3390/nu13082493 (accessed on 16th July 2025).

20. O'Driscoll, B. R., Howard, L., Earis, J. E., & Mak, V. (2017). British Thoracic Society guideline for oxygen uses in adults in healthcare and emergency settings. *BMJ Open Respiratory Research, 4*, e000170–e000170. https://doi.org/10.1136/bmjresp-2016-000170 (accessed on 16th July 2025).

21. Patel, N., Chong, K. K. L., & Baydur, A. (2022). Methods and applications in respiratory physiology: Respiratory mechanics, drive and muscle function in neuromuscular and chest wall disorders. *Frontiers in Physiology, 13*. https://doi.org/10.3389/fphys.2022.838414 (accessed on 16th July 2025).

22. Preusser, M., Silvani, A., Le Rhun, É., Soffietti, R., Lombardi, G., Sepúlveda-Sánchez, J. M., Brandal, P., et al. (2021). Trabectedin for recurrent WHO grade 2 or 3 meningioma: A randomized phase II study of the EORTC Brain Tumor Group (EORTC-1320-BTG). *Neuro-Oncology, 24*, 755–767. https://doi.org/10.1093/neuonc/noab243 (accessed on 16th July 2025).

23. Priebe, H. (2016). High versus low technology in assessment of endotracheal tube position. *Anesthesiology, 125*(6), 1246–1247. https://www.semanticscholar.org/paper/d022a536429e06a584a3f6c4b5968ec72afaccb4 (accessed on 16th July 2025).

24. Ramli, M. I., Hamzaid, N. A., Engkasan, J. P., & Usman, J. (2023). Respiratory muscle training: A bibliometric analysis of 60 years' multidisciplinary journey. *BioMedical Engineering OnLine, 22*. https://doi.org/10.1186/s12938-023-01103-0 (accessed on 16th July 2025).

25. Rohrig, S., Lancé, M., & Malmstrom, M. F. (2020). Surgical intensive care–current and future challenges? *Qatar Medical Journal, 2019*. https://www.semanticscholar.org/paper/a44f7f9cea040d0870d8c043ce8a1494eb429ad8 (accessed on 16th July 2025).

26. Rolfe, S. (2019). The importance of respiratory rate monitoring. *British Journal of Nursing, 28*, 504–508. https://doi.org/10.12968/bjon.2019.28.8.504 (accessed on 16th July 2025).

27. Rotevatn, A. Ø., Eagan, T., Tangedal, S., Husebø, G., Ostridge, K., & Nielsen, R. (2025). Gut microbiota in chronic obstructive pulmonary disease varies by CT-verified emphysema status. *European Clinical Respiratory Journal, 12*. https://www.semanticscholar.org/paper/78d06ad52b612d4ef30b28284e3ed5bb5a86446f (accessed on 16th July 2025).

28. Schnell, J., Beer, M., Eggeling, S., Gesierich, W., Gottlieb, J., Herth, F. J. F., Hofmann, H. S., et al. (2018). Management of spontaneous pneumothorax and post-interventional pneumothorax: German S3 guideline. *Respiration, 97*, 370–402. https://doi.org/10.1159/000490179 (accessed on 16th July 2025).

29. Shadmi, E., Chen, Y., Dourado, I., Faran-Perach, I., Furler, J., Hangoma, P., Hanvoravongchai, P., et al. (2020). Health equity and COVID-19: Global perspectives. *International Journal for Equity in Health, 19*. https://doi.org/10.1186/s12939-020-01218-z (accessed on 16th July 2025).

30. Taplitz, R., Kennedy, E. B., Bow, E. J., Crews, J. R., Gleason, C., Hawley, D. K., Langston, A., et al. (2018). Outpatient management of fever and neutropenia in adults treated for malignancy: American Society of Clinical Oncology and Infectious Diseases Society of America clinical practice guideline update. *Journal of Clinical Oncology, 36*, 1443–1453. https://doi.org/10.1200/jco.2017.77.6211 (accessed on 16th July 2025).

31. Thillai, M., Atkins, C., Crawshaw, A., Hart, S. P., Ho, L. P., Kouranos, V., Patterson, K., et al. (2020). BTS clinical statement on pulmonary sarcoidosis. *Thorax, 76*, 4–20. https://doi.org/10.1136/thoraxjnl-2019-214348 (accessed on 16th July 2025).

32. van Stralen, D., & Mercer, T. (2021). Common sense high reliability organizing (HRO) in the response to COVID-19. *Neonatology Today, 16*, 90–102. https://doi.org/10.51362/neonatology.today/2021716790102 (accessed on 16th July 2025).

33. Vetrugno, L., Baciarello, M., Bignami, E., Bonetti, A., Saturno, F., Orso, D., Girometti, R., et al. (2020). The "pandemic" increase in lung ultrasound use in response to COVID-19: Can we complement computed tomography findings? A narrative review. *The Ultrasound Journal, 12*. https://doi.org/10.1186/s13089-020-00185-4 (accessed on 16th July 2025).

34. Younes, S., Ahmed, N., Ahmed, I., & Hassan, E. (2022). Effect of multimodality chest physiotherapy interventions on prevention of ventilator associated pneumonia among mechanically ventilated patients. *Alexandria Scientific Nursing Journal, 24*, 36–46. https://doi.org/10.21608/asalexu.2022.246005 (accessed on 16th July 2025).

CARDIOVASCULAR SYSTEM ASSESSMENT IN NURSING

11

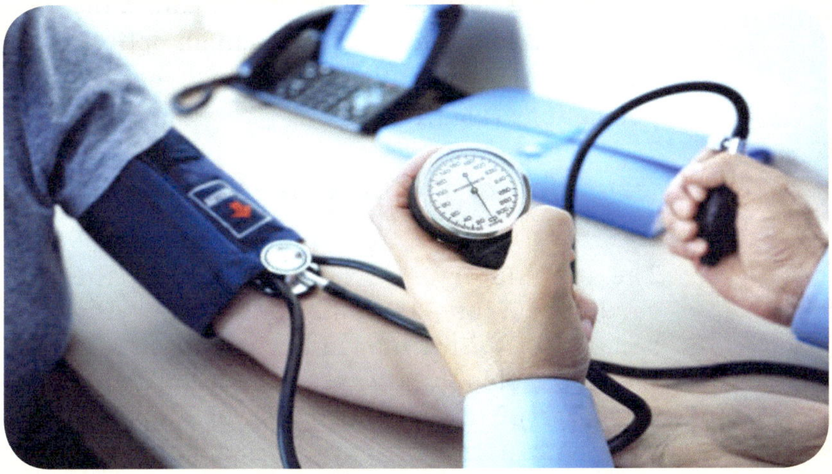

LEARNING OBJECTIVES

After studying this chapter, you will be able to:

1. Illustrate the anatomy of the cardiovascular system;
2. Elaborate the physiology of the cardiovascular system;
3. Give importance of cardiovascular assessment;
4. Explain the techniques for cardiovascular assessment;
5. Identify the common cardiovascular conditions;
6. Explore the nursing interventions in cardiovascular care.

Introduction

The cardiovascular system is at the center of human physiology and is integral to maintaining homeostasis and overall organ function. In nursing practice, thorough assessment of the cardiovascular system is integral to early detection of potential health issues, particularly with the high prevalence of cardiovascular disease in a wide variety of populations. Cardiovascular assessment comprises a set of evaluations that are utilized to assist clinicians in assessing heart health as well as confirm diseases that are likely to place patients at risk of developing critical illnesses, such as heart failure or myocardial infarction. The nursing practitioners must be proficient in utilizing both the clinical data and assessment techniques in monitoring and caring for patients' cardiovascular health. These efforts are essential in the regions where cardiovascular disease is prevalent, like Saudi Arabia, where risk factors like hypertension and obesity are horrifyingly prevalent (Clark et al., 2012). Also, understanding the unique demographic factors influencing cardiovascular health is a must in nursing assessment. For instance, sex variations have been noted in the prevalence and risk of cardiovascular disease, which necessitates a sex-specific approach to management and assessment. Women, particularly in certain cultures, may face specific impediments to receiving cardiovascular health care and thus become under-diagnosed and poorly managed for their illness. The intersection of gender, culture, and disease prompts nurses to conduct cardiovascular assessment with culturally sensitive care.

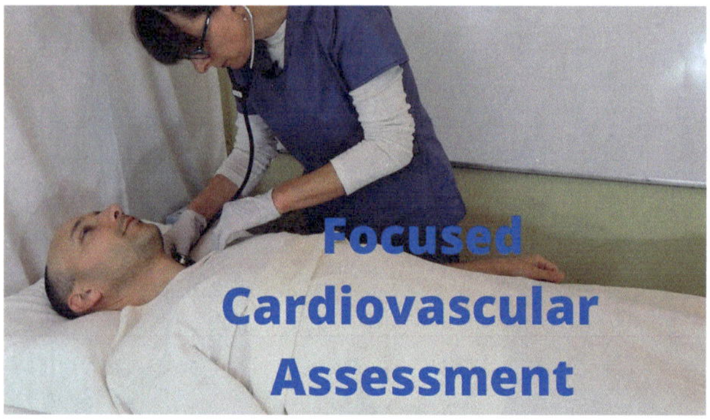

Figure 11.1. Focused cardiovascular physical assessment.

Source: https://i.ytimg.com/vi/qFTuK_rscyY/maxresdefault.jpg.

This comprehension is crucial since it directly influences clinical decision-making and enables healthcare providers to properly address the nuances of cardiovascular health among multiethnic groups (Clark et al., 2012). In addition to cultural considerations, the integration of evidence-based practice is the key to the advancement of cardiovascular assessment in nursing. Applying guidelines established via consensus statements from specialist panels has the potential to streamline and standardize assessment protocols such that nursing examinations are in compliance with modern best practices. Applying such evidence-based guidelines can make a big difference in improving patient care quality, particularly for complex cases such as community-acquired pneumonia patients who are most likely to develop cardiovascular complications. By grounding nursing assessments in evidence-based research and professional consensus, nurses are able to not only deliver effective patient management but also guide the broader conversation when it comes to cardiovascular health. This comprehensive process culminates in improved health outcomes, which affirm the global mission of nursing to maintain optimal well-being across all categories of patient populations (Figure 11.1).

Definition of the Cardiovascular System

The circulatory system, or rather the cardiovascular system, maintains the homeostasis of the human body. It consists of the blood, blood vessels, and the heart and is in charge of the collective task of supplying cells with nutrients, oxygen, and hormones and eliminating waste products such as carbon dioxide and metabolic byproducts. The heart is the organ employed in the transport of blood, which is based on a complex rhythm of relaxation and contraction, otherwise known as the cardiac cycle. Blood vessels, including arteries, veins, and capillaries, constitute a vast network employed to distribute and return blood to the body, demonstrating the dynamic and integrated nature of this system. Aside from its general role in circulation, the cardiovascular system is tightly interlinked with other physiological variables and conditions, and thus is of considerable relevance to the focus of nursing study. For instance, prevalence of multimorbidity patterns, particularly those with cardiovascular and metabolic diseases, is commonly seen in daily clinical practice, and thus it is essential to identify relationships among diseases and their impacts on patients (Shawn et al., 2021). Cardiovascular health is affected by a multitude of factors such as genetics, lifestyle, and the environment that may give rise to such pathologies as hypertension, coronary artery disease, and heart failure. Therefore, nursing diagnostics need not only ascertain the cardiovascular system's physiological status but also incorporate these broader determinants of health in order to deliver holistic care. Effective cardiovascular system assessment entails the use of various diagnostic techniques and clinical guidelines that enable nursing clinicians to identify abnormalities and prepare patients' care effectively. Clinical practice guidelines, such as those in the critical care setting, enhance complete understanding of the cardiovascular function in facilitating treatment decisions (John et al., 2018). This entails auscultation, the recording of electrocardiograms (ECGs), and vital sign monitoring in an attempt to assess heart sounds. Through the provision of the definitions as well as functions of the cardiovascular system to nursing practitioners, they are able to enhance patient outcomes through early detection and treatment of cardiovascular diseases, thus enhancing improved quality of care in most healthcare institutions.

Importance of Cardiovascular Assessment in Nursing

A thorough cardiovascular assessment is crucial for nurses because it directly influences patient outcomes and the quality of care itself. By systematically assessing heart function as well as the cardiovascular system overall, nurses can identify health issues before they become serious, so they can initiate interventions early enough not to cause additional complications. The integration of cardiovascular assessment skills into clinical practice not only enhances clinical judgment but also encourages the holistic model of care so critical in the nursing profession as well. The use of standardized models of assessment, such as the core curriculum developed to direct nurse education in the cardiovascular setting, enables nurses to weigh their assessments based on the most current best practices. As it is explained in newer evidence, the stronger learning foundation in these assessments is correlated with increased patient mortality rates, hence highlighting the need for proper training in this significant branch of nursing education (Astin et al., 2015). Moreover, the understanding of the intricacies of cardiovascular diseases is imperative for nurses, especially when caring for complex patients with chronic diseases. In heart failure, for instance, comprehensive assessment allows nurses to recognize appropriate plans of care and facilitate the informed discussion of end-of-life decisions, an issue that is at times sensitive and warrants expertise. Outcomes of a quality improvement project indicate that nurses reported higher intention to utilize knowledge of assessment effectively in practice, and its prominence is underscored (Battah et al., 2016). Such education not only empowers nurses with the confidence to address patient symptoms but also enhances their ability to provide supportive care appropriate to the unique needs of each patient and that ultimately leads to enhanced health outcomes. In addition, cardiovascular assessment is inherently intertwined with the larger goals of nursing, including patient education and advocacy. By excelling in cardiovascular assessment, nurses can empower patients with information on disease and risk factor management as well as motivate patients to self-manage and follow treatment regimens. The education role is crucial since it gives patients the empowerment, they need to be actively involved in their own health care decisions, taking a sense of agency in their cardiovascular care. Also, as more nurses are involved in multidisciplinary teams, cardiovascular assessment skills may become central to the overall health plan so that cardiovascular disease prevention strategies are used in the clinic. By bridging the gap between initial education for nurses and advanced practice through comprehensive training in cardiovascular assessment, nursing practice can significantly enhance outcomes of patients in care and aid in further tackling the management of cardiovascular disease (Astin et al., 2015) (Figure 11.2).

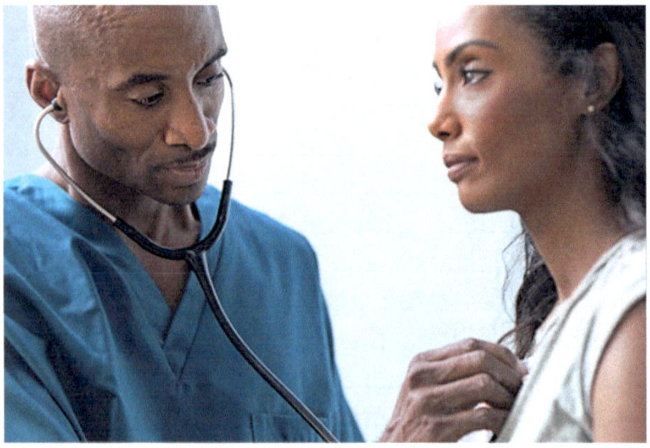

Figure 11.2. Cardiovascular assessment in nursing.

Source: https://external-content.duckduckgo.com/iu/?u=https%3A%2F%2Fwww.optum.com%2Fcontent%2Fdam%2Fo4-dam%2Fimages%2Fprofessionals%2Flife-sciences%2Fnurse-listening-to-heart-1080x720.jpg&f=1&nofb=1&ipt=5c94b2d5b7d0efd799ba1a98b3ef27a1fa90b36325c3acb9729fd3179b91bbed.

11.1. Anatomy of the Cardiovascular System

Learning Outcome

1. Major Components: Heart, Blood Vessels, and Blood
2. Function of the Heart and Its Chambers
3. Role of Arteries, Veins, and Capillaries

Understanding the anatomy of the cardiovascular system is essential for nursing practitioners who conduct patient assessment and management. The complex system comprises the heart, blood vessels, and blood, which plays an integral role in maintaining the body in a state of homeostasis. The muscular organ of the heart consists of four chambers, including the right atrium, right ventricle, left atrium, and left ventricle. Each one of these chambers has various functions in circulating blood, such as the right side of the heart directing deoxygenated blood to the lungs and the left side delivering oxygenated blood to the body. This information about these structures and how they work can be used by nurses in effectively assessing cardiac function and identifying potential abnormalities, which will ultimately lead to timely interventions that can save patients. Apart from the heart, the cardiovascular system consists of a humongous amount of blood vessels categorized into arteries, veins, and capillaries. Arteries carry blood away from the heart under high pressure, whereas veins carry blood to the heart under low pressure. Capillaries are where the exchange of gas and nutrients between tissues and blood takes place. Nurses ought to be able to recognize the significance of such blood vessels and the implication of their structural role. For example, atherosclerosis, characterized by plaque deposition along the walls of arteries, can lead to significant cardiovascular events such as myocardial infarction or stroke. Thus, knowledge of the anatomy and physiology of such vascular structures is crucial for effective assessment and management in clinical nursing practice. Besides, the understanding of cardiovascular system anatomy and physiology will help a nurse recognize deviations from the norm, which is essential during patient assessment. For instance, understanding the electrical conduction system of the heart, including sinoatrial and atrioventricular nodes, is essential in recognizing arrhythmias. Nurses so trained can recognize such a symptom as palpitations or syncope and go on to perform appropriate assessments and interventions. Furthermore, because the prevalence of cardiovascular disease continues to rise, particularly among the elderly, greater expertise in cardiovascular assessment becomes increasingly requisite. To meet this requirement, standardized training programs must be implemented. Such programs may enhance the competency of nursing practitioners in conducting echocardiography and other diagnostic examinations, eventually enhancing patient care (Hanekom et al., 2017; Moon et al., 2017) (Figure 11.3).

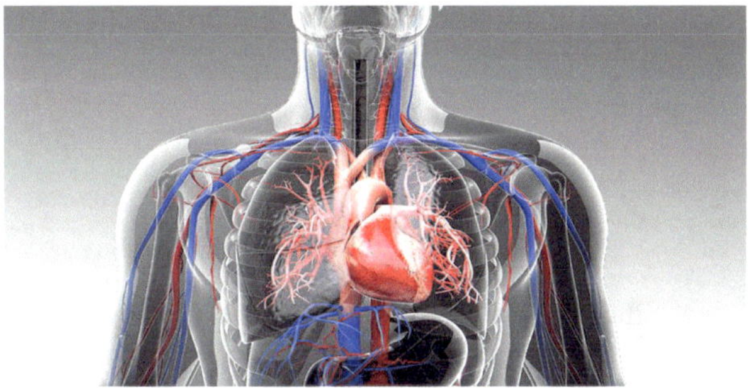

Figure 11.3. Anatomy of the cardiovascular system.

Source: https://external-content.duckduckgo.com/iu/?u=https%3A%2F%2Fbiologicallyblog.files.wordpress.com%2F2020%2F09%2Fcardiovascular-system.png&f=1&nofb=1&ipt=d61d5ce02829935aa7383e6e437867fab0bc120d8b7b7c232354bf8aa7ae7522.

11.1.1. Major Components: Heart, Blood Vessels, and Blood

The cardiovascular system is essentially composed of three major components: the heart, blood vessels, and blood, and they are each crucial for maintaining physiological homeostasis. The heart is a muscular pump organ that delivers blood to every area of the body. By executing rhythmic contractions, it ensures oxygenated blood reaches tissues as well as facilitates the return of deoxygenated blood to the lungs to become reoxygenated. The intricate structure of the heart, like its valves and chambers, is vital to the delivery of unidirectional blood flow. When assessing cardiovascular wellbeing as nursing practice, these structural and functional features need to be addressed as nursing professionals both to recognize potential abnormalities and to intervene early, thereby improving patient outcomes (Herman et al., 2025). Blood vessels include arteries, veins, and capillaries, and these are channels through which blood is conveyed in the circulatory system. Arteries carry oxygenated blood away from the heart, and veins return deoxygenated blood. Capillaries provide for the exchange of oxygen, carbon dioxide, nutrients, and waste products between tissue and blood. Central to the understanding of cardiovascular dynamics, assessment of the health and function of blood vessels is significant in nursing practice. For instance, the assessment of blood pressure and investigation for signs of vascular diseases can aid in the diagnosis of diseases such as atherosclerosis or peripheral artery disease. This assessment not only aids in the diagnosis of cardiovascular diseases but also helps in developing personalized treatment plans as per the individual needs of the patients (Ranjan et al., 2025). Another essential part of the circulatory system is blood, comprised of red blood cells, white blood cells, platelets, and plasma. All these elements work together to perform functions such as the delivery of oxygen, immune function, and clotting. While conducting nursing tests, it is necessary to test blood parameters like hematocrit levels, hemoglobin levels, and white blood cell count to assess overall health and detect potential problems. With every new technological advancement, new devices such as wearable technology and smart phone applications become inevitable to monitor the blood parameters in real time. Such technologies enhance the ability of nurses to provide prophylactic care, especially in those high-risk cardiovascular complication patients, ultimately leading to better health care management strategies (Herman et al., 2025; Ranjan et al., 2025) (Figure 11.4).

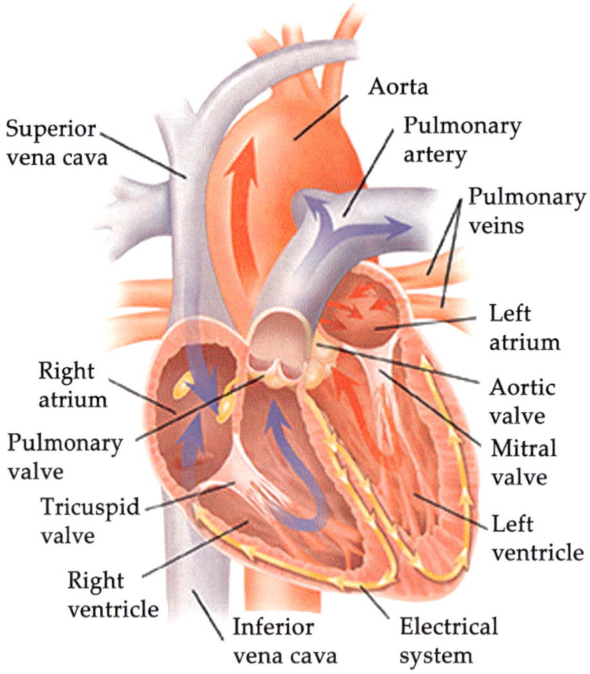

Figure 11.4. Major components: Heart, blood vessels, and blood.

Source: https://api.kramesstaywell.com/Content/ea71e7eb-cb87-49b4-826a-a5b60118a08f/medical-illustrations/Images/P01761_2.

11.1.2. Function of the Heart and Its Chambers

The heart is the central organ of the cardiovascular system, orchestrating the complex series of pumps that allow for the flow of blood throughout the body. Composed of four chambers—two atria and two ventricles—the heart functions by receiving deoxygenated blood from the body by way of the right atrium, which then transfers it to the right ventricle. The right ventricle sends this blood to the lungs to be oxygenated through the pulmonary arteries. This initial phase of the cardiac cycle is significant in ensuring adequate oxygen supply in the blood, which is needed for cellular function and overall metabolic processes. Proper understanding of heart anatomy and function is thus significant in nursing practice to allow clinicians to assess potential cardiovascular disease appropriately and understand their impacts on patient health and treatment interventions. In addition to facilitating oxygen exchange, the heart chambers also work synergistically in the mechanism of blood circulation to facilitate efficient systemic perfusion. Having been oxygenated in the lungs, oxygenated blood returns to the left atrium before being pumped into the left ventricle, which is the main pumping chamber of the heart. The left ventricle creates the greatest pressure of all the chambers, and this enables it to eject blood throughout the body via the aorta. The chambers function according to a series of physiological factors, including preload, afterload, and myocardial contractility. Nurses play a critical role in monitoring such factors, knowing how they affect heart functions, especially among patients with pre-existing cardiovascular disease or those on medication that may exacerbate such illnesses.

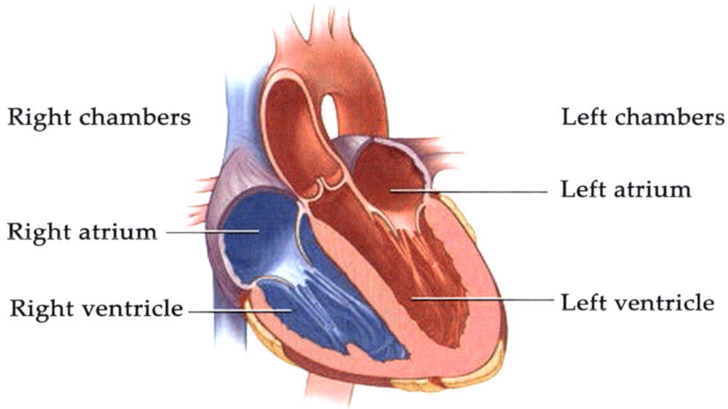

Figure 11.5. Function of the heart and its chambers.

Source: https://content.ca.healthwise.net/resources/14.2/en-ca/media/medical/hw/h9991324_001.jpg.

In addition, the intricate interaction between the hearts' chambers and systemic hemodynamics highlights the importance of an integrated approach to cardiovascular assessment in nursing. Nurses also need at their disposal a knowledge of the structural components of the heart but also of the functional implications of any dysregulation that is observed, for instance, in heart failure or arrhythmias. Interventions like are dedicated to the actions of drugs on the renin-angiotensin-aldosterone system (RAAS) and are essential to maintaining myocardial function and avoiding damage caused by heart failure.

For instance, studies have shown that angiotensin receptor antagonists may be employed to prevent myocardial dysfunction arising from tumors, highlighting how systemic interventions can benefit heart chamber function and cardiovascular stability in general (Bicer et al., 2015). Thus, a comprehensive knowledge of the function of the heart is critical for nurses when they screen and intervene against cardiovascular diseases in their clients (Figure 11.5).

11.1.3. Role of Arteries, Veins, and Capillaries

The cardiovascular system's intricate network of arteries, veins, and capillaries plays a vital role in the regulation of homeostasis and normal functioning of the body. The function of arteries is to transport oxygenated blood from the heart to various tissues for cellular metabolism purposes. The pressure-containing arteries facilitate the conditions to allow for rapid blood transport to supply needed nutrients and oxygen.

When the arteries are divided and narrowed, they then become arterioles, or blood regulators, which are constricted or dilated based on physiological demands. This regulation is necessary during the activities or exercises wherein tissues require more oxygen and nutrients in order to sustain high metabolic rates, a testament to the adaptability of the arteries to the body's needs. Conversely, veins play a vital role in returning deoxygenated blood to the heart for circulation completion. Unlike arteries, veins have less pressure and larger lumens, which enable them to hold varying volumes of blood. Venous valves prevent backflow so that blood flows against gravity, especially in the legs. The pump of skeletal muscle also drives venous return; when the skeletal muscles contract, they pump on the veins, forcing blood towards the heart.

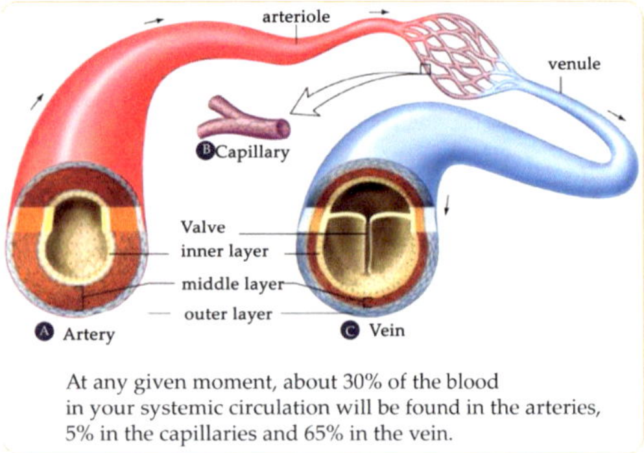

Figure 11.6. Role of arteries, veins, and capillaries.

Source: https://biology-igcse.weebly.com/uploads/1/5/0/7/15070316/9479447_orig.png.

This incredible venous system has to be functioning properly to deliver adequate preload and cardiac output, especially in disease where shifts in blood volume can make a significant impact on circulatory efficiency. Thus, venous function and its measurement are paramount aspects of cardiovascular assessment in nursing practice. Capillaries, the body's smallest blood vessels, are sites of exchange between the blood and tissues.

The thin walls, composed of one cell layer of endothelial cells, are permeable for free diffusion of oxygen, carbon dioxide, nutrients, and waste products.

The complex network of capillaries provides maximum exchange area, delivering tissues with necessary supplies required for cellular functions while at the same time removing metabolic waste. Also, the metabolic needs of the local tissue and blood flow dynamics influence capillary perfusion. Detection of color changes, temperature, and refill time in capillary refill on nursing assessment identifies underlying circulatory compromise because these are signs of the health of the capillary beds.

An excellent understanding of capillary function is thus paramount in defining clinical findings of impaired tissue perfusion and offering early interventions, thereby enhancing patient outcomes in the cardiovascular scenario (Figure 11.6).

Test Your Knowledge

1. What are the major structures of the cardiovascular system, including the heart, blood vessels, and circulation pathways, and how do they function together?
2. How does understanding the anatomy of the cardiovascular system assist in identifying abnormalities during assessment?

11.2. Physiology of the Cardiovascular System

Learning Outcome

1. Blood Circulation Process
2. Cardiac Cycle and Its Phases
3. Regulation of Heart Rate and Blood Pressure

The cardiovascular system is an orderly network that maintains homeostasis in the body. It comprises the heart, blood vessels, and blood, each with a specific function in the circulation of oxygen, nutrients, and waste products. The heart is a muscular pump that contract-rhythmically to pump blood through a highly ordered network of capillaries, veins, and arteries. It not only guarantees oxygen supply to tissues but also helps in carbon dioxide and metabolic waste removal. It is important for nursing professionals who assess cardiovascular health as any abnormality may be a reflection of underlying pathophysiologies that require intervention. Secondly, proper knowledge of cardiovascular mechanics also allows nurses to recognize normal vs. abnormal findings during tests, maximizing their ability for good patient care and better clinical outcomes. The structure of hearts is the key to its functioning, as the distinct form of the atria, ventricles, valves, and conduction system all contribute to good blood flow. The atrioventricular and semilunar valves control one-way blood flow, and the electrical conduction system, which consists of the sinoatrial and atrioventricular nodes, controls the rhythms of the hearts. These structures work collaboratively to supply a uniform cardiac output needed to sustain body functions. Nurses must be skilled in the detection of possible interference with this complex balance, such as arrhythmias or valve dysfunction, which can cause diminished patient well-being. As acknowledged in existing research, greater understanding of combined medical knowledge regarding cardiovascular physiology is crucial for nurses in order to appropriately interpret information from tests and make proper clinical judgments regarding patient care (Hanekom et al., 2017). Additionally, the interface between the cardiovascular system and other bodily systems further emphasizes its significance in overall health. The cardiovascular system is closely interwoven with the respiratory system where gas exchange occurs and with the endocrine and renal systems for blood pressure and volume control.

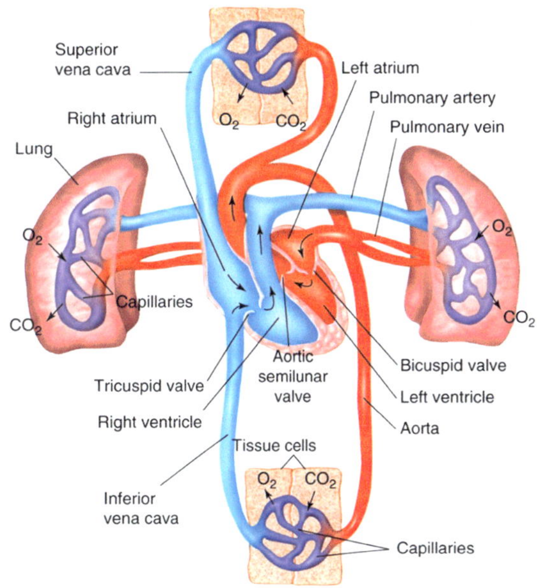

Figure 11.7. Physiology of the cardiovascular system.

Source: https://www.accessscience.com/binary/mheasworks/e2808a329af3607e/d8ddfceae18ba1859ae07bd6d2c020028d4dce0b146b6797e9600681f4b2af08/109900FG0050.jpg.

Defects in this system have important implications for patient management. For instance, chronic heart failure leads to fluid accumulation involving several organ systems and thus requires a multidimensional assessment approach to nursing care. As nurses play a core role in monitoring hemodynamic status of patients and managing complications, understanding the physiology of cardiovascular is crucial. This helps nurses to provide holistic care that respects the complexity of their patients' conditions, as would be desirable in guidelines for continued professional practice and interprofessional collaboration in critical care settings (Aristarán et al., 2016) (Figure 11.7).

11.2.1. Blood Circulation Process

Circulation of blood is the cornerstone of the functioning of a cardiovascular system, and it is a significant aspect in patient assessment in a clinical practice. Circulation of blood is an ongoing process by which oxygenated blood is carried from the heart through arteries to tissues and organs and then deoxygenated blood is returned to the heart through veins. This dynamic process is directly responsible for the exchange of oxygen and carbon dioxide, thereby guaranteeing cellular metabolism and overall homeostasis. Nurses are primarily responsible for monitoring this process because they are often the first medical staff to identify possible circulatory disruptions, including those caused by hypovolemic shock or cardiovascular disease. Understanding the intricacies of circulatory blood allows nurses to provide effective interventions and patient education, especially in the critical issue of lifestyle modification that affects cardiovascular health. Through a deep understanding of circulatory blood, there is a direct correlation with the promotion of exercise as a healthy behavior and is most important in preventing chronic disease.

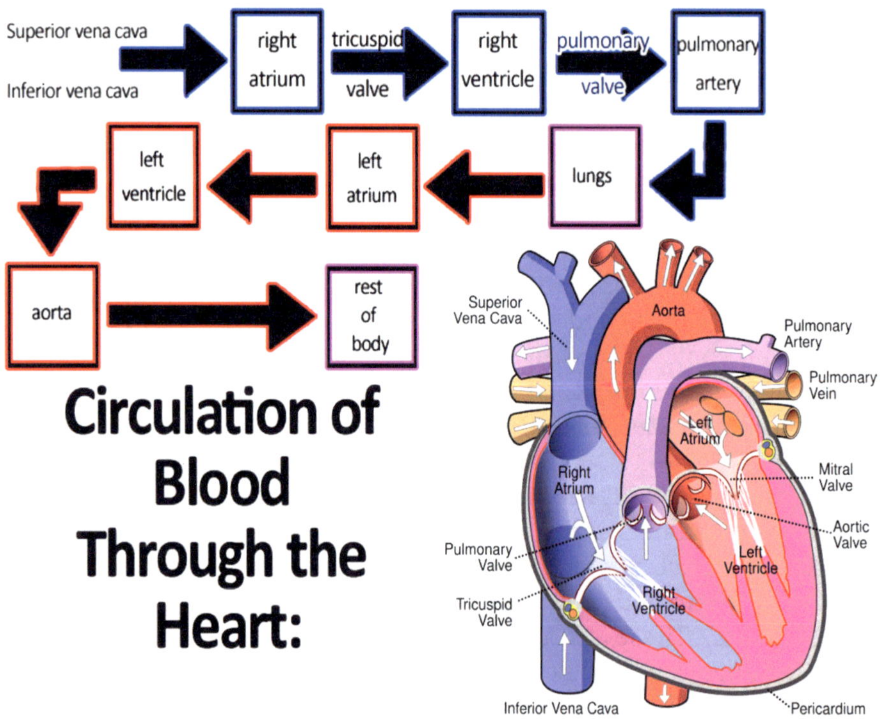

Figure 11.8. Blood circulation process.

Source: https://study.com/cimages/multimages/16/circulation_of_blood_through_the2680280700669290105.jpg.

The modifiability of the cardiovascular systems is highly facilitated by regular physical exercise, which optimizes blood circulation efficiency. Supported by evidence, acute care nurses can integrate patient education regarding the necessity for physical exercise as guidelines provide recommendations for exercising for 30 minutes on most weekdays (Bayles et al., 2012). However, a significant percentage of nurses consider counseling on physical activity to be less important compared to other forms of care. This indicates the need for additional training and emphasis on the significance of physical exercise in nursing education, such that nurses are adequately equipped to counsel patients and comprehend the implications of circulation dynamics on overall health outcomes. In more complex clinical situations, such as the care of patients with significant burn injuries, information on blood circulation is all the more important. Burned patients, as discussed in case studies, typically experience significant alterations in circulation due to the loss of fluid and consequent inflammatory reaction to such injury (Cox et al., 2015). Such a combination of variables demonstrates how imperative it is to rapidly and accurately evaluate blood circulation as part of nursing care. Nurses must be competent to detect signs of impaired circulation, i.e., changes in blood pressure, heart rate, and perfusion, in order to trigger immediate interventions. They must also intervene against the risk of complications such as infection and wound healing impairment that can arise due to impaired circulation. Thorough evaluation of the cardiovascular system thus becomes the fulcrum in delivering high-quality nursing care, particularly for high-risk patient groups (Figure 11.8).

11.2.2. Cardiac Cycle and Its Phases

Cardiac cycle is a series of events that the heart undergoes during one complete heartbeat, such as diastole and systole during both atria and ventricles. Ventricular filling, isovolumetric contraction, ventricular ejection, and isovolumetric relaxation are the major phases of the cardiac cycle. One has to be aware of each phase in order to perform nursing assessment as small abnormalities can hint towards associated cardiovascular diseases. During diastole, the heart muscles are able to relax, and the chambers will be filled with blood—contracting atria pump blood into the ventricles, basically preparing the heart for the subsequent strong contraction. This is a vital period of filling since it sets the tone for the stroke volume and cardiac output during systole when the heart contracts to pump oxygenated blood to the body tissues. Deep analysis of these phases can be of great help in identifying patient health and potential heart problems. The isovolumetric contraction phase follows diastole when ventricles begin to contract without changing volume because all heart valves are shut off. This phase is crucial as it generates pressure necessary to open aortic and pulmonary valves through which the blood can be forced out of the ventricles. In nursing assessment, it is important to evaluate the contractility and time of this contraction since it can help identify such pathologies as left ventricular hypertrophy or other issues that compromise contractility. To observe changes within this phase, therefore, guarantees early detection of potential heart failures or blockages. Similarly, the subsequent ventricular ejection period can provide valuable information in terms of cardiac performance, as any deviation may be indicative of mechanical dysfunction or impaired cardiac output, which will need subsequent diagnostic tests within a clinical setting. Finally, the cardiac cycle is concluded by isovolumetric relaxation, whereby the ventricles relax following blood ejection. This period is important in allowing the chambers to ready themselves for the subsequent filling cycle. When taking patient assessment, nurses must monitor the effectiveness with which the heart transitions from these cycles—here, impairments may reveal such conditions as diastolic dysfunction. Proper interpretation of clinical signs at stages of the cardiac cycle is paramount to the assessment of risk factors for cardiac failure, as highlighted in nursing literature. As an example, research emphasizes the clinical relevance of teaching interventions to improve heart failure care, a field supported in turn by an understanding of these cardiac dynamics (McCord et al., 2017). Overall, detailed knowledge of cardiac phases guides nursing assessment and enhances early identification and treatment of cardiovascular disease (Despins et al., 2019) (Figure 11.9).

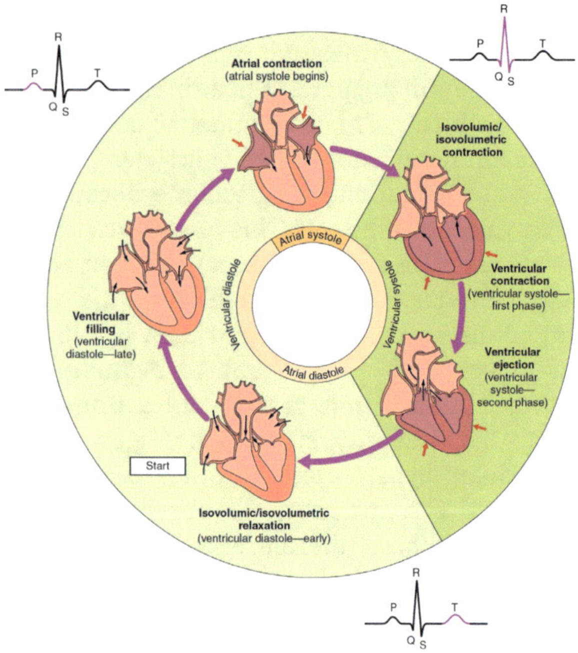

Figure 11.9. Cardiac cycle and its phases.

Source: https://upload.wikimedia.org/wikipedia/commons/3/38/2027_Phases_of_the_Cardiac_Cycle.jpg.

11.2.3. Regulation of Heart Rate and Blood Pressure

Regulation of blood pressure and heart rate is a very complex process that is involved in the maintenance of homeostasis within the cardiovascular system. The autonomic nervous system is accountable for it, and both the sympathetic and parasympathetic divisions act in opposite directions. Sympathetic nervous system increases heart rate and contractility through the discharge of catecholamines, predominantly epinephrine and norepinephrine, which stimulate beta-adrenergic receptors. Conversely, the parasympathetic nervous system, via the vagus nerve in particular, reduces heart rate through the release of acetylcholine. This tension and relaxation dynamic sees the body's response to either stress or relaxation and illustrates how heart rate changes in accordance with both physiological demand and emotional states. Sufficient perfusion of critical organs is maintained through efficient regulation, helping to prevent dysregulatory complications such as hypertension or heart failure. This is something to take into account while evaluating the cardiovascular system in practice nursing. Blood pressure regulation is also significant and involves several mechanisms, that is, neural, hormonal, and renal mechanisms. Baroreceptors in the carotid arteries and aorta detect changes in blood pressure and transmit signals to the central nervous system that elicit reflexive responses immediately. Hormones such as aldosterone, renin, and angiotensin also regulate long-term blood pressure through control of vascular resistance and fluid balance. For instance, the renin-angiotensin-aldosterone system (RAAS) is activated by falling blood pressure and results in sodium retention, which increases blood volume. Furthermore, physical exercise, diet, and psychological state may influence these regulatory systems. Understanding these mechanisms underlies effective nursing assessment in cardiovascular health, as they help identify risks and tailor appropriate interventions for hypotension- or hypertension-affected patients. In reality, cardiovascular screening and blood pressure checking are not technical, per se, processes but a significant overall assessment of cardiovascular function. The addition of extended cardiovascular testing such as resting electrocardiograms (ECG) and thorough health histories allows nurses to identify underlying abnormalities such as arrhythmias or hypertrophic cardiomyopathy that can lead to sudden cardiac death in athletes (Basavarajaiah et al., 2010). Furthermore, recognition of the impact of cardiovascular risk factors such as diabetes and hyperlipidemia is key in individualized care provision. Nurses are not only required to monitor these parameters but also understand their implications in relation to specific patients' health status. This holistic approach can aid early intervention and lifestyle change education to patients, hence enhanced cardiovascular health outcomes and overall well-being (Adlard et al., 2005).

Test Your Knowledge

1. How do cardiac output, heart rate, and vascular resistance work together to maintain adequate tissue perfusion?
2. What physiological mechanisms regulate blood pressure and blood flow in the body?

11.3. Importance of Cardiovascular Assessment

Learning Outcome

1. Early Detection of Cardiovascular Diseases
2. Monitoring Patient Health Status
3. Guiding Treatment and Intervention Strategies

Accurate cardiovascular assessment is most critical in the practice of nursing because it is a fundamental component utilized in identifying potential health issues before they turn into complicated diseases. Nurses have the crucial task of carrying out thorough assessments that involve taking a patient's history, conducting a physical examination, and using diagnostic tools. The well-being of a person's cardiovascular system may be an indication of that individual's general health, and thus early identification of abnormalities is essential. Strong assessment skills enable nurses to identify risk factors, such as hypertension or arrhythmias, which may lead to severe complications if not controlled. Through systematic approaches to cardiovascular assessment, nurses contribute to the provision of preventive care, compliance with healthcare guidelines, and improved patient outcomes, reflecting nursing's foundational mission to improve comprehensive health. Cardiovascular assessment is even more crucial in specialist groups, such as critically ill or athletic populations. In intensive care situations, for instance, precise assessments are central to the management of complicated health conditions, such as those of community-acquired pneumonia patients. Evidence indicates that expert consensus has noted the significance of stringent physiotherapy and assessment methods in these situations, describing the extremely interdependent nature of cardiovascular and respiratory medicine (Braun et al., 2018). Similarly, young athletes must undergo rigorous screening for potential cardiovascular defects which can lead to sudden cardiac death, which points towards the appropriateness of employing instruments like resting 12-lead electrocardiogram as an evaluation tool (Basavarajaiah et al., 2010). All these are illustrations of the utility of cardiovascular examination in multiple clinical scenarios, having significant impact on both short-term and long-term health outcomes. Other than improving patient care, cardiovascular assessment facilitates evidence-based nursing practice culture among nurses. By integrating results of prior research and clinical guidelines into daily assessments, nursing decision-making is improved. For example, the utilization of standardized tools to assess heart sounds or blood pressure not only improves consistency in care but also permits greater reliability in detecting abnormal results. These habits play a significant function in shaping a firm foundation for interventions that are specific to patient need. Further, professional and continuing cardiovascular education equip nurses with high-level competencies for effectively representing their patients. Through embracing an all-encompassing and evidence-based process of cardiovascular assessment, nurses are capable of directly impacting patients' health, corroborating the significance of this practice within the greater nursing framework (Figure 11.10).

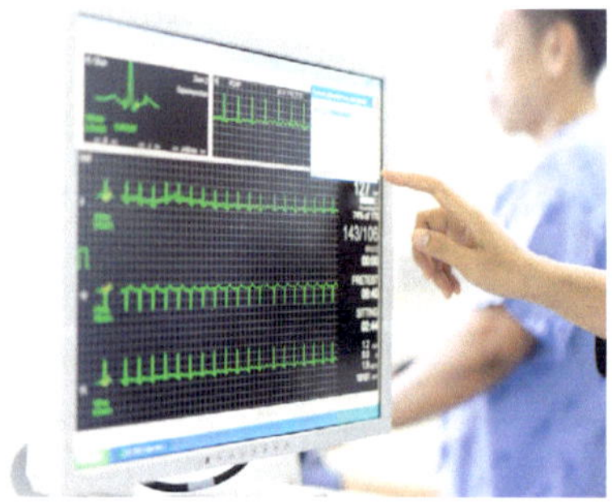

Figure 11.10. Importance of cardiovascular assessment.

Source: https://www.practicenursing.com/media/qbiai0bs/assessment-and-examination-of-the-cardiovascular-system.jpg.

11.3.1. Early Detection of Cardiovascular Diseases

Early detection of cardiovascular diseases (CVD) is an essential feature in the nursing practice because it directly relates to better patient outcomes and reduced healthcare costs. Early intervention comes about through early detection, and thus, the disease is prevented from progressing. Nurses play a major role in this through conducting thorough assessments, for example, physical assessment and patient history assessment. Their experience equips them with the ability to recognize early warning features of cardiovascular distress in the form of dyspnea, chest pain, or arrhythmias. Early detection processes involving family histories and lifestyle assessments might also enable anticipatory intervention that is imperative in detecting at-risk populations. Whereas scholars debate that improved education and understanding of cardiovascular wellness are essential to boost the rates of early detection among patients, ultimately to lead towards more effective nursing processes and improved public health outcomes (N/A, 2023), technology advancements have further significantly contributed towards the processes of early detection of CVD. The integration of telemedicine and telehealth services has provided nursing practitioners with improved devices to monitor patients on a regular and real-time basis. Remote patient monitoring systems are able to offer constant monitoring of vital signs, enabling nurses to identify deviant patterns that indicate cardiovascular issues. At the onset of the COVID-19 pandemic, the use of telehealth became especially widespread, demonstrating its value in maintaining contact with patients while constantly monitoring cardiovascular health (Rashid et al., 2020). This technological advancement facilitates a participatory approach between patients and healthcare professionals, where data exchange is uncomplicated and swift, facilitating the whole process of detection. Hence, integrating these technologies in nursing practices can significantly augment early detection ability, leading to timely intervention and hospitalization reduction. Health literacy and education also play critical roles in early detection of cardiovascular diseases. Informed patients with knowledge of risk factors, signs and symptoms, and requirements for early assessment are more likely to be actively involved in their health care management. Nurses, therefore, have the role of educating patients on lifestyle modifications, such as diet and physical activity, to minimize risk factors for CVD. Promotion of health through activities like community outreach sessions and personal counseling sessions educates patients about signs and symptoms and seeks care when necessary. Besides, a good understanding of cardiovascular health enables decision-making by the patient through education, thus establishing an interprofessional practice between healthcare workers and patients, which is central to successful disease management. Utilization of patient health literacy approaches can result in impressive early detection intervention enhancement, thus building towards a healthy population (N/A, 2023).

11.3.2. Monitoring Patient Health Status

Monitoring patient health status is a vital part of nursing practice, particularly for cardiovascular system assessment. Accurate monitoring allows for continuous evaluation of a patient's cardiovascular status and facilitates timely interventions that can prevent complications. With various methods such as measurement of blood pressure, checking heart rate, and symptom observation, nurses can gather essential information that will be used in making clinical judgments. Besides, integration of technology in tracking health—either telehealth system or mobile health apps—improves the follow-up of patient recovery post-discharge. This transition towards technologically aided practice has been effective in improving patient outcomes, as evidenced from research where patients utilizing a web-based tool showed better control of chronic heart disease during early post-discharge weeks (Brown et al., 2010). Using these sophisticated tools, more tailored care can be delivered to patients, and ultimately, better health status results. The assessment of cardiovascular health status also emphasizes patient self-management in extended care. Research shows that active engagement by the patient with self-monitoring methods has a discernible effect on improved health outcomes. Self-management interventions have been proven to make patients more independent with their own health, particularly for individuals who have chronic illness such as heart disease. Health policy interventions for the promotion of health awareness on self-monitoring behavior have been linked to enhanced symptom control and quality of life in patients (Brown et al., 2010). However, there remains a broad gap in health policy regarding the promotion of self-management interventions in practice. Closing these gaps is likely to lead to more effective coordination of care and health interventions that make the most efficient use of interventions in response to patient-specific needs. Support of patient-centered models of care is thus important in advancing the nursing profession and improving cardiovascular health outcomes. Beyond this, having an integrated approach to patient monitoring of health status includes full communication between healthcare providers and patients. An assessment is not just the accumulation of quantitative information but qualitative understanding acquired from patient consultations. Patient interviews can be given useful information on lifestyle elements, mental status, and adherence to treatment regimens that can degrade cardiovascular status. Through an open discussion environment, nurses are better placed to appreciate the challenges facing patients in managing conditions. This information is particularly crucial in discussing self-management goals and resources for achieving them (Brown et al., 2010). In addition, the implementation of evidence-based policy supporting self-management and palliative care for older people can bridge the gap between research and practice to equip patients and carers with the tools to maintain the optimum health outcomes. These multidirectional efforts underscore the importance of monitoring for health status as a mutual effort, one that is central to effective cardiovascular nursing practice (Figure 11.11).

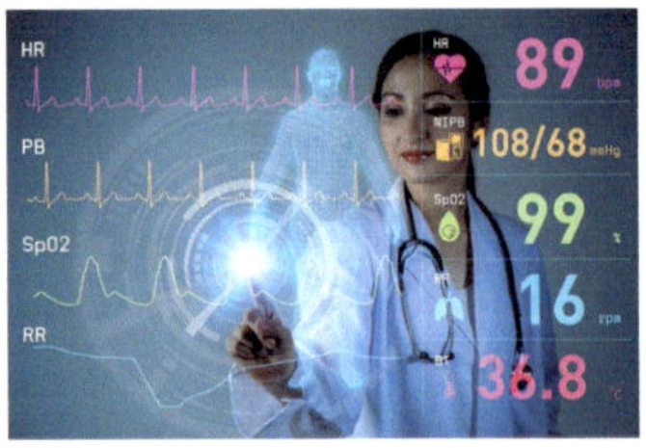

Figure 11.11. Monitoring patient health status.

Source: https://vantagemedtech.com/wp-content/uploads/patient-monitoring-system.jpg.

11.3.3. Guiding Treatment and Intervention Strategies

Effective intervention and treatment processes in cardiovascular nursing depend on comprehensive assessments and evidence-based practice that respond to individual patient needs. Nurses play a pivotal role in the delivery of care that responds to the individuality of each patient's health status, like their history and symptomatology. A significant aspect of this process is aligning nursing interventions with current best practices to ensure care that is both effective and responsive to changing patient conditions. Community nurses, for instance, must have knowledge in models of case management that promote collaboration and coordination among health professionals. These models, just like community nursing interventions, point out the necessity of ongoing learning that translates evidence into actionable measures and therefore optimizes patient outcomes in cardiovascular care (Gray et al., 2010). Moreover, informing intervention and treatment planning quite often needs the use of biomarkers in directing clinical practice. This is best exemplified by the GUIDE-IT study as they researched the level of NT-proBNP as a mechanism to tailor heart failure management. Through the provision of prognostic information, higher levels of natriuretic peptides enable clinicians to more specifically direct therapies, potentially decreasing mortality and hospitalization. The evidence indicates a trend toward biomarker-guided care resulting in an enhancement of the quality of care being given, thereby leading to an optimized use of medical resources. These approaches not only improve the determination of risk factors but also contribute to the formation of tailored treatment regimens that are aligned with existing guidelines for cardiovascular nursing (Adams et al., 2014). The implementation of these directive treatment strategies necessitates proactive responses by nurses engaged in community practice, emphasizing the necessity for continuous education and interprofessional working. In the backdrop of the evolving scenario in cardiovascular care, nurses must be geared to take on both generalist and specialist roles, particularly in fields like chronic heart care management. Real life solution-based projects in the community reveal the pitfalls in the skill transfer process and movement towards new care models. Through investment in learning which addresses the requirements of current challenges in cardiovascular assessment and intervention, nurses are positioned to significantly enhance the quality of patient care. Lastly, the integration of the new methods of evaluation and evidence-based intervention strategies has the impact of enabling nurses to address the complexities entailed in cardiovascular health while maintaining the concerns of patient care at the forefront of nursing practice (Gray et al., 2010).

Test Your Knowledge

1. Why is regular cardiovascular assessment essential for early detection of heart and vascular diseases?
2. How can assessment findings guide clinical decision-making and patient management?

11.4. Techniques for Cardiovascular Assessment

Learning Outcome

1. Patient History and Physical Examination
2. Use of Diagnostic Tools: ECG, Echocardiogram, and Blood Tests
3. Interpretation of Assessment Findings

Careful assessment of the cardiovascular system plays a crucial role in nursing practice, particularly patient identification and management at risk of heart disease. Among the fundamental methods employed are patient history review and physical assessment, which enable nurses to gather full information about the patient's cardiovascular status. The essential component of this assessment is awareness about the patient's medical history, i.e., previous cardiovascular events, risk factors such as hypertension, diabetes, or cardiovascular disease family history. In addition to this, physical examination includes vital signs, heart sounds, and peripheral pulses, which can provide information on abnormal patterns indicative of underlying cardiovascular disease. Detection of issues early helps in intervention at the right time, which is necessary to allow improved patient outcomes. Therefore, an integral means of gathering clinical information is necessary to preserve effective cardiovascular assessment in nursing practice. In addition to standard assessment processes, more recently developed techniques such as electrocardiograms (ECGs) and echocardiograms significantly enhance the nurses ability to evaluate cardiovascular function. An ECG is necessary to identify arrhythmias, ischemic alterations, or signs of previous myocardial infarction, which provides vital information concerning the electrical activity of the heart. Its expedient and non-invasive nature make ECG a valuable resource in acute care. Echocardiography takes this assessment further by examining cardiac structures and assessing hemodynamic function. it is capable of revealing invaluable information regarding chamber size, abnormalities in wall motion, and valve function, which aids in decision-making. This multifaceted approach further develops nurses' capacity for evidence-based practice, ultimately leading to improved cardiovascular management and patient safety. Further, the role of patient education in cardiovascular assessment practices cannot be overstated. Nurses are pivotal in teaching patients about risk factors and prevention measures in cardiovascular health. These include counseling patients on lifestyle modification such as diet change, exercise, and smoking cessation, compliance with medication and return visits.

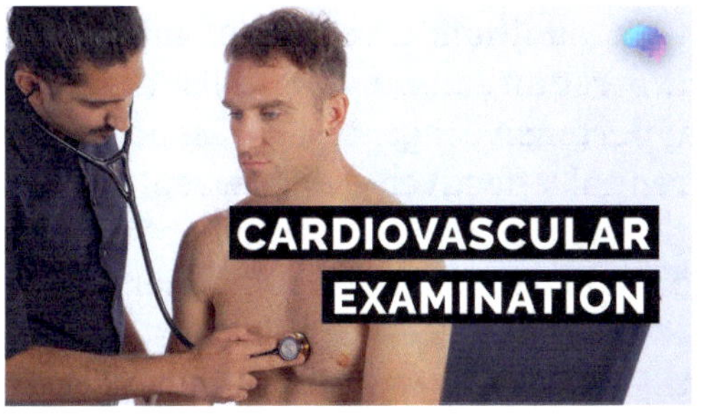

Figure 11.12. Techniques for cardiovascular assessment.

Source: https://i.ytimg.com/vi/rqdQV2M60ec/hq720.jpg?sqp=-oaymwEhCK4FEIIDSFryq4qpAxMIARUAAAAAGAElAADIQj0AgKJD&rs=AOn4CLDfAmKcZrvS4G9rHC2galGILquekQ.

By engaging patients in their own care, nurses help foster responsibility and knowledge that can lead to healthier outcomes. As cardiovascular diseases remain one of the primary contributors to morbidity and mortality worldwide, it is essential to employ a holistic strategy that encompasses not just technical skills of assessment but also patient education. Finally, this combined approach is appealing in light of the growing emphasis on prevention and management initiatives that are attuned to the complexities of cardiovascular health, as recognized in contemporary studies with culturally appropriate concerns over health practices and conduct, particularly in mixed populations (Clark et al., 2012) (Figure 11.12).

11.4.1. Patient History and Physical Examination

A thorough patient history is essential in assessing the cardiovascular system since it lays the foundation for acquiring information on the patients overall state of health and risk factors. Patient medical histories tend to yield vital information regarding their cardiovascular status, including previous diseases of hypertension, hyperlipidemia, or diabetes, all of which significantly impact the health of the heart. In addition, a record of medication is specific requirement; it entails that certain antihypertensive agents are associated with differential effectiveness between population groups, such as in the illustration of the varying response in African American patients (Allman et al., 2015). Awareness of family history can also identify inherited conditions that predispose to cardiovascular complications, highlighting the importance of genetic factors in patient assessment. By fully taking a patient history, nurses can identify red flags that need to be explored further, which eventually leads to the design of an individualized care plan. The physical examination supplements the patient history by conducting an objective assessment of the cardiovascular system. During this process, vital signs like blood pressure and heart rate are taken with care in order to detect any abnormalities. As an example, the presence of elevated systolic blood pressure (SBP) can indicate impending hypertension, which is prevalent in heterogeneous groups, like older African American individuals, with greater mean SBP compared to their white counterparts (Allman et al., 2015). Furthermore, head-to-toe assessments, like heart sounds auscultation and palpation of the peripheral pulses, allow nurses to obtain valuable information about cardiac performance and circulating blood. Anomalies such as unusual noises of the heart or arrhythmias can be signs of underlying cardiovascular diseases, which must be dealt with in urgency. So, physical examination becomes a significant tool for the overall cardiovascular assessment, with subsequent timely interventions. Physical examination and patient history combined offer an integrated view of one's cardiovascular status and allow for informed clinical decisions. The interplay between subjective data gathered through interviews with the patient and objective data obtained through physical examination becomes the basis of effective nursing practice. By a holistic attitude, nurses are provoked not just to consider the physiological aspects of cardiovascular health but also the broader psychosocial context. For instance, the patient's lifestyle and stress level can affect their cardiovascular status since studies have been conducted to prove that behavior and psychosocial components are quite significant in older African American adults for SBP (Allman et al., 2015). By integrating information from both patient history and physical examination, nurses can take an active stand in advocating for more patients and ensuring that any and all cardiovascular risks are met in full. This integrated strategy is important to achieve maximum patient outcomes and enhance the quality of care in nursing practice.

11.4.2. Use of Diagnostic Tools: ECG, Echocardiogram, and Blood Tests

The utilization of diagnostic tools such as the electrocardiogram (ECG) is important when it comes to nursing diagnosis of the cardiovascular system. An ECG provides valuable information about the heart's electrical activity, allowing for arrhythmias, ischemic alterations, and other cardiac anomalies to be determined. The non-invasive procedure records the rhythm and conduction of the heart, allowing nurses to identify early detection of potential cardiac events. By interpreting ECG findings, nurses can efficiently triage patients in such a way that patients with an urgency for treatment are treated accordingly. Additionally, inclusion of ECG in standard assessment is aligned with evidence-based practice in which early diagnosis of cardiovascular disease is optimized, lowering patient morbidity and mortality in the long term (Halvorsen et al., 2022). In addition to the ECG, echocardiography is an equally valuable diagnostic tool in cardiovascular assessment. This imaging technique employs ultrasound waves to generate detailed images of the structure and function of the hearts and assess cardiac chambers, valves, and overall myocardial function.

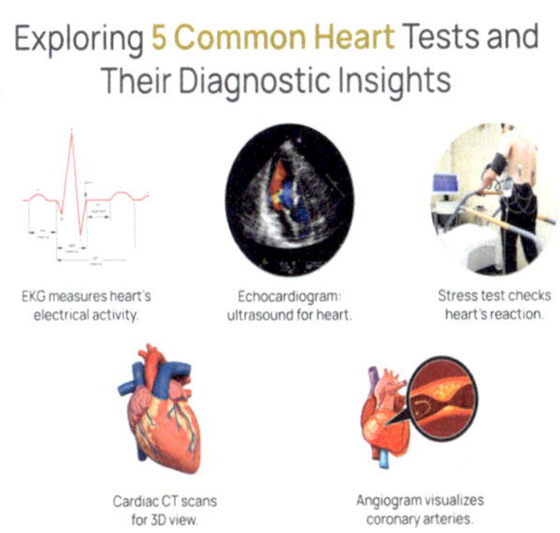

Figure 11.13. Diagnostic tools.

Source: https://sunfox.in/wp-content/uploads/2024/04/exploring-5-Common-Heart-Tests-and-Their-Diagnostic-Insights-2048x1152.jpg.

Echocardiograms can show abnormalities in keeping with heart failure, valve disease, or congenital abnormalities. For nurses, it is important to understand echocardiographic findings as they assist in interpretation and communicate pertinent information to the healthcare team. This collaborative approach assists in the development of patient-specific care plans based on the specific cardiovascular condition of patients and promotes enhanced interprofessional communication (Bryan et al., 2021). Laboratory blood tests are a vital part of cardiovascular examination, providing information regarding many biomarkers indicating cardiac status. These markers include troponin levels, brain natriuretic peptide (BNP), and lipid profile through which nurses assess myocardial injury, risk of heart failure, and total cholesterol, respectively. The emergency assessment of these blood markers is crucial in distinguishing between different types of cardiac disease and guiding treatment. Not only do nurses order such markers, but they also inform patients about their implications and significance. By creating a general impression of the results, nurses facilitate decision-making processes that assist in well-informed practices, allowing patients to maintain an effective control over their cardiovascular health (Halvorsen et al., 2022) (Figure 11.13).

11.4.3. Interpretation of Assessment Findings

Interpretation of test findings within the cardiovascular system is a crucial aspect of effective nursing practice, particularly in identifying the presence of underlying health issues and informing clinical decision-making. Systematic observations allow nurses to gain such vital information as heart rate, blood pressure, and the absence or presence of any abnormal murmurs or sounds upon auscultation. The findings provide a foundation for clinical judgment and inform interventions tailored to each patient's specific needs. Because the cardiovascular disease is multifactorial in nature, the ability to properly interpret these test results can make a significant difference in a patient's treatment plan. Additionally, inputs such as patient history and risk profiles should also be integrated during assessment to enhance clinical understanding and deliver comprehensive care. This integrative process not only improves the patient's outcome but also improves the continuous development of nursing competencies and application of evidence-based practice within cardiovascular care. One of the distinguishing aspects of the interpretation of results from cardiovascular assessment is the application of standard frameworks that allow for the establishment of clinical boundaries. For instance, consensus by experts on assessment and treatment protocols, such as those in physiotherapy for intubation patients, provides proof for best practice when evaluating cardiovascular status in diverse populations. Practitioner use of findings from research such as that discussed by Braun et al. (2018) is encouraging practitioners to adopt a consistent procedure when evaluating cardiovascular status, offering a complete report both subjective and objective. With the utilization of systematic reporting of assessment findings, nurses not only facilitate good communication with interprofessional teams but also enhance their professional practice in the future, thereby enhancing patient safety and care. Furthermore, ongoing education and training play an imperative role in the interpretation of cardiovascular system-related assessment findings. Nursing education still lays emphasis on the integration of clinical judgment and critical thinking skills in a manner where the students are able to make appropriate judgments and interpretations regarding cardiovascular complicated data. Efforts geared towards enhancing community nursing intervention have established the significance of the utilization of professional knowledge in cardiovascular care as referenced by Gray et al. (2010). By engaging in continuous professional development, nurses are able to refine their assessment competencies, remain updated on new findings, and accommodate revised clinical practice guidelines. Given that cardiovascular wellness is a concern globally, complying with refining better methods of assessment through evidence-based practices ultimately allows nurses to deliver quality patient care and improves the outcomes of health among different populations.

Test Your Knowledge

1. What assessment techniques are used to evaluate heart sounds, pulses, blood pressure, and circulation?
2. How can inspection, palpation, percussion, and auscultation be systematically applied to detect cardiovascular abnormalities?

11.5. Common Cardiovascular Conditions

Learning Outcome

1. Hypertension and Its Implications
2. Heart Failure and Its Management
3. Coronary Artery Disease and Risk Factors

Cardiovascular diseases represent a heterogeneous collection of heart and blood vessel disorders that fundamentally affect global health. A few of the most prevalent diseases are coronary artery disease (CAD), heart failure, arrhythmias, and hypertension. CAD, most commonly a result of atherosclerosis, leads to decreased blood supply and oxygenation of the heart muscle and significantly predisposes to myocardial infarction. Conversely, heart failure, characterized by the malfunction of the hearts to pump, is a complex problem that requires specialist nursing assessment for symptom management and education of patients. Nurses should be well-acquainted with these common conditions since they have a mandate for routine cardiovascular assessments, employing the diagnostic apparatus and the patient's history to identify early indicator signs of deterioration to ensure intervention in time and improved patient outcomes. Hypertension, also known as the silent killer, is now a significant risk factor for many cardiovascular conditions. Aside from the causative role it plays in the etiology of CAD and heart failure, high blood pressure is also implicated in the development of stroke and renal disease. The multicausal etiology of hypertension mandates the use of an integrated assessment approach, such as lifestyle, family history, and comorbidities. Nurses have a pivotal role to detect such diversified risk factors, counseling patients regarding lifestyle modification, and facilitating effective management practices. Through the implementation of evidence-based practice guidelines, for example, by the European Society of Cardiology, nurses are better able to equip patients with knowledge and skills required to properly manage their blood pressure and thereby reduce healthcare systems' burden from cardiovascular disease (Astin et al., 2015). A second common cardiovascular condition worthy of consideration is arrhythmia, which is defined by irregular heartbeats that may compromise cardiac efficiency.

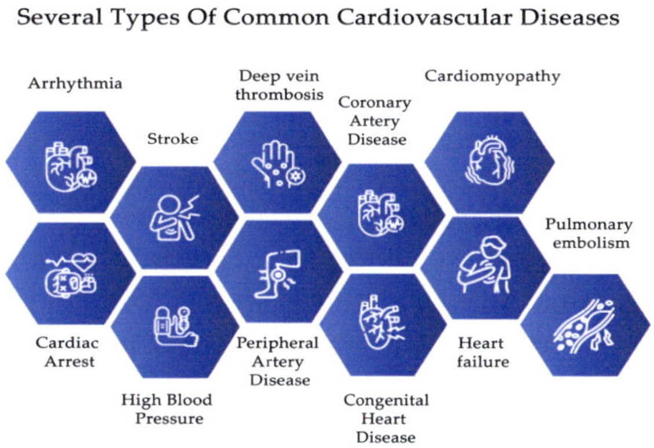

Figure 11.14. Common cardiovascular conditions.

Source: https://assets.delveinsight.com/blog/wp-content/uploads/2022/02/01102955/Several-Types-Of-Common-Cardiovascular-Diseases-01-01-01-01.png.

Disease conditions such as atrial fibrillation and ventricular tachycardia can lead to severe morbidity and mortality if not managed adequately. The nursing intervention in arrhythmia assessment involves close cardiac rhythm monitoring through electrocardiogram (ECG) trends, along with recognition of patient symptoms such as palpitations or dizziness. Given the frequency of arrhythmias in the elderly and those with prior cardiovascular disease, nursing assessment should focus not only on diagnostic diagnosis but also on patient education regarding lifestyle changes and medication adherence. By integrating these critical nursing skills into nursing curricula, as new curriculum models suggest, nurses can take a decisive role in ongoing prevention and control of adverse cardiovascular outcomes (Clark et al., 2012) (Figure 11.14).

11.5.1. Hypertension and Its Implications

Hypertension or the silent killer is a severe cardiovascular disease condition that needs to be evaluated comprehensively and controlled. Hypertension is characterized by elevated blood pressure levels that could progress to such severe complications as stroke, heart attack, and kidney failure. An effective assessment of hypertension is not only a measurement of blood pressure but also understanding the patients' overall health profile, including lifestyle, family history, and comorbidity. All these need to be incorporated into nursing practice because nurses play a key role in early detection and education of patients. Moreover, hypertension is conditioned by social factors, including cultural beliefs regarding diet and physical activity, and is affected by health behaviors at the societal level that ultimately create disease outcomes, particularly among diverse populations like Saudi women, who possess unique cardiovascular disease risk factors (Clark et al., 2012). The implications of hypertension are far-reaching beyond immediate health effects, as they reach into a wider category of social and economic consequences. Patients with inadequate control of their hypertension are likely to require ongoing medical attention, which can strain health resources and put enormous burdens on individuals and health systems. Effective management interventions, including lifestyle adjustments and adherence to prescribed pharmacotherapy, are necessary in reducing such risks. In addition, exercise cannot be overemphasized for its importance in hypertension. Current guidelines recommend at least 30 minutes of moderate physical activity most days of the week as a means of lowering blood pressure and improving cardiovascular health (Bayles et al., 2012). Nurses must be competent and informed to advise patients regarding these guidelines and to help them incorporate physical activity into daily activities. In terms of nursing education, hypertensions implications must be comprehended so as to create a workforce competent in responding to the cardiovascular care requirements. Continuing education programs must emphasize the importance of hypertension control, teaching nurses not only assessment skills but patient involvement complexities and health promotion complexities. In furtherance of this, specialized training in culturally responsive intervention can assist in providing better care to vulnerable groups such that nurses can address hypertension prevalence and treatment disparities. With hypertension being very prevalent in most populations, nursing education has to prepare future practitioners for comprehending the etiologically multifactorial nature of the disease and preparing patient-specific plans. Through such learning activities, nurses may significantly influence the outcomes of antihypertensive control, ultimately improving the quality of cardiovascular care (Clark et al., 2012).

11.5.2. Heart Failure and Its Management

The prevalence of heart failure is a clinical issue in the healthcare sector, which should be tackled by effective management strategies. Heart failure, which refers to the failure of the hearts to pump sufficient blood to meet the body's needs, can be presented with an array of underlying illnesses like coronary artery disease and high blood pressure. Effective management constitutes a multidisciplinary approach encompassing pharmacotherapy, lifestyle modifications, and patient education. Nurses are also vital to the team, not only with medication management but also with monitoring patients for side effects and symptoms and educating self-management techniques. With development of a positive nurse-patient relationship, health care providers may improve patient compliance with treatment and enhance outcomes, thereby decreasing re-admission to hospitals and enhancing quality of life for individuals with heart failure. The challenge of treating heart failure is generally in terms of needing to develop customized care plans adaptable to the specific clinical profile of every patient. This entails careful assessment of heart function through varying diagnostic tests, such as echocardiograms and biomarkers, to inform treatment. The treatment methods may also differ widely according to geographic and socioeconomic factors, such as varying health outcomes in different populations. For instance, in areas of limited access to health facilities and resources, such as rural settings, treatment-access inequalities can exacerbate the course of disease and the outcomes of morbidity. This emphasizes the necessity of specialized nursing curricula that educate nursing practitioners to address the specific demands of diverse populations, as laid out in the fundamental curriculum developed by the European Society of Cardiology and the Council on Cardiovascular Nursing and Allied Professions (Astin et al., 2015).

Moreover, effective handling of heart failure extends beyond clinical care to include more inclusive approaches that recognize psychological and social dimensions of the patient's well-being. Educational interventions for heart failure self-management can empower patients with the capacity to recognize early symptoms, make lifestyle changes, and understand medication regimens. Such empowerment is critical to improve patient outcomes and reduce the health burden of heart failure on healthcare systems, especially among diverse populations where standard care protocols might not be readily translatable. For example, cultural beliefs that impact health behaviors must be known, as these can influence quite a significant amount on treatment compliance and resultant health outcomes (Clark et al., 2008). By including these factors, nurses can provide not only clinically effective treatment but also culturally sensitive treatment, thereby enhancing the care of heart failure as a whole (Figure 11.15).

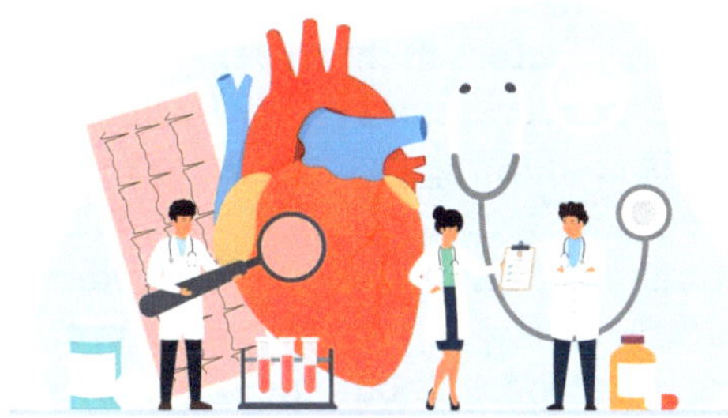

Figure 11.15. Heart failure and its management.

Source: https://external-content.duckduckgo.com/iu/?u=https%3A%2F%2Fpcna.net%2Fwp-content%2Fuploads%2F2023%2F01%2FiStock-1363685371-2-1.jpg&f=1&nofb=1&ipt=d04499c77fd7b0da0490f879ff039fcaa568d1ce8659f2f3e4ef8758b12ccf95.

11.5.3. Coronary Artery Disease and Risk Factors

The prevalence of coronary artery disease (CAD) is highly modifiable by a number of risks factors and hence warrants comprehensive cardiovascular assessment in nursing. The key modifiable risk factors include smoking, hypertension, diabetes mellitus, and dyslipidemia, all of which are involved in the process of atherogenesis. Smoking introduces harmful chemicals into the bloodstream that increase endothelial damage, leading to plaque formation in coronary arteries. Apart from that, hypertension also increases arterial stiffness and shear stress, which further augment the risk of atherosclerosis. According to an American College of Cardiology (ACC) and American Heart Association (AHA) report, detection and management of these risk factors are crucial to prevent cardiovascular morbidity and mortality (Paul et al., 2017). Given that nurses are in the frontline of healthcare, they play a central role in conducting thorough assessment to identify individuals at risk so that early intervention can stop the progression of CAD. Lifestyle choices also predominantly dictate the fate of coronary artery disease. Physical inactivity, poor nutrition, and excessive alcohol intake are contributory factors in the development of CAD. Changing conversations with patients about lifestyle is something that can help them make improved decisions to reduce their risk. Health education programs need to be implemented, particularly among high-risk groups, in an effort to raise awareness about the value of regular exercise and a heart-healthy diet. Effectively explaining these lifestyle changes, backed by clinical guideline evidence, can enhance patients' health literacy and support compliance with recommended changes (Tom et al., 2016). Work with patients to establish a working relationship in practice nursing can allow for the delivery of patient-specific interventions aimed at the individual circumstances and possible change barriers. In addition to risk factors in the individual, genetic susceptibility is also implicated in coronary artery disease risk. CAD family history can demonstrate higher risk, with increased screening and management in these risk patients. The interaction between lifestyle factors and genetics, however, simply mirrors the multifactorial pathophysiology of CAD. Appreciation of this dualism is necessary for clinical assessment nurses, where detailed cardiovascular examination would have to incorporate both familial and lifestyle interrogation. Additionally, beyond this, ACC/AHA guidelines also emphasize the necessity for tailored care methods that are sensitive to both genetic and environmental factors (Paul et al., 2017). By integrating these observations into their practice, nurses can employ their professional role to encourage preventive measures that target not only modifiable risk factors but also recognize inherent vulnerabilities in their patient populations.

Test Your Knowledge

1. What are common cardiovascular conditions, such as hypertension, heart failure, and arrhythmias, and what are their typical assessment findings?
2. How can early recognition of cardiovascular disorders impact patient outcomes and treatment plans?

11.6. Nursing Interventions in Cardiovascular Care

Learning Outcome

1. Patient Education and Lifestyle Modifications
2. Medication Management and Adherence
3. Emergency Response and Critical Care

Effective nursing intervention is imperative in the management of cardiovascular disease patients, and an assessment plays a pivotal role. The utilization of the Roy Adaptation Model (MAR) is highly beneficial because it allows patient care to be tailored individually depending on the adaptive responses an individual exhibits when they are exposed to the state of being diseased. Nurses can examine the patient's emotional and physiological condition, which is central to developing appropriate care measures. The case of a male patient with coronary artery disease who underwent successful post-CABG surgery is an ideal one; the particular requirements and circumstances in his case were addressed using the MAR framework.

Such interventions not only guarantee better outcomes but also empower the patient to be in a position to engage in their recovery process, with a reminder that holistic care begins with thorough assessment (Muatarobin et al., 2020). In addition to the application of theoretical models, the role of a nurse involves identifying and managing cardiovascular disease risk factors. In the majority of regions, including Saudi Arabia, cardiovascular disease rates reflect overall health concerns within society, such as sedentary behavior and overweight (Clark et al., 2012). Patients need to be educated about the risk factors by nurses while creating habits that are conducive to cardiovascular health. This includes an active education plan for the patient, promoting discussion of lifestyle changes, including exercise regimens, dietary modifications, and quitting smoking. By transferring patients with the education and competencies necessary for preventive care, nurses are able to effectively reduce the incidence of cardiovascular complications. The synergy of education and intervention is one of the most important aspects where the overall quality of cardiovascular care can be improved by nurses. In addition, continuous assessment and evaluation are the foundation of nursing interventions in cardiovascular care, hence ensuring that patient needs are met at every stage of the care continuum. Ongoing monitoring of vital signs, medication compliance, and emotional status allows nurses to identify potential complications at an early stage, permitting timely interventions. For example, when a patient shows evidence of diminishing cardiac output, the quick adoption of targeted interventions by the nurse can prevent further deterioration in health. The use of standardized nursing diagnoses using frameworks such as NANDA can enhance effective communication among healthcare providers, culminating in better patient outcomes. Such integrative care strategies emphasize the importance of nursing assessments in aiding the improvement of the understanding of individual patients' requirements in cardiovascular care (Muatarobin et al., 2020). With responsive and flexible nursing interventions, patients' cardiovascular health can be significantly improved, reflecting the pivotal function of nursing in healthcare (Figure 11.16).

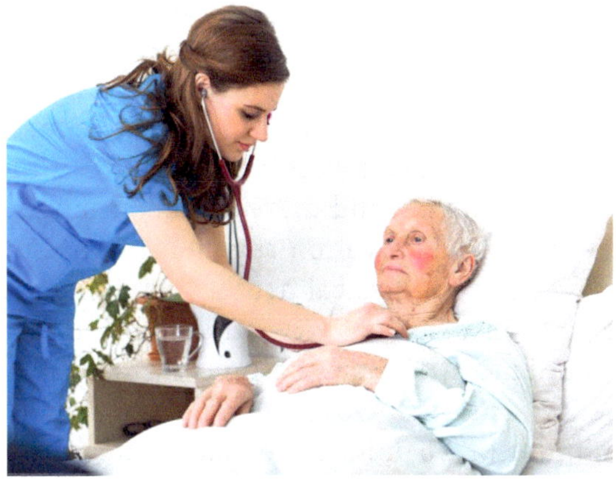

Figure 11.16. Nursing interventions in cardiovascular care.

Source: https://external-content.duckduckgo.com/iu/?u=https%3A%2F%2Fwww.registerednursing.org%2Fwp-content%2Fuploads%2F2017%2F03%2FCardiac-Care-Nurse-Image-768x604.jpg&f=1&nofb=1&ipt=17a412d1f8b5c2a8c8c310adfa4893e52450a2d1fcdb6f25cb9e50fe683c565b.

11.6.1. Patient Education and Lifestyle Modifications

Effective patient education and lifestyle modification are the key components of managing cardiovascular health, particularly in diagnosed patients such as those with congestive heart failure (CHF). Upon discharge from the hospital, the patient is faced with various challenges typical of self-management, requiring a substantial shift in the routines and practices of a daily nature. Empowering patients with adequate knowledge regarding their status and lifestyle changes they need to make can go a long way in enhancing their health outcomes and overall well-being. Specifically, using tools like the Patient Knowledge of Self-care activities in Congestive Heart Failure© (PaKSAC) questionnaire can help healthcare professionals understand areas where patients lag, and therefore, targeted education ultimately leads to curtailing the demand for acute care services. Such a proactive approach not only empowers patients but also encourages greater adherence to recommended lifestyle modifications that can minimize symptoms of CHF (Tovar et al., 2016). Lifestyle modifications are vitally significant far beyond mere dietary change or adherence to medication regimens. Consistent engagement in physical activity, as defined by current physical activity guidelines, is vital for patients who have chronic cardiovascular disease. Patients would ideally engage in a minimum of 30 minutes of moderate activity on the majority of weekdays. Nurses have the ability to be change leaders in the discussion of physical activity within an acute care setting, providing a climate that would support healthy behavior change. Considerable as there has been recognition of physical activity as a vital health behavior, it has been demonstrated in research that it is difficult for most nurses to integrate this counseling into practice. Therefore, greater emphasis on the role of exercise in patient education can enhance nursing care by giving nurses the knowledge to guide patients towards improved ways of living (Bayles et al., 2012). In addition, patient education must continue beyond discharge but be continued along the health trajectory of a patient. Reiterating certain principles of symptom control, dietary restriction, and recognition of warning signs can be important in preventing exacerbations and emergency inpatient admissions. By forming robust discharge plans with precise education tailored to the needs of each patient, clinicians not only fulfill an essential role in cardiovascular disease management but also enhance a culture of patient self-efficacy. By recognizing gaps in patient knowledge and employing gap-filling techniques, nurses can create a care method that ultimately addresses the multifaceted aspects of lifestyle change necessary for optimal cardiovascular status (Tovar et al., 2016).

11.6.2. Medication Management and Adherence

Optimal drug management is paramount within cardiovascular therapy, wherein strict adherence to prescribed regimens determines patient outcomes. Non-adherence to medication is a multifaceted problem, especially among older patients who are more likely to be exposed to polypharmacy and comorbidities of chronic illnesses. Research reveals that myriad interventions—ranging from simple reminders to highly codified support systems—have been investigated to increase the degree of adherence. However, studies indicate that few interventions are theory-driven, and in most cases, do not consider patient-specific preferences and obstacles. There was a systematic review that identified dominant themes to encompass the individual's personal perspectives towards medication and the interaction among lifestyle factors, which all affect adherence in significant ways. This serves to emphasize the importance for healthcare providers, particularly nurses, in establishing an environment of open communication in which patients are enabled to air their experiences and challenges regarding medication use (Banning et al., 2009). Pharmacists, nurses, and healthcare providers play a crucial role in encouraging compliance with medication regimens. These prescribers are not only responsible for dispensing medications but also for teaching patients about their significance and possible side effects. Under motivational interviewing, health practitioners are able to assist patients in resolving ambivalence and developing intrinsic motivation towards healthier behaviors, such as medication compliance. Motivational interviewing is also focus on the importance of culturally sensitive communication, which plays a critical role in addressing specific barriers encountered by diverse groups. Engaging community leaders to assist in identifying such barriers can lead to interventions that are patient-specific and more significant, finally leading to an environment conducive to behavioral change. By incorporating such interventions into day-to-day practice, healthcare professionals are able to effectively increase adherence rates, thereby leading to better health outcomes in cardiovascular care environments (N/A, 2020). Finally, understanding the theoretical models underlying medication adherence interventions is crucial for formulating nursing practices in cardiovascular care. Patient-specific barriers, including drug misconceptions and effects of lifestyle choices, emphasize the call for individualized strategies. The majority of intervention trials reveal insufficient operational definitions of non-adherence, which hinders their evaluation of efficacy. More effort in forthcoming studies should go towards establishing clear frameworks linking strategy of intervention with observed outcomes and incorporating qualitative approaches that can detect complexity in patient experience. By building a more robust theoretical framework, nurses shall be in a better position to navigate the intricate landscape of drug management, leading to greater compliance and improved cardiovascular outcomes. These findings from research must be integrated into nursing education programs as well as guidelines for practice for evidence-based approaches to medication management (Banning et al., 2009).

11.6.3. Emergency Response and Critical Care

It is the convergence of critical care and emergency response within nursing practice that is of major concern, particularly when cardiovascular assessment is being considered. Nurses are central to acute patient management during cardiac emergencies and thus require extensive understanding of both the pathophysiology behind such events as well as emergent intervention required. Rapid assessment of cardiovascular status using the likes of ECG interpretation, blood pressure monitoring, and the detection of life-threatening symptoms forms the essence of quality emergency care. The ability to detect changes in patients vital signs can prove to lead to early interventions, which are crucial in an effort to restore further physiological deterioration. Actually, as literature discusses, emphasis on early identification of cardiovascular issues is in direct proportion with improved patient outcomes under emergency conditions, justifying the importance of rigorous training and readiness among nursing personnel for effective management of cardiac emergencies. In the context of emergency management, enforcement of evidence-based policies serves a critical function in delivering quality care to the patient. The application of best practices in emergency settings, especially with regard to prevention and coordination of care, has been supportive, particularly among the elderly who are high-risk patients. Patient self-management and palliative care programs are essential but not frequently applied based on recent findings. Nurses should promote these evidence-based practices within the clinical context to ensure comprehensive emergency care that considers long-term effects. Also, the urgent need for supportive policies reducing barriers in access to more resources—labs and drugs, for example—cannot be overemphasized, especially in free clinics for the uninsured, as referenced in review of resource constraints preventing healthcare service expansions (Morton et al., 2015; Tammy, 2011). The roles of family caregivers and healthcare workers are also worthy of note in the argument on emergency response and critical care within nursing. As healthcare systems evolve, the role of family members in chronic cardiovascular disease management becomes stronger by the day, and the inclusion of family caregivers in care plans not only aids the patient but also alleviates some burden from emergency healthcare systems. Nursing actions that promote effective communication and patient education to patients and their families can lead to better self-care and compliance with treatment interventions, reducing the use of emergency departments. Additionally, raising awareness and prevention of staff and resource limitations in emergency departments is crucial in order to enhance the quality of care and preparedness to respond suitably to cardiovascular emergencies. Thus, the establishment of nursing education and policy reform in such fields becomes critical in ensuring effective emergency response systems within a dynamic healthcare setting.

Test Your Knowledge

1. What nursing interventions can help manage patients with cardiovascular conditions and prevent complications?
2. How can nurses educate patients on lifestyle modifications, medication adherence, and monitoring for cardiovascular health?

SUMMARY

An analysis on the cardiovascular system in nursing discusses the importance of holistic practice in patient care. Effective nursing care calls for proper knowledge about the cardiovascular system, including awareness of various conditions such as hypertension. Experts with an understanding of typical vascular conditions, symptoms, and interventions can have a critical impact on patient outcomes. This integrated approach involves not only physiological assessment but lifestyle as well as psychosocial determinants of cardiovascular disease. For instance, evidence of focused nursing care on hypertension families underscores how education and support enable families to manage health conditions and make well-informed decisions about their care. Besides, collaboration between families, health practitioners, and the healthcare system is crucial in controlling cardiovascular disorders. Effective nursing practice is dependent on establishing effective lines of communication that facilitate the provision of critical health information to families. Encouraging open communication enhances the capacity of families in detecting and controlling symptoms of hypertension and other cardiovascular conditions. This strategy can alleviate acute pain in cardiovascular illnesses and minimize the risk of recurring recurrences due to inadequate health management among families. This collaboration not only maximizes patient care but also promotes a supportive atmosphere that inspires proactive seeking of health care among patients. Lastly, implementation of expert consensus in nursing practice can direct cardiovascular assessment management strategies. Evidence-based guidelines, established through clinical practice and scholarly research, offer templates that have the potential to enhance the quality of nurse interventions. Based on research, the creation of best practices in cardiovascular treatment can promote effective patient evaluation as well as customized treatment. By grounding nursing care in proven evidence and professional opinions, nurses can ensure that their interventions are responsive and adaptive to evolving cardiovascular patient needs. As such, the impact of such practice leads to improved patient outcomes, increased knowledge in cardiovascular health, and a closer association with holistic care nursing.

The assessment of the cardiovascular system in nursing is an integrated approach, with equal weightage given to theoretical and practical aspects. The most vital areas to focus on are the necessity for precise cardiovascular assessment, which is critical in determining potential health issues in patients. Nurses must be proficient in making proper assessments, including but not limited to heart rate, blood pressure, and hearing of heart sounds. Proficiency in the skills enables nurses to recognize abnormal results at the earliest stage, with effective interventions that impact patient outcomes substantially. Additionally, familiarity with the underlying pathophysiology underpinning various cardiovascular ailments enhances nurses' capability to provide patient-tailored care, aligning treatment aims against individual patient requirements. Cardiovascular nursing education has emerged into prominence recently with the attempt made to standardize curricula across Europe. The development of a core curriculum highlights the significance of educating nurses with in-depth, customized knowledge suitable for cardiovascular settings so that they are able to meet complex patient needs effectively. Eight main themes were achieved as being essential elements of this curriculum, representative of the art and science of cardiovascular care. This structured framework is not just a resource for initial education but also a tool for ongoing professional development in specialist practice. In filling the gap between educational opportunities at the foundational level and specialist knowledge, the curriculum is framed to enhance the standard of overall care delivered in cardiovascular nursing and, indirectly, patient outcomes and death rates due to cardiovascular disease (Astin et al., 2015). Moreover, best practice knowledge in assessment and treatment remains paramount in cardiovascular nursing. Recent evidence, including expert consensus activities, demonstrates a cumulative approach in developing effective physiotherapeutic interventions in treating complicated patients, including those resulting from community-acquired pneumonia. Expert panels have established consensus statements as guidelines of best practice, thereby facilitating more consistent care for patients in critical settings. The potential application of this research extends beyond acute clinical practice; it opens the door for follow-up studies aimed at determining the effectiveness of various treatment interventions. Such evidence-based practice not only enhances nursing practice but also augments the universal dream of reducing the burden of cardiovascular disease globally (Braun et al., 2018).

KEY TERMS FROM THIS CHAPTER

- Heart Sounds
- Apical Pulse
- Pulse Rate
- Blood Pressure
- Hypotension
- Capillary Refill
- Auscultation
- Carotid Artery
- Murmur
- Peripheral Pulse
- Pulse Rhythm
- Hypertension
- Heart Apex
- Edema
- Precordium
- Jugular Venous Distention (JVD)

CRITICAL THINKING QUESTIONS

1. **Which of the following assessment findings indicates a normal peripheral pulse?**
   a. Weak, thready, and irregular
   b. Bounding and rapid
   c. Regular, 2+ strength
   d. Absent
2. **The nurse auscultates a whooshing sound over the carotid artery. This is called:**
   a. Bruit
   b. Murmur
   c. Thrill
   d. Rub
3. **During cardiovascular assessment, the nurse notes a heart rate of 55 beats per minute in a healthy adult. This is documented as:**
   a. Tachycardia
   b. Bradycardia
   c. Arrhythmia
   d. Normal
4. **Jugular vein distension (JVD) is an important indicator of:**
   a. Right-sided heart failure
   b. Left-sided heart failure
   c. Peripheral arterial disease
   d. Myocardial infarction
5. **Which of the following heart sounds is associated with closure of the mitral and tricuspid valves?**
   a. S1
   b. S2
   c. S3
   d. S4

Short Answer Questions

1. What are the main components of the cardiovascular system that should be assessed during a physical examination?
2. Describe the proper technique for assessing heart rate, rhythm, and quality of the pulse.
3. What are the anatomical landmarks for auscultating the heart sounds, and what does each site correspond to?
4. Explain the differences between S1 and S2 heart sounds and their clinical significance.
5. What are common abnormal heart sounds (e.g., murmurs, clicks, rubs), and what conditions might they indicate?

Answer to Critical Thinking Questions

1. (c) 2. (a) 3. (b) 4. (a) 5. (a)

REFERENCES

1. Abi Muhlisin, H. M., & Rahmawati, R. (2015). Asuhan keperawatan pada keluarga Tn. I dengan gangguan sistem kardiovaskuler: Hipertensi pada Ny. S di Desa Kebon Baru Kartasura. https://core.ac.uk/download/148605893.pdf (accessed on 16th July 2025).
2. Accettola, E., Bogdan, A., Callahan, S., et al. (2023). *Introduction to Health Assessment for the Nursing Professional: Part II.* https://core.ac.uk/download/622362029.pdf (accessed on 16th July 2025).
3. Adams, K. F., Ahmad, T., Anstrom, K. J., et al. (2014). Rationale and design of the GUIDE-IT study: Guiding evidence-based therapy using biomarker intensified treatment in heart failure. https://core.ac.uk/download/83049374.pdf (accessed on 16th July 2025).
4. Adlard, A., Anton, A., Attwell, B., Baumbach, B., Bierman, B., et al. (2005). Exercise, cognition and Alzheimer's disease: More is not necessarily better. https://core.ac.uk/download/pdf/12940806.pdf (accessed on 16th July 2025).
5. Allen, T. J. (2011). Addressing resource gaps in the U.S. health care safety net: An assessment of the free clinic network. https://core.ac.uk/download/71357645.pdf (accessed on 16th July 2025).
6. Allman, R. M., Clay, O. J., Crowther, M., et al. (2015). Race and sex differences in correlates of systolic blood pressure in community-dwelling older adults. https://digitalscholarship.unlv.edu/cgi/viewcontent.cgi?article=1269&context=jhdrp (accessed on 16th July 2025).
7. Alzheimer's Association. (2023). 2023 Alzheimer's disease facts and figures. *Alzheimer's & Dementia, 19*, 1598–1695. https://doi.org/10.1002/alz.13016 (accessed on 16th July 2025).
8. Aristarán, M., Guevara, M. R., Hartmann, D., et al. (2016). The research space: Using the career paths of scholars to predict the evolution of the research output of individuals, institutions, and nations. http://arxiv.org/abs/1602.08409 (accessed on 16th July 2025).
9. Astin, F., Carroll, D. L., Hinterbuchner, L., et al. (2015). A core curriculum for the continuing professional development of nurses: Developed by the Education Committee on behalf of the Council on Cardiovascular Nursing and Allied Professions of the ESC. https://core.ac.uk/download/30732812.pdf (accessed on 16th July 2025).
10. Banning, M. (2009). A review of interventions used to improve adherence with medication in older. https://core.ac.uk/download/335823.pdf (accessed on 16th July 2025).
11. Basavarajaiah, S., Giese, E. A., International Olympic Committee Medical Commission, & Ingle, L. (2010). Pre-participation cardiac screening in young athletes: Models and criteria. https://core.ac.uk/download/29019018.pdf (accessed on 16th July 2025).
12. Bashshur, R. L., Doarn, C. R., Frenk, J., Kvedar, J. C., & Woolliscroft, J. O. (2020). Telemedicine and the COVID-19 pandemic, lessons for the future. *Telemedicine Journal and e-Health, 26*, 571–573. https://doi.org/10.1089/tmj.2020.29040.rb.
13. Battah, C. (2016). End-of-life heart failure education with staff nurses: A quality improvement project. https://core.ac.uk/download/162578694.pdf (accessed on 16th July 2025).
14. Bayles, C., Hoffman, L., Jakicic, J., et al. (2012). Examination of acute care nurses' ability to engage in patient education related to physical activity as a health behavior. https://core.ac.uk/download/12212129.pdf (accessed on 16th July 2025).

15. Bicer, S., Clark, Y., Devine, R. D., et al. (2015). Losartan treatment attenuates tumor-induced myocardial dysfunction. https://core.ac.uk/download/213059445.pdf (accessed on 16th July 2025).

16. Braun, V., Dennis, D., Hodgson, C., Hsu, C. C., McMillan, S. S., & Portney, L. G. (2018). Expert consensus for respiratory physiotherapy management of mechanically ventilated adults with community-acquired pneumonia: A Delphi study. https://core.ac.uk/download/213607876.pdf (accessed on 16th July 2025).

17. Brown, R. L., Burke, L., Casper, G., et al. (2010). Technology-enhanced practice for patients with chronic cardiac disease: Home implementation and evaluation. https://core.ac.uk/download/213077805.pdf (accessed on 16th July 2025).

18. Clark, R., Davidson, P., Driscoll, A., et al. (2008). Heart failure nursing in Australia: Challenges, strengths, and opportunities. https://core.ac.uk/download/10904833.pdf (accessed on 16th July 2025).

19. Clark, R., Rawas, H., Windsor, C., et al. (2012). Cultural challenges to secondary prevention: Implications for Saudi women. https://core.ac.uk/download/10909715.pdf (accessed on 16th July 2025).

20. Cox, A. (2015). Thermal burns and smoke inhalation injuries. https://core.ac.uk/download/58826490.pdf (accessed on 16th July 2025).

21. Cox, C. L., Evans, P., Gibbons, H., et al. (2011). HLA-B27 positivity: Associated health implications. https://core.ac.uk/download/9983108.pdf (accessed on 16th July 2025).

22. Despins, L., Enayati, M., Guidoboni, G., et al. (2019). Cardiovascular function and ballistocardiogram: A relationship interpreted via mathematical modeling. https://core.ac.uk/download/228101928.pdf (accessed on 16th July 2025).

23. Devlin, J. W., Skrobik, Y., Gélinas, C., Needham, D. M., Slooter, A. J. C., Pandharipande, P. P., Watson, P. L., et al. (2018). Executive summary: Clinical practice guidelines for the prevention and management of pain, agitation/sedation, delirium, immobility, and sleep disruption in adult patients in the ICU. *Critical Care Medicine, 46*, 1532–1548. https://doi.org/10.1097/ccm.0000000000003259 (accessed on 16th July 2025).

24. Gray, C. M., James, B., Lauder, W., et al. (2010). Developing community nursing practice: Promoting case management and skill enhancement to support shifting the balance of care. https://core.ac.uk/download/110605.pdf (accessed on 16th July 2025).

25. Halvorsen, S., Mehilli, J., Cassese, S., Hall, T. S., Abdelhamid, M., Barbato, E., De Hert, S., et al. (2022). 2022 ESC guidelines on cardiovascular assessment and management of patients undergoing non-cardiac surgery. *European Heart Journal, 43*, 3826–3924. https://doi.org/10.1093/eurheartj/ehac270.

26. Hanekom, S., Patman, S., Plani, N., et al. (2017). Developing minimum clinical standards for physiotherapy in South African ICUs: A qualitative study. https://core.ac.uk/download/213606949.pdf (accessed on 16th July 2025).

27. Herman, H., Annafii, M. N., Biddinika, M. K., & Fitriah, F. (2025). Human digital twin modeling for cardiovascular system. *Scientific Journal of Informatics.* https://www.semanticscholar.org/paper/e44eedffdd028eec80ff8c6a716fa8962b204d09 (accessed on 16th July 2025).

28. McCord, E. (2017). Improving heart failure education prior to discharge: An Emmi implementation project. https://core.ac.uk/download/84120327.pdf (accessed on 16th July 2025).
29. Moon, S. (2017). Echocardiography curriculum development for physician assistants using entrustable professional activities. https://core.ac.uk/download/215924737.pdf (accessed on 16th July 2025).
30. Morton, S., & Dunn, W. (2015). Addressing the health needs of an aging America: New opportunities for evidence-based policy solutions. https://core.ac.uk/download/75783019.pdf (accessed on 16th July 2025).
31. Muatarobin, M. (2020). Nursing analysis in disorder patients with cardiovascular system approach: The model of the Roy adaptation theory. https://core.ac.uk/download/478597871.pdf (accessed on 16th July 2025).
32. N/A. (1986). 216 Jewish Hospital of St. Louis. https://core.ac.uk/download/70380870.pdf (accessed on 16th July 2025).
33. N/A. (2020). Motivational interviewing impact on cardiovascular disease. https://core.ac.uk/download/322838243.pdf (accessed on 16th July 2025).
34. Rajoo, S. S., Wee, Z. J., Lee, S., Wong, F. Y., & Lee, E. S. (2021). A systematic review of the patterns of associative multimorbidity in Asia. *BioMed Research International, 2021*, 1–10. https://doi.org/10.1155/2021/6621785.
35. Ranjan, S., Shingare, S., Umesh, D. H., & Rohith, G. N. (2025). Implementation paper on contactless heart-beat detection using image processing. *Indian Journal of Computer Science and Technology*. https://www.semanticscholar.org/paper/d4b473150e7365fa4d3d22a21143f666d6014e69 (accessed on 16th July 2025).
36. Schneider, B. J., Naidoo, J., Santomasso, B., Lacchetti, C., Adkins, S., Anadkat, M. J., Atkins, M. B., et al. (2021). Management of immune-related adverse events in patients treated with immune checkpoint inhibitor therapy: ASCO guideline update. *Journal of Clinical Oncology, 39*, 4073–4126. https://doi.org/10.1200/jco.21.01440 (accessed on 16th July 2025).
37. Tomás, C., Oliveira, E., Sousa, D. C. F., Chupel, M. U., Furtado, G. E., Rocha, C., Teixeira, A., et al. (2016). *Proceedings of the 3rd IPLeiria's International Health Congress. BMC Health Services Research, 16*. https://doi.org/10.1186/s12913-016-1423-5 (accessed on 16th July 2025).
38. Tovar, N. (2016). The effects of patient education and knowledge of CHF patients as evaluated by the PakSAC survey. https://core.ac.uk/download/84119719.pdf (accessed on 16th July 2025).

ABDOMINAL ASSESSMENT IN NURSING

12

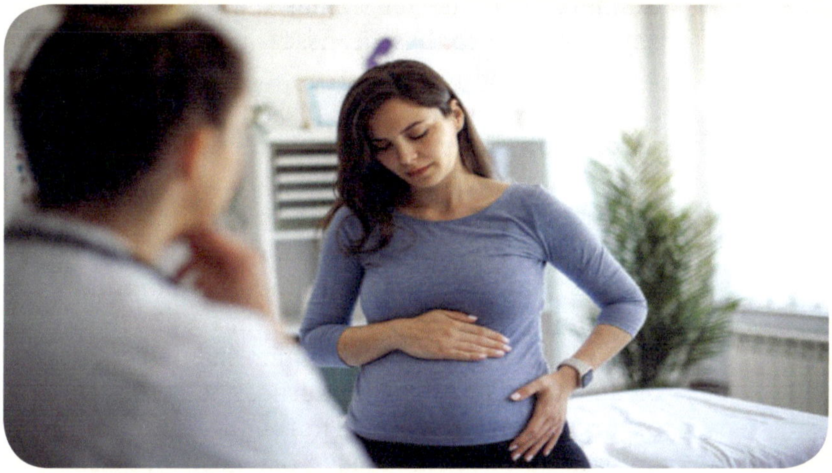

LEARNING OBJECTIVES

After studying this chapter, you will be able to:

1. Understand the anatomy of the abdomen;
2. Explain the techniques of abdominal assessment;
3. Identify the common abdominal conditions;
4. Explore the cultural considerations in abdominal assessment;
5. Discuss the documentation and reporting;
6. Focus on the challenges in abdominal assessment.

Introduction

In practice, accurate abdominal assessment is the bedrock of patient assessment and care. Abdominal assessment not only facilitates the identification of gastrointestinal diseases but is also critical to the assessment of overall health. An understanding of the anatomy and physiology of the abdominal region enables nurses to detect abnormalities that signify underlying health problems, hence creating avenues for early interventions. Proficiency in assessment skills of inspection, auscultation, percussion, and palpation is essential to ensure proper diagnosis and treatment. The ability to interpret results of these assessments can make a significant contribution to patient outcomes and interventions in nursing and hence is a relevant skill for nursing practitioners. Abdominal assessment is much more intricate than physical examination; it's an eclectic approach that involves patient history, presenting complaints, and potential psychosocial participation. For instance, the prevalence of conditions such as fecal incontinence, which affects just over 1% of noninstitutionalized adults, highlights the need for targeted assessment techniques that are tailored to an individual patient's needs (Chelvanayagam et al., 2000). Nurses must employ good communication skills to gain comprehensive patient histories, which they can then use to formulate suitable plans of care. This combined strategy not only aids in identification, but also aids in a therapeutic relationship that encourages disclosure of sensitive health information among patients, hence enhancing the accuracy of the assessment process.

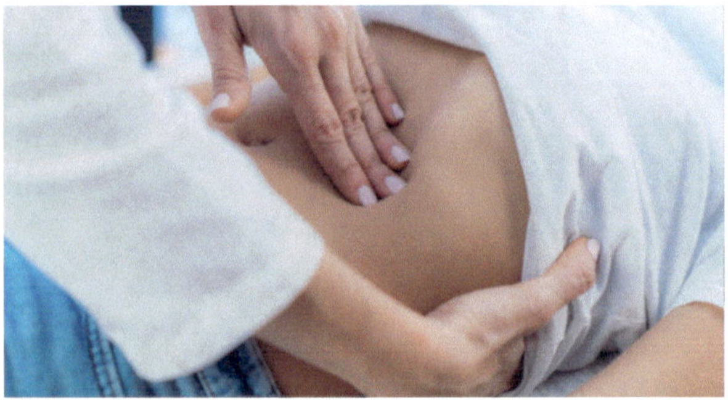

Figure 12.1. Abdominal assessment nursing.

Source: https://www.springerpub.com/media/.renditions/wysiwyg/blog/Doctor_examining_abdominal_Blog_Image_1200x630_1.png.

Moreover, the science of abdominal assessment has expanded to encompass evidence-based practices that optimize patient care and outcomes. Innovative approaches to managing specific conditions, such as the incorporation of spontaneous maternal bearing down during childbirth, have been shown to provide excellent physiologic benefits to the mother and baby (Hanson et al., 2009). These observations serve to illustrate the interactive, dynamic nature of nursing practice in which incorporation of constant education and sensitivity to new discoveries is paramount. Also, the use of newer technological tools and assessment models can increase the validity and efficacy of abdominal examination. Therefore, this introduction to abdominal examination in nursing provides a comprehensive foundation to later explain more detailed methods and techniques that underpin more effective patient care in a variety of clinical environments (Figure 12.1).

Definition of Abdominal Assessment

Abdominal assessment is an integral part of nursing practice that entails thorough examination of the abdominal cavity to identify any potential health issue. Assessment is usually conducted both subjectively and objectively through a systematic process involving inspection, auscultation, palpation, and percussion. Nurses begin the process by taking pertinent patient history, e.g., gastrointestinal symptomatology, surgical history, and lifestyle factors that could influence abdominal well-being. Subsequent to that, physical examination techniques facilitate the detection of abnormalities like tenderness, distension, or organ enlargement. Thorough abdominal examination not only aids in diagnosis but also acts as a baseline for subsequent care, thereby enhancing the efficacy of total treatment. Abdominal examination importance lies in the fact that symptom focus that may result in underlying pathology is included in it. For example, constipation is also classically linked to straining on the bowel or with a sensation of incomplete evacuation, which is relevant to the efficacy of colonic transit (Gardiner et al., 2016). The ability to recognize such clinical presentation through focused abdominal examination by the nurse can go a long way to addressing the needs of the patients adequately. Further, understanding these symptoms in relation to the general health of the gastrointestinal tract allows nurses to use appropriate interventions. Abdominal examinations, therefore, are not only diagnostic tools but also as critical components that facilitate patient-centered care through holistic assessment and individualized treatment planning. Within the scope of nursing education broadly speaking, abdominal assessment importance is being viewed more and more as necessary to prepare future nurses for the reality of clinical practice. As health care evolves further, particularly through expansion in biomedical sciences, nursing degree curricula increasingly prioritize the integration of multidisciplinary competencies, such as advancing fields such as omics (Cindy et al., 2015). As such an evolving learning environment requires, more emphasis needs to be placed on discovering how abdominal assessment relates to overall patient health, influencing immediate management as well as long-term result. Through skills acquisition in this discipline, nursing practitioners can enhance effectiveness in healthcare interventions by addressing both physiological and contextual patient needs, thereby solidifying their role as chief caregivers in the healthcare system.

Importance in Nursing Practice

The value of abdominal examination in nursing cannot be overestimated, as it is a critical component in the diagnosis of various health issues that may impact patients. Through accurate evaluation of the abdomen, nurses can diagnose abnormalities such as tenderness, distension, or organ enlargement, which may be indicative of underlying conditions such as appendicitis or liver disease. It is particularly vital in acute settings, as early treatment has implications for patient outcomes. Understanding the worth of palpation, auscultation, and inspection enables nurses to establish a baseline for patients' health and guide future care strategies. Because of their position as primary care providers, nurses must have the knowledge and expertise to perform comprehensive abdominal examination and be able to refer findings to the appropriate medical team to guarantee patient safety and health optimization. Moreover, education and ongoing nurse training to enhance nurses' competency in abdominal assessment is an essential part of nursing practice. Through initiatives such as workshops or quality improvement efforts, healthcare professionals can stay up to date on best practice and emerging guidelines related to abdominal assessment. For instance, clinical intervention for screening for metabolic syndrome among users of second-generation antipsychotic medication increased the knowledge and adherence motivation of providers (Moreno et al., 2016). Improved adherence to evidence-based practice not only enhances the accuracy of tests but also allows nurses to report results more effectively to interprofessional teams, thus encouraging interprofessional practice in patient care. The combination of complementary methods, such as the application of dzikir as therapy, can further improve nursing outcomes related to abdominal assessments.

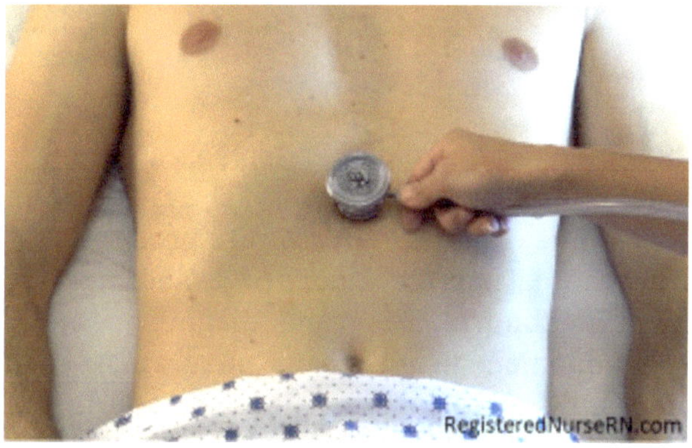

Figure 12.2. Abdominal assessment in nursing practice.

Source: https://www.registerednursern.com/wp-content/uploads/2017/12/abdominal-assessment-01-300x186.png.

Research has shown that the use of dzikir during postoperative care can significantly and meaningfully reduce patients' pain levels (Misnawati et al., 2015). It brings together spiritual care and physical examination such that nurses are able to address the general health needs of their patients and foster comfort and well-being in the challenging health process. Such a multi-faceted approach reflects the worthiness of full-spectrum nursing practice, whereby extensive abdominal examination is carried out not only to determine potential health issues but also to address the psychological and emotional requirements of patients. Thus, nurses are positioned to offer client-focused care that respects and responds to individual values and socio-cultural preferences (Figure 12.2).

12.1. Anatomy of the Abdomen

Learning Outcome

1. Major Organs Located in the Abdominal Cavity
2. Anatomical Regions of the Abdomen
3. Relationship Between Anatomy and Assessment Techniques

An understanding of the abdomen's anatomy is essential for accurate abdominal evaluation in nursing, as it provides healthcare professionals with the background knowledge necessary to identify abnormalities and diagnose illness. The abdomen includes four quadrants—each consisting of crucial organs and structures that can exhibit a wide range of symptoms when disrupted. For instance, the gallbladder and liver are located in the right upper quadrant, while the stomach and spleen are located in the left upper quadrant.

This anatomical knowledge enables the nurse to palpate and check for masses, distension, or tenderness, thus enabling the identification of conditions such as gastrointestinal bleeding or liver disease. By the accurate mapping of these areas, nurses are able to streamline their testing procedures and enhance patient outcome, not missing evidence of underlying pathology. In abdominal anatomy assessment, however, an understanding of the mesentery's functional role as a fold of peritoneum which attaches and fixes the intestines is also important. The mesentery has within it blood vessels, lymphatics, and nerves that are essential to intestinal function and immunity. Immunohistochemical differentiation of the significance of the mesentery also makes nurses sensitive to how conditions of the intestines, say inflammatory bowel disease, can present in an assessment. The relative closeness of abdominal organs to each other also proves the intricacies and inter-relatedness of multiple systems; for instance, renal system issues can present as abdominal pain that will mislead clinicians. Comprehension of such anatomical relations is supported by the importance of the global outlook in abdominal assessment, allowing nurses to comprehend the multifaceted nature of the patient's condition and allow holistic patient care. Furthermore, special attention is called for in the pelvic region, particularly because myofascial pelvic pain (MFPP) causes considerable impacts on the abdomens global function. The condition is characterized by trigger points in the pelvic floor muscles that may lead to chronic pain referred to adjacent areas, complicating the assessment process and typically resulting in misdiagnosis. Accurate identification and treatment of MFPP need an interdisciplinary strategy, which is crucial to eliminate patient distress. Myofascial trigger point release and biofeedback are some of the treatment strategies that may be deeply engaged, which makes the knowledge of abdominal and pelvic anatomy dynamics critical for nurses. The acknowledgment of the complexity of MFPPs emphasizes the importance of nurses being expert in anatomical expertise as well as in the greater connotations of pelvic pain to gut health, thereby enhancing patient management practices and assessment skills (Katzman et al., 2012) (Figure 12.3).

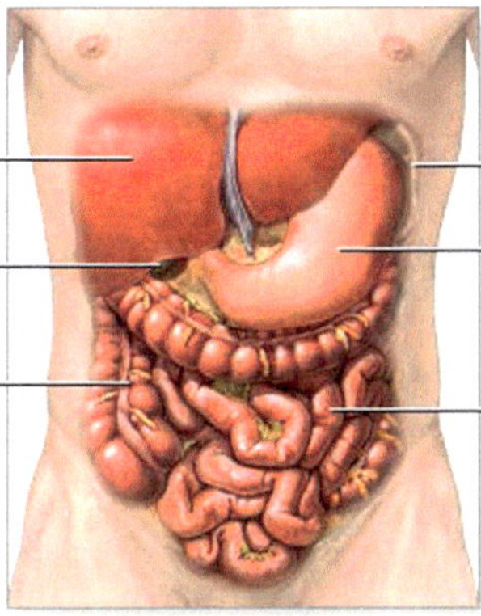

Figure 12.3. Anatomy of the abdomen.

Source: https://medlineplus.gov/ency/images/ency/fullsize/10083.jpg.

12.1.1. Major Organs Located in the Abdominal Cavity

The abdominal cavity is to provide space for some of the vital organs responsible for digestion, metabolism, and the proper functioning of the body in general. The cavity is bordered by the diaphragm above and the pelvic brim below and contains vital organs like the stomach, intestines, liver, and pancreas. The stomach initiates the digestion process by breaking down food with gastric acids, while the intestines, including small and large intestines, are responsible for nutrient absorption and waste removal. This information is vital to nursing assessment as any irregularities in these organs will lead to significant clinical presentations, impacting patient health and treatment plans. Additionally, the knowledge of the anatomical positioning of these organs is helpful in assessing symptoms such as abdominal pain or distension, which are frequent complaints in clinical practice. The liver, an abnormally large abdominal cavity organ, has many roles to play in metabolism, detoxification, and synthesis of proteins involved in blood clotting. Nurses must be able to assess liver health, particularly for those who have risk factors for liver disease such as alcohol abuse or viral hepatitis. Not only does the liver play a metabolic function, but its contribution to the production of bile for digestion further accentuates the importance of the liver in the digestive process. Nurses also commonly undertake palpation of the liver in routine examination because an enlarged liver or other unusual findings can indicate associated conditions warranting further study. A sound familiarity with the roles of the liver and the potential pathology is thus not only a development of nursing assessment but also of patient education and treatment.

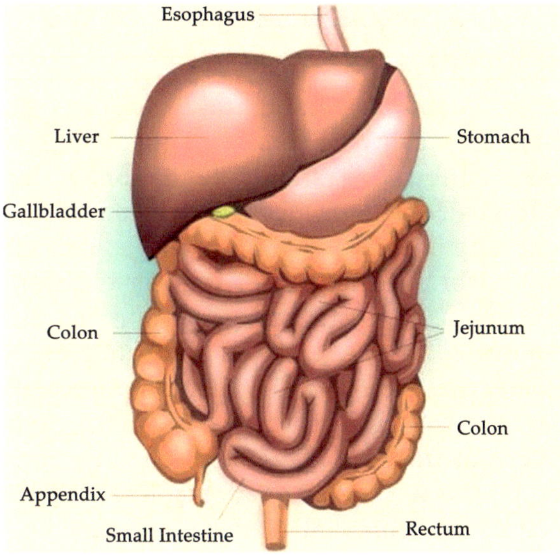

Figure 12.4. Major organs located in the abdominal cavity.

Source: https://biologydictionary.net/wp-content/uploads/2017/03/Digestive-organs.jpg.

The pancreas is yet another vital organ that is located within the abdominal cavity and is involved in the digestive as well as the endocrine system. It secretes enzymes for the digestion of carbohydrates, proteins, and fats along with the livers bile. Its role in insulin production also highlights its significance in glucose metabolism, a basic process for health. During nursing assessments, it is important to monitor for signs of pancreatic impairment since pancreatitis has severe consequences and necessitates urgent medical management. Knowledge of the anatomical and physiological complexities of the pancreas thus equips nurses with the necessary knowledge to undertake effective assessment and management practices in diabetes or other metabolic disorder patients. Collectively, the organs are fundamental to body physiological functioning and hence their assessment is essential in nursing practice in the context of comprehensive abdominal assessments (Figure 12.4).

12.1.2. Anatomical Regions of the Abdomen

Understanding the anatomical divisions of the abdomen is a critical component of abdominal assessment in nursing. The abdomen has traditionally been divided into four quadrants: right upper quadrant, left upper quadrant, right lower quadrant, and left lower quadrant. Each quadrant contains specific organs and structures, and it is crucial for nurses to identify these during assessment. For instance, the liver and gallbladder occupy the right upper quadrant while the stomach and spleen occupy the left upper quadrant. Knowing the position and function of these organs allows the nurse to identify probable causes of pain or discomfort and make more informed diagnoses and intervention strategies. Also, knowing all this helps nurses to perform comprehensive physical examination and ensure that they provide holistic care to patients who present with varying abdominal complaints. In addition to the four-quadrant scheme, the abdomen can also be divided into nine regions, allowing for additional specificity needed in clinical assessment. The method divides the abdomen into distinct regions: right hypochondriac, epigastric, left hypochondriac, right lumbar, umbilical, left lumbar, right iliac, hypogastric, and left iliac regions. Each region corresponds to distinct anatomical structures, allowing for additional specificity in localizing pathologic processes. For instance, right iliac pain would imply appendicitis, while left hypochondriac discomfort would mean problems with the stomach or spleen. Nurses familiar with this nuanced approach are better able to convey information to the treatment team, which contributes to a more cohesive care effort and better patient outcomes. Furthermore, it is not possible to overemphasize the importance of anatomical landmarks when considering the abdominal examination.

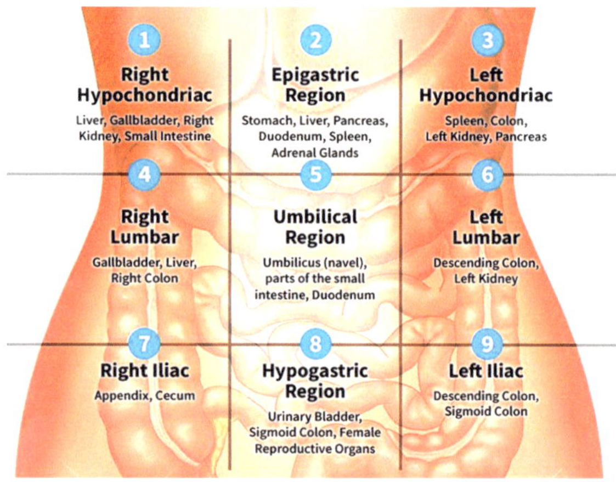

Figure 12.5. Anatomical regions of the abdomen.

Source: https://samarpanphysioclinic.com/wp-content/uploads/2022/10/abdominal-regions-1200x900.jpg.

Identifying key structures, such as the linea alba and costal margins, helps nurses orient themselves during examinations. Furthermore, methods of palpation used in various regions of the abdomen may differ based on structures below. As an example, assessment of tenderness in the right lower quadrant commonly involves checking the appendix, while palpation of the left upper flank can identify splenic enlargement. In addition, an understanding of population differences in anatomy can more specifically adapt the assessment process. As a critical consequence, a comprehensive understanding of abdominal anatomy is totally necessary for nurses who perform abdominal assessments to make appropriate judgments and deliver effective care to patients (Figure 12.5).

12.1.3. Relationship Between Anatomy and Assessment Techniques

The abdominal anatomy and evaluation techniques of abdominal nursing are associated with quality patient assessment. Thorough understanding of the abdominal anatomy enables the nurses to make particular evaluations, noticing abnormalities from normal findings that may be indicative of pathology. The abdominal cavity houses vital organs such as the liver, spleen, kidneys, and intestines, each with particular anatomical landmarks. By the application of inspection, palpation, percussion, and auscultation methods, nurses utilize their anatomical knowledge to interpret weak signs of pain, swelling, or organ dysfunction. The anatomical structure guides the practitioner on how to perform optimal methods of assessment and interpreting the results accurately. As a result, accurate anatomical information not only enhances the process of assessment but also serves as the foundation of clinical judgment and nursing practice decision-making. Methods of assessment are directly related to the anatomical structures under assessment, which points toward the paramount significance of such a relationship in nursing practice. By way of illustration, a nurse may use palpation to check for tenderness over the location of the liver in the right upper quadrant of the abdomen. The ability to locate organs and determine their normal size and shape is crucial, because variations can be an indicator of underlying pathology such as hepatomegaly or splenomegaly. Furthermore, in appendicitis, anatomical relation also helps determine referred pain to the abdomen and therefore inform proper interventions in a timely manner. Training in abdominal anatomy, therefore, allows nurses to hone their assessing abilities in a way that they are able to spot the abnormalities early enough and initiate the corresponding care pathways, resulting in improved patient outcomes. With enhanced care complexity, the incorporation of anatomy-based assessment techniques is even more crucial in nursing care. The increasingly fuller integration of medical information into practice means that nurses need to have knowledge of the latest guidelines and best practice in order to maximize their assessment ability. For instance, advanced imaging technologies and advancing surgery have changed the body's anatomical terrain, so nurses must adapt their assessment skills accordingly. Continued professional learning and continued learning in anatomy form the basis of nurses' ability to apply assessing skills effectively in different clinical contexts, particularly where conditions such as Fontan circulation are present, and potentially could present unique challenges and complexities (Rychik et al., 2019). Knowledge of anatomy, thus, not only develops assessing skills but also empowers nurses with the ability to give high-quality care tailored to individual patient needs.

Test Your Knowledge

1. What are the major organs and structures of the abdomen, and how are they organized within the abdominal quadrants?
2. How does understanding abdominal anatomy assist in identifying normal versus abnormal assessment findings?.

12.2. Techniques of Abdominal Assessment

Learning Outcome

1. Inspection Methods
2. Palpation Techniques
3. Auscultation Procedures

The processes of abdominal assessment are central to nursing, enabling health professionals to evaluate and diagnose a range of gastrointestinal and systemic conditions. Observation is normally the first step to any proper assessment, whereby the abdomen is examined for any abnormalities in shape, scarring, or coloration. Careful attention is given to searching for contours and movement of the abdomen, representing signs of subproblems such as distension or peristalsis. Upon inspection, palpation is utilized to assess tenderness, tension of muscles, or masses and provide significant information on organ size and abnormality. Auscultation, in most instances completed before percussion to avoid the disruption of bowel sounds, allows nurses to perceive normal and abnormal sounds of intestinal activity. With these fundamental skills, nurses can collect significant data to direct clinical decisions and patient-care planning in a rational manner. Palpation, one of the basic techniques of abdominal examination, can be subdivided further into light palpation and deep palpation, both with different objectives. Light palpation is carried out with light pressure, which is applied to explore surface pathology and to assess for the presence of sensitivity or tenderness over the abdominal wall. Deep palpation is used to explore deeper structures and can detect abnormalities in liver or kidney size that can indicate pathologies such as hepatomegaly or nephromegaly. Moreover, specific techniques may be used to particular maneuvers targeting certain organs or regions to enhance overall diagnostic competency. For instance, Murphys sign is employed to diagnose inflammation of the gallbladder, while rebound tenderness may indicate appendicitis. As techniques of abdominal examination get developed, they enhance both diagnostic capacity as well as patient confidence and trust during investigations. Moreover, utilization of complementary therapy alongside traditional assessment tools is gaining popularity in nursing practice.

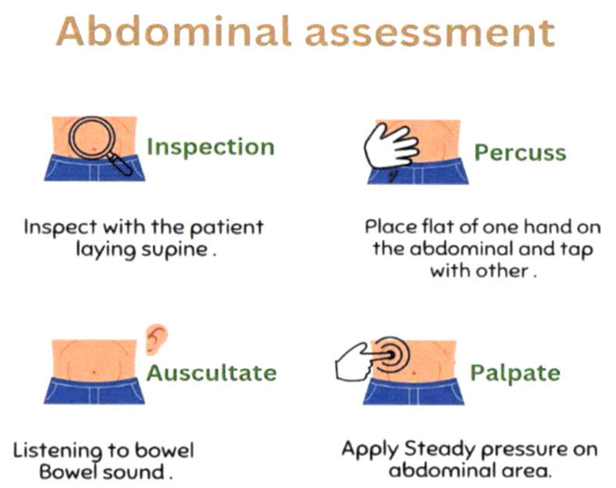

Figure 12.6. Techniques of abdominal assessment.

Source: https://encrypted-tbn0.gstatic.com/images?q=tbn:ANd9GcT7ZDauSDu50my0RYGzYGEQfee93JgqvcHcvA&s.

Techniques such as *dzikir*, a meditation and mindfulness exercise, have been found to have therapeutic impacts on pain management, particularly among postoperative patients. Recent studies have demonstrated that patients who used the *dzikir* experienced lower pain intensity after surgery compared to those that did not utilize the practice. The use of such integrated approaches gives considerable emphasis to the engagement of nurses not just in respect of physical assessment competence but also with a focus on psychological and spiritual well-being in patient care. The combination of stringent abdominal assessment practices with such integrated approaches facilitates a greater understanding of the unique need of each patient, hence enhancing the overall quality of nursing care provided within various healthcare settings (Figure 12.6).

12.2.1. Inspection Methods

Inspection methods constitute an integral part of the abdominal examination within nursing practice as the initial approach to the process of general assessment. By visual inspection, the nurses gain necessary information regarding the condition of the abdomen and identify abnormalities such as distension, scars, or color alteration. By the application of this method, the practitioner is capable of examining the contour, symmetry, and movement in and out of inspiration of the abdomen. As an example, an abdominal distension may be suggestive of underlying pathologies such as fluid overload or bowel obstruction and requires further investigation. Also crucial is the ability to observe by the nurse because they must be able to identify normal anatomical variations versus pathological signs. This heightened vigilance during the inspection phase is crucial because it sets the tone for the subsequent checks of palpation and auscultation. Following visual inspection, palpation is then important in the abdominal examination process, allowing health professionals to assess tenderness, tone, and potential masses located in the abdominal cavity. The method supplements the use of touch to the assessment that might be lacking in visual inspection. Through sequential palpation of the different quadrants of the abdomen, nurses can detect pathologies such as enlargement of the organs or masses or fluid presence. The nurse needs to apply the appropriate pressure in order to get clear information on deeper structures without compromising patient comfort and upholding an empathetic style of assessment. Combining information gathered through palpation with initial visual examination optimizes diagnostic accuracy. Nursing practitioners should also be adequately trained in these techniques because their skill has a direct impact on the quality of care. Apart from palpation and visual inspection, auscultation is also an important factor in determining the health of the abdomen, particularly bowel sounds. It allows nurses to listen for the characteristic sound of gastrointestinal movement that is indicative of normal or abnormal function. Hyperactive or active sounds might be suggestive of gastrointestinal obstruction or inflammation, while reduced or absent sounds might be suggestive of severe diseases such as ileus. Auscultation requires careful technique, for the nurse must distinguish between various sounds and listen for patterns of rhythm heard.

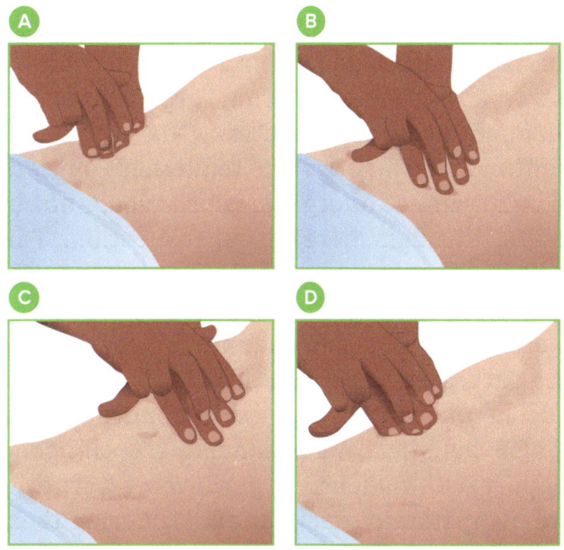

Figure 12.7. Inspection methods of abdominal assessment.

Source: https://cdn.lecturio.com/assets/abcd-showing-percussion-of-all-4-quadrants-1200x1137.png.

Additionally, combining the results of auscultation with visual inspection and palpation creates an extended assessment model. In multifactorial diseases such as myofascial pelvic pain, effective inspection skills will aid healthcare practitioners in making appropriate diagnosis decisions, as would be highlighted in the imperative multidisciplinary treatment of such diseases (Katzman et al., 2012). Nursing practitioners can play a critical role in patient outcomes using optimal and accurate abdominal examination, enhancing maximization of a patient-directed approach to treatment. In addition, a systematic approach towards maintaining hygienic practice between consecutive inspection processes is most critical in-patient safety terms, similar to food safety within healthcare facilities as depicted by HACCP regulations (Buzby et al., 2025) (Figure 12.7).

12.2.2. Palpation Techniques

Palpation abilities are at the fore of the abdominal assessment process, providing the nursing professional with important information about a patient's internal organ function. Through ordered palpation, the nurse can identify abnormalities like tenderness, masses, or enlargement of organs, which would not be visible through mere visual inspection. This technique involves pressure being applied on the abdomen with fingers or hands to specific areas in order to assess pain or abnormal consistency. The successful execution of palpation not only aids in diagnosing the likely conditions but is also beneficial in enhancing the clinicians rapport with patients by performing a truthful and sympathetic examination. Mastering these skills is important for nursing students who are getting ready to handle the intricacies of patient care without compromising comfort and trust throughout the assessment process. Proper palpation skills need both theoretical and practical knowledge and demonstrate a holistic approach towards nursing education. The integration of clinical insight, as prioritized in materials written for nursing students, allows practitioners to evaluate the abdominal area with acuteness, directing attention toward the information observed during palpation. Nurses improve their performance in addressing indications of clinical decline with increasing mastery of these skills, thus improving outcomes for patients. Besides, the education emphasizes cultural sensitivity in testing practices to allow nurses to address various patient populations. Not only does this improve clinical skill, but it also identifies the divergence of patients' backgrounds in order to bring about more inclusive communication and treatment strategies, as emphasized by the education courses in the field (Accettola et al., 2023). This collaborative effort between nursing educators to strengthen palpation and assessment skills reinforces evidence-based practice for nursing. According to the consensus report on conservative management of female pelvic floor dysfunction, the outlining of distinct terminology and approaches contributes to clarity in clinical practice (Abramov et al., 2016). Such emphasis on standardization allows nursing specialists to apply their knowledge capably and consistently in different clinical settings. Through constant revision and revision of clinical guidelines, nursing education programs can equip prospective providers with the competencies necessary to perform full abdominal exams. Not only does this empower the foundation of nursing practice, but also enhances patient safety and quality of care, as it exemplifies the inextricable link between education and successful health outcomes (Figure 12.8).

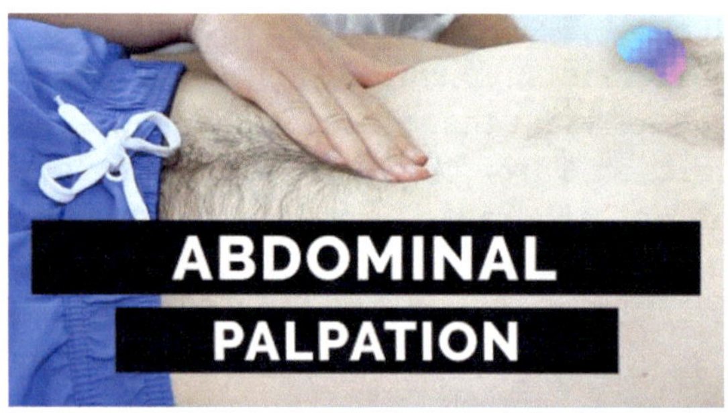

Figure 12.8. Palpation techniques of abdominal assessment.

Source: https://i.ytimg.com/vi/b6xfeF5usK0/hqdefault.jpg.

12.2.3. Auscultation Procedures

Auscultation is a critical component of abdominal examination in nursing and gives a window into the physiological state of the gastrointestinal tract. Nurses must utilize a stethoscope and implement a rational method of auscultation that begins with the patient relaxing in a comfortable, supine position. The abdominal area must be exposed properly without compromising the dignity and warmth of the patient. Large areas, the four quadrants of the abdomen inclusive, are examined for bowel and vascular sounds and for abnormalities. The presence or absence of bowel sounds, whose intensity and frequency can vary, can be evidence of gastrointestinal function or dysfunction. Nurses need to interpret these sounds accurately and realize that a recent surgery and medication can significantly influence their nature. Incorporating auscultation guidelines is among evidence-based practices that enhance nursing interventions. Research finds that labeling normal and abnormal bowel sound is vital in establishing the appropriateness of further investigation and intervention. For instance, decreased or absent bowel sounds can stimulate examinations for underlying conditions such as ileus or bowel obstruction. According to Kitsiou et al. (2013), the ability to detect these variations is a reflection of the clinical knowledge of a nurse. Furthermore, the auscultation of vascular sounds will also reflect possible complication in the form of abdominal aortic aneurysm or vascular stenosis, hence the need for comprehensive assessment approaches. With the integration of auscultation techniques with clinical reasoning, patients' outcomes may be improved through early interventions that are underpinned by accurate assessment. In addition, ongoing education and training play a significant role in enhancing auscultation skills among nurses. Emphasized by Tipton et al. (2019), evidence-based practice in abdominal well-being observation directly impacts efficient procedures like nasogastric tube insertion, where precise measurement of the position of feeding tubes during insertion must be carried out. Enhancing auscultation competencies not only benefits immediate patient assessment but also enhances nursing education about gastrointestinal wellness. Finally, competency in abdominal auscultation equips nurses to provide holistic care where interventions applied are appropriate and timely, highlighting the correlation between appropriate assessments and improved clinical outcomes among nursing practice (Figure 12.9).

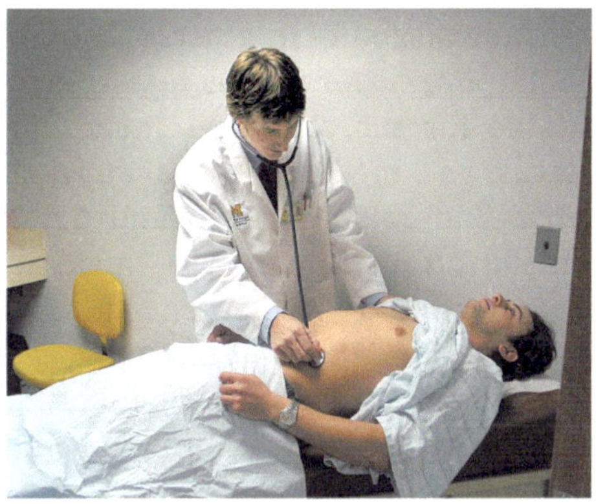

Figure 12.9. Auscultation procedures of abdominal assessment.

Source: https://upload.wikimedia.org/wikipedia/commons/6/6d/Standardized-Patient-Program-examining-t_he-abdomen.jpg.

Test Your Knowledge

1. What are the key techniques for abdominal assessment, including inspection, auscultation, percussion, and palpation, and why is the order important?
2. How can proper positioning and technique improve the accuracy of abdominal assessment findings?

12.3. Common Abdominal Conditions

Learning Outcome

1. Gastrointestinal Disorders
2. Urinary Tract Issues
3. Reproductive System Concerns

In nursing, assessing endemic abdominal conditions is a vital component of care in the patient. A detailed knowledge of such conditions results in enhanced patient assessment and management. Among all types of abdominal conditions, constipation is one of the most frequent issues to be encountered in clinical practice as well as in the community. Offering slow bowel movements, straining, and a sense of incomplete evacuation, constipation can lead to significant disability in a person's quality of life. It is important for nurses to assess factors accountable for the condition, including diet, fluid status, and medication use. Physiological mechanisms in colonic transit and defecation mechanism allow for nursing practice by allowing nurses to implement appropriate management modalities, enhancing patient outcomes (Gardiner et al., 2016). Identification and treatment of constipation are integral parts of abdominal assessment to ensure appropriate care for this common disease. Another vital abdominal disease that most likely requires nursing assessment is myofascial pelvic pain (MFPP), a common presentation of chronic pelvic pain (CPP). This disorder is often overlooked, leading to prolonged patient suffering and loss of quality of life. MFPP is characterized by myofascial trigger points in the pelvic floor muscles, which refer pain to areas above them. Diagnosis for nurses consists of recognizing the hallmark of MFPP as evaluation for these trigger points and observation of the patients pattern of pain and associated symptoms. Early identification is necessary because there are effective treatment modalities available, including myofascial trigger point release and biofeedback therapy. Besides, MFPP multidisciplinary management is essential since the collaboration of clinical practitioners may lead to better overall care and effective patient management (Katzman et al., 2012). Furthermore, identification of MFPP complexity enables nurses to make specific interventions to counteract this incapacitating condition. Additionally, conditions such as irritable bowel syndrome (IBS) further emphasize the necessity of tight abdominal investigations in clinical practice.

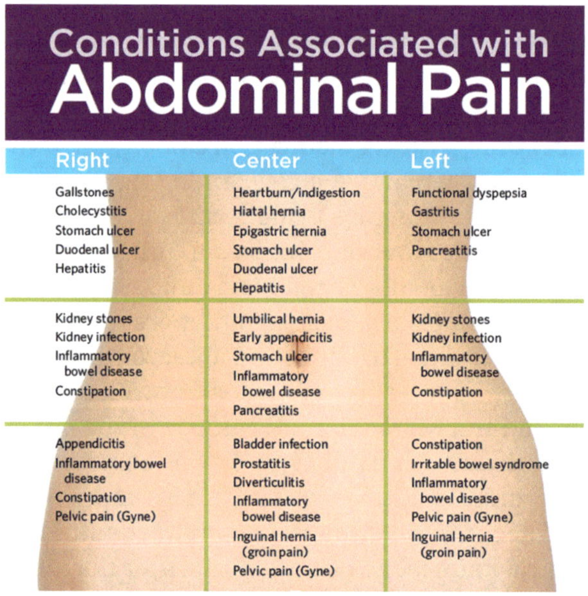

Figure 12.10. Common abdominal conditions.

Source: https://medicaldialogues.in/wp-content/uploads/2015/09/stomach-pain-infographic.png.

IBS has many symptoms like pain, distension, and change in bowel habits and brings great distress to the patients. It is essential that the multifactorial nature of the etiology of IBS is considered for nursing care assessment, such as dietary, psychological, and disorders of gastrointestinal motility. A thorough assessment consists of taking a detailed patient history, physical exam, and symptom description, which allows the nurses to develop tailored management plans addressing body and mind. Patient education on lifestyle modification, diet modification, and potential pharmacotherapy can significantly improve symptom control in IBS patients. Lastly, effective assessment and management of a variety of common abdominal complaints such as constipation, MFPP, and IBS are the core of nurses' delivery of cohesive and effective patient-centered care (Figure 12.10).

12.3.1. Gastrointestinal Disorders

The importance of proper abdominal examination in nursing cannot be overstated, particularly when it comes to dealing with gastrointestinal conditions. These conditions, which encompass a wide range of conditions including irritable bowel syndrome, gastroesophageal reflux disease, and inflammatory bowel disease, have significant implications on the quality of life of a patient. Prompt diagnosis and effective management of gastrointestinal conditions require the application of comprehensive assessment techniques, including taking comprehensive patient histories and performing physical assessments. Through understanding the subtle signs that are connected with these disorders, nurses can differentiate between probable underlying conditions and implement appropriate interventions that best fit individual patients. This highlights the very important role of nurses not just in diagnosing gastrointestinal disorders but also interpreting results that would suggest more serious health conditions. Biofeedback has been shown to be a promising non-invasive treatment for gastrointestinal disorders, particularly in managing bowel dysfunction, as present studies reveal. This is a method that instructs patients to control different body functions, and these can be used for pain management such as constipation or fecal incontinence. In a retrospective study by Chelvanayagam et al., some patients were reported to have improved outcomes using the application of biofeedback therapy. Notably, the therapy is of particular applicability to those patients who are likely to have secondary psychiatric disorders, such as anorexia nervosa, highlighting the complex interdependence of physical and mental health. Nurses play a leading role in the detection of such disorders and modifying settings that can be supportive of including such therapies within care plans as a whole, thereby supporting wholesome care of patients and enhancing the efficacy of treatment (Chelvanayagam et al., 2012). Gastrointestinal illnesses are often exacerbated by developmental and psychiatric diseases, which make them challenging to manage in children. People with autism spectrum disorder usually experience gastrointestinal issues that require close observation and management.

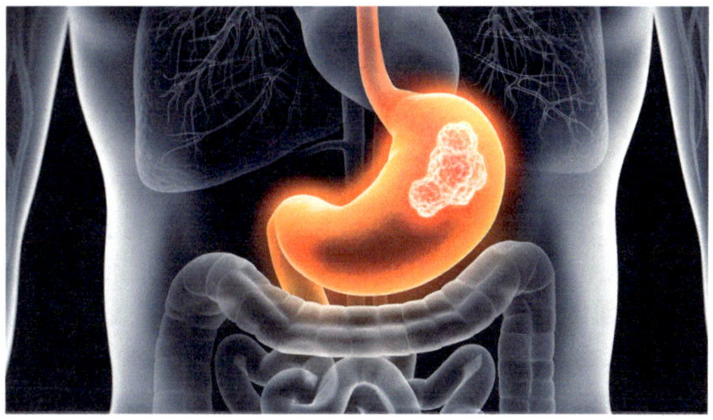

Figure 12.11. Gastrointestinal disorders.

Source: https://www.pharmacy-network.co.uk/images/view/21c9bc821c454625de712d520a56da1a.jpg.

Nurses and healthcare providers need to be equipped with best practices in providing evidence-based care in order to help manage these challenges effectively by family members. They should understand how autism-related behaviors can render routine activities and also healthcare interactions more challenging. Through the use of focused evaluations and interventions, nurses are able to instruct families on maximizing care and improving the overall health outcomes of their child. The incorporation of family-focused recommendations into gastrointestinal disorder care not only reduces symptoms but also empowers those who care for them, supporting them as they navigate the nuances found in their child's health (Bultas et al., 2016) (Figure 12.11).

12.3.2. Urinary Tract Issues

It is necessary for nursing professionals conducting abdominal assessment to understand urinary tract diseases since they directly contribute to the safety and well-being of patients. The urinary system, including the kidneys, ureters, bladder, and urethra, is susceptible to various dysfunctions like infections, obstructions, and birth defects. Symptoms typically present themselves as changes in urination habits, pain, or discomfort. Early detection and intervention of such signs are necessary to prevent complications such as renal damage or systemic infection. Nurses therefore have a significant function to monitor such signs during abdominal examination to plan appropriate care and interventions related to detected urinary conditions. Apart from infections and anatomical disorders, urinary tract disorders are often multifactorial in origin and therefore require detailed nursing assessments. For instance, bladder cancer, neurogenic bladder dysfunction, and chronic inflammatory conditions can complicate a patient's urinary situation. Nursing assessments therefore must take into account a broader perspective of the patient's medical history, present medications, and lifestyle. Such data enable nurses to identify not only presenting urinary symptoms but also potential causative factors. The urinary system's integration with other intra-abdominal organs highlights the need for comprehensive evaluation in order to provide holistic and systematic nursing care addressing all aspects of the patients' health, such as the most important details outlined in consensus statements on pelvic floor dysfunction (Abramov et al., 2016). Surgical interventions may also be pivotal in managing severe urinary tract complications, particularly when conservative treatment is not sufficient. Surgical interventions such as repair of the bladder or diversion surgery necessitate extensive pre-surgical assessment to ensure optimal results (Cody et al., 2012). Nurses have an important role to play in informing patients about potential risks, benefits, and post-surgical activities of surgical interventions in such assessments. Moreover, postoperative management requires vigilant observation for difficulties like infection or change in urinary function. As urinary tract dysfunction has a direct effect on patients quality of life, nurses are advised to use their assessment to provide holistic care ensuring both physical healing as well as psychological well-being, hence validating the relevance of exhaustive abdominal assessment for nursing practice (Figure 12.12).

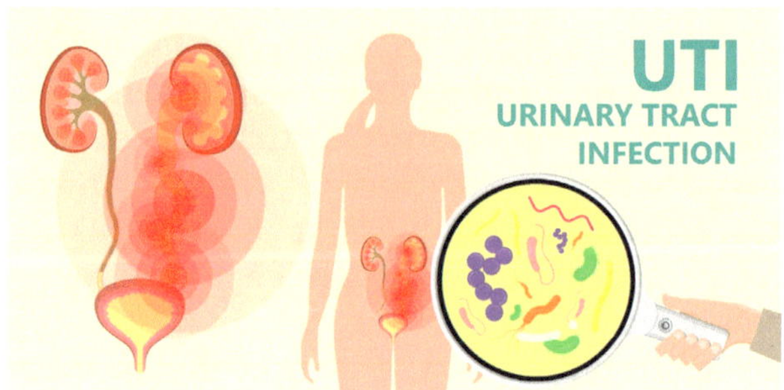

Figure 12.12. Urinary tract infection.

Source: https://www.news-medical.net/images/Article_Images/ImageForArticle_553_16620069160399362.jpg.

12.3.3. Reproductive System Concerns

The evaluation of the reproductive system is a vital part of abdominal examination in nursing, particularly in managing conditions related to chronic pelvic pain (CPP). Myofascial pelvic pain (MFPP) is a significant etiology of CPP and is characterized by the existence of myofascial trigger points on the pelvic floor muscles leading to referred pain in adjacent areas. Identification of these trigger points is crucial to ensure good care and to ensure pain management interventions succeed. Wholistic approaches that include physical exams and histories are able to discover hidden factors not made distinctly evident by standard assessments. Hence, an evident understanding of MFPP facilitates nursing experts to make a contribution towards patient health by integrating various modes of treatment and with multidisciplinary teams, requiring the right diagnosis and tailored interventions in addressing the problems of the reproductive system as part of intensive abdominal examination (Katzman et al., 2012). Moreover, such specific disorders as polycystic ovary syndrome (PCOS) illustrate the complexities of reproductive system problems described in abdominal examinations. During clinical practice, identification of PCOS symptoms and signs can significantly enhance patient outcomes. Nurses must be aware that patients with bowel dysfunction tend to have an increased incidence of PCOS and thus proper assessments must extend beyond the normal evaluation of reproduction. The use of innovative technologies, such as biofeedback, yields optimistic results in managing conditions on the periphery of reproductive health, as indicated by research that evaluates the efficacy of such an approach in clinical settings. Engaging with patients holistically and paying attention to their reproductive health history not only boosts the assessment process but also fosters a supportive environment for patients grappling with complex reproductive health issues (Chelvanayagam et al., 2012). Standard abdominal checks involving reproductive system evaluations can therefore be a revolutionary influence in addressing women's health concerns. These comprehensive practices create regular checks chances for close awareness of patients reproductive status. With well-structured processes that incorporate observation, symptom checking, and inter-disciplinary collaboration, nursing professionals can effectively speak on behalf of patients health interests and preference. Understand that the intertwined issues of pelvic and abdominal health positions nurses to more effectively advocate for interventions that address both quality of life and outcomes of health for assorted populations. As nursing is becoming more forward-thinking, incorporating reproductive system screenings into routine assessment will become increasingly essential, which will result in enhanced patient engagement and whole-person care processes with the goal of resolving multifaceted reproductive problems (Chelvanayagam et al., 2012; Katzman et al., 2012).

Test Your Knowledge

1. What are common abdominal conditions, such as appendicitis, liver disease, or bowel obstruction, and what assessment findings indicate each?
2. How can early recognition of abdominal conditions impact patient outcomes?

12.4. Cultural Considerations in Abdominal Assessment

Learning Outcome

1. Variations in Abdominal Anatomy
2. Cultural Beliefs Affecting Assessment
3. Communication Barriers in Diverse Populations

Cultural aspects are at the core of the abdominal assessment conducted by nurses, influencing both intervention methods used and patient-healthcare professional communication. Awareness of cultural backgrounds allows nurses to comprehend the complex meanings accorded to abdominal symptoms and to sex, thereby providing a complete examination process. For instance, certain cultures may have particular convictions concerning gastrointestinal complaints as indicators of spiritual illness rather than physical illness. This cultural belief can be critical in affecting patient response, compliance with diagnostic testing, and cooperation with the delivery of pertinent health information. Therefore, culturally appropriate nursing practice hinges on sensitivity to these paradigms so that nurses can adjust their assessment approach to the patient-specific setting of each patient, facilitating enhanced health results as well as patient satisfaction. Moreover, the language used in conducting abdominal exams may be significantly influenced by cultural variations in health literacy and pain or discomfort representation. Patients with diverse backgrounds can describe abdominal issues in terms or lingo that deviate from clinical speak, thereby complicating the assessment process. This emphasizes the importance of applying simple, culturally relevant communication methods. Nurses not only need to be instructed on the technical skills of abdominal exams but also on the art of communicating effectively with patients with diverse backgrounds. The utilization of culturally conscious words and ensuring that patients understand the questions asked can help fill up any gaps in understanding. This manner, medical professionals are capable of optimizing the validity of their findings and establishing a therapeutic relationship founded upon respect and trust of cultural diversity, which are the fundamental building blocks of effective nursing care. Cultural considerations extend to where the abdominal examinations are conducted as well.

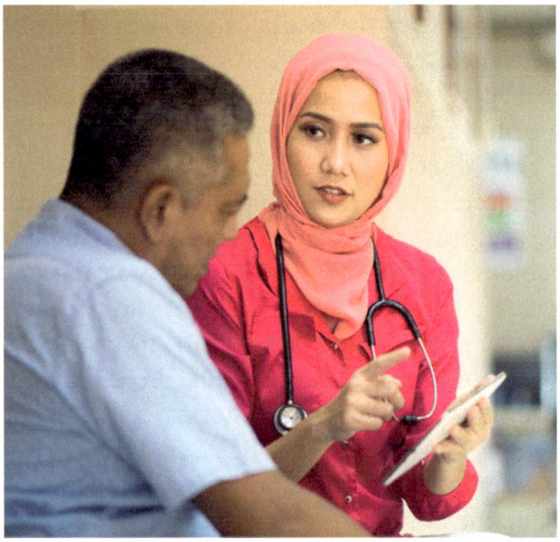

Figure 12.13. Cultural considerations.

Source: https://external-content.duckduckgo.com/iu/?u=https%3A%2F%2Fmrctcenter.org%2Fhealth-literacy%2Fwp-content%2Fuploads%2Fsites%2F3%2F2019%2F10%2Fbest-practice-resources-cultural-considerations-2.jpg&f=1&nofb=1&ipt=881a23c2c4191f3bae583358caaedf9fd30f580df3452c4c19f943678439270e.

The setting must adapt to accommodate patients' cultural norms, which could encompass such factors as anonymity during tests or the presence of family. For example, inclusion of the family in healthcare decision-making is important in some cultures since this will align with their overall beliefs. This can be particularly relevant with abdominal assessments, where patients would feel exposed or vulnerable. Also, the choice of methods of assessment may be needed to be adjusted; for instance, certain methods may be insensitive or taboo in specific cultures. The nurses, therefore, must be responsive and flexible, ensuring their methods of assessment are respectful and sensitive to different patients' cultural beliefs. Such a focus increases the depth of the patient experience and makes nursing practice in diverse clinical settings much more efficient, as noted in successful nursing practice and education literature (Rivera-Hernandez et al., 2017; Tanyi, 2017) (Figure 12.13).

12.4.1. Variations in Abdominal Anatomy

It is necessary for nursing practitioners who perform abdominal assessment to understand the variations of abdominal anatomy. The intricate composition of abdominal structures within the abdominal cavity can be quite different from one individual to another depending primarily on genetic, developmental, and environmental factors. Such anatomical variations can be present in the location, size, and orientation of such vital organs as the liver, kidneys, and spleen, complicating diagnosis and treatment. For instance, ectopic kidneys may appear in the lower abdomen instead of where they normally occur, and variations in vasculature can impact blood flow and complicate surgery. Through the identification of these variations, nurses can become more precise in assessment, make informed decisions, and anticipate potential complications that may arise in the process of caring for a patient and, in doing so, improve the level of clinical practice. In addition, the significance of such anatomical differences crosses over into imaging and diagnostic processes. For instance, the accuracy of an ultrasound or CT scan can be jeopardized if anatomical variations are not taken into consideration. Such awareness enables nurses to better interpret imaging findings, whether results of observed anomalies are due to pathological changes or merely anatomical variations. Such awareness is particularly pertinent in acute abdomen pain cases, in which a misperception could lead to inappropriate interventions or delayed treatment. When integrated into nursing education through courses on anatomical differences, such readiness of future professionals to approach abdominal assessments with greater confidence and skepticism, emphasizing the importance of patient-specific care in nursing practice, can be highly beneficial. Finally, the relationship between patient outcomes and anatomical variation warrants intensive training for nursing professionals. As medical doctors, nurses must understand that variations can drastically influence clinical presentations and responses to treatments. For instance, certain variations can predispose patients to conditions like hernias or bowel obstruction that must be handled with immediate care. Admitting an in-depth understanding of variation in abdominal anatomy into clinical practice supports holistic observation and enables nurses to modify their practice based on patient history and anatomy. Such attention does not merely add quality to care being provided but also develops a culture in which nurses feel compelled to voice for effective treatment plans that reflect specific patient requirements. With the progression of nursing, anatomical information will continue to serve as the key to ensuring the best patient outcomes.

12.4.2. Cultural Beliefs Affecting Assessment

Cultural beliefs have a strong impact on nursing assessment attitude and perception. The patient's cultural background may affect their perceptions of health, illness, and even the healthcare system. Cultural beliefs can, for instance, affect perceptions of abdominal pain and the readiness of patients to disclose symptoms to healthcare professionals during abdominal examination. Certain cultures may view illness and pain as indications of spiritual or moral transgressions, thus affecting patients receptiveness during assessment. In effect, nurses must navigate the cultural dynamics with care to be in a position to communicate and understand accordingly. Such cultural sensitivity is not only crucial for accurate assessment but also for trust and rapport development between patients and healthcare professionals as they grapple with various worldviews of well-being and health. Furthermore, the process of cultural safety in nursing is significant in facilitating that these ingrained health inequalities be confronted, which are established on cultural misconceptions and biases. It is necessary that medical practitioners are mindful of their personal cultural bias and values because these may inadvertently affect their practice of assessment. Lack of considerations for these forces may lead to misdiagnosis or missing significant health issues in terms of abdominal examinations, particularly in a multicultural population. By prioritizing cultural safety, nursing education and practice can be constructed to include training in cultural competency, where practitioners not only learn about different cultural beliefs but also learn about power relationships within healthcare relations. These measures encourage practitioners to reflect on critiquing dominant power relations that would otherwise marginalize some cultural viewpoints within clinical practice (Curtis et al., 2019). Moreover, hearing patients of varying cultural backgrounds as part of the assessment process is necessary to acknowledge in attempts to enhance healthcare practices. Studies indicate that prescriber decisions are also informed not only by clinical guidelines but by prescribers' own assumptions about a patient's background and needs (Anderson et al., 2014). It is thus equally crucial to understand cultural beliefs during the time of abdominal exams, wherein symptom interpretation and decision-making may be varied by culture. An understanding of such differences makes possible a more individualized care approach, not just respecting patients' beliefs but also for building a more tolerant healthcare setting. This overall point of view improves patient satisfaction as well as medical advice compliance, ultimately resulting in equity in healthcare delivery (Figure 12.14).

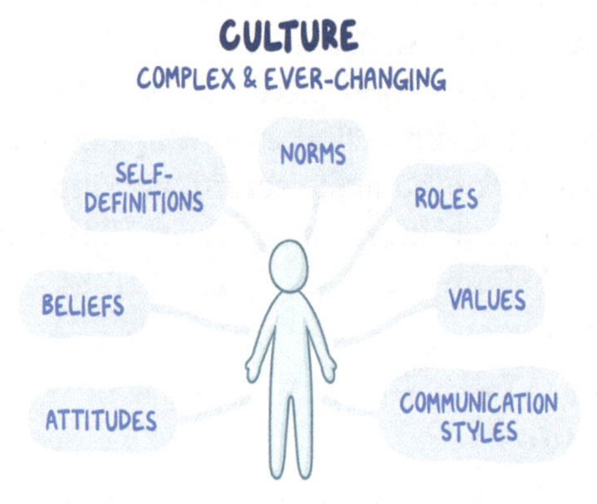

Figure 12.14. Concepts of cultural assessment.

Source: https://external-content.duckduckgo.com/iu/?u=https%3A%2F%2Fosmose-it.s3.amazonaws.com%2FfMTi55EORjWeCtUz7Y9eF_B2QGeVuEqW%2F_.jpg&f=1&nofb=1&ipt=7d8f05d35a016e1ffd91c93da81b87cf1794bf87ea6263b6549bbce124e0c947.

12.4.3. Communication Barriers in Diverse Populations

Effective communication is a guideline for effective nursing practice, particularly in conducting abdominal examinations where proper conversation is paramount in accurate diagnosis. However, barriers to communication are prevalent among healthcare providers and a wide range of populations. These barriers can be caused by language differences, cultural misunderstandings, as well as variations in health literacy. For instance, low English language speakers will not be able to describe their symptoms, leading to inadequate information gathering during examinations. Furthermore, assumptions about culture and illness and health may affect how patients describe their problems or define medical vocabulary, hence complicating the process of nursing assessment. Such challenges are resolved through a certain method of blending linguistic competencies and sensitivity to culture in nursing practice to ensure that assessments yield relevant and useful information required for patient care (Piotrowski et al., 2003). In addition to the linguistic challenges, social determinants of health can exacerbate communication barriers in multi-cultural populations. Socioeconomic status, education, and healthcare availability all potentially influence how effectively patients will be able to describe their illnesses. The patient from the disadvantaged segment might be unacquainted with normal medical practices or medical lingo, so he or she will be less likely to talk about his or her gastrointestinal issue. In addition, stringent time constraints within clinical settings may hamper the ability of nurses to foster an open communication setting. These constraints deter patients from describing health experiences in detail, and this ultimately leads to misdiagnosis or delayed treatment. Nurses, through the understanding of the broader environment of patients' lives, can enhance effective mechanisms of communication, thereby enhancing the quality of abdominal examination and subsequent treatment (Asian American Pacific Islander Nurses Association, 2016). Having effective means to break communication barriers is imperative in order to achieve an extensive nursing evaluation. Interventions such as employing interpreters, utilizing visual aids, and empathizing may tremendously enhance nurses' and patients' comprehension of one another. Training nursing staff to recognize and value cultural differences will also optimize communication for a more holistic abdominal evaluation. Engaging patients in question-probing and confirming dialogue also enables them, leading to greater health literacy and active participation in their own health care. Last but not least, transcending communication barriers through reflective practice not only improves the quality of abdominal exams but also leads to a strong therapeutic relationship, which is fundamental to successful nursing practice. Prioritizing these strategies will enable healthcare professionals to offset the dangers of miscommunication and enable all portions of the population to take advantage of the highest available standard of care (Piotrowski et al., 2003).

Test Your Knowledge

1. How can cultural differences in diet, body shape, or health beliefs affect abdominal assessment findings?
2. Why is it important to be culturally sensitive when interpreting abdominal symptoms and patient responses?

12.5. Documentation and Reporting

Learning Outcome

1. Importance of Accurate Documentation
2. Standardized Reporting Formats
3. Legal Implications of Documentation Errors.

Quality documentation and report writing are also important in nursing, particularly when it comes to abdominal assessment. Documentation is a form of communication that is very vital in facilitating care continuity and fostering shared understanding among healthcare providers. This is important in order to maintain the safety and wellbeing of a patient. For instance, when nurses report in detail during their abdominal assessment, they create in-depth records that optimize the clinical decision-making process. Such records not only indicate results of physical evaluations but also capture subjective data contributed by the patient. Through both perspectives, nurses can develop a comprehensive picture of the patients' health conditions, which in turn determine treatment strategies. Moreover, parent and caregiver opinions in pediatric settings cannot be ignored, as research findings have shown with regard to the need for aligning documentation with observed symptoms. In a previous study, parents had documented symptoms in infants that were not always present in the medical records and which could delay best end-of-life care (Switala et al., 2016). Such a gap emphasizes the importance of nurses, recognizing and incorporating family observations into their documentation. By offering recorded results along with responding to parental issues, nurses can enhance the quality of care considerably, rendering the plans for treatment responsive to the actual perceptions and symptoms which parents report. Another critical aspect of documentation and reporting is good pain control, particularly in emergency situations. A study of presentations to emergency departments concluded that a significant percentage of patients presented with pain but many patients had not had adequate analgesia prior to presentation (Fry et al., 2012). This suggests that nurses must report in detail the pain assessments and interventions against pain during abdominal examinations. By documenting pain measurements, patient reports, and treatment responses in a methodical manner, nurses can ensure better pain control and less unnecessary suffering. Such meticulous recording not only allows for instant clinical interventions but also forms the groundwork for subsequent research and adjustments in pain management policy within clinical settings (Figure 12.15).

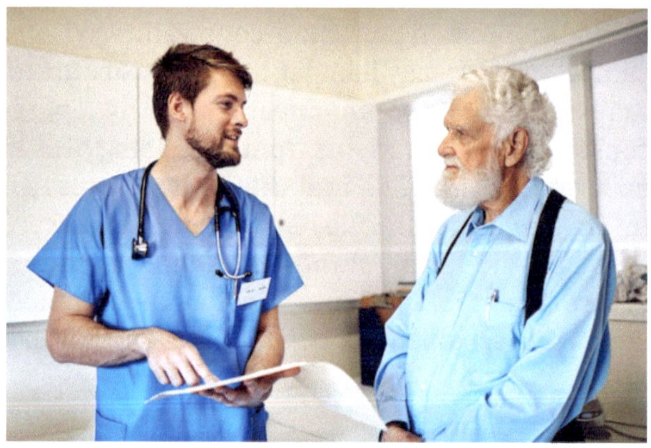

Figure 12.15. Documentation and reporting during health assessments.

Source: https://img.freepik.com/premium-photo/senior-man-nurse-with-documents-healthcare-consultation-medical-diagnosis-test-results-elderly-patient-doctor-health-report-recovery-treatment-planning-assessment-clinic_590464-451347.jpg.

12.5.1. Importance of Accurate Documentation

Accurate documentation is an adjunct to good practice in quality nursing, and therefore especially crucial in the assessment of the abdomen, where precise information gathering can be of considerable consequence to the outcome of the patient. Adequate documentation not only serves as a legal record of care provided, but also enhances communication among the health team members. In the nursing practice, especially in critical care or psychiatric settings, each piece of information written has the potential to guide better decision-making. For instance, early identification of metabolic side effects among severely mentally ill patients on second-generation antipsychotics will depend largely on meticulous documentation of vital signs and symptoms. As mentioned in the quality improvement project for metabolic syndrome, improved provider awareness facilitated through accurate record-keeping can enhance screening behavior and subsequently result in improved long-term patient outcomes for health, hence emphasizing the extreme significance of documentation within nursing care (Moreno et al., 2016). Furthermore, the urgency of correct documentation is again emphasized by its use in guaranteeing patient safety. In abdominal tests, precise and repeatable documentation allows nurses to detect changes in the status of an individual in a timely fashion. Such close observation allows for easy recording of divergences from normal results and treatment, which ultimately prevents complications. For example, in labor tests, detection of the nuances of signs may lead to timely intervention, a feature that is most critical in high-risk groups. Results from the qualitative study of pregnant women show that the inability to correctly interpret abdominal feelings can cause delay in required medical treatment. Therefore, when healthcare practitioners carefully document what they observe, it increases their capacity to communicate efficiently regarding a patient's condition, leading to timely action and diminishing the potential for negative outcomes (Harris et al., 2002). Finally, in the practice of advanced nursing, the interaction of specific documentation with evidence-based guidelines captures the balance between clinical expertise and patient care. Documented abdominal results can guide treatment and serve as a reference for future care. Educational interventions reported on in the setting of metabolic screening illustrate how adherence to current guidelines—along with accurate documentation—can lead to improved adherence among health care providers. Through documenting their observations accurately, nurses deliver an accurate report that not only meets regulation but also contributes to the body of research. Such ongoing accumulation of knowledge results in ongoing enhancement of nursing practice, which enhances the overall quality of care delivered for cases of complex health issues like those encountered during abdominal examination (Moreno et al., 2016).

12.5.2. Standardized Reporting Formats

Adoption of standard reporting formats in nursing practice goes a long way towards enhanced efficiency and accuracy in abdominal examinations. For nursing, these formats facilitate the gathering of information in a systematic way, with essential patient information being documented and communicated accurately. This is most critical in shift changes or handovers, where mishandling of information would have negative outcomes on the care of patients. The standardized formats exclude any confusion, making it easy for nurses to quickly comprehend important information regarding the patients abdominal condition and interventions that have already begun. Improved clarity and organization in the reporting also improve continuity of care and assist in improving overall patient safety, highlighting the need for having a common protocol across all healthcare settings (Tasseri et al., 2013). Further, standardized reporting formats are an important aspect of the quest for quality improvement in nursing practice. Using a common technique, nursing staff can carry out more efficient benchmarking and quality assurance. In abdominal examination, this involves the determination of typical risks and complications that can occur, such as acute abdominal pain or post-operative complications. Having a standard format ensures that such complications are reported and addressed in a logical sequence, and that leads to improved patient outcomes. Furthermore, this standardized reporting is consistent with other healthcare practices that are meant to mitigate risks, such as hospital-acquired venous thromboembolism (VTE), which is seen to perform well with standard reporting practices. These kinds of initiatives have produced better compliance with prevention measures, finally reducing morbidity and mortality due to typical hospital-acquired conditions (Maynard et al., 2009). The advantages of standard report form templates are not limited to direct patient care but influence educational and training activities as well. The educational curriculum for students in nursing more and more incorporates such templates, equipping up-and-coming nurses with the resources to deliver high-quality, safe care. By encouraging an appreciation of systematic reporting, nursing students form an appreciation for thorough abdominal assessments and fill the theory to practice gap. Enhanced reporting techniques contribute to developing critical thinking and clinical judgment, which effective nursing practice is based on. Regular professional learning opportunities in standardized formats can promote a culture of ongoing improvement within the nursing workforce as well. Encouraging compliance with reporting standards is not only in the patient's best interest but also reinforces the collective responsibility of nursing professionals to uphold patient safety and quality service (Tasseri et al., 2013).

12.5.3. Legal Implications of Documentation Errors

Sound documentation is the backbone of nursing practice, particularly in the case of abdominal assessments where accuracy is capable of influencing patient outcomes. Misdocumenting findings can lead to serious legal consequences, as failure to accurately document information may result in misdiagnosis or mismanagement. This can trigger legal action against health care professionals when patients experience untoward outcomes resulting from such inaccuracies. Moreover, the validity of patients medical record can also be challenged during litigation, where inaccuracies in documentation could be considered as negligence. Therefore, nurses should exercise caution regarding maintaining accurate and detailed records, as deviations could not only jeopardize patient safety but also have the clinician become vulnerable to potential legal liability in the event of a lawsuit. The. handover. complexity. in. healthcare. environments. sheds. light. on. the. importance. of. documentation. consistency. An analysis of handover failures among emergency department studies considers that time pressure and organizational influences reduce the transmission of necessary patient information, such as previous abdominal examinations (Chessum et al., 2014). Poor documentation during handovers might precipitate misunderstandings or omissions, influencing patient care continuity. Such reliance on verbal communication may compound this issue even further, with critical information not included in patients medical record, at risk of compromising treatment outcomes and malpractice lawsuits. Appreciation of the subtleties of documentation mistakes in patient handover therefore highlights the necessity for effective guidelines in place for proper handover of information amongst nursing personnel. Furthermore, the general implications of documentation errors are extensive and encompass institutional accountability as well as legal mandates for nursing practice. Where strict compliance with documented protocols is mandatorily sanctioned by law, all deviations are susceptible to attract regulation or professional disciplinary measures from nursing boards. Litigation has established that poor or erroneous documentation has incurred considerable penalties to medical facilities, impacting their operational integrity and financial sustainability (N/A, 2017). Emphasizing the legal implications associated with inaccurate documentation during abdominal examinations helps to underscore the necessity of continuing education and training for nursing professionals. By implementing a culture of care and respect for precise documentation, hospitals are able to enhance patient safety, reduce the risk of legal action, and ultimately provide a higher standard of care (Figure 12.16).

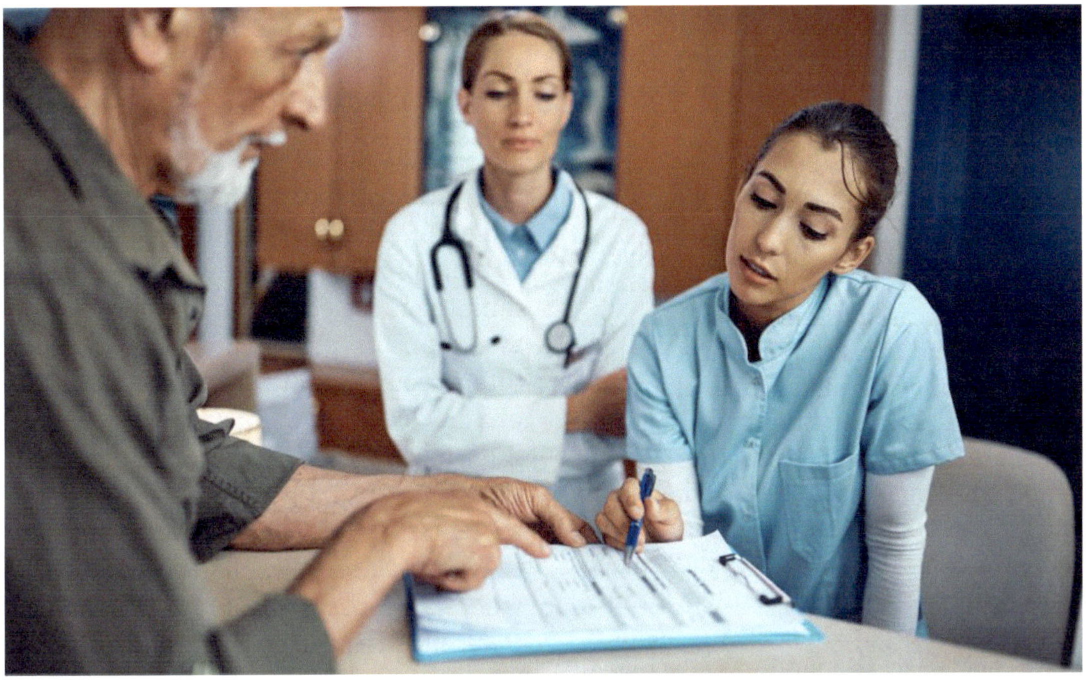

Figure 12.16. Legal implications of documentation errors.

Source: https://www.gammacompliance.com/media/magefan_blog/GammaComplianceSolutions-249522-Medical-Documentation-Mistakes-Blogbanner1.jpg.

Test Your Knowledge

1. How should normal and abnormal abdominal assessment findings be documented to support patient care and continuity?
2. What key details should be included when reporting abdominal assessment findings to the healthcare team?

12.6. Challenges in Abdominal Assessment

Learning Outcome

1. Patient-Related Factors
2. Environmental Influences
3. Limitations of Assessment Techniques

Nursing abdominal assessment encompasses some of the challenges that have far-reaching effects on patient outcomes. Among the primary challenges are inherent patient variation in presentation, such as anatomical differences or pathological conditions that obscure normal signs and symptoms. For instance, in assessing abdominal pain, factors of patient age, sex, and comorbid status could influence the clinical presentation, thus making nurses adjust their approach in assessing. This measure can be misunderstood, especially when standardized assessment protocols are implemented without regard for the specific patient contexts. Inability to quickly recognize acute conditions, like bowel obstruction or appendicitis, leads to delays in treatment and incites a requirement for nurses to possess skill and critical thinking in order to adequately deal with such problems. The other major obstacle is the connection between the psychological status of the patient and the abdominal assessment process. Patients tend to be fearful or apprehensive about having abdominal assessments done, which can be followed by muscle guarding, hence masking underlying pathology. This poses a challenge to palpation and auscultation, two of the key maneuvers in the assessment. Furthermore, patients exhibit different pain tolerance and tolerance of discomfort, which brings another layer of challenge in the assessment process. Strategies aimed at the reduction of anxiety, such as providing reassurance and conducting assessment in a relaxed environment, may improve true evaluation. The potential for psychological and emotional barriers to influence the assessment highlights the importance of utilizing a holistic care system that includes management of the patient's emotional status. Lastly, environmental factors can pose significant obstacles to effective abdominal assessment, especially in the prehospital or emergency context. The location where the assessment is done can be small, noiseful, or inadequately lit, posing challenges to thorough investigations.

For instance, in emergency medical service, the paramedics have to conduct assessments while in transit, which poses a great limitation to them providing a thorough assessment. These limitations are echoed in studies which indicate variation in prehospital cannulation rates often results from environmental limitations on the practice of paramedics (Iqbal et al., 2008). Moreover, failure to surmount these environmental limitations can also lead to unnecessary procedures or interventions in that nurses will employ invasive techniques where a full assessment is not entirely feasible. Determination of these environmental limitations remains a crucial part of nursing practice for ensuring patient safety and accurate diagnosis.

12.6.1. Patient-Related Factors

In nursing, and indeed in abdominal assessment, patient-related factors cannot be overemphasized. Patient-related factors encompass a broad range of such things as the patient's medical history, psychology, and social surroundings, all of which may have an influence on the assessment. It is important to comprehend patients existing health issues because previous gastrointestinal issues or operations may have an effect on current symptoms and affect intervention strategies. In addition, the consideration of social determinants such as socioeconomic status and healthcare resource access helps in the formulation of individualized nursing interventions. With the integration of this comprehensive perspective, nurses can ensure that their assessments and corresponding care plans accurately mirror the unique context of every patient, ultimately enhancing their global health and wellness. Psychological determinants such as anxiety and depression are also prevalent among patient-related factors in nurse assessments. These have been shown to forecast post-operative outcomes by affecting a patient's experience of pain and recovery. Specifically, the patients who are operated upon with high anxiety will have prolonged post-operative anxiety and heightened pain perception and worsen the overall recovery process (Abiodun et al., 2005).

Thus, these psychological factors need to be addressed in abdominal assessments to encourage patient comfort and cooperation. By incorporating strategies for minimizing anxiety through patient education and reassurance, nurses can assist in fostering a therapeutic environment that supports more positive recovery patterns and engages patients in their care. In addition, effective communication remains an important component of revealing patient-associated factors in the course of abdominal exams. Building rapport and trust allows nurses to obtain accurate information from patients, a precursor to constructing an overall nursing diagnosis. With illnesses like fecal incontinence, obtaining a good history becomes essential, as patients may be shy to discuss their symptoms and hence there is underreporting (Chelvanayagam et al., 2000). Nurses therefore must be sensitive in handling the situation, making an environment for open discussion. This not only helps in assessing appropriately but also encourages patients to be active participants in their care. By recognizing and addressing the psychological and the communicative barriers, nursing practice can be made significant in giving rise to more effective abdominal assessments (Figure 12.17).

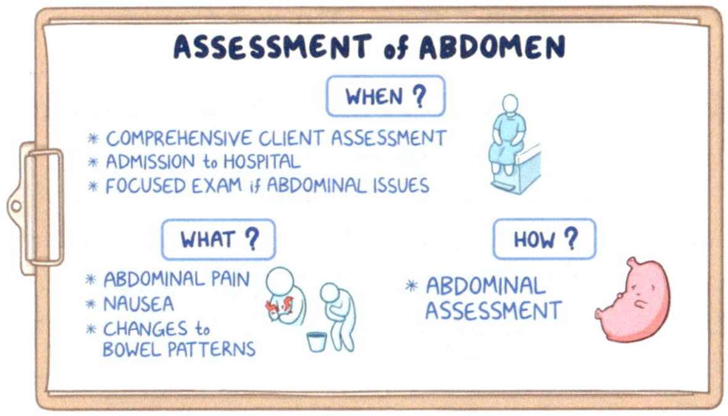

Figure 12.17. Patient-related factors concerning abdominal assessment.

Source: https://www.osmosis.org/_next/image?url=https%3A%2F%2Fd16qt3wv6xm098.cloudfront.net%2F_yHvZSQXQB6oKQbvg3-kkDKXSZqxwIMn%2F_.jpg&w=3840&q=75.

12.6.2. Environmental Influences

Environmental interactions with abdominal well-being are crucial in nursing assessments. Toxin exposure, lifestyle, and diet are of the highest significance in understanding the onset and development of gastrointestinal disease. Up-to-date evidence identifies dietary consumption as key environmental influences for conditions such as inflammatory bowel disease (IBD), which has seen its incidence increase exponentially. Specifically, research by the D-ECCO working group identifies dietary exposure as being central to the etiology of IBD, inferring that environmental stimuli act independently on gut microbiota in genotypically susceptible individuals. Nurses then need to incorporate nutritional assessment as part of abdominal examination to identify potential risk factors that would worsen the condition of patients. By being aware of these influences, nurses can modify dietary recommendations and aid interventions conducive to gastrointestinal well-being and facilitating improved clinical results. More than diet, environmental factors encompass broader lifestyle behaviors that affect abdominal wellbeing as well. Inactive lifestyle behavior, so widespread in modern times, has been linked to various gastrointestinal diseases, including obesity, which increase the risk of becoming ill with conditions such as type II diabetes significantly. The importance of this trend is particularly elevated in pediatric populations; there is emerging evidence for a sudden rise in pediatric presentation of type II diabetes, and it is critical that specific interventions follow. To this end, nursing assessments must move beyond physiological examination to include assessment of lifestyle and exercise. Understandings of environmental factors like sedentary living on abdominal well-being place nurses in a position to aid in effective prevention and good lifestyle modifications that benefit patient groups. Lastly, the integration of this comprehensive assessment into practice instills improved management of gastrointestinal health complications. In addition to that, nurses' roles are also used to educate patients on how their environment affects abdominal well-being.

Effective dissemination of information on precautionary measures against environmental toxins as well as the benefit of remedial lifestyle habits is required. Increased public awareness about how environmental pollutants, diet, and lifestyle factors contribute to abdominal health allows more patient-centered care with more responsible patients who can actively collaborate in their own management. Moreover, as indicated in present-day research, assessment of nutritional status and supportive nutrition therapy is crucial for patients who have conditions like IBD in order to curb symptoms effectively. As more evidence continues to be provided citing environmental factors' interaction in disease pathology, nursing practice ought to adapt to include such findings. Lastly, patient awareness of the environmental factors involved in nursing assessments will not only enhance patient outcomes but also spur further research into preventive care that is essential to the advancement of public health initiatives in relation to abdominal well-being.

12.6.3. Limitations of Assessment Techniques

Inappropriateness of the methods used in assessment in nursing, notably for abdominal assessment, has the capacity to impact patient outcomes significantly. One of the largest challenges is the lack of consistency in terms of methods used by practitioners. Different practitioners apply various techniques based on their education, practice experience, and personal interpretation of the findings. The inconsistency has the potential to create inconsistencies in diagnoses and the related treatment plans devised. Furthermore, the majority of evaluation techniques lack standardized procedures, and therefore gaps in care may exist. For example, in some healthcare environments, failure to have standardized guidelines would lead to overreliance on specific evaluation modalities at the expense of others, which would consequently obscure the clinical findings. This inconsistency reveals the need for standardized assessment techniques in order to ensure that nursing practitioners all possess the same fundamental skill sets in abdominal evaluations. Additionally, assessment techniques often exclude patient variation, including age, gender, and preexistent medical conditions. These physiological and demographic variations could strongly influence abdominal symptoms, and uniform assessment techniques would be less effective. For instance, a good assessment technique for one subset of patients may not yield valid results in another set due to differences in anatomy or preexistent comorbidity. As reviewed in the literature, studies have shown the deficiency of certain measuring tools in their application to various populations and can lead to missed diagnosis or improper treatment (Cunen et al., 2016). This limitation highlights the importance of tailoring the measuring instruments to the subject patient according to their own personality and health history in an effort to enhance diagnostic precision and enhance the efficacy of the treatment. Besides, the need for subjective interpretation and the susceptibility to human error add to the complexity of assessment method efficacy in abdominal assessment. Nurses' clinical judgment is very critical when it comes to interpreting results of assessment, but differences in experience and personal bias may generate inconsistent results. The problems can arise due to the misinterpretation of sounds heard on auscultation of the abdomen or flawed palpation techniques. Studies have revealed considerable inconsistencies in the results of assessment outcomes depending on these factors, rendering the provision of valid criteria of nursing assessment challenging (Iqbal et al., 2008). With these challenges, education and training are essential to ensure the highest reliability of the assessment techniques in nursing. Deliberate emphasis on the incorporation of evidence-based practice could in the long term eradicate the limitation of subjective assessment and promote more standardized patient care.

Test Your Knowledge

1. What factors, such as patient obesity, pain, or anxiety, can make abdominal assessment difficult?
2. How can nurses overcome challenges to ensure accurate and thorough abdominal evaluation?

SUMMARY

A nursing study of abdominal assessment, identification of the complex aspect of this essential skill in clinical practice must be present. Abdominal assessments are not a routine procedure but a critical diagnostic aid that assists in the detection of anything ranging from gastrointestinal illness to systemic disease. Effective performance of such examinations requires careful knowledge of anatomy, physiology, and pathology and acute observation skills. Nurses play an important role in the same, combining their observations with patient history to provide a comprehensive picture of the patient's health. A good understanding of abdominal assessment can thus contribute significantly to the quality of patient care, allowing for early intervention and potentially better health outcomes. Furthermore, the significance of continued education and adherence to established standards cannot be overlooked in the process of abdominal examinations. Education programs aimed at enriching the capability and confidence of nursing practitioners in the performance of abdominal examinations are indispensable for the building of capability and confidence in performing abdominal examinations. In accordance with recent studies, education interventions yield significant improvement in the willingness and capability of healthcare providers to implement assessment schemes. These interventions also ensure not only clinicians' understanding of the physiological effects of their outcomes but also stimulate evidence-based practice uptake. It is for this purpose that ongoing professional development becomes integral to maintaining nursing practice in line with the latest health advancements, thus promoting patient well-being. The implications of enhanced abdominal assessment skill extend beyond isolated nursing practice to also encompass the larger healthcare dynamics. All these advancements can be translated into enhanced communication and collaboration among medical practitioners, eventually optimizing patient care pathways. The use of evidence-based guidelines and continuous professional education helps facilitate the development of an environment where nurses are capable of adequately advocating for their patients when they interface with multidisciplinary teams. Secondly, by becoming skilled at the early presentation of emergent health complications, nurses can become part of preventive care planning that minimizes issues even before they spiral out of control. This proactive role positions nursing as the first line in patient health addressing, strengthening the credibility of abdominal examination within holistic nursing care patterns rooted in evidence indicating sensitization works to significantly improve treatment outcomes and overall quality of care (Moreno et al., 2016; Switala et al., 2016).

In nursing practice, an effective assessment of the abdomen is important in a diagnosis and treatment of various kinds of health issues. It is an orderly process that incorporates inspection, palpation, percussion, and auscultation to assess the gastrointestinal system. The full evaluation not only enables nurses to identify abnormalities but also assists in having a clearer idea about the general state of well-being of the patients. Recognition of such signs as pain, tenderness, or distension allows for timely intervention and improved patient outcomes. The assessment must then be tailored to the individual presentation of the patient, and this necessitates clinical judgment and critical thinking to allow for full assessment. Emphasis on the psychological aspects of patient care is also important. Through research, it has been established that preoperative anxiety at a high level can directly affect postoperative experience, particularly in abdominal surgeries. In a study by Abbott et al. (2006), there was also an association between anxiety levels and postoperative pain, thus highlighting the importance of addressing psychological factors in the entire process of nursing. In addition, by appreciating the emotional factors, nurses can implement effective interventions to reduce anxiety and improve coping measures. By managing anxiety in anticipation, nurses can enhance the quality of care and satisfaction of patients, justifying the belief that mental health is as vital as physical examination. Multidimensional care is essential to ensure optimal care of patients, especially when evaluating the abdominal area. Integrating psychological and physical evaluation can provide a better picture of the states of the patients. In Abiodun et al. (2005), evidence is presented that not only does preoperative anxiety affect postoperative pain, but that high psychological distress can also negatively impact recovery. This correlation highlights the necessity for incorporating mental health concerns into nursing care. By way of patient education, empathetic communication, and offering complete information, nurses can achieve a reduction in anxiety levels, thus improving patient assessment efficacy and ultimately patient outcomes. This is indicative of the changing face of nursing, where comprehension of the intricate relation between mind and body leads the way to offering high-quality care.

KEY TERMS FROM THIS CHAPTER

Abdomen	Quadrants
Regions	Bowel Sounds
Hyperactive Sounds	Hypoactive Sounds
Absent Sounds	Auscultation
Percussion	Palpation
Light Palpation	Deep Palpation
Organs	Liver Span
Spleen	Abdomen Contour
Tenderness	Distension
Guarding	Rebound Tenderness

CRITICAL THINKING QUESTIONS

1. **The nurse auscultates high-pitched, tinkling bowel sounds. This may indicate:**
   a. Normal bowel activity
   b. Early bowel obstruction
   c. Constipation
   d. Peritonitis
2. **When performing an abdominal assessment, the correct sequence is:**
   a. Palpation → Percussion → Inspection → Auscultation
   b. Inspection → Palpation → Percussion → Auscultation
   c. Inspection → Auscultation → Percussion → Palpation
   d. Auscultation → Inspection → Palpation → Percussion
3. **A firm, rigid abdomen with guarding is most consistent with:**
   a. Normal variation
   b. Peritonitis
   c. 1Gas distension
   d. Constipation
4. **The nurse palpates the liver edge just below the right costal margin. This is:**
   a. A normal finding if smooth and non-tender
   b. Always abnormal
   c. Indicative of liver failure
   d. Sign of splenomegaly
5. **Rebound tenderness (pain upon release) is a sign of:**
   a. Gastritis
   b. Appendicitis or peritoneal irritation
   c. Peptic ulcer disease
   d. Constipation

Short Answer Questions

1. What are the key anatomical regions of the abdomen used during assessment, and why are they important?
2. Describe the correct sequence of abdominal assessment techniques and explain why this order is recommended.
3. What characteristics of bowel sounds should a nurse assess, and what do abnormal findings indicate?
4. How is abdominal palpation performed, and what differences exist between light and deep palpation?
5. What signs and symptoms might indicate abdominal tenderness or guarding?

Answer to Critical Thinking Questions

1. (b) 2. (c) 3. (b) 4. (a) 5. (b)

REFERENCES

1. Abbott, R., Aksoy, M., Allen, C., Altman, D., Appleton, S., Aronson, J., Astedt-Kurki, P., et al. (2006). Patterns and frequency of anxiety in women undergoing gynecological surgery. https://core.ac.uk/download/75117.pdf (accessed on 16th July 2025).
2. Abiodun, O. A., Andrews, F. M., Aylard, P. R., Barczak, P., Barriball, K. L., Beck, C. T., Bergen, A., et al. (2005). Patient experiences of anxiety, depression and acute pain after surgery: A longitudinal perspective. https://core.ac.uk/download/76097.pdf (accessed on 16th July 2025).
3. Abramov, Y., Almeida, F. G., Berghmans, B., Bo, K., et al. (2016). An International Urogynecological Association (IUGA)/International Continence Society (ICS) joint report on the terminology for the conservative and nonpharmacological management of female pelvic floor dysfunction. https://core.ac.uk/download/293861075.pdf (accessed on 16th July 2025).
4. Accettola, E., Bogdan, A., Callahan, S., Chawda, H., et al. (2023). Introduction to health assessment for the nursing professional: Part II. https://core.ac.uk/download/622362029.pdf (accessed on 16th July 2025).
5. Ahmad, K., Al-Nasser, M., Andronikou, S., Andronikou, S., Andronikou, S., Andronikou, S., Andronikou, S., et al. (2009). Advances in imaging chest tuberculosis: Blurring of differences between children and adults. https://core.ac.uk/download/pdf/9417669.pdf (accessed on 16th July 2025).
6. Alewijnse, D., Alewijnse, M., Alhasso, A., Alves, S., Amaro, J. L., Balshem, H., Bastian, H., et al. (2016). Conservative interventions for urinary incontinence in women: An overview of Cochrane systematic reviews. https://core.ac.uk/download/293881644.pdf (accessed on 16th July 2025).
7. Allan, P., Fiorino, G., Gatti, S., Gerasimidis, K., et al. (2017). Research gaps in diet and nutrition in inflammatory bowel disease: A topical review by D-ECCO Working Group (Dietitians of ECCO). https://core.ac.uk/download/84340703.pdf (accessed on 16th July 2025).
8. Anderson, C. M., Lyon, D. E., McCarthy, D., Corwin, E. J., Taylor, J. Y., Voss, J., Gregory, K. E., et al. (2015). Educating future nursing scientists: Recommendations for integrating omics content in PhD programs. https://core.ac.uk/download/213074828.pdf (accessed on 16th July 2025).
9. Anderson, K., Stowasser, D. A., Freeman, C., & Scott, I. (2014). Prescriber barriers and enablers to minimizing potentially inappropriate medications in adults: A systematic review and thematic synthesis. *BMJ Open, 4*, e006544–e006544. https://doi.org/10.1136/bmjopen-2014-006544 (accessed on 16th July 2025).
10. Asian American Pacific Islander Nurses Association. (2016). Proceedings of the 2015 Asian American/Pacific Islander Nurses Association conference: Biological measures: A role in nursing self-management research. https://digitalscholarship.unlv.edu/cgi/viewcontent.cgi?article=1017&context=apin (accessed on 16th July 2025).
11. Baumgartner, H., De Backer, J., Babu-Narayan, S. V., Budts, W., Chessa, M., Diller, G. P., Lung, B., et al. (2020). 2020 ESC guidelines for the management of adult congenital heart disease. *European Heart Journal, 42*, 563–645. https://doi.org/10.1093/eurheartj/ehaa554 (accessed on 16th July 2025).

12. Benato, L., & Hammond, J. (2018). Rabbit neutering in primary-care education: Insights from a surgical clinic. https://core.ac.uk/download/74231223.pdf (accessed on 16th July 2025).

13. Borg Cunen, N., Borg Xuereb, R., Jomeen, J., Poat, C., et al. (2016). A narrative review of interventions addressing the parental-fetal relationship. https://core.ac.uk/download/151162916.pdf (accessed on 16th July 2025).

14. Buissink, C., Hogg, P., & Thompson-Hogg, R. (2016). Optimizing image quality for medical imaging. https://core.ac.uk/download/77067051.pdf (accessed on 16th July 2025).

15. Bultas, M. W., Burkett, K., Johnson, N. L., et al. (2016). Translating research to practice for children with autism spectrum disorder: Part 2: Behavior management in home and health care settings. https://core.ac.uk/download/213081290.pdf (accessed on 16th July 2025).

16. Buzby, J. C., Crutchfield, S. R., Lin, C. T. J., Ollinger, M., et al. (2025). Economic assessment of food safety regulations: The new approach to meat and poultry inspection. https://core.ac.uk/download/pdf/6459734.pdf (accessed on 16th July 2025).

17. Chelvanayagam, S., & Norton, C. (2000). A nursing assessment tool for adults with fecal incontinence. https://core.ac.uk/download/20321232.pdf (accessed on 16th July 2025).

18. Chelvanayagam, S., Collins, B., Duncan, J., O'Brien, C., et al. (2012). Uncovering anorexia nervosa in a biofeedback clinic for bowel dysfunction. https://core.ac.uk/download/20321227.pdf (accessed on 16th July 2025).

19. Chessum, P., Cooke, M., Cross, S., Fitton, L., et al. (2014). Clinical handover within the emergency care pathway and the potential risks of clinical handover failure (ECHO): Primary research. https://core.ac.uk/download/19882629.pdf (accessed on 16th July 2025).

20. Cody, J. D., Dublin, N., McClinton, S., Nabi, G., et al. (2012). Urinary diversion and bladder reconstruction/replacement using intestinal segments for intractable incontinence or following cystectomy. https://core.ac.uk/download/20454622.pdf (accessed on 16th July 2025).

21. Coward, J., De Labouchere, S., Lowe, J., Mercer, C., et al. (2017). Optimax 2016: Peer observation of facilitation. https://core.ac.uk/download/82896178.pdf (accessed on 16th July 2025).

22. Curtis, E., Jones, R., Tipene-Leach, D., Walker, C., Loring, B., Paine, S. J., & Reid, P. (2019). Why cultural safety rather than cultural competency is required to achieve health equity: A literature review and recommended definition. *International Journal for Equity in Health, 18*. https://doi.org/10.1186/s12939-019-1082-3 (accessed on 16th July 2025).

23. Foering, A. (2018). Pediatric type II diabetes mellitus: Examining the upward trend. https://core.ac.uk/download/158970346.pdf (accessed on 16th July 2025).

24. Fry, M., Hearn, J., & McLaughlin, T. (2012). Pre-hospital pain management patterns and triage nurse documentation. https://opus.lib.uts.edu.au/bitstream/10453/18465/1/2011005764.pdf (accessed on 16th July 2025).

25. Gardiner, A., & Hilton, A. (2016). Managing constipation in adults with co-morbidities. https://core.ac.uk/download/151161237.pdf (accessed on 16th July 2025).

26. Hanson, L. (2009). Second-stage labor care: Challenges in spontaneous bearing down. https://core.ac.uk/download/213073254.pdf (accessed on 16th July 2025).

27. Harris, S., Saks, N. P., & Weiss, M. E. (2002). Resolving the uncertainty of preterm symptoms: Women's experiences with the onset of preterm labor. https://core.ac.uk/download/213077034.pdf (accessed on 16th July 2025).

28. Iqbal, M., Shaw, D., Siriwardena, A. N., Spaight, R., et al. (2008). To cannulate or not to cannulate? Variation, appropriateness and potential for reduction in cannulation rates by ambulance staff. https://core.ac.uk/download/55503.pdf (accessed on 16th July 2025).

29. Katzman, W. B., & Pastore, E. A. (2012). Recognizing myofascial pelvic pain in the female patient with chronic pelvic pain. https://core.ac.uk/download/305124272.pdf (accessed on 16th July 2025).

30. Kitsiou, A., Caforio, A. L. P., Porta-Sanchez, A., Vahanian, A., Iung, B., Carrera, C., Szymanski, C., et al. (2013). ESC core curriculum for the general cardiologist (2013). https://core.ac.uk/download/55756305.pdf (accessed on 16th July 2025).

31. Maynard, G., & Stein, J. (2009). Designing and implementing effective venous thromboembolism prevention protocols: Lessons from collaborative efforts. https://core.ac.uk/download/pdf/81053541.pdf (accessed on 16th July 2025).

32. Misnawati, M., Wiwik, W., & Ropyanto, C. B. (2015). The effect of dzikir concerning to pain level after surgical operation reduction internal fixation (ORIF). https://core.ac.uk/download/76929262.pdf (accessed on 16th July 2025).

33. Moreno, A. (2016). Metabolic syndrome screening in seriously mentally ill patients: A quality improvement project. https://core.ac.uk/download/286607497.pdf (accessed on 16th July 2025).

34. N/A. (1985). Focal Spot, Fall 1985. https://core.ac.uk/download/129069250.pdf (accessed on 16th July 2025).

35. N/A. (1986). 216 Jewish Hospital of St. Louis. https://core.ac.uk/download/70380873.pdf (accessed on 16th July 2025).

36. N/A. (2017). Iowa Board of Nursing Newsletter November, December 2017 – January 2018, Vol. 36, no. 4. https://core.ac.uk/download/95086520.pdf (accessed on 16th July 2025).

37. Piotrowski, A., Chen, A. H., Jacobs, E. A., Hardt, E. J., & Agger-Gupta, N. (2003). Language barriers in health care settings: An annotated bibliography of research literature. https://core.ac.uk/download/71352611.pdf (accessed on 16th July 2025).

38. Rivera-Hernandez, M., Rahman, M., Mor, V., & Trivedi, A. (2017). Skilled nursing facilities that disproportionately serve Medicare beneficiaries in the U.S. *Innovation in Aging, 1*, 793–793. https://www.semanticscholar.org/paper/28b9fc1c3db5a09daf692041b0924550f3a89812 (accessed on 16th July 2025).

39. Rychik, J., Atz, A. M., Celermajer, D. S., Deal, B. J., Gatzoulis, M. A., Gewillig, M., Hsia, T. Y., et al. (2019). Evaluation and management of the child and adult with Fontan circulation: A scientific statement from the American Heart Association. *Circulation, 140*. https://doi.org/10.1161/cir.0000000000000696 (accessed on 16th July 2025).

40. Switala, M. (2016). Parent perceptions of infant symptoms at end-of-life in the NICU. https://core.ac.uk/download/286359999.pdf (accessed on 16th July 2025).

41. Tanyi, V. E. (2017). Assessing the components of mentoring in nursing practice placements: A mixed study approach. *IOSR Journal of Nursing and Health Science, 06*, 86–102. https://www.semanticscholar.org/paper/0ed749cfc246bdb16e1a51298927889ab81afb05 (accessed on 16th July 2025).

42. Tasseri, A., Malekzadeh, J., Mazluom, S. R., & Etezadi, T. (2013). A standardized shift handover protocol: Improving nurses' safe practice in intensive care units. https://core.ac.uk/download/pdf/26788131.pdf (accessed on 16th July 2025).
43. Tipton, B. L. (2019). Practice vs. evidence: Predicting insertion length and verifying placement of feeding tubes in neonates. https://core.ac.uk/download/227560096.pdf (accessed on 16th July 2025).

MUSCULOSKELETAL SYSTEM ASSESSMENT IN NURSING

13

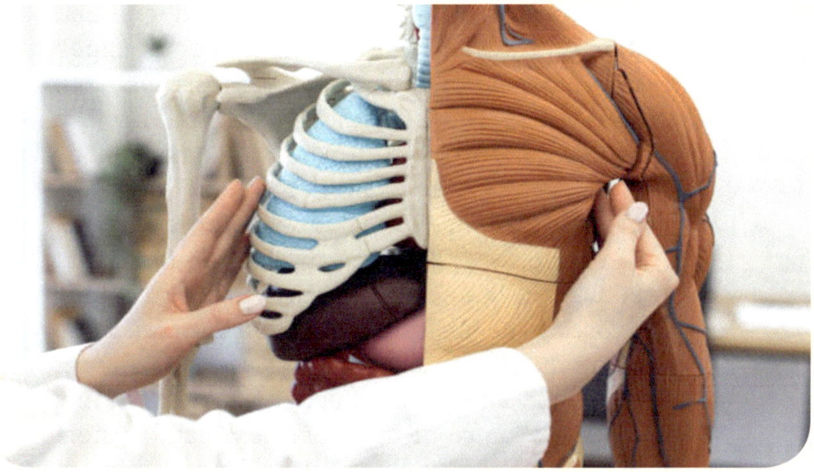

LEARNING OBJECTIVES

After studying this chapter, you will be able to:

1. Explain the anatomy of the musculoskeletal system;
2. Describe the assessment techniques;
3. Identify the common musculoskeletal disorders;
4. Discuss about patient history and interview;
5. Elaborate the documentation and reporting;
6. Explore the nursing interventions..

Introduction

The musculoskeletal system is critical in human health because it includes the bones, muscles, joints, and connective tissues that enable movement as well as the upkeep of body functions. In nursing, this system should be assessed to identify various disorders in health, evaluate pain, and guide interventions. Comprehensive assessment of the musculoskeletal system is crucial not only in diagnosing pathology but also in ensuring effective patient care. As medical practitioners, nurses are spearheading this process of evaluation and therefore should possess the technical skills as well as clinical knowledge to recognize deviations from the norm. This introduction indicates the applicability of musculoskeletal assessments, paving the way for an in-depth analysis of their methodology, implications, and impact in nursing practice. Effective musculoskeletal assessment is a systematic process involving the integration of patient history, physical examination, and relevant diagnostic procedures. Nurses must conduct proper evaluations to detect musculoskeletal disorders in the initial stages, enhancing treatment outcomes significantly. Musculoskeletal injury and disorders are induced by age, lifestyle, and occupational hazards, requiring a guided assessment plan according to individual patient needs. In addition, ergonomic significance takes precedence since traditional work practices will not take into consideration human variability and individualized needs placed on healthcare professionals. With the help of tools such as OWAS, REBA, and RULA, nurses can quantify levels of risk in relation to musculoskeletal injury and formulate strategies for injury reduction and enhanced overall patient care (Case et al., 2013).

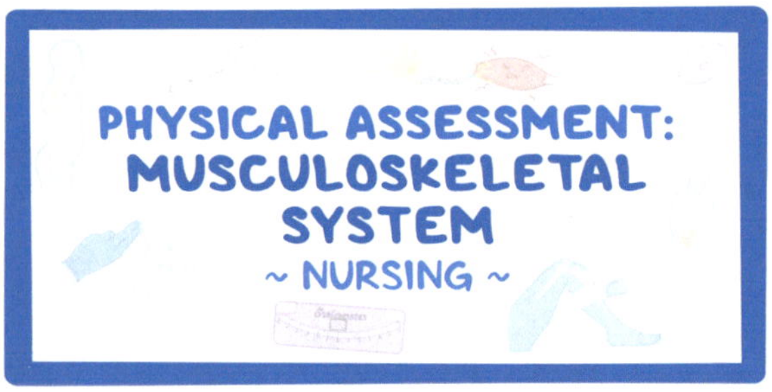

Figure 13.1. Physical assessment – musculoskeletal system.

Source: https://osmose-it.s3.amazonaws.com/O5uyADptR4eVKqIhVWYwyFOGRdOSA5qs/_.jpg.

Thus, mastering the nuances of musculoskeletal examination is crucial in creating a safe and successful health facility. Psychological aspects of musculoskeletal disorders cannot be ignored in nursing practice either. Stress and burnout among healthcare workers can aggravate musculoskeletal conditions, highlighting the intricate interplay between body and mind. Holistic practices, such as yoga and stress management, can enhance resilience, as well as physical and emotional health among nurses (Cocchiara et al., 2019). This approach, which is multi-faceted in nature, not only benefits healthcare professionals but also enhances the quality of care offered to patients. As we continue in the intricacies of musculoskeletal system assessments in nursing, it is important to view the connection between physical assessment, injury prevention strategies, and mental health treatment to foster a holistic model of patient and practitioner wellness (Figure 13.1).

Definition of the Musculoskeletal System

The musculoskeletal system is an integral and dynamic system in the human body made up of bones, muscles, cartilage, tendons, and ligaments. The system is essential for the structural integrity, locomotion, as well as protection of vital organs in the body. The bones provide a framework of support for the weight of the body, while muscles generate force that enables walking and other activities of the body to occur. The intricate interaction between these components facilitates an incredible amount of motion and physical activity, demonstrating the importance of the musculoskeletal system for health as well as daily functioning. In addition, an understanding of this systems complexity is critical to effective evaluation in practice for nursing because this knowledge is the foundation necessary to identify potential disorders and diagnose related diseases that will be manifested in patients during clinical setting evaluations. A comprehensive examination of the musculoskeletal system is particularly relevant in nursing practice because it involves the examination of structural as well as functional components. Nurses are tasked with identifying signs of musculoskeletal disorders, including pain, swelling, deformity, or limitation of motion. Proper assessment must not only be aware of anatomy but also familiar with normal musculoskeletal disorders like arthritis, fractures, and tendonitis. Further, incorporation of standard assessment tools, e.g., the Nordic Musculoskeletal Questionnaire, can assist nurses in quantifying patients' symptoms and enhancing care plans. Definitiveness of musculoskeletal symptomatology is particularly relevant to nurse education, as deduced from studies pointing towards the prevalence of musculoskeletal symptoms amongst nursing students themselves (Antunes et al., 2019). In treating the pain management issues of the musculoskeletal system in pain managements' contemporary settings, nursing professionals must meet the effectiveness of intervention with the need to minimize the dependence on pharmacological interventions, particularly opioids. The shift towards nonpharmacological intervention of pain management has been necessitated by the increasing misuse of opioids' prescriptions, prompting national agencies to redirect treatment guidelines (Swezey et al., 2018). This paradigm also calls on nurses to keep abreast of other interventions, such as lifestyle modifications and physical therapy, for the management of musculoskeletal pain. An understanding of the complexity of the musculoskeletal system gives nurses crucial information about patient care, enabling them to deal with not only symptoms but also causative factors of conditions. Thus, a solid foundation in musculoskeletal health is required for nursing practitioners to provide patient-centered, holistic care.

Importance of Assessment in Nursing

Nursing evaluation, or musculoskeletal system evaluation, is a fundamental practice with direct influence on clinical judgment and patient outcome. One of the strengths of total assessment is the potential to reveal latent underlying disorders which are otherwise not so readily apparent. Nurses conducting thorough musculoskeletal symptom evaluations, for instance, can detect nascent symptoms of disorders, which, left untreated, can lead to grave patient morbidity. It is an active process not just to identify conditions but also to facilitate the generation of effective intervention strategies that are tailored to the patient. Secondly, global assessments facilitate better communication among interdisciplinary teams to ensure that all team members understand the patient's condition as well as the treatment plan, hence facilitating care in collaboration. Optimal delivery of patient care requires strict compliance to protocols of assessment before it can be done, especially when examining musculoskeletal disorders. Research stresses the need for reliable measurement tools in determining exercise compliance among patients with such conditions. Accurate assessment requires utilization of scientifically proven instruments that are capable of ascertaining the degree and experience of patients regarding adherence to exercise regimens, as recent studies (Williams et al., 2014) have indicated. This does not only enable tracking of the effectiveness of exercise programs but also identifies compliance barriers so interventions can be clearly directed at increasing patient compliance and participation. An intensive understanding of these features enhances the delivery of holistic care by nurses and guides the modification of treatment plans when needed, thus leading to improved patient health outcomes. Furthermore, the integration of concept analysis in nursing education can significantly facilitate the evaluation skills of nursing students. As evidenced through more recent evaluations of undergraduate nursing students' symptomology of the musculoskeletal system, understanding basic concepts—pain, discomfort, as well as the use of measuring tools like the Nordic Musculoskeletal Questionnaire—is paired with improvement in assessment practice (Antunes et al., 2019). With the inclusion of such understanding in nursing education curriculum, educators equip future nurses with the skills necessary to conduct comprehensive examination of the musculoskeletal system. This early learning not only aids in critical thinking but also equips learners to enter patient assessments with increased confidence and ability. Ensuring nurses are adequately trained in assessment techniques will ultimately lead to better patient care, addressing the evolving requirements of those with musculoskeletal conditions (Figure 13.2).

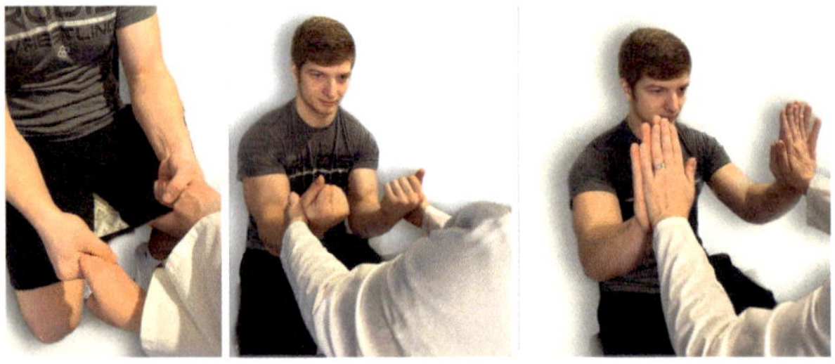

Figure 13.2. Assessment in nursing.

Source: https://wtcs.pressbooks.pub/app/uploads/sites/29/2020/09/Assessing-Hand-grips-1024x424.png.

13.1. Anatomy of the Musculoskeletal System

Learning Outcome

1. Major Components: Bones, Muscles, and Joints
2. Functions of the Musculoskeletal System
3. Common Anatomical Terms Used in Assessment

The musculoskeletal system is a complex system comprising bones, muscles, tendons, ligaments, and connective tissues. Nursing staff should be well aware of the musculoskeletal system since it is an essential component of movement, stability, and general body functioning. Bones not only serve as the supports for structural stability but also serve as a protective sheath for some organs, and muscles generate movement by contracting and relaxing. Tendons connect muscles to bones, facilitating the transfer of force, and ligaments stabilize joints by connecting bones to each other. Nurses must be familiar with assessing this intricate process for identifying abnormalities or trauma that might inhibit a patient's mobility or lifestyle. Comprehensive knowledge of anatomical landmarks, joint kinematics, and muscle dynamics directs the process of nursing assessment and results in improved outcomes of care in musculoskeletal function. In clinical practice, examination of the musculoskeletal system is done by a methodical process, like inspection, palpation, and functional assessment. Inspection enables the nurses to check for symmetrical alignment, swelling, or deformity that can indicate pathological conditions. Through palpation, nurses can determine tenderness or variations in temperature that can indicate underlying inflammation or injury. Functional testing, such as range of motion testing, quantifies the operation of muscles and joints and helps to classify any deficiency or pain associated with movement. In combination, these methods provide an overall profile of a patient's musculoskeletal status. Understanding the anatomical etiology of common conditions, such as piriformis syndrome, is central to the recognition of clinical findings such as buttock pain or greater sciatic notch tenderness, leading ultimately to effective nursing intervention and referral for additional management (Chantraine et al., 2010). Nurses should remain current with recent studies and advances in the understanding of musculoskeletal disorders in order to maintain high-quality musculoskeletal assessments. For instance, writings about conditions like piriformis syndrome emphasize the need for more study of the relationship between specific clinical characteristics and pathologies. As emphasized by studies looking into prevalent symptoms and diagnostic problems, an additional exploration of the musculoskeletal system is essential to the development of proper care measures (N/A, 1985). Nurses therefore play a central role in not only assessing the musculoskeletal system but also in educating patients on preventive measures and lifestyle modifications that enhance musculoskeletal health. By creating a general appreciation of the anatomy and physiology of the system, nursing practitioners can thus go a long way towards improving patient outcomes and quality of care in musculoskeletal care (Figure 13.3).

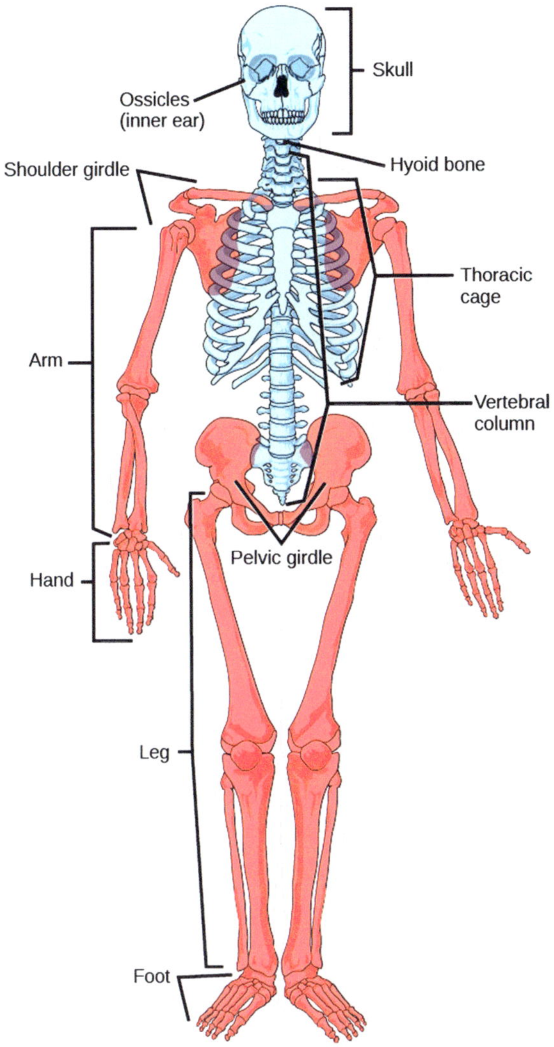

Figure 13.3. Anatomy of the musculoskeletal system.

Source: https://open.lib.umn.edu/app/uploads/sites/261/2019/08/Figure_16_05_01.jpg.

13.1.1. Major Components: Bones, Muscles, and Joints

Musculoskeletal system is a highly intricate system consisting primarily of bones, muscles, and joints that all function together in order to allow for locomotion and posture. Bones not only supply the body's rigid support system but also carry out a variety of vital functions in defending organs, Mineral storage, and hematopoiesis resulting in the formation of blood cells. Human bone is composed of 206 bones in adulthood of particular shapes and function based on age, sex, and amount of physical activity. Nursing assessment is commonly aimed at the condition of bones in patients, particularly older adults, as they have an elevated risk of developing disorders such as osteoporosis that decreases bone mass and increases the risk of fractures. From their understanding of the anatomical and physiological roles of bones, nurses can better evaluate and monitor musculoskeletal condition in patients, guiding interventions aimed at preventing injury and improving bone strength. Muscles are also a key component of the musculoskeletal system, which facilitate movement by contracting and relaxing. Comprising various types of muscles—skeletal, smooth, and cardiac—only skeletal muscles are voluntary and directly connected to the bones by tendons. Muscle strength and function testing is an important part of musculoskeletal evaluation in nursing practice. Diseases such as sarcopenia, in which progressive loss of muscle mass and strength occurs with increasing age, are also expected to decrease mobility as well as the overall quality of life in older patients. Furthermore, nurses should be vigilant when assessing muscle tone and strength because these symptoms can exhibit underlying illnesses or the effectiveness of interventions in rehabilitation. Nurses can prepare for patient mobility and independence setbacks through an understanding of the significance of muscle health. Joints, the body components where two or more bones meet, play a fundamental role in facilitating movement while stabilizing the skeleton. The complexity of the joints ranges from the fixed sutures of the skull to the highly mobile ball-and-socket hip and shoulder joints. Joint health is essential in ensuring a healthy active lifestyle. For the elderly, for example, diseases like osteoarthritis become common. Osteoarthritis, which is cartilage degeneration with subsequent arthralgia, can severely impact locomotion as well as decrease the quality of life in the affected individuals. Nursing assessments should include assessing joint mobility, pain level, and the ability to function, particularly in patients who experience joint pain. Nurses must be aware of how joint health is associated with the rest of the musculoskeletal system because whole assessments form the groundwork for effective care plans, like physical therapy and prevention programs for injuries, to enhance patients' mobility and overall quality of life (Hagino et al., 2016; Ntolopoulou et al., 2017) (Figure 13.4).

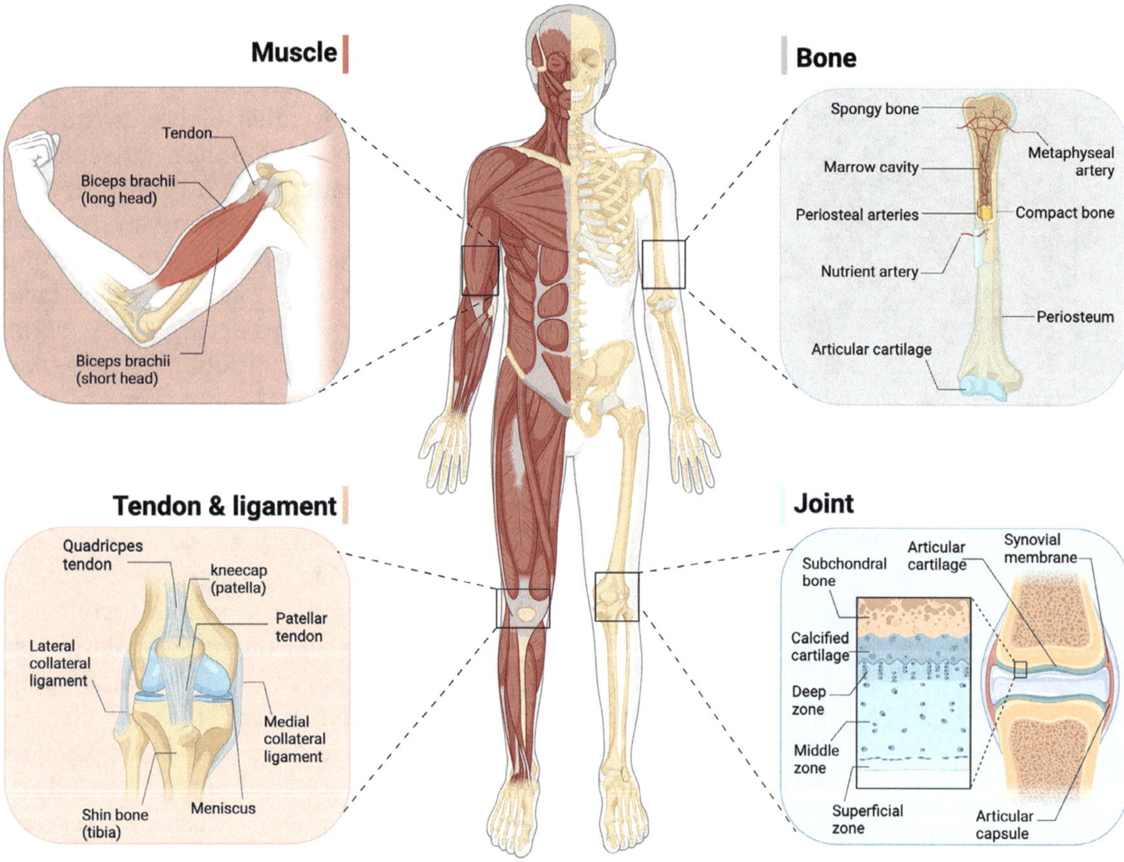

Figure 13.4. Bones, muscles, and joints of the musculoskeletal system.

Source: https://www.researchgate.net/publication/379024668/figure/fig3/AS:11431281303672866@1736934568036/Schematic-diagram-of-the-MSK-system-and-key-components-including-muscles-bones.png.

13.1.2. Functions of the Musculoskeletal System

The musculoskeletal system plays an important role in the structural support of the human body since it is the system that supports and protects essential organs. The skeleton, muscles, cartilage, tendons, and ligaments are components that make up the musculoskeletal system which enables a variety of functions critical to daily living. The skeletal system gives structure and support and even serves as protective armor for organs such as the heart and lungs. Also, the bones produce blood cells in the bone marrow, highlighting their core function in the hematopoietic process.

Nursing practitioners need to identify the core functions of the musculoskeletal system to address the assessment and evaluation of any abnormality or dysfunction that may impact a patient's general health status and quality of life, particularly in chronic ill patients (Amirpour et al., 2023). Other than support and protection, the musculoskeletal system plays a crucial role of facilitating movement through the action of muscles. The skeletal muscles work with the skeleton to provide leverage, thus facilitating a significant range of movements from simple walking to sophisticated sporting performance. This active musculoskeletal part relies on neuromuscular coordination, with the requirement for exact interaction between the central nervous system and the musculoskeletal parts to be able to function optimally. Nurses must be able to assess the range of motion and strength of the muscles, assess any restrictions or injuries that may cause limitations in mobility or deterioration of current conditions. This responsibility reflects the significance of holistic knowledge of the musculoskeletal system in patient care because mobility is involved in the healing and rehabilitation process (Argent et al., 2017). Moreover, the musculoskeletal system provides homeostasis through mineral storage and metabolic processes. Bones also store needed minerals, such as calcium and phosphorus, which can be released into the circulatory system to assist in regulating body functions such as muscle contraction and nerve impulse transmission. Additionally, the interdependency of bone density and overall health is a vital focus of nursing assessments, especially in the context of older individuals who also have a higher risk factor for osteoporosis and fractures. Understanding these biochemical functions helps the nurses in the provision of targeted education and interventions to patients to promote lifestyle habits that optimize musculoskeletal health. By patient education and appropriate assessment, nursing professionals are able to help prevent musculoskeletal disorders and enhance musculoskeletal function across a broad spectrum of patient populations (Amirpour et al., 2023) (Figure 13.5).

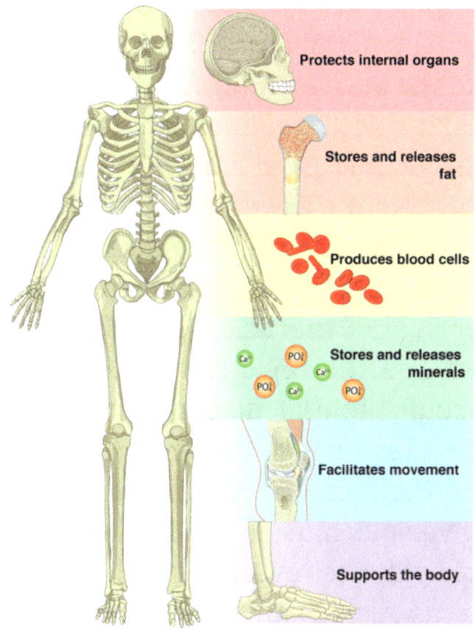

Figure 13.5. Functions of the musculoskeletal system.

Source: https://open.oregonstate.education/app/uploads/sites/157/2019/07/mineral_storage_revised-838x1024.png.

13.1.3. Common Anatomical Terms Used in Assessment

In the practice of nursing, particularly in musculoskeletal system examination, the use of standard anatomical terms enhances communication and understanding among the health professionals. Use of appropriate terminology is essential in accurate labeling of pain locations, assessment of the extent of musculoskeletal disorders, and forming appropriate treatment plans. Anatomical terms like "proximal" and "distal" differentiate locations in relation to the center of the body, enabling accurate expression of examination findings. Besides, the application of words such as "medial" and "lateral" is crucial during the evaluation of joint or soft tissue pathology that requires focused intervention. Application of such terms simplifies patient assessment, improves documentation, and supports interprofessional communication, where all stakeholders have a shared knowledge of patients' status and treatment interventions. Familiarity with common anatomical terms is also important in evaluating musculoskeletal complaints, particularly in measuring pain prevalence and site involvement in disorders. Specific examples of these include terms such as "cervical," "thoracic," and "lumbar" which address specific regions of the spine involved in musculoskeletal disorders. Localization of pain on these specified sites directs nurses in labeling the location of pain and differentiating among various musculoskeletal disorders. A key body of evidence reveals typical musculoskeletal symptoms such as lower back and neck pain are usually associated with specific anatomical sites, situating the patients clinical presentation in the broader framework of their lifestyle determinants and medical history. Thus, employing the use of specific anatomy ensures complete examinations and aids in effective clinical decision-making practices in nursing practice. Furthermore, the impacts of the correct application of universal body terms do not remain confined to the initial patient assessments to risk factors and potential treatment outcomes. Assessing pain in the various regions of anatomy, the shoulder complex or knee joint, typically reveals existing risk factors—lifestyle or conditions. For example, knee and hip pain diagnosis might be associated with pain in other regions like the leg or ankle, justifying a general view of the musculoskeletal systems interconnectedness (Antunes et al., 2019). Not only do these assessments define the engaged regions but also guide nurses on the decision-making related to symptom intensity and if additional diagnostic workup or referral could be needed. Such multifaceted evaluation allows health practitioners to deliver patient-centered interventions and improve musculoskeletal health outcomes (Antunes et al., 2019).

Test Your Knowledge

1. What are the major components of the musculoskeletal system, including bones, muscles, joints, and ligaments, and what are their primary functions?
2. How does understanding musculoskeletal anatomy assist in identifying abnormalities during assessment?

13.2. Assessment Techniques

Learning Outcome

1. Inspection and Palpation Methods
2. Range of Motion Evaluations
3. Special Tests for Musculoskeletal Conditions

In nursing, particularly in the assessment of the musculoskeletal system, various approaches are employed to obtain a proper insight into the patient's health. One of the most advanced approaches is shear wave elastography (SWE), which is a high-tech ultrasound technique that assesses the elastic properties of biological tissues. The elastic properties are significant in identifying the functionality of muscles, tendons, and joints. With its benefits of quantitative measurement and real-time inspection, SWE has increasingly had a role in musculoskeletal examinations. Not only does the method advance the accuracy of diagnostic protocols, but it also allows clinicians to see conditions evolve over time, making it a valuable resource in acute and chronic settings. The seamless integration of SWE into clinical practice is an indicator of the ongoing evolution of assessment strategies aimed at improving patient outcomes in nursing practice. In addition to technology-dependent approaches, observational strategies remain crucial in the evaluation of musculoskeletal disorders. These strategies form a robust foundation for the identification of functional impairment and potential risks of musculoskeletal injury. For instance, observational testing, such as the Key Indicator Method Whole-Body Forces (KIM-BF), allows practitioners to understand the body forces of performing tasks, which might be important in preventing musculoskeletal disorders among nurses. It has been shown through research that the use of a combination of direct observation and biomechanical data enhances the reliability of assessments. However, the effectiveness of such observational assessments can be influenced by subjective factors like the experience and competency of the assessor. These factors indicate the need to standardize observation procedures for ensuring the highest level of assessment accuracy in nursing. Furthermore, the integration of technology with traditional forms of assessment underlines the need for a holistic approach in musculoskeletal assessments. Although quantifiable measurement techniques, such as those employing body-worn sensors and force plates, are extremely revealing of physical stresses faced by nursing procedures, their use can be tiresome and labor-intensive. Studies show a moderate level of reliability in measurements made using biomechanical models, which means that although they may provide accurate measurements, reliance on these measures alone without contextual examination may lead to false conclusions about the musculoskeletal health of a nurse. It was essential to weigh up high-tech testing with realistic observation approaches so as to create an overall knowledge of musculoskeletal dangers to health within the practice contexts of nursing, finally contributing towards a safer and more effective practice (Figure 13.6).

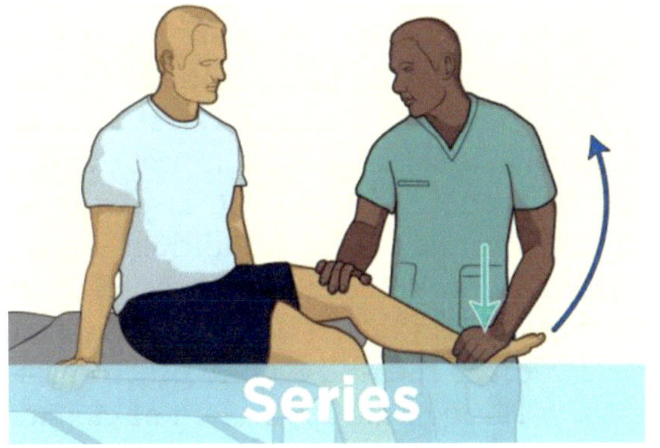

Figure 13.6. Assessment techniques of the musculoskeletal system.

Source: https://cdn.ps.emap.com/wp-content/uploads/sites/3/2024/10/PracProc-Musculoskeletal-492x328.jpg.

13.2.1. Inspection and Palpation Methods

In the overall assessment of the musculoskeletal system, inspection and palpation skills are rudimentary nurse abilities. Inspection involves accurate visual assessment of the muscles, joints, and overall skeletal system of a patient for asymmetry, edema, redness, and deformity. This procedure allows nurses to identify abnormal states or potential pathologies before proceeding on to more invasive diagnostics. Successful inspection requires a discerning eye for detail, as small variations in one's musculoskeletal appearance can indicate underlying pathology. Additionally, the significance of the original assessment cannot be overestimated, as it can be utilized to affect subsequent diagnostic procedures and interventions. Through coming to a certain baseline by means of inspection, nurses are able to maximize clinical judgment and affect a more particular focus for the care of the patient, providing better patient outcomes.

Palpation is utilized alongside inspection to provide information by touch that supplements the musculoskeletal system evaluation. Palpation allows nurses to assess temperature, texture, and tenderness of joint and muscle through slow and gentle palpation. Palpation may provide crucial signs regarding inflammation or trauma. Palpation on some points, for instance, may indicate myofascial trigger points not visible on visual inspection. This method is particularly applicable in diagnosing conditions such as myofascial pelvic pain (MFPP), where myofascial trigger points in the musculature of the pelvic floor can cause referred pain to other parts of the body. Through the application of palpation during diagnosis, nurses are able to develop a general idea of the patient's musculoskeletal status, thus better planning management and treatment regimes. Through combination of both inspection and palpation, nurses are able to produce a detailed picture of each patient's unique presentation. Combination of inspection and palpation not only enhances the nurse's own clinical expertise but also their reporting of findings within an interdisciplinary health team. Working critically together with other members of the healthcare team is especially crucial, especially in managing complex musculoskeletal presentations. For instance, where nurses find abnormal findings by palpation and observation, they are in a position to collaborate with physical therapists or pain specialists to provide targeted interventions. This multi-professional collaboration is particularly valuable in managing cases such as MFPP, where there are effective treatments but would be at risk if not coordinated within and between disciplines. By preserving such interprofessional relationships and proper use of inspection and palpation, nursing professionals can play a great role in patient outcomes and overall quality of healthcare, thus fostering an integrated and holistic approach to the assessment of health (Accettola et al., 2023; Katzman et al., 2012) (Figure 13.7).

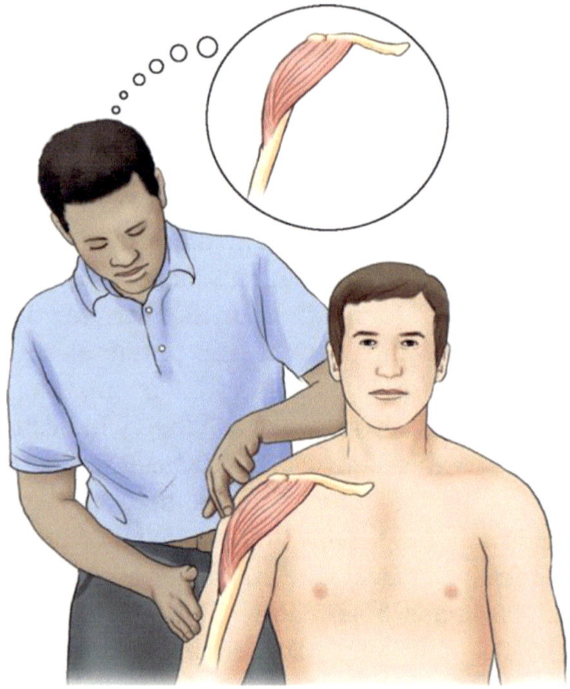

Figure 13.7. Inspection and palpation methods.

Source: https://musculoskeletalkey.com/wp-content/uploads/2016/08/F500108f04-01-9780323086844.jpg.

13.2.2. Range of Motion Evaluations

Range of motion examinations are an integral part of the general evaluation of the musculoskeletal system in nursing practice. Range of motion examinations are used to determine patients' function and limitations, which are essential for creating tailored care plans. By measuring the amount of motion at several joints, health professionals can obtain valuable information about underlying disease, the effectiveness of rehabilitation, and needs for future intervention. Of particular interest, accurate range of motion measurement not only directs diagnosis and treatment but also enhances the quality of patient care overall as nurses are able to monitor for changes and alter therapeutic modalities accordingly. In musculoskeletal exams, some techniques such as goniometry are used to ensure precision in measurement of angles of joints. This method provides quantitative data, and comparisons can be made to normative values and displaying any deviation that may indicate musculoskeletal disorders. Nurses need to be mindful to notice factors that influence these measurements, such as pain, swelling, and weakness of the muscles, all of which influence range of motion.

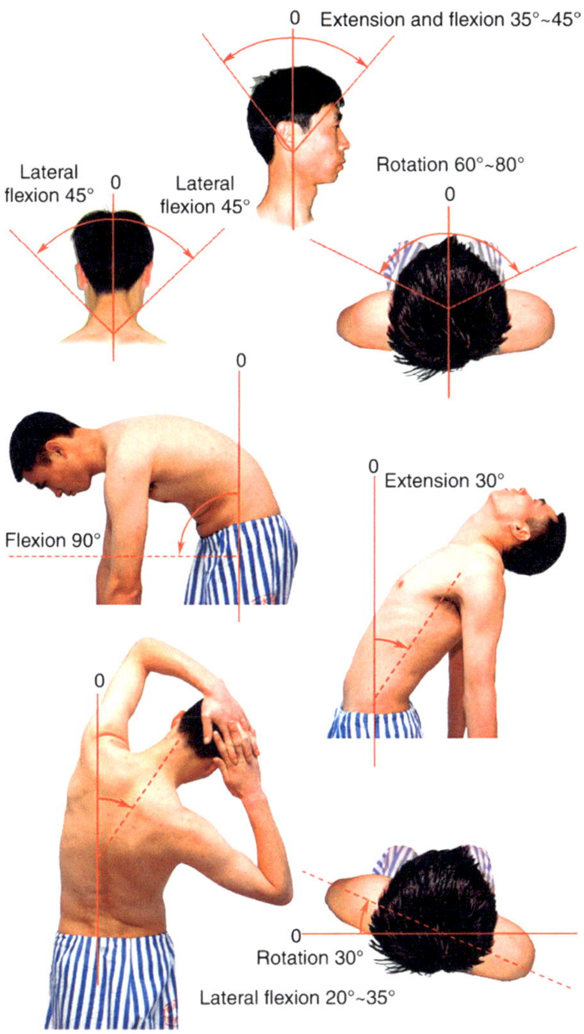

Figure 13.8. Range of motion evaluations of the musculoskeletal system.

Source: https://media.springernature.com/lw685/springer-static/image/chp%3A10.1007%2F978-981-13-7677-1_48/MediaObjects/457552_1_En_48_Fig2_HTML.png.

Besides, understanding the significance of restricted movement is important, for instance, the restricted range of motion of cervical spine can be related to cervical spine radiculopathy, as evidenced by studies indicating dramatic improvement of cervical mobility by targeted interventions like cervical rotation-traction manipulation, thus signifying the significance of such an assessment in clinical practice (Feng et al., 2024). Additionally, the application of ergonomic methods and assistive devices can be significantly effective in fostering patient mobility and safety, particularly in high-risk populations such as the elderly or individuals with serious impairments. Recent studies have claimed that advances in assistive technology can enhance risks of caregiving by reducing the physical load on caregivers and improving overall transfer efficiency and safety (Shantanu et al., 2024). These findings underscore the critical intersection of range of motion evaluation with overall musculoskeletal health strategy. Accordingly, hospital musculoskeletal system examination in nursing must continually evolve to incorporate not only traditional assessment techniques but also innovative solutions with functional mobility consideration and safeguarding care for nurses and patients alike (Figure 13.8).

13.2.3. Special Tests for Musculoskeletal Conditions

Assessment of musculoskeletal disorders in the nursing practice involves a range of special tests that are used to diagnose several disorders effectively. Special tests like joint stability, range of motion, and functional tests provide a good picture of the factors underlying the musculoskeletal system. For instance, special tests like the Lachman test or the McMurray test are specifically constructed to assess the stability of the knee joint so that medical practitioners may identify ligamentous trauma or meniscal rupture.

Through the administration of these tests, nurses can facilitate appropriate interventions and refer patients to physical therapy or orthopedic services, thereby improving the outcomes of patients. The employment of special tests in nursing assessment underscores the importance of extensive assessments in handling musculoskeletal disorders, which are frequent and mostly affect patients quality of life, hence making these assessments an essential component of nursing practice. Understanding the rationale of every special test is requisite for effective assessment and diagnosis in musculoskeletal disorders. These subtleties of the tests also provide data not just regarding structural defects but also regarding the patient's functional capacity. The Valgus stress test, for example, evaluates the stability of the ulnar collateral ligament of the elbow, which is significant in taking into account a patient's athletic activity or work capacity. Special testing can also capture potential compensatory mechanisms the patients will use due to pain or dysfunction. This knowledge enables nurses to educate patients on the implication of their results and reflection on their care plan, thereby patient activation on care. By giving emphasis on the educative aspect of such measures, nurses can help patients make informed decisions regarding their care plan and lifestyle interventions. Besides, as the practice setting for pain management keeps evolving, utilization of special tests in musculoskeletal examination becomes increasingly important. With greater concern for nonpharmacologic methods for managing pain, as recent trends towards reducing opioid prescriptions have highlighted, findings from these tests can serve as the basis for implementing targeted therapeutic interventions. For instance, identification of a patient's range of motion deficits can guide clinicians in the formulation of individualized exercise programs to maximize function and decrease pain. A reaction towards the need for adequate pain management with minimal medication dependency is at the core, as evidenced by the shift toward holistic health care. This change not only reduces risks for opioid use but also imposes the importance of thoroughly assessing musculoskeletal conditions in order to make timely and appropriate interventions (Swezey et al., 2018). Adding these special tests to nursing assessment emphasizes the contribution of nurses towards improved musculoskeletal health outcomes.

Test Your Knowledge

1. What techniques are used to assess the musculoskeletal system, including inspection, palpation, range of motion (ROM), and strength testing?
2. How can a systematic approach to musculoskeletal assessment improve the accuracy of findings?

13.3. Common Musculoskeletal Disorders

Learning Outcome

1. Osteoarthritis and Its Implications
2. Rheumatoid Arthritis and Assessment Challenges
3. Fractures and Their Assessment Protocols

It is critical for nursing practitioners to have an appreciation of common musculoskeletal disorders (MSDs) since they make major contributions to patients' functionality and quality of life. MSDs are a compendium of conditions, including arthritis, tendinitis, and low back pain, each with varied etiology, symptoms, and management. These disorders can be due to repetitive strain, injury, and degenerative changes, where risk factors such as age, lifestyle, and occupational risk are of utmost significance in their occurrence. Further, the interplay between physical, psychological, and social factors influences their occurrence and severity, which necessitates a comprehensive appraisal approach in nursing practice. With these complexities being understood, nurses can employ appropriate assessment tools and interventions to best manage and rehabilitate patients with MSDs. The Nordic Musculoskeletal Questionnaire (NMQ) is a standard clinical practice and research tool used to assess musculoskeletal symptoms and measure their impact on one's life. Systematic evaluation with the NMQ can identify the very areas of discomfort and pain, which ultimately result in individualized nursing interventions. This survey not only reveals the prevalence of MSDs among different groups but also aids in assessing psychosocial and occupational hazards related to these disorders (Callejón et al., 2017). Clinical use of NMQ encourages the comprehension of the different presentations by which MSDs present and affect the overall health of patients. To nursing professionals, the ability to accurately diagnose musculoskeletal symptoms makes them ready to educate patients on self-management strategies, thereby optimizing patient outcomes with fewer implied complications resulting from neglected musculoskeletal health needs. Musculoskeletal symptomology has implications extending beyond immediate clinical practice, like the impact on students, healthcare professionals, and general workplace environments.

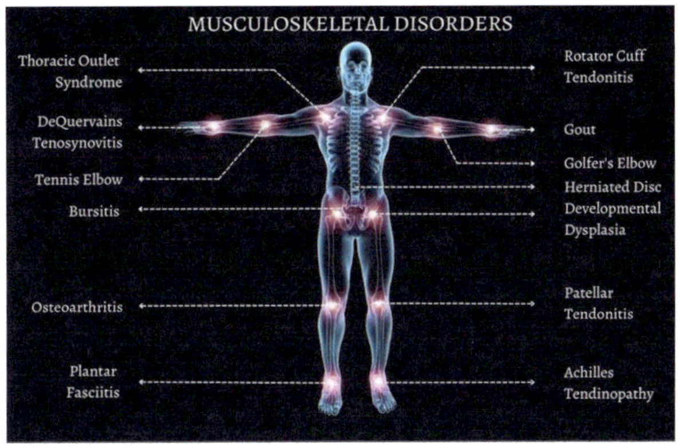

Figure 13.9. Common musculoskeletal disorders.

Source: https://media.medlegal360.com/wp-content/uploads/2023/12/27094016/types-of-musculoskeletal-disorders-know-how-to-manage-them-1-1024x576-1.webp.

Research has indicated that nursing students experience specific musculoskeletal-related problems, including pain and discomfort that hinder their academic and clinical training experience (Antunes et al., 2019). The implications for nursing education are, therefore, tremendous; curricula must address the importance of awareness regarding musculoskeletal health and preventive measures. By including musculoskeletal disorder principles in the education of nurses, future health professionals will be more able to comprehend the significance of bodily health and the psychosocial consequences that accompany such disorders. Perhaps most importantly, increased awareness about common MSDs not only equips nursing students with professional development but also guarantees the sustainability of healthcare service through employee well-being and efficiency (Figure 13.9).

13.3.1. Osteoarthritis and Its Implications

Osteoarthritis (OA) is the most prevalent form of arthritis and is a serious condition in the musculoskeletal system evaluation conducted in nursing. Characterized by joint cartilage wear and tear and the involved bone, OA generally manifests itself as pain, stiffness, and reduced movement. Not only do these deteriorate patients quality of life, but they also complicate the patients overall health status. Nurses must be capable of identifying the symptoms of OA through appropriate assessments, including patient history and physical examination. The course and ramifications of OA allow health care professionals to utilize proper management measures, with a primary focus on pain relief and maintenance of joint function. Since OA has a multifocal impact on patients in both psychological distress and physical disability, the identification of this is essential for devising complete treatment plans that address the physical and emotional aspects of the disease. To osteoarthritis are attached connotations beyond those of joint pain; they encompass significant socio-economic demands. OA often translates to increased healthcare spending in terms of frequent doctor visits, imaging, and potential surgery such as joint replacement.

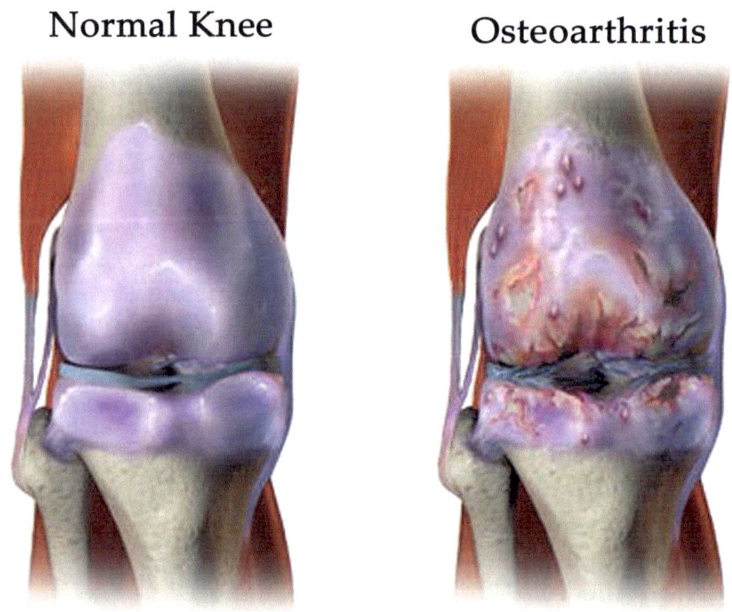

Figure 13.10. Osteoarthritis.

Source: https://www.physio-pedia.com/images/thumb/d/da/Osteoarthritis.png/399px-Osteoarthritis.png.

OA also tends to limit sufferers from activities, leading to lost productivity and income. Nurses play a crucial role in educating patients regarding lifestyle modifications that can reduce these economic costs. Through counseling regarding weight management, activity regimens tailored to the person's function, and pain control techniques, nursing professionals are able to assist patients in better managing their condition and minimizing the economic burden of advanced osteoarthritis. In addition, awareness of public health issues surrounding OA can spur nursing advocacy for more effective healthcare policy aimed at resource allocation and research funding. In the instance of a nursing assessment for osteoarthritis, it is essential to emphasize individualized treatment and ongoing patient education. Nurses can best guide patients by knowledge of their condition and treatments that can include pharmacologic therapy and non-pharmacologic interventions like physical therapy or alternative therapies. Evidence shows that an aggressive approach of repeated monitoring and reassessment of the patient's condition can lead to significantly improved outcomes. This ongoing evaluation enables nurses to detect alterations in function or symptomatology that may necessitate changes in treatment modalities. In addition, promoting an interdisciplinary setting with other healthcare providers secures a holistic care strategy that takes into account the complex nature of osteoarthritis and how it affects the daily life of a patient, thereby reiterating the significant impact of nursing in chronic musculoskeletal disorder management (Figure 13.10).

13.3.2. Rheumatoid Arthritis and Assessment Challenges

Rheumatoid arthritis (RA) measurement is linked with a great number of problems that require the integration of clinical experience, diligent patient assessment, and understanding of the diseases multi-dimensionality. The numerous dimensions of RA are not only induced by its intricate symptomatology but also by the need for proper communication between the health care team and patients. Measurements are key to the early diagnosis of inflammatory arthritis, which can significantly improve long-term results.

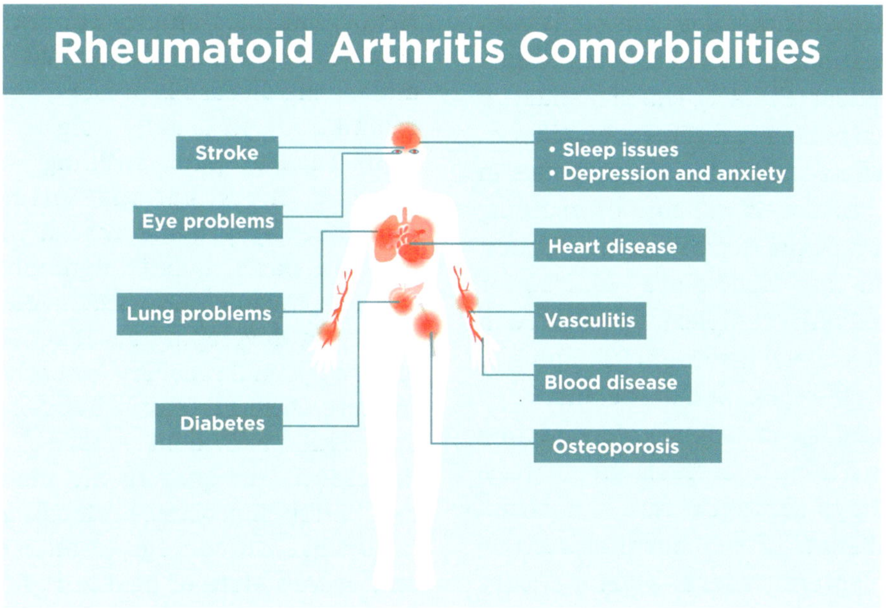

Figure 13.11. Rheumatoid arthritis.

Source: https://external-content.duckduckgo.com/iu/?u=http%3A%2F%2Fcreakyjoints.org%2Fwp-content%2Fuploads%2F0619_Rheumatoid-Arthritis-Comorbidities.jpg&f=1&nofb=1&ipt=8d4d9d8e0368563dd22fe22b70881bf908306b09ea1f82471479942d5cb4df28.

Patients are likely to present with a variety of signs and symptoms, including joint ache, fatigue, and stiffness, which can lead to diagnostic overshadowing in which other diseases are forgotten. The nurse's capacity to identify these symptoms within a broader context of musculoskeletal pathology is core to the delivery of effective diagnoses and on-time referrals for secondary care where necessary, as identified in the actions of Tier 2 services to increase patient satisfaction and care quality (Ball et al., 2007). Moreover, the physical and emotional impacts of RA serve to complicate the assessment process. Patients of rheumatoid arthritis usually also have other conditions like depression, which can significantly influence the levels of medication adherence and general well-being. Little acknowledgment of the role of such conditions of mental illness exists on physical outcomes, and this often results in a cycle of challenging behavior to treat. Effective nursing assessments must include psychosocial elements that are consistent with the recommendations of the European League against Rheumatism (EULAR), which mandate a holistic approach to the management of patients. The inclusion of mental health professionals in rheumatology practice is capable of enabling better resolution of these cross-cutting issues, since integrated care models are required for the management of the complexities involved in chronic musculoskeletal disorders (Chipping et al., 2016). Lastly, the transition of rheumatology care from secondary to primary care setting has implications for the assessment process. The change aims to decongest care and curtail excessive utilization of the hospital setting, providing a system where primary care practitioners can effectively perform initial assessment. Challenges remain in equipping these practitioners with the appropriate training and support for them to cope effectively with the nuances of RA. Educating nurses in primary care with advanced skills training in musculoskeletal examination not only enhances patient care but also enables early detection and intervention strategies. Lastly, an organization based, multidisciplinary plan is necessary to conquer the assessment problems inherent in rheumatoid arthritis and give patients continuous and comprehensive care through any healthcare environment (Ball et al., 2007) (Figure 13.11).

13.3.3. Fractures and Their Assessment Protocols

In nursing practice, it is important to know about fractures and their assessment protocols for appropriate patient care. Fractures are divided according to severity, location, and type and have several challenges that need thorough investigation and tailor-made treatment. Assessment protocols usually include comprehensive patient history, physical examination, and imaging techniques. History includes inquiry about the mechanism of injury, patient's age, and whether any underlying disease is present. Focused physical examination is usually able to reveal typical signs such as pain, swelling, and deformity. Imaging investigations, primarily X-rays, subsequently provide crucial information on fracture pattern and alignment. Integration of these various assessment elements assists nurses in developing an effective care plan to ensure optimal recovery for each patient with a fracture. Once a fracture has been confirmed, the application of evidence-based clinical protocols is essential in guiding the management and rehabilitation process. Protocols may differ with factors like patients age, location of the fracture, and overall state of health. For older patients, in particular, stringent protocols pay attention not only to the treatment of fractures but also to rehabilitation methods to restore functioning and aid a return to daily life. Effective programs are likely to include interdisciplinary models that address the physical rehabilitation as well as the psychological impact of injury. For instance, in one study, it was stressed that an interdisciplinary treatment increased health-related quality of life (HRQOL) following hip fracture in older patients, showing that proper assessment and individualized rehabilitation procedures significantly enhance the outcomes of the process of recovery (Adunsky et al., 2010). This brings to the fore the imperative for an interdisciplinary model of fracture assessment and management. Furthermore, physiological deterioration with advancing age also complicates fracture management, necessitating heightened alertness in assessment techniques. Bone density alterations, loss of muscle mass, and decreased physical function are processes of aging that necessitate anticipatory measures of assessment to counteract risks of recurrent fracture. Elderly have been observed to exhibit patterned muscle strength decline and bone mineral density, depending on which regular evaluation and tailored interventions become the need of the hour (Cauley et al., 2020). Not only is the immediate care for fracture to be evaluated in the field, but longer-term monitoring must also be included that addresses the patients' long-term mobility and overall musculoskeletal well-being. In conclusion, thorough assessment of fractures, together with regard for the individual patient's requirements and the family as a support, is essential to optimizing outcomes in musculoskeletal health care in nursing (Figure 13.12).

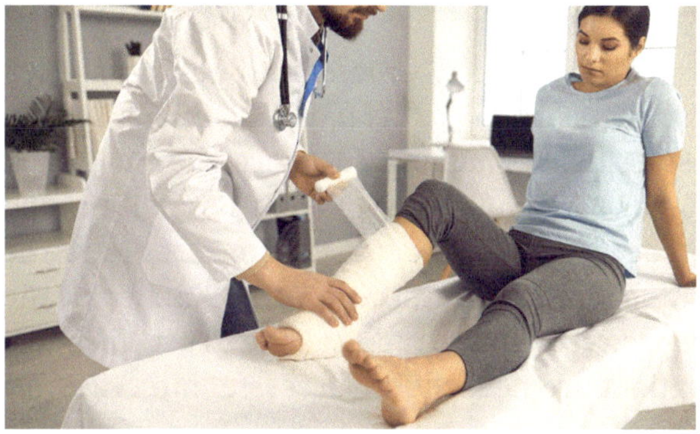

Figure 13.12. Fractures and their assessment.

Source: https://cdn.prod.website-files.com/64605f825e4b02b72c87a9f6/6624dab1399a5db334d48cad_Untitled%20(Brand%20Board)%20(5).png.

Test Your Knowledge

1. What are some common musculoskeletal disorders, such as arthritis, osteoporosis, and fractures, and what are their typical assessment findings?
2. How can early recognition of musculoskeletal disorders impact patient mobility and overall health outcomes?.

13.4. Patient History and Interview

Learning Outcome

1. Importance of a Thorough Patient History
2. Key Questions to Ask During Assessment
3. Understanding Patient-Reported Symptoms

The interview process and patient history are an essential part of musculoskeletal system assessment in nursing. They form the foundation for understanding the patient's condition and direct further diagnostic and therapeutic management. Both technical skill and the capacity to build rapport and trust with the patient are needed for successful interviewing. The rapport and trust facilitate open discussion, allowing patients to offer more detailed histories. Key aspects of the musculoskeletal history include previous injury, operations, and chronic disease, all of which inform the nurses assessment. Furthermore, familiarity with a patient's pain level, range of movement limitations, and functional ability provides a key background for the ensuing physical assessment. As has been elucidated in patient-centered care models, thorough history taking is essential in order to be able to provide interventions that are individually specific to the needs of the patient and maximize effective health outcomes. Also, the process of interviewing serves as a tool for educating patients by nurses. This is a critical element, particularly in musculoskeletal assessment where patients are not sensitive to how their lifestyle and behavior are causing them pain or loss of movement. From a discussion of occupation, leisure activities, and activity levels, nurses can discern lifestyle modifications that can help in preventing musculoskeletal problems. Second, integrating patient teaching with taking history introduces the possibility of informed treatment decision-making. For instance, options could range from the use of assistive devices to exercises that can be employed to strengthen the musculoskeletal system. Such discussions not only empower patients, but they also foster a collaborative atmosphere that induces quality care and adherence to treatment plans. Finally, the incorporation of information gathered when interviewing the patient directs the nursing care plan and subsequent assessment interventions. Employing models such as Marjory Gordon's functional health patterns allows the nurse to categorize and rank the gathered information by examining functional issues regarding the musculoskeletal system.

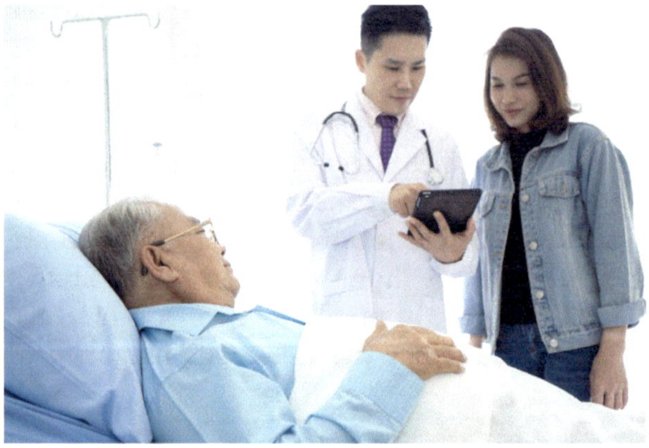

Figure 13.13. Patient history and interview.

Source: https://blogger.googleusercontent.com/img/b/R29vZ2xl/AVvXsEgv8a8ukK_-0zhx9AWpv0o7X4kUv_m1fbXFQ7dUtMCrmb26oY-D5SzFMChVDtXapdZr7BXCI9IgEXB8CEX01V5R3cgJYpNe3dIgq4ulLRMsQ7p2aymRuiyifIlmKEyymUwzl5k3P_F39TyoFjoYwfUtpTcWjmOtWuoselGwhOnTBxMkdTX47cik0mXq/s1000/Data%20To%20Be%20Obtained%20In%20Patient%20Medication%20History%20Interview.jpeg.

For instance, establishing change in mobility or chronicity of pain may yield nursing diagnoses that address these phenomena directly, e.g., risk for injury or impaired physical mobility. Effective application of this method supports timely and relevant nursing interventions. In accordance with evidence-based practice, patient outcome and response evaluation against established goals are essential, eventually leading to optimization of care delivery and enhanced patient well-being, reflected in studies on pediatric musculoskeletal disorder care (Jeny et al., 2024) and the role of good history taking in appreciating subtleties of health (İçim et al., 2024) (Figure 13.13).

13.4.1. Importance of a Thorough Patient History

An entire patient history is at the core of the evaluation of the musculoskeletal system since it is crucial for establishing context regarding a patient's condition. Effective evaluation relies on obtaining a thorough report of the patients' medical background, including previous injuries, surgeries, and any chronic diseases that may influence the musculoskeletal system. Additionally, aspects of the patient's lifestyle such as activity levels, work requirements, and even their psychological state can all affect musculoskeletal well-being. Establishing these aspects can assist nurses in identifying potential risk factors or susceptibility to musculoskeletal disorders. By not having such a basis, healthcare providers stand to overlook critical indicators that can inform diagnosis and treatment and therefore undermine patient care. Also, the inclusion of a patients entire history enhances the validity of clinical assessments, particularly with regard to a condition such as myofascial pelvic pain (MFPP). MFPP, characterized by trigger points, is prone to go undetected since it is multidimensional. By learning pertinent information through a thorough patient history, nurses can identify certain trigger points and related symptoms, which play a critical role in devising successful interventions. Interestingly, multidisciplinary approaches through physical therapy interventions such as trigger point release or biofeedback are also most effective if nursing assessment is comprehensive. Not only does this comprehensiveness enhance communication between care teams, but patients are also provided with holistic and targeted treatments, eventually achieving improved outcomes in musculoskeletal examinations and interventions (Katzman et al., 2012). Finally, obtaining a total patient history is at the core of formulating an educated and shared process of decision-making in musculoskeletal care. Variation in practice in the instance of community-acquired pneumonia makes informed process necessary. Similarly, in musculoskeletal assessment, patients' history adds to clinical decision-making. Expert consensus statements for physiotherapy, to which clinical practice is guided, are rooted in comprehensive patient histories that inform appropriate interventions (Braun et al., 2018). By incorporating patient history into evidence-based practice, nurses can optimize their assessment and interventions to achieve a holistic approach toward effective musculoskeletal disorder management. Ultimately, the inclusion of complete patient histories enhances care for specific patients as well as enhances overall goals of nursing practice within musculoskeletal health.

13.4.2. Key Questions to Ask During Assessment

When performing an extended musculoskeletal system assessment, the nurses have to make sure that the key questions are asked to get vital information regarding the patient's mobility and functional capacity. The key area to ask about is the patient's baseline ability to walk. Questions regarding their usual mobility patterns, previous injuries that have affected their performance, and reliance on the use of assistive devices assist in finding out their current level of functioning. These questions can aid in projecting future recovery needs and discharge planning because it has been demonstrated that enhanced baseline walking function correlatively enhances the prospects of home discharge post-operatively

(Borja et al., 2022). Therefore, incorporating mobility-related items to the assessment not only helps with planning but also helps nurses tailor interventions that enhance patient outcomes. Just as important to the knowledge of a patients musculoskeletal status is the addressing of their support structures. Inquiry about the presence of a postoperative caretaker can assist in determining the degree of support the patient will receive after discharge. Determining whether patients are dependent upon community support, including meal delivery systems, can also shed light upon levels of vulnerability during rehabilitation (Borja et al., 2022). In addition, these questions can help nurses identify individuals at greatest risk for complications so that extra resources or referral can be initiated early. Questioning about community supports promotes a complete understanding of the patient's care setting, thus enhancing discharge planning and overall safety in the recovery process. Lastly, it should be assessed how much patients understand and perform regarding their musculoskeletal health, particularly in prevention and occupational safety.

Questions that can be crucial include inquiring how they understand body mechanics, the way they properly perform lifting, and the utilization of supportive devices. It has been proven via studies that education trends significantly improve nursing interns knowledge and practices regarding occupational health. Thus, an assessment of the patient's awareness enables special education, which in musculoskeletal disorders is much more significant. By providing specially tailored educational interventions that respond to questions that have been acquired, nurses can enable enhanced self-management skills that maximize patient compliance and reduce future harm, and hence achieve better health outcomes in the musculoskeletal system (Figure 13.14).

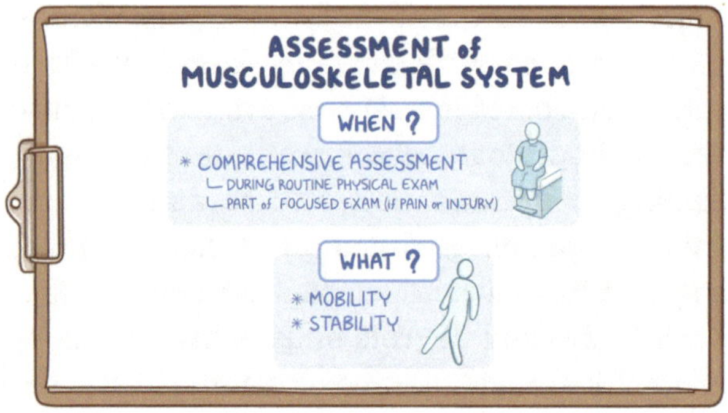

Figure 13.14. Key questions to ask during musculoskeletal system.

Source: https://www.osmosis.org/_next/image?url=https%3A%2F%2Fd16qt3wv6xm098.cloudfront.net%2FjZ6doovjRsiOoCPwZ9OQqFBWTtWoNDIH%2F_.jpg&w=3840&q=75.

13.4.3. Understanding Patient-Reported Symptoms

In the case of nursing, in the assessment of the musculoskeletal system, awareness of patient-reported symptoms is becoming a requirement for effective diagnosis and treatment. Patient-reported symptoms provide relevant information that can frequently reveal the impact of musculoskeletal disorders on the quality of life of the patient. Through diligent assessment that considers the patient's perspective, clinicians are more likely to realize not only the physical manifestations of pain but the emotional and psychosocial consequences these illnesses can induce. For example, patients with chronic pain may also report fatigue and anxiety in addition to pain and which can complicate their management. Therefore, the integration of patient-reported outcomes into practice can facilitate an integrated model with patients' needs and experiences as a priority that eventually enhances treatment efficacy and satisfaction. Moreover, the significance of clearly documenting patient-reported symptoms is highlighted by several studies citing discrepancies between clinical assessment and patients' actual experiences. Differential reporting can take place where healthcare practitioners focus primarily on clinical data and overlook subjective complaints that hold key information about the patient's condition. According to existing literature, not giving attention to these subjective experiences can lead to ineffective treatment plans. An appreciation of patient-report symptom sensitivity forms the foundation for enhanced patient-provider communication, which is fundamental in the development of personalized care plans. This process not only empowers patients but also helps nurse practitioners better recognize more effective intervention methods to cure musculoskeletal issues, thus helping to contribute positively to patient outcomes and the overall effectiveness of nursing interventions. Furthermore, the difficulty of being able to effectively translate patient-reported symptoms into effective nursing interventions cannot be overemphasized. The empirically based patient-reported quality of symptoms creates a demand that healthcare practitioners receive continuous education on a variety of conditions affecting the musculoskeletal system. For instance, evidence confirms that patients suffering from conditions such as fibromyalgia tend to produce heterogenous symptom reports that are not necessarily in concordance with clinical diagnoses, as noted by Claire et al. (2024). This disagreement emphasizes the importance of applying standard assessment tools and evidence-based treatment to improve the comprehension of patient-reported outcomes. Through their application, a link is established between clinical findings and subjective complaints and thus nursing assessments become complete and comprehensive. In the end, prioritizing the understanding of patient-reported symptoms in musculoskeletal evaluations promises significantly to enhance patient care by relating treatment modalities to the needs and situation of those involved (Figure 13.15).

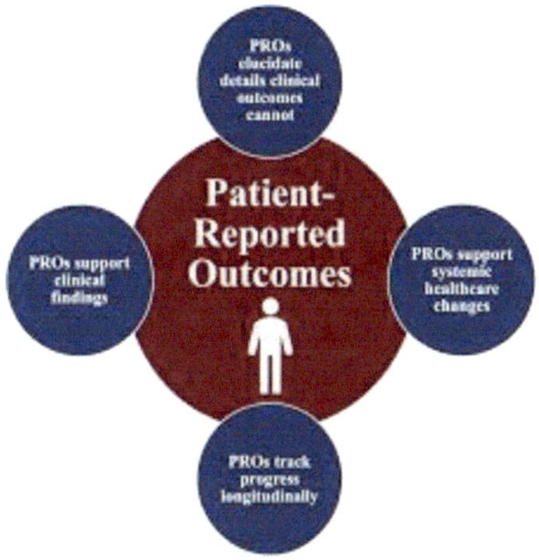

Figure 13.15. Understanding patient-reported symptoms.

Source: https://encrypted-tbn0.gstatic.com/images?q=tbn:ANd9GcRAvRvxzYhg8fIEpKPvJZlPYAkAJqQ5iWFVZg&s.

Test Your Knowledge

1. What questions should be included in a patient history to identify risk factors or previous musculoskeletal injuries?
2. How can patient-reported symptoms, such as pain, stiffness, or limited mobility, guide further assessment and care planning?

13.5. Documentation and Reporting

Learning Outcome

1. Importance of Accurate Documentation
2. Standardized Assessment Tools and Forms
3. Communicating Findings to the Healthcare Team

Effective documentation and reporting are critical cornerstones of musculoskeletal system assessment in nursing practice as they facilitate holistic patient care and promote patient safety. Accurate documentation yields effective data collection that reflects patients' musculoskeletal status, including any deformities, injuries, or fall histories. This is particularly significant due to the high incidence of falls among older individuals, which may have undesirable health implications and influence their overall independence. By methodically recording outcomes of tests such as the get up and go test (GUGT), nurses can provide essential data that guides clinical assessment and patient-specific care plans. Incorporating fall risk assessment into routine documentation reinforces the nursing process by allowing all key signs of health status to be continuously examined and monitored, thereby reducing potential risks from musculoskeletal issues and enhancing patient outcomes (Hermoso et al., 2009). Documentation is not merely confined to the direct observation of patients but extends to the general implications of recorded data in research and quality improvement initiatives. Through researching trends and patterns during musculoskeletal assessments under rigorous reporting, healthcare professionals are able to identify areas where the administration of care can be enhanced. This process of analysis can be employed in establishing better protocols to reduce fall risk and optimize patient mobility. Furthermore, accurate documentation facilitates tracking across time of the effect of various interventions. Through data-driven decision-making, practitioners can contribute to a wider body of knowledge about musculoskeletal health with relevance for individualized care and public health policy. Such evidence-based understanding is eventually applied to inform policy and resource allocation in nursing care (Kriebel et al., 2011). Moreover, proper documentation and reporting ensure legal and ethical standards are upheld in nursing practice. Where patients experience adverse outcomes with respect to musculoskeletal complications, thorough documentation is needed for legal protection and accountability. They offer evidence of the devotion of the nurse to prevailing standards of care and thoroughness of assessments carried out. Such importance warrants the ethical role of nurses in ensuring correct and standard documentation processes. With an alteration in nursing education, giving preference to training on documentation skills continues to be a priority, ensuring that those who will work in the future are equipped with the skills to properly document and communicate musculoskeletal examination findings. Elevating the status of documentation thus is not merely a matter of compliance but also a means of instilling a culture where patient-centered care thrives (Hermoso et al., 2009).

13.5.1. Importance of Accurate Documentation

Proper documentation is central to the nursing practice, particularly in regard to musculoskeletal system assessment. Documentation becomes a means of creating an accurate patient assessment record, interventions, and response to treatment. It assists in communication throughout the multidisciplinary care team as well as supports continuity of care. Nurses can employ accurate records to identify trends among patients' conditions, quantify the adequacy of care plans, and adjust treatment interventions accordingly. With quality and detailed documentation, it minimizes the chances of making mistakes that would lead to adverse consequences. As has been suggested from results obtained through physical therapy outcome studies, inadequate documentation can hinder the tracking of patients' recovery journeys, which can impact their general healthcare experience and discharge location decisions, ultimately impacting their quality of life and safety (Cortney et al., 2017). The impact of effective documentation goes beyond short-term clinical practice; they involve legal as well as ethical implications. Careful note-taking is a significant line of defense in court proceedings because it can establish that appropriate care was provided based on a thorough examination of the musculoskeletal system. Poor records could jeopardize the legal standing of nursing professionals should there be concerns raised about the care of patients. Accurate record-keeping not only protects the nurse but also ensures that the integrity of the healthcare organization is upheld through responsibility and transparency. Importantly, adequate records produce crucial information for performance reviews, quality improvement, and compliance, ensuring organizations uphold standards of care (Street A et al., 2025). Proper documentation of musculoskeletal examination also fosters improved clinical outcomes via enhanced quality management. Through routine documentation of patient assessments and interventions, nurses assist in creating a database that can be analyzed for global effectiveness and efficiency in musculoskeletal care. This evidence-based system enables healthcare institutions to establish practices based on supported patient outcomes, thus optimizing delivery pathways for future patients. Further, express documentation facilitates ongoing staff training and education by establishing areas for enhancement. As healthcare continues to develop with reforms such as Payment by Results, the role of thorough documentation in demand management and effective resource utilization becomes increasingly significant. Ultimately, effective documentation fosters a culture of continuous quality improvement in nursing so that patient care is both effective and safe (Cortney et al., 2017) (Figure 13.16).

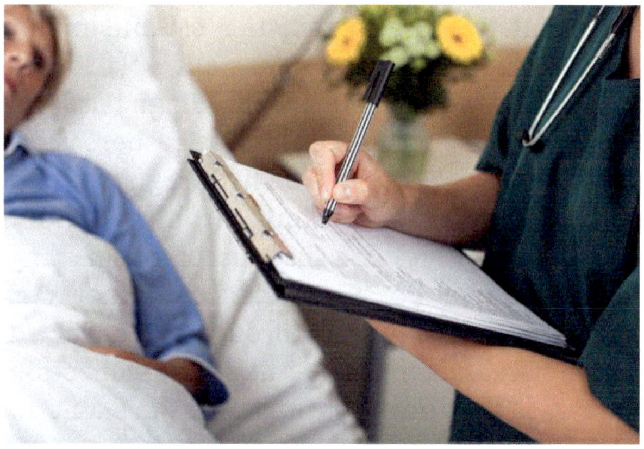

Figure 13.16. Accurate documentation is fundamental to nursing practice.

Source: https://nursingeducation.org/wp-content/uploads/2024/04/nursing-education.jpg.

13.5.2. Standardized Assessment Tools and Forms

Implementation of standardized test forms and instruments in nursing practice is of critical significance to ensure that the utmost accuracy and validity are achieved in musculoskeletal system evaluations. They enable a systematic approach of assessing fundamental musculoskeletal aspects, such as strength, range of motion, and sensitivity to pain. An example is the Nordic Musculoskeletal Questionnaire (NMQ), which is greatly established as a reliable instrument for assessing musculoskeletal disorders (MSDs) among various populations globally. This survey is an indirect assessment tool for MSDs and is often used alongside other standardized tools to achieve an accurate assessment of psychosocial and occupational determinants of these disorders. Utilizing standardized assessments such as the NMQ, nursing practitioners are then able to collect equivalent information that supports interdisciplinary care planning, ultimately leading to enhanced patient outcomes and greater workplace sustainability among healthcare institutions (Callejón et al., 2017). In pediatric populations, the establishment of standardized measurement protocols has played a key role in the diagnosis and treatment of musculoskeletal disorders. The creation of a comprehensive registry and database of childhood idiopathic inflammatory myopathies (IIMs) is a case in point regarding the need for uniform data collection methods in a clinical setting. It is through standardized patient assessment forms and data collection processes that health practitioners are able to decongest the process of evaluation to enable collection of such crucial data concerning patient demographics, clinical presentation, and biological samples in a systematic way. It not only facilitates harmony in interdependence among different care centers but also enhances the richness and validity of research findings, thereby informing treatment protocols as well as improving patient care strategies for complex musculoskeletal conditions (Bohan et al., 2011). Use of standardized instruments in assessment leads not only to direct management of musculoskeletal disorders but also to the broader context of clinical science and public health. By the utilization of instruments such as the NMQ in industries such as healthcare and manufacturing, nurses can identify trends related to MSDs that may go unrecognized. This information is able to direct proactive action taken to reduce injuries within workplaces and enhance conditions among affected populations. Further, conclusions derived from standardized assessments can direct policymakers and health administrators toward effective preventive interventions and resource allocation. Finally, their integration into practice nursing is vital in order to maximize both patient-specific and overall aims for public health sustainability in the management of musculoskeletal well-being (Callejón et al., 2017).

13.5.3. Communicating Findings to the Healthcare Team

Clear result communication to the healthcare team is a crucial process step in nursing, particularly in musculoskeletal system evaluations. Not only does the process facilitate informed decision-making, but interdisciplinary collaboration too is facilitated by this process, which is a cornerstone in the improvement of patient outcomes. Through the application of structured communication models like SBAR (Situation, Background, Assessment, Recommendation), nurses are empowered with the tools of articulating assessment findings clearly and concisely. These models have been seen to enhance the standard of communication, improving handovers by as much as 85%, thus reducing cases of miscommunication between teams. Through the implementation of these practices, nursing professionals can greatly improve the level of care offered to patients through the proper dissemination of information pertaining to musculoskeletal findings, thus improving patient safety and general care dynamics. In addition, because nursing staffing shortages are difficult to healthcare provision, innovative models of communication are necessary. Virtual forms of nursing are modern solutions for such staffing issues, where professional nursing care can be provided from afar. Communication of outcome measures in a virtual environment requires familiarity with various technological tools and platforms. This requires nurses to possess adequate skills and knowledge to efficiently utilize these systems, with ease of communication with the healthcare team while optimizing technology for effective delivery of care. For instance, remote monitoring devices can provide instant data for musculoskeletal assessment, lending more strength to the quality of feedback nurses can provide to other nurses. These advancements not only facilitate easier mitigation of nursing shortages but also enhance the continuum of care by rendering crucial information exchanged timely and effectively. In general, the ability to share findings effectively with the healthcare team is directly proportionate to the quality of musculoskeletal system assessments in nursing. Barriers such as cultural resistance and limitations imposed by dominant practices can hinder effective communication, pointing to the need for systematic approaches. The use of new ideas such as simulation-based training and electronic communication aids can be the steppingstone in overcoming these barriers. These measures have been contended to enhance team dynamics and interpersonal trust among health professionals, developing teamwork culture eventually leading to enhanced patient care. By focusing on effective communication, particularly in musculoskeletal examinations, healthcare teams can ensure complete, safe, and quality-based patient outcomes in an increasing more complex health care environment (Figure 13.17).

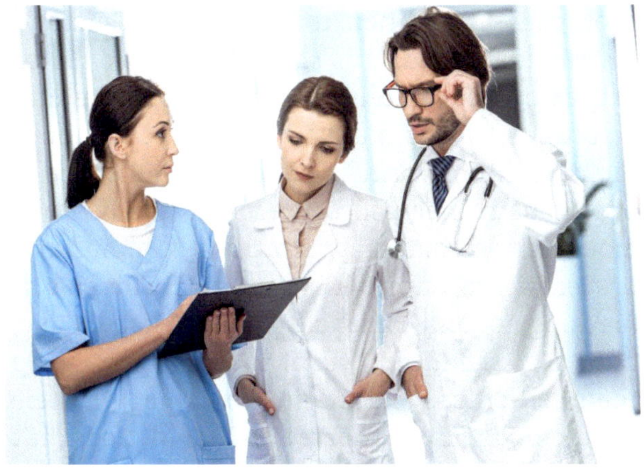

Figure 13.17. Communicating findings to the healthcare team.

Source: https://wtcs.pressbooks.pub/app/uploads/sites/31/2020/08/Shutterstock-Image-1322557028-huge-1024x683.jpg.

Test Your Knowledge

1. How should musculoskeletal assessment findings, including ROM and strength measurements, be accurately documented?
2. What details are essential when reporting abnormal musculoskeletal findings to other healthcare providers?

13.6. Nursing Interventions

Learning Outcome

1. Pain Management Strategies
2. Rehabilitation and Physical Therapy Referrals
3. Patient Education on Musculoskeletal Health

Nursing care is at the core of total assessment and care of musculoskeletal disorders (MSDs). Nursing care targets several aspects of a patient's condition, not only pain relief but also overall functionality and quality of life. A part of it is physical assessment, through which nurses evaluate joint movement, muscle power, and pain. According to the recent evidence, effective interventions are best achieved through a multi-factorial approach that considers interaction among physical and psychosocial mechanisms influencing patient outcomes (Paul et al., 2024). Moreover, the nursing professionals should personalize such interventions in line with the specific needs of patients to develop an interdisciplinary care plan that fosters patient involvement and adherence to treatment protocols. In addition to physical assessment, instructional measures should be employed to empower the patients with musculoskeletal disorders. Nurses must educate patients about their conditions, bringing out the significance of proper body mechanics, exercises, and lifestyle modifications that may improve symptoms and prevent aggravation of the condition. This role in teaching not only enhances patients' knowledge, but it also significantly contributes to enhancing their self-efficacy in relation to managing their conditions, as supported by evidence that educated patients can fully participate in their care processes (Herlinah et al., 2024). Through developing a learning environment, nurses are capable of reinforcing regular follow-up and adherence to prescribed therapies, thereby contributing to enhanced patient outcomes in musculoskeletal health. Finally, interdisciplinary collaboration plays a key role in managing the complexities entailed in musculoskeletal assessment and management. Nurses must coordinate with physiotherapists, occupational therapists, and other medical professionals to develop integrated care plans incorporating both physical and psychosocial rehabilitation care. Interdisciplinary collaboration has the potential to lead to improved interventions through the alleviation of work-related risk factors and maximization of active patient participation in rehabilitation programs (Paul et al., 2024). Integrating evidence from all of the disciplines not only enriches the care process but also highlights the necessity of having a multidisciplinary approach to health that values the many influencing factors of musculoskeletal disorders. With research being conducted in the field continuously, the use of these nursing interventions will be fundamental in improving the quality of patient care and enhancing overall musculoskeletal health outcomes.

13.6.1. Pain Management Strategies

Effective pain management methods are central to nursing assessment and treatment of musculoskeletal system conditions, particularly in view of the intricate relationship among physical pain, psychological well-being, and functional loss. In addition to assessing the site and intensity of the pain, a proper evaluation will also encompass assessing the patient's mental status and pain's impact on his or her daily activities. For instance, adolescents and children living with major depressive disorder (MDD) are known to exhibit somatic symptoms such as musculoskeletal pain, thus complicating their treatment. The nursing clinicians are required to understand that the pain experienced by these groups has strong long-term consequences, for instance, increased suicide risk and worsened social and family relationships (Forman-Hoffman et al., 2016). Thus, the inclusion of mental health screenings in pain management protocols can improve overall patient outcomes and direct more extensive therapeutic care. Among a number of methods to be offered through pain management, non-pharmacologic therapy has gained widespread use in nursing practice due to its effectiveness and minimal side effects. Techniques such as physical therapy, cognitive-behavioral therapy (CBT), and alternative therapies like Guasha have been found effective in treating musculoskeletal pain. Guasha, a traditional scraping modality that is intended to relieve the stagnation of blood, has been the target of recent research. Although data from studies reflect conflicting outcomes in pain relief, these forms of therapy can be beneficial as adjuvant therapy to conventional medical treatments. There is a need for nurses to critically assess potential benefits of such treatments in the context of the patient's unique situation and preferences (Lee et al., 2010). This encourages patient-specific care with a focus on intensive treatment and evidence-based practice. Pharmacological options continue to be at the core of pain management protocols in nursing, particularly for severe or chronic musculoskeletal pain. The employment of analgesics, NSAIDs, and if needed, opiates can be of immense relief to patients. Nurses do need to be cautious for the risk of dependence on these drugs, especially in adolescents, with appropriate education to the patient and concern about risks. Further, pain management together with the psychological illnesses, such as MDD, is important since the absence of treatment of depression can exacerbate the experience of pain and vice versa (Forman-Hoffman et al., 2016). It is therefore imperative to apply a multi-disciplinary treatment plan in consultation with mental health professionals in conjunction with pain management practices to enhance patient outcomes and maximize the efficacy of nursing interventions in the assessment of the musculoskeletal system (Figure 13.18).

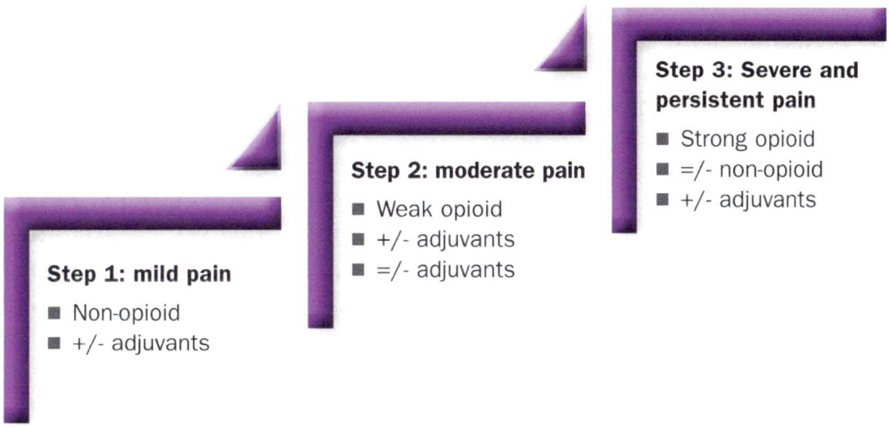

Figure 13.18. Pain management strategies in the nursing assessment.

Source: https://www.britishjournalofnursing.com/media/wmpgqk5v/bjon2024335246_f03.jpg.

13.6.2. Rehabilitation and Physical Therapy Referrals

Rehabilitation and physical therapy referrals are also critical in the comprehensive care of patients who undergo musculoskeletal system evaluation in nursing. The inclusion of physical therapy in rehabilitation processes can significantly enhance patients' recovery and functional outcomes. For instance, patients with fracture are at increased risk for further fracture, particularly those with osteoporosis, on their musculoskeletal health (Meryl et al., 2022). Nurses must also be mindful of these patients and coordinate early referral to physical therapists, who can provide customized programs of rehabilitation aimed at strengthening the surrounding musculature and enhancing balance. A multidisciplinary approach is required in order to prevent recurrent injury and optimize long-term mobility. Thus, the integration of nursing and physical therapy not only complements the rehabilitation process but addresses the root peril of musculoskeletal disorders. Physical therapists use evidence-based examination to determine patients mobility and impairments in function, providing a priceless complement to nursing assessment. Through the rehabilitation process, physical therapy can institute systematic interventions that focus on increasing strength, flexibility, and overall musculoskeletal well-being. For example, some exercises are intended to manage the noted functional deficits in patients with orthopedic surgeries or injuries (Thomas et al., 2020). Such interventions might include manual therapy techniques, therapeutic exercises, and posture and body mechanics training. Thus, through the application of physical therapists' expertise, nurses can offer more integrated patient care with confidence that all rehabilitation aspects of musculoskeletal rehabilitation are addressed. The integrated effort therefore ultimately results in efficient recovery arrangements for the patients, promoting autonomy and facilitating their return to usual activities. Another area where the formation of effective referral pathways between physical therapy and nursing can play a significant role in streamlining patient care is with the conditions such as osteoporosis, where there is high risk of the fracture and resulting complication (Meryl et al., 2022). Nurses must be educated with adequate screening material to identify patients who can be helped with physical therapy because early intervention can prevent deterioration of the patients status. Additionally, with the changing challenges such as those faced during the COVID-19 pandemic, adequate guidelines on referral processes can assist in managing care in acute care settings effectively (Thomas et al., 2020). Therefore, enhanced communication pathways and interprofessional collaboration among healthcare teams are essential for maximizing patient outcomes for musculoskeletal rehabilitation. This integrated approach can lead to improved global health status and reduced long-term disability for musculoskeletal-impaired patients (Figure 13.19).

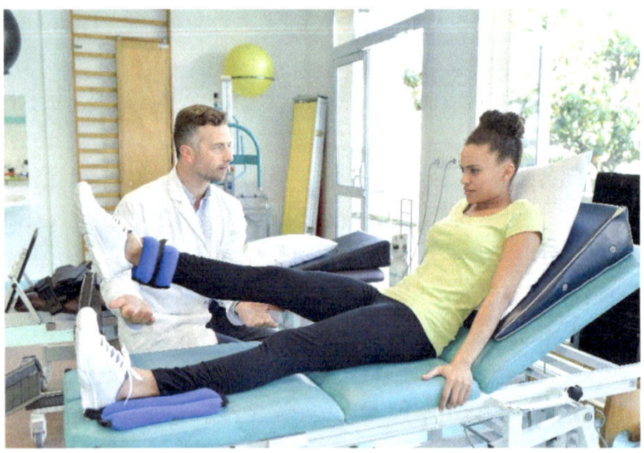

Figure 13.19. Rehabilitation and physical therapy referrals in the nursing assessment.

Source: https://blog.rehabselect.net/hubfs/rehab%20terms.jpeg.

13.6.3. Patient Education on Musculoskeletal Health

Effective patient education is at the heart of musculoskeletal health, particularly for nursing. Nurses often serve as the first contact healthcare professionals who can influence patients' knowledge and management of their condition. Nurses can empower patients to become participants in their own health care by teaching them about anatomy, common musculoskeletal disorders, and risk factors. With education on their conditions provided to the patients, they can then more fully engage in shared decision-making and self-management techniques. Active participation not only enhances treatment adherence but also increases a better understanding of the role that lifestyle changes, such as exercise and diet, have in maintaining musculoskeletal health into old age. The integration of patient education in nursing practice is instrumental in limiting the impact of musculoskeletal disorders on individual well-being and in enhancing the overall quality of healthcare. Furthermore, the application of various educational tools can optimize the efficacy of patient education concerning musculoskeletal health. With the increasing dissemination of online information via sources like YouTube, patients have a tendency to use digital media to acquire information regarding their health conditions. Even though this is the case, the quality and accuracy of such information may vary significantly. A study looking into the quality of internet information on musculoskeletal diseases shows a disparity between academic literature developed by health professionals and sub-academic sources of lower quality. Nurses need to guide patients to accurate online information while supplementing education with evidence-based textbooks and live demonstrations in an effort to prevent misinformation. Emphasis on using trusted sources enhances patients' ability to identify correct information, promoting well-informed decision-making regarding their health. Finally, it is important to reflect on the role of interdisciplinary teamwork in enhancing patient education on musculoskeletal health. Nurses have a tendency to work in conjunction with physical therapists, occupational therapists, and physicians, developing an integrative care strategy that addresses different needs of patients. Such collaboration also guarantees the sharing of experience and resources, thereby increasing learning opportunities for patients. Secondly, programs offered by contributions from a variety of healthcare professionals guarantee that different aspects of musculoskeletal health, from pain management through rehabilitation of functions, receive coverage. This all-inclusive approach not only equips patients with broader knowledge but also guarantees a network that facilitates continuous learning. By putting emphasis on the collaborative method of patient education, the nurse can lead efforts to significantly raise awareness and management of musculoskeletal health among their patients, thus enhancing quality of life and functional outcomes.

Test Your Knowledge

1. What nursing interventions can help maintain or improve musculoskeletal function in patients with mobility limitations?
2. How can nurses educate patients on exercises, ergonomics, and preventive measures to reduce the risk of musculoskeletal disorders?

SUMMARY

In nursing exploration of the musculoskeletal system evaluation, an understanding of the critical role that assessment has in optimizing patient outcomes is crucial. Nurses can uncover underlying causes of chronic pain and functional deficit through the application of careful evaluation techniques. Evidence indicates that interventions such as an exercise and psychological combined intervention have far-reaching impacts on both pain measures and central sensitization (Deegan et al., 2024). The implication of this testing, therefore, goes far beyond diagnosis; it guides individualized interventions that are able to improve patients' quality of life and allow for active participation in their recovery processes. Besides, the prevalence of musculoskeletal disorders (MSDs) among various categories of healthcare professionals accentuates the importance of effective assessment methods in nursing practice. Studies have established that a majority of nursing staff suffer from MSDs due to ergonomic risk factors, such as prolonged standing and repetitive motion (Mahajan et al., 2023). Thus, there is a dire need for nursing education programs to have a strong emphasis on highlighting the importance of musculoskeletal assessment. It should impart skills to practitioners that allow them to recognize risk factors and implement prevention. The highlight does not just benefit nurses but also clinical practice, patient care and outcomes. At the end of the day, integrating musculoskeletal system assessments into practice is at the core of ensuring holistic patient-centered care. It enables nurses to identify not only current conditions but also potential risks which can create future health complexities. As stressed by recent research, proactive care by way of good assessment can establish the tone for better patient management measures (Deegan et al., 2024; Mahajan et al., 2023). Thus, nursing training and continuing professional development must prioritize musculoskeletal assessment training so that nurses are capable of handling such complicated cases with skill and assurance and ultimately create better health outcomes in communities.

A complete musculoskeletal system evaluation is at the heart of nursing practice, providing vital information about a patient's overall condition and ability to function. Nurses are at the heart of the assessment process, employing a methodical process to evaluate posture, gait, and range of movement. Understanding these dynamics provides the means to identify anomalies which are not always apparent and facilitates early intervention and management. In addition, the inclusion of occupational history in evaluations is more stressed, as it can reveal significant indicators of musculoskeletal-related issues of a patient's work environment. Nevertheless, problems exist in the effective collection of this information, such as privacy and time issues within high-speed clinical environments. These challenges underscore the significance of standardized procedures for occupational history taking, as noted in research that explores the integration of occupational and public health systems to promote assessment practice improvement for better patient outcomes (Paek et al., 2024). Emerging technologies, particularly computerized decision-support systems, are significant contributors to enhancing efficiency and accuracy in musculoskeletal assessment in nursing. The intersection of deep learning software facilitates the processing of enormous amounts of medical data, including automation of diagnosis functions. These technologies enhance nurses ability to understand somatoscopic measurements, which serve as the basis for valid descriptions of patients musculoskeletal status. Through precise identification of landmark anatomical points on patients images, nursing evaluations are not only expedited but also improved in terms of diagnostic subtlety. Use of automated systems minimizes subjective errors made during manual assessment, thereby enhancing the quality of care delivered. As the need for accuracy increases in musculoskeletal assessment, use of advanced information technologies is a necessity in nursing practice and education (Poplavskyi et al., 2024). Lastly, the ongoing evolution of musculoskeletal system assessment in nursing highlights the balance between ancient ways and new technological advancements. The nurses are compelled to continuously redesign their competence sets to leverage the benefits of the innovations to complete and effectively make patients' assessments. Enhanced training programs incorporating the use of computerized decision aids and standardized occupational history approaches will prepare nurses to conduct more knowledgeable assessments. These systems approach not only improves the understanding of individual patient needs but also supports improved health outcomes through targeted intervention. Through the integration of sound assessment methods and advanced technology, nursing practice can much better respond to musculoskeletal health disorder management and promote the overall goal of patient care and evidence-based practice.

KEY TERMS FROM THIS CHAPTER

Bones	Joints
Muscles	Ligaments
Tendons	Range of Motion (ROM)
Active ROM	Passive ROM
Muscle Strength	Muscle Tone
Gait	Posture
Spinal Alignment	Crepitus
Swelling	Deformity
Kyphosis	Lordosis
Scoliosis	Atrophy

Critical Thinking Questions

1. **Which of the following is an example of a synovial joint?**
   a. Skull sutures
   b. Vertebrae
   c. Knee joint
   d. Sternum
2. **During musculoskeletal assessment, the nurse asks the patient to bend the elbow. This is testing:**
   a. Flexion
   b. Extension
   c. Abduction
   d. Adduction
3. **Muscle strength is graded on a scale from 0 to 5. A grade of 3 indicates:**
   a. No muscle contraction
   b. Full range of motion against gravity only
   c. Full range of motion against resistance
   d. Slight contraction
4. **A nurse notes swelling, redness, and tenderness in a patient's joint. This is most consistent with:**
   a. Osteoporosis
   b. Arthritis
   c. Muscular dystrophy
   d. Tendonitis
5. **When assessing posture and gait, the nurse observes a patient walking with a shuffling gait. This may indicate:**
   a. Normal variation
   b. Parkinson's disease or neurological disorder
   c. Strong leg muscles
   d. Healthy aging

Short Answer Questions

1. What are the major components of the musculoskeletal system that should be assessed during a physical examination?
2. Describe the steps for assessing posture, gait, and mobility in a patient.
3. How is joint range of motion (ROM) assessed, and what is the difference between active and passive ROM?
4. What signs of musculoskeletal abnormalities (e.g., swelling, deformity, tenderness) should a nurse look for during inspection and palpation?
5. How can muscle strength be evaluated, and what grading system is typically used?

Answer to Critical Thinking Questions

1. (c) 2. (a) 3. (b) 4. (b) 5. (b)

REFERENCES

1. Accettola, E., Bogdan, A., Callahan, S., Chawda, H., et al. (2023). Introduction to health assessment for the nursing professional: Part II. https://core.ac.uk/download/622362029.pdf (accessed on 16th July 2025).
2. Adunsky, A., Randell, A. G., Moseley, A. M., Samuelsson, B., McHorney, C. A., McHorney, C. A., Wu, C. C., et al. (2010). An interdisciplinary intervention for older Taiwanese patients after surgery for hip fracture improves health-related quality of life. https://core.ac.uk/download/pdf/8609596.pdf (accessed on 16th July 2025).
3. Amirpour, A., Eckerblad, J., Thorell, A., Bergman, L., & Nilsson, U. (2023). Usability and feasibility of a digital cognitive screening tool measuring older adults' early postoperative neurocognitive recovery: A protocol for a pilot study. *BMJ Open, 13*. https://www.semanticscholar.org/paper/cb4712ab7469983d99694fc80354291b32848b15 (accessed on 16th July 2025).
4. Antunes, A. V., Firmino, C. F., Marques, F. M., Marques, A. P., et al. (2019). Sintomatología musculoesquelética en estudiantes de enfermería: Un análisis de concepto. https://core.ac.uk/download/232112844.pdf (accessed on 16th July 2025).
5. Argent, K., & Cronin, M. (2017). Working with families. https://www.semanticscholar.org/paper/65ffab8a04232efb84b4134453b2eb122322b6f6 (accessed on 16th July 2025).
6. Ball, E., & Critchley, S. (2007). Patient and practitioner views of a new rheumatology (Tier 2) primary care service. https://core.ac.uk/download/1661487.pdf (accessed on 16th July 2025).
7. Bohan, A., Brown, D., Chinoy, H., Christen-Zaech, S., Pilkington, C. A., et al. (2011). A national registry for juvenile dermatomyositis and other pediatric idiopathic inflammatory myopathies: 10 years' experience; the Juvenile Dermatomyositis National (UK and Ireland) Cohort Biomarker Study and Repository for Idiopathic Inflammatory Myopathies. https://core.ac.uk/download/10413.pdf (accessed on 16th July 2025).
8. Borja, A., Farooqi, A. S., Golubovsky, J. L., Glauser, G., Strouz, K., Burkhardt, J., McClintock, S. D., et al. (2022). Simple and actionable preoperative prediction of postoperative healthcare needs of single-level lumbar fusion patients. *Journal of Neurosurgery: Spine*. https://www.semanticscholar.org/paper/46e6c198c40bc7edafb42b168fbdeab53e10a8c2 (accessed on 16th July 2025).
9. Braun, V., Dennis, D., Hodgson, C., Hsu, C. C., McMillan, S. S., & Portney, L. G. (2018). Expert consensus for respiratory physiotherapy management of mechanically ventilated adults with community-acquired pneumonia: A Delphi study. https://core.ac.uk/download/213607876.pdf (accessed on 16th July 2025).
10. Callejón Ferre, Á. J., Gómez Galán, M., López Aragón, L., & López Liria, R., et al. (2017). Applications of the Standardized Nordic Questionnaire: A review. https://core.ac.uk/download/286590648.pdf (accessed on 16th July 2025).
11. Case, K., Hussain, A., Marshall, R., Summerskill, S., et al. (2013). Achieving workplace inclusiveness by using ergonomics risk assessment. https://core.ac.uk/download/42143922.pdf (accessed on 16th July 2025).
12. Cauley, J. A., Cawthon, P. M., Cummings, S. R., Drieling, R. L., et al. (2020). Individual and joint trajectories of change in bone, lean mass and physical performance in older men. https://core.ac.uk/download/323072203.pdf (accessed on 16th July 2025).

13. Chantraine, A., Hulbert, A., Ku, A., Miller, A., Filler, A. G., Freiberg, A. H., Freiberg, A. H., et al. (2010). The clinical features of the piriformis syndrome: A systematic review. https://core.ac.uk/download/2780274.pdf (accessed on 16th July 2025).
14. Chen, Y., Gui, Y., Yu, X., Ma, H., Guo, J., Liu, B., Cheng, Y., et al. (2025). Application and research progress of real-time shear wave elastography in quantitative assessment of musculoskeletal system. *International Journal of Public Health and Medical Research*. https://www.semanticscholar.org/paper/edd66f0a94d6fe9f5508c09de64b3b47f6728826 (accessed on 16th July 2025).
15. Chipping, J., Macgregor, A. J., & Mooney, J. (2016). The benefits of syndication of mental health nurses within rheumatology out-patient departments: A narrative discussion. https://core.ac.uk/download/77027872.pdf (accessed on 16th July 2025).
16. Cocchiara, R. A., Guerra, F., La Torre, G., Mannocci, A., et al. (2019). The use of yoga to manage stress and burnout in healthcare workers: A systematic review. https://core.ac.uk/download/195777145.pdf (accessed on 16th July 2025).
17. Cortney, C., Lutjens, K., & Raines, K. (2017). Disposition and success of patients following discharge in the acute setting. https://digitalscholarship.unlv.edu/cgi/viewcontent.cgi?article=3927&context=thesesdissertations (accessed on 16th July 2025).
18. Deegan, O., Fullen, B., Segurado, R., & Doody, C. (2024). The effectiveness of a combined exercise and psychological treatment programmed on measures of nervous system sensitization in adults with chronic musculoskeletal pain–A systematic review and meta-analysis. *BMC Musculoskeletal Disorders, 25*. https://www.semanticscholar.org/paper/5552da0dcf233d8933709f302360be0d10ee5593 (accessed on 16th July 2025).
19. Díaz-Pacheco, J., & Cabanillas-Chávez, M. T. (2024). Nursing process applied to a preschooler with spinal muscular atrophy and chronic respiratory failure. *Multidisciplinary (Montevideo)*. https://www.semanticscholar.org/paper/c7ca40f0b8c183ae2f05dbcc22702cd2bdbb2825 (accessed on 16th July 2025).
20. El Mehdi, A., & Lahiala, A. (2025). Enhancing communication and patient safety in anesthesia nursing: A review of the SBAR method. *International Journal of Research and Innovation in Social Science*. https://www.semanticscholar.org/paper/ecc80bcde5a1eb8f7175e685b03421a854df4a53 (accessed on 16th July 2025).
21. Feng, T., Wang, X., Bu, H., Sun, K., Qin, X., Xie, R., Zhu, L., et al. (2024). Cervical rotation-traction manipulation for cervical radiculopathy: A systematic review and meta-analysis of randomized control trials. *Journal of Pain Research, 17*, 4055–4070. https://www.semanticscholar.org/paper/b9b94b966dc4f2c68854ad238c7c196a24110b5f (accessed on 16th July 2025).
22. Forman-Hoffman, V., McClure, E., McKeeman, J. L., Wood, C., Middleton, J., Skinner, A., Perrin, E. M., et al. (2016). Screening for major depressive disorder in children and adolescents: A systematic review for the U.S. Preventive Services Task Force. *Annals of Internal Medicine, 164*, 342–349. https://www.semanticscholar.org/paper/a0da04d57415ae7ef5db7e778b4341a0c9443268 (accessed on 16th July 2025).
23. Gökkaya, İ., Özceylan, Ö. F., Çolak, B., Renda, G., Duman, M., & Duman, E. (2024). Assessment of physicians' knowledge, thoughts, and attitudes regarding the phytovigilance system. *Expert Opinion on Drug Safety*. https://www.semanticscholar.org/paper/f5e60d0dd134994f82b562053d2b8d7306b1b95b (accessed on 16th July 2025).

24. Hagino, H., Kobayashi, E., Matsumoto, H., Wada, Y., et al. (2016). Locomotive syndrome presents a risk for falls and fractures in the elderly Japanese population. https://core.ac.uk/download/pdf/82325797.pdf (accessed on 16th July 2025).

25. Herlinah, L., Khasanah, U., Syamsir, S. B., & Badriah, S. (2024). The role of community-based nursing interventions on knowledge, self-efficacy, and blood pressure control among elderly people with hypertension. *Malahayati International Journal of Nursing and Health Science*. https://www.semanticscholar.org/paper/58b9501336b1e6ef020b6b9a644c372112ab800a (accessed on 16th July 2025).

26. Hermoso, M. E. (2009). The use of the Get Up and Go Test as the initial screening measure for fall risk with community dwelling seniors. https://core.ac.uk/download/223074305.pdf (accessed on 16th July 2025).

27. Katzman, W. B., & Pastore, E. A. (2012). Recognizing myofascial pelvic pain in the female patient with chronic pelvic pain. https://core.ac.uk/download/305124272.pdf (accessed on 16th July 2025).

28. Khairat, S. S., Morelli, J., Edson, B. S., Aucoin, J., & Jones, C. B. (2024). Needs assessment of virtual nursing implementation using the Donabedian Framework. *CIN: Computers, Informatics, Nursing, 43*. https://www.semanticscholar.org/paper/3ed6a6fe9c3f7be727a0f4cee58bbb68ac8e23c2 (accessed on 16th July 2025).

29. Klussmann, A., Nasir, J., Jost, M., Tolg, B., & Popp, J. (2024). P-618 Risk assessment of work-related musculoskeletal exposures. Are measurements better than observations? Results from the "EVERBA-study." *Occupational Medicine*. https://www.semanticscholar.org/paper/bf2d53af3bcb57d0ccd6123c1965cfd2e8fb32e2 (accessed on 16th July 2025).

30. Kriebel, D., Tickner, J., Jacobs, M., & Markkanen, P. (2011). Lessons learned: Solutions for workplace safety and health. https://core.ac.uk/download/71352756.pdf (accessed on 16th July 2025).

31. LeBoff, M. S., Greenspan, S. L., Insogna, K., Lewiecki, E. M., Saag, K. G., Singer, A., & Siris, E. S. (2022). The clinician's guide to prevention and treatment of osteoporosis. *Osteoporosis International, 33*, 2049–2102. https://doi.org/10.1007/s00198-021-05900-y (accessed on 16th July 2025).

32. Lee, M. S., Choi, T., Kim, J. I., & Choi, S. M. (2010). Using Guasha to treat musculoskeletal pain: A systematic review of controlled clinical trials. *Chinese Medicine, 5*, 5. https://www.semanticscholar.org/paper/82051ec97384b94fd13fba858baa04fb0bbeb1ba (accessed on 16th July 2025).

33. Mahajan, D., Gupta, M. K., Mantri, N., Joshi, N., Gnanasekar, S., Goel, A., Srinivasan, S., et al. (2023). Musculoskeletal disorders among doctors and nursing officers: An occupational hazard of overstrained healthcare delivery system in western Rajasthan, India. *BMC Musculoskeletal Disorders, 24*. https://www.semanticscholar.org/paper/f0247c6f035f5527f012a2fe6664507f86e6623a (accessed on 16th July 2025).

34. N/A. (1985). Focal Spot, Fall 1985. https://core.ac.uk/download/129069250.pdf (accessed on 16th July 2025).

35. Ntolopoulou, M. (2017). Biomechanics of assisted locomotion in elderly osteoarthritis patients. https://core.ac.uk/download/83926247.pdf (accessed on 16th July 2025).

36. Paek, D., Zoh, K., Kim, Y., Kang, M. Y., Kim, J., Yoon, J. H., Choi, E., et al. (2024). P-094 Taking occupational history into electronic database in public health, the key to the integration of two different systems; occupational versus public health. *Occupational Medicine*. https://www.semanticscholar.org/paper/94bfe566a5675ea3b7b07931931683960cda9d02 (accessed on 16th July 2025).
37. Paul, P., Kuijer, F. M., van der Wilk, S., Evanoff, B., Viikari-Juntura, E., & Coenen, P. (2024). What have we learned about risk assessment and interventions to prevent work-related musculoskeletal disorders and support work participation? *Scandinavian Journal of Work, Environment & Health, 50*, 317–328. https://www.semanticscholar.org/paper/42a476216cdf762713e82512e9c5300a4e19976c (accessed on 16th July 2025).
38. Pita-Fernández, S., Raposo-Vidal, I., Rodríguez-Romero, B., Seoane-Pillado, M. T., et al. (2011). Prevalence, co-occurrence, and predictive factors for musculoskeletal pain among shellfish gatherers. https://core.ac.uk/download/61916771.pdf (accessed on 16th July 2025).
39. Poplavskyi, O. A., Shkuratov, O., Kolisnyk, S., Poplavska, A. A., & Yovenko, D. (2024). Methodological foundations of somatoscopic research in automated decision support systems. *Management of Development of Complex Systems*. https://www.semanticscholar.org/paper/d7e6f0819e9a87e5c382e372f9ee1fa1ab4ff4fa (accessed on 16th July 2025).
40. Ravi, T., Johnson-Esparza, Y., Hernandez, J. F., Andry, N., Ali, F., Montanez Villacampa, M. D. P., Rincon, R., et al. (2024). Clinical assessment and patient education of chemical intolerance. *International Journal of Community Medicine and Public Health*. https://www.semanticscholar.org/paper/a86ade0f5e4a10c829e0e8fed0b50bef09d51a08 (accessed on 16th July 2025).
41. Satpute, S. A., Uribe, K. J., Olaore, O. O., Iizuka, M., McCumber Gandara, I. C., Schoy, W. J., Kulkarni, R. A., et al. (2024). Time efficiency and ergonomic assessment of a robotic wheelchair transfer system. *Sensors (Basel, Switzerland), 24*. https://www.semanticscholar.org/paper/813242a06b2570be2de44ff52ac28804b48445e4 (accessed on 16th July 2025).
42. Schneider, B. J., Naidoo, J., Santomasso, B., Lacchetti, C., Adkins, S., Anadkat, M. J., Atkins, M. B., et al. (2021). Management of immune-related adverse events in patients treated with immune checkpoint inhibitor therapy: ASCO guideline update. *Journal of Clinical Oncology, 39*, 4073–4126. https://doi.org/10.1200/jco.21.01440 (accessed on 16th July 2025).
43. Street, A., & Mannion, R. (2025). Payment by results and demand management: Learning from the South Yorkshire laboratory. https://core.ac.uk/download/pdf/6833648.pdf (accessed on 16th July 2025).
44. Swezey, L. (2018). Pain management: A flowsheet for providers. https://core.ac.uk/download/213462537.pdf (accessed on 16th July 2025).
45. Thomas, P., Baldwin, C., Bissett, B., Boden, I., Gosselink, R., Granger, C. L., Hodgson, C., et al. (2020). Physiotherapy management for COVID-19 in the acute hospital setting: Clinical practice recommendations. *Journal of Physiotherapy, 66*, 73–82. https://doi.org/10.1016/j.jphys.2020.03.011 (accessed on 16th July 2025).
46. Todd, C. L., Johnson, E., Stewart, F., Wallace, S. A., Bryant, A., Woodward, S., & Norton, C. (2024). Conservative, physical and surgical interventions for managing fecal incontinence and constipation in adults with central neurological diseases. *The Cochrane Database of Systematic Reviews, 10*, CD002115. https://www.semanticscholar.org/paper/a9c6703c6320d10ed38f0d7ac06a69a54e94c49a (accessed on 16th July 2025).

47. Williams, A., Beswick, A. D., Woolf, A. D., Martin, C., Terwee, C. B., Terwee, C. B., Abrams, D., et al. (2014). Recommendations for exercise adherence measures in musculoskeletal settings: A systematic review and consensus meeting (protocol). https://core.ac.uk/download/19553903.pdf (accessed on 16th July 2025).

48. Xue, S., He, L., & Zhang, M. (2021). Study on the effect of Green's Education Model in improving the knowledge, attitude and practice of occupational protection in chemotherapy among nursing interns. *International Journal of Clinical and Experimental Medicine Research*. https://www.semanticscholar.org/paper/298fb0d0e1e92991a9f20b2c68a94b2e3ecacc3f (accessed on 16th July 2025).

49. Yahya, M. H. (2023). Bladder agenesis: A systematic review. *Cureus, 15*. https://www.semanticscholar.org/paper/4880015cb29c3205b72501c62358d2e9d7ab0db1 (accessed on 16th July 2025).

50. Yemeshev, Y., Bekaryssova, D., & Koçyiğit, B. (2025). Assessment of the quality and reliability of YouTube videos related to teleradiology in musculoskeletal and rheumatic diseases: A cross-sectional study. *Rheumatology International, 45*. https://www.semanticscholar.org/paper/0e8e847f2e5e4769628b251828fa864a9c3e0379 (accessed on 16th July 2025).

NEUROLOGICAL SYSTEM ASSESSMENT IN NURSING

14

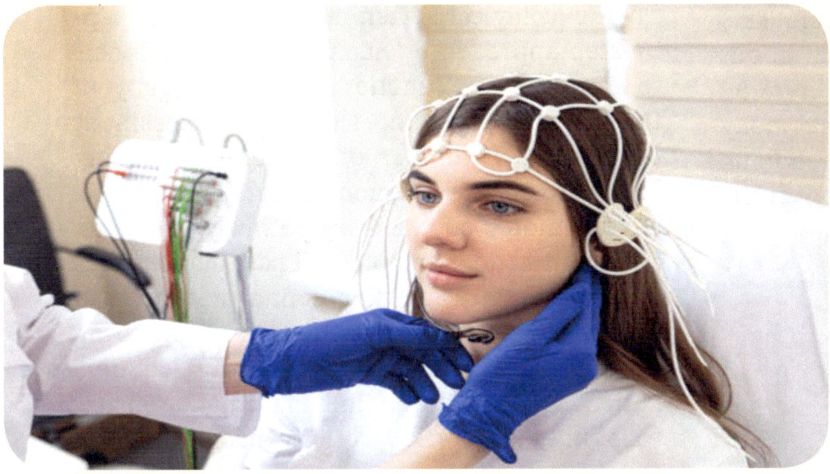

LEARNING OBJECTIVES

After studying this chapter, you will be able to:

1. Illustrate the anatomy of the neurological system;
2. Describe the common neurological assessment techniques;
3. Define the neurological assessment in different patient populations;
4. Explore the interpretation of neurological assessment findings;
5. Identify the documentation and communication of assessment results;
6. Focus on the challenges in neurological assessments.

Introduction

The complex and pivotal role of the neurologic system within the human organism justifies the necessity of thorough and systematic assessment in nursing practice. Neurologic assessment in health care is not only a method employed to test cognitive and motor functions but also pivotal strategies for early diagnosis and intervention. This is all the more significant in light of increasing rates of neurological illness and injury, much of which remains undiagnosed or misdiagnosed in the general practice setting. For instance, the prevalence of traumatic brain injuries (TBIs) necessitates that primary care providers, including nurse practitioners, be competent at making effective use of efficient screening tools to diagnose such conditions at an early age through reliable exams encompassing patient history, neurological checks, and ancillary testing options (Bizon et al., 2017). Nursing practice is at the forefront in treating patients with neurological disorders and is therefore quintessential that their assessment skills be paramount.

Neurologic function is a comprehensive system that affects all aspects of human function, ranging from motor function to sensory perception. Competent assessment by nurses has the potential to provide useful information about neurological status, facilitating timely intervention and improved patient outcomes. Standardized screening instruments, such as the Mini Mental Status Exam and Montreal Cognitive Assessment, have been cited for their utility but highlight a disconcerting trend of variability among practitioners in their application. This variance in practice raises question about whether training and education that nursing personnel receive are sufficient given that many of them report not feeling confident in making neurological disorder diagnoses (Bizon et al., 2017).

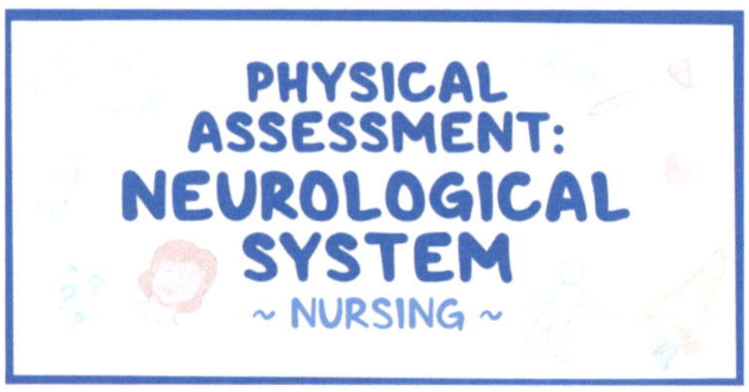

Figure 14.1. Physical assessment – neurological system.

Source: https://osmose-it.s3.amazonaws.com/NCB2u_uSQ1_QYhTIiFBRcLciSI6whJUI/_.jpg.

The integration of evidence-based procedures into neurological examination has the potential to enhance clinical efficacy and thus patient care in a significant manner. Familiarity with the best methods for neurological health assessment is an emerging area of contemporary research, leading to recommendations to advance screening practice in addition to the education of healthcare providers. The evolving landscape of neurological assessment demands nurses and other health professionals to dedicate themselves to continuous learning and transformation, ensuring that they are up-to-date with the latest developments and technology needed for optimal patient assessment. With the increasing use of new screening techniques, nursing professionals must keep themselves current and engaged in advocating best practice to enhance the early detection and management of neurological conditions (Figure 14.1).

Definition of Neurological System Assessment

The neurological system assessment is a step-by-step approach by health care professionals to evaluate the functioning and integrity of the nervous system. Thorough assessment consists of a number of elements, including consciousness assessment, function of cranial nerves, motor and sensory pathways, reflexes, and coordination. Neurological examination helps in the identification of potential neurological illnesses, severity of injury, and planning for treatment. Painstaking observation of a patient's mental status, limb movement, sensory response, and reflex activity provide useful information about their neurological health. The combination of clinical knowledge and practical skills is required for effective assessment in order to allow health practitioners to build an integrated picture of the state of a patient and the mechanisms involved. Underlying the neurological examination is the capacity for the diagnosis of several diseases and nervous system conditions. Clinicians can use standardized equipment and well-defined procedures to enhance reliability and validity of their findings. The Glasgow Coma Scale (GCS), for instance, is widely used in the measurement of levels of consciousness, enabling nurses to monitor changes over time appropriately. Moreover, specific tests such as the Babinski reflex help identify neurological integrity among both pediatric and adult groups. These evaluations not only facilitate the creation of knowledgeable diagnostic decisions but also inform discussions between multidisciplinary teams of possible interventions. Ensuring quality and consistency with neurological evaluations ultimately improves patient outcomes by encouraging timely intervention where aberrations exist. Additionally, examination of the neurological system goes beyond identifying deficits; it adds significantly to continuity of care, especially when transferring patients from one environment to another within the health-care system. This aspect is of utmost significance in palliative care, wherein transition from child to adult services often presents unique difficulties. Evidence indicates that there is commonly a lack of standardized transition frameworks within care systems, and this leads to disjointed care and potential compromise in continuity of care (Adi et al., 2009). The same holds true for disorders such as autism, wherein a lack of adequate knowledge possessed by emergency care providers can hinder appropriate management strategies (Miller et al., 2015). Through making the neurological assessment processes more streamlined and having clear-cut guidelines, doctors are better positioned to cope with the complexities of patient requirements as unique individuals, rendering care holistic in approach and responsive to changing conditions over time.

Importance of Neurological Assessments in Nursing

Neurological assessments are core components of nursing practice that provide valuable information regarding a patient's neurological status and overall health. They enable nurses to identify deviation from baseline function, facilitating intervention in a timely and effective manner. Regular monitoring of neurological function can reveal early signs of serious conditions such as stroke, traumatic brain injury, or neurological disease. The ability to identify such changes immediately is essential because delays in treatment can lead to catastrophic morbidity or death. The nuances of conducting an extensive neurological assessment make it possible for nurses not only to evaluate physical presentation but also to engage in therapeutic communication, which allows for improved patient care to be addressed in a more holistic way. Therefore, the nursing practice of incorporating routine neurological evaluations underscores the nursing profession's contribution to the delivery of whole-person care that addresses immediate clinical needs in addition to enhancing patient outcomes. Incorporating systematic neurological evaluations into the nursing practice contributes to enhanced plans for managing patients more effectively, which highly benefits neurologically affected patients. For instance, applying observational tools and specific evaluation guidelines has the potential to facilitate the identification of issues related to motor function, sensation, and intellectual abilities. This information cycles back into nursing interventions focusing on rehabilitation and self-care, encouraging patient independence and enhancing quality of life. Another study had previously termed the utilization of mirror therapy as a nursing intervention for stroke hemiparesis patients in an effort to increase muscle power and bodily mobility. While there was little short-term success, necessity for using standardized measures in measuring progress in such therapy is evident (Widiawati et al., 2025). This continuous monitoring allows nursing staff to adapt care strategies based on patient reactions, again reinforcing the need for neurological evaluations in efficient patient-focused care. The emphasis on neurological evaluations is also likely to enhance more profound therapeutic relationships between patients and health workers. Informing patients regarding their own neurological conditions promotes greater patient involvement and adherence to treatment protocols. The nurse educator role during the assessment process is vital as they not only perform assessments but also open lines of communication that empower patients to own their health. Through case studies, nursing professionals are able to learn a great deal about successful patient assessment methods, which illustrate how these assessments are instrumental in delivering better health outcomes for individuals with neurological disorders (Teixeira, 2024). Lastly, integration of comprehensive neurological assessment into practice improves clinical effectiveness and demonstrates the overarching mission of the profession to promote patient well-being (Figure 14.2).

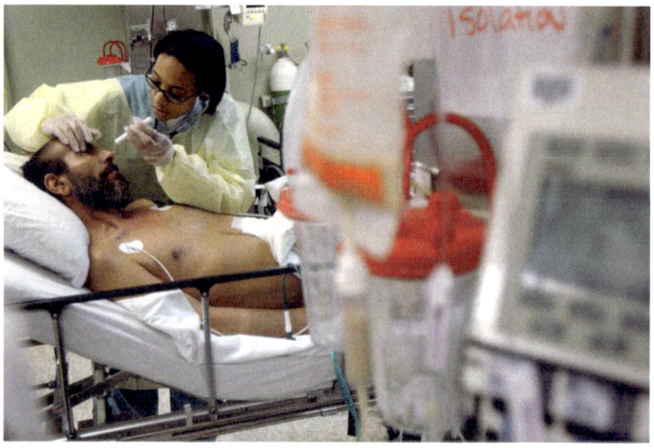

Figure 14.2. Neurological exam.

Source: https://wtcs.pressbooks.pub/app/uploads/sites/29/2020/09/US_Navy_030424-N-6967M-240_Lt._j.g._Elavonta_Thomas_conducts_a_routine_check_on_one_of_the_patients_in_the_Intensive_Care_Units_ICU_aboard_USNS_Comfort_T-AH_20-1024x667.jpg.

14.1. Anatomy of the Neurological System

Learning Outcome

1. Central Nervous System Components
2. Peripheral Nervous System Components
3. Functional Roles of Different Neurological Structures

It is significant to know the anatomy of the neurological system in order to perform effective nursing assessments. The neurological system consists of the brain, spinal cord, and peripheral nerves that are all responsible for significant roles to facilitate the communication between the body and the central nervous system. The brain is divided into various regions with different functions such as cognition, motor function, and sensory perception. The spinal cord is the central route of transmission of signals between the brain and the rest of the body and allows coordinated response to stimuli. Peripheral nerves beyond this extend throughout the body, conducting reflex action and sensation. As neurological examination is conducted by nurses, it is essential to have extensive knowledge of this anatomical foundation to allow precise assessments, more easily detecting deviation from normal function and guiding patient care tactics. The depth of understanding in the intricate aspects of the neurological system directs practice at the clinical level, particularly in nursing. Recent developments have focused on integrating anatomy and physiology into nursing education as a means of enhancing students' competence on exams. For instance, simulated skill practice has been successfully incorporated with theory to enhance a more integrated learning process. This integration allows nursing students to apply anatomical information to real-world situations, ultimately making their own assessment skills and confidence more effective when interacting with patients. By filling in the gap between theory and practice, nursing education can more effectively teach more thoroughly on neurological function and its relevance for patient management. These innovations in education highlight the significance of incorporating anatomy and functional pathology into clinical practice in nursing in line with evolving perspectives in health care education (Dougherty et al., 2015). Besides, assessment of the neurological system in practice calls for a structured approach, utilizing anatomy as an evaluation framework. The assessments are conducted by nurses for the identification of anomalies that could indicate underlying neurological disease. Through qualitative and quantitative methods, these tests might involve testing reflex arcs, testing sensory pathways, and cognitive functions.

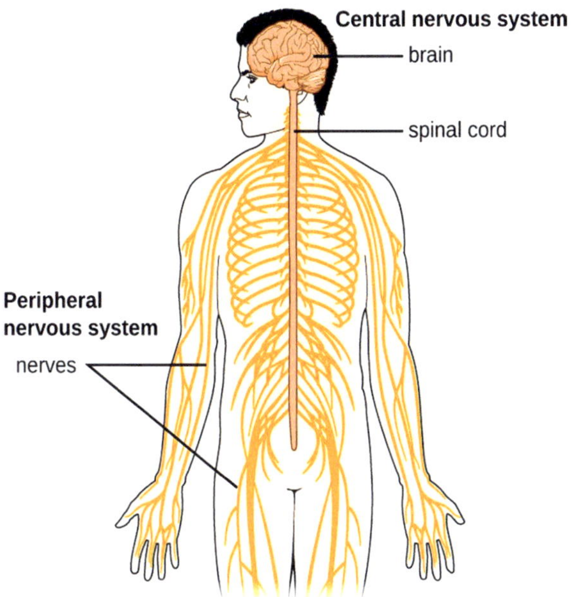

Figure 14.3. Anatomy of the neurological system.

Source: https://s3-us-west-2.amazonaws.com/courses-images/wp-content/uploads/sites/1094/2016/11/03175856/OSC_Microbio_26_01_NervSys.jpg.

Due to the anatomical basis of such tests, nurses need to possess abilities in the identification of deviances between normal and abnormal findings. Effective communication about anatomy structures and their functions can also enhance inter-professional collaboration, which ultimately results in integrated patient-centered care. By regularly refreshing their knowledge of the neurological system, nurses are able to ensure they provide prompt and accurate assessments, thereby improving healthier results for their patients (Kitsiou et al., 2013) (Figure 14.3).

14.1.1. Central Nervous System Components

The central nervous system (CNS) has two structures: the brain and spinal cord, which are both responsible for maintaining body functions and supporting higher mental functions. The brain, commonly known as the body's control center, becomes the overall controller of processing sensory information, regulating emotions, and directing voluntary movements. Within the brain, numerous regions such as cerebrum, cerebellum, and brainstem communicate with one another to execute complex functions from thinking to balance. The spinal cord is also the information superhighway connecting the brain to the rest of the body and passing on messages while executing the reflex actions. Nurses must learn these components as they conduct neurological assessments, allowing for early identification of potential disorders and immediate intervention. A holistic neurological assessment in nursing is not merely familiarity with the CNS anatomy; it includes familiarity with the physiological functions coupled with each component. Normal CNS activity guarantees homeostasis via autonomic regulation, dictating the involuntary as well as voluntary reaction to internal and external stimuli. Nurses must evaluate patients' neurological condition by levels of consciousness, sensory perception, and motor function, which reflect the CNS status. Abnormal findings during these tests could reflect potential complications, such as stroke or other cerebrovascular diseases, and that is why it is important to implement in-depth tests in the clinical field. To substantiate this, neurological evaluation recommendations increasingly highlight the necessity to value the complexities of the CNS in diagnosing various pathologies on evidence-based practices clinically relevant to nursing. Apart from structure and function knowledge, a comprehensive neurological assessment would also need to consider the impact of various disorders on the elements of the CNS. Diseases such as stroke, traumatic brain injury, and multiple sclerosis may severely affect cognitive and motor functions and require accurate and timely interventions on the part of medical professionals. The scenario of a patient with symptoms of a stroke, an all-too-common yet emergent scenario, relies on the ability to identify changes in consciousness, speech, and motor function in a timely fashion. A study shows that having well-established standards in the conduct of neurological examination greatly improves patient outcome, reiterating the nurse's position in the acute setting because they monitor patients with neurological disorders (Honkala et al., 2017). Therefore, extensive knowledge of the CNS components is imperative not only for proper examination but also to utilize accurate client-centered interventions in order to achieve a better recovery process (Figure 14.4).

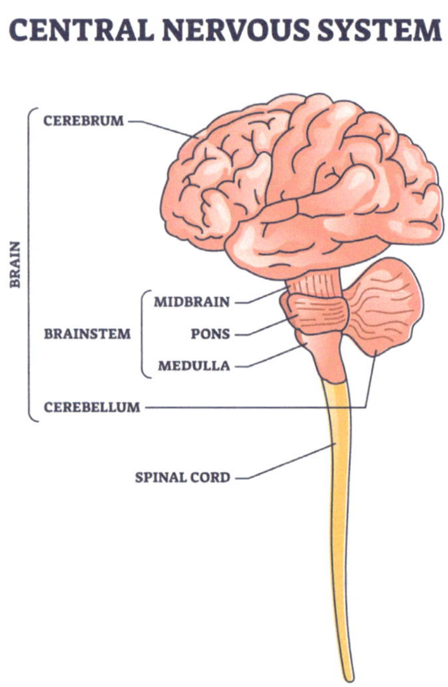

Figure 14.4. Central nervous system components.

Source: https://www.simplypsychology.org/wp-content/uploads/central-nervous-system.jpeg.

14.1.2. Peripheral Nervous System Components

The peripheral nervous system (PNS), which is important in the communication of the central nervous system with the rest of the body, consists of numerous parts that form a complex network. Comprising sensory nerves, motor nerves, and ganglia, the PNS is tasked with carrying sensory information from other parts of the body to the brain and passing motor commands from the brain to muscles. Such bidirectional exchange of information is essential for homeostasis and appropriate response to environmental stimuli. Nurses with an understanding of the elements of PNS are better positioned to assess neurological function, identify abnormalities, and implement appropriate care interventions. It is through understanding the organization and operation of the PNS that the entire process of nursing assessment becomes fortified, such that timely intervention within acute clinical situations, where the swift determination of peripheral nerve injury can be life-saving, is facilitated. Understanding the structure of the PNS is crucial in the correct conduct of neurological assessment, especially within acute care situations where timely intervention is essential. Major features such as the cranial and spinal nerves facilitate important functions such as reflex response and coordinating sensory inputs. For example, spinal nerves emerging from the spinal cord give rise to sensory and motor fibers, enabling voluntary movement and reflexes. Cranial nerves, with their twelve pairs, have different functions ranging from vision to mastication. The knowledge of these components aids nurses to carry out comprehensive examinations that include testing muscle strength, sensory perception, and reflexes—each of which may reveal concealed pathologies. The thorough examination of these PNS components ensures nurses are well equipped to respond to neurological emergencies and provide proper follow-up care that conforms to evidence-based requirements (Honkala et al., 2017). Recent developments serve to emphasize the importance of short-term neurological evaluations in nursing interventions due to the significant impact that such processes have on the outcomes of patients. Identification of the key components in a neurological evaluation—history taking, the level of consciousness, and motor assessment—ensures complete evaluation of the status of a patient. This becomes particularly pertinent in the case of cerebrovascular disorders where timely and accurate evaluation is most critical (Molina-Aroca et al., 2019).

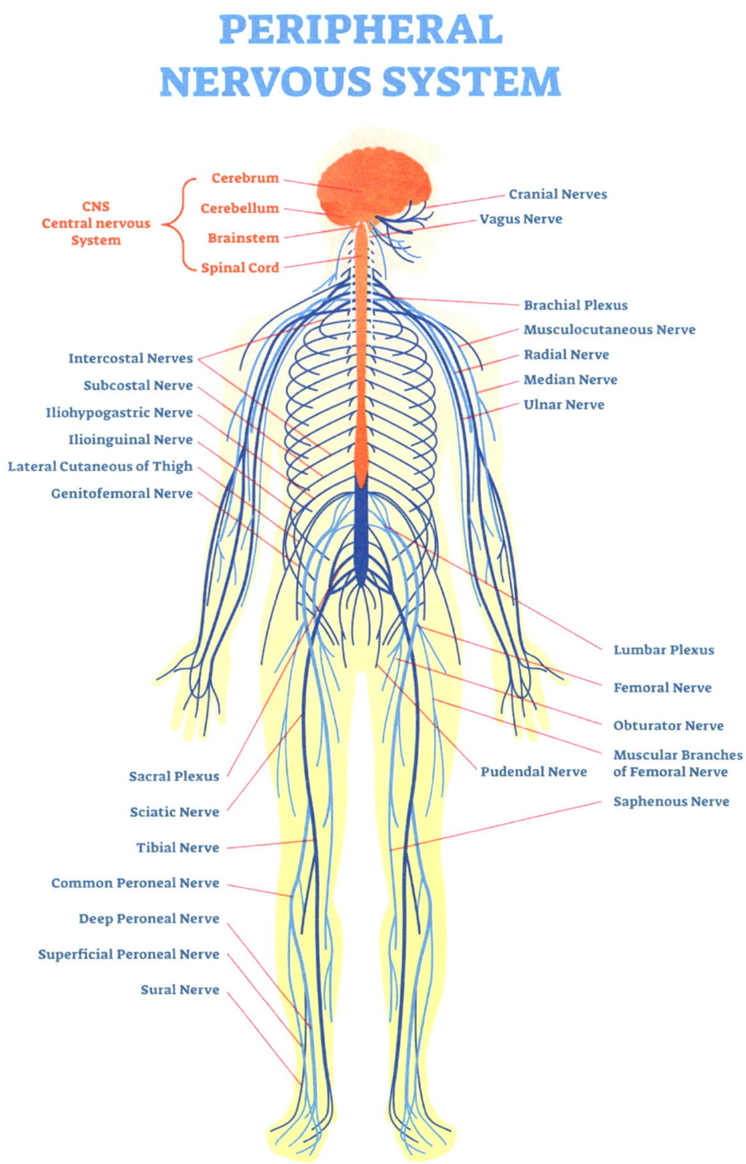

Figure 14.5. Peripheral nervous system components.

Source: https://www.simplypsychology.org/wp-content/uploads/peripheral-nervous-system.jpeg.

Moreover, incorporating newer methods and technologies of therapy, such as mechanical horse-riding simulators, offers new means of improving patients mobility and balance, particularly among those with neurological impairments. By understanding such developments, nurses are able to implement evidence-based outcomes in order to enhance practice and support higher-quality patient care. Overall, the ability to assess and comprehend the PNS components effectively is at the heart of nursing practice and patient health improvement for neurological patients (Figure 14.5).

14.1.3. Functional Roles of Different Neurological Structures

The intricate neurological apparatus has many different structures serving various different functional purposes in ensuring and maintaining body function and regulation. The central nervous system (CNS), composed of the brain and spinal cord, serves as the regulator of these functions. In the brain, various regions, such as the frontal, parietal, occipital, and temporal lobes, permit various cognitive functions—such as decision-making, sensory perception, and memory. For instance, the frontal lobe has a vital function in executive functions, with implications for personality and behavior, whereas the occipital lobe is specialized in processing visual information. Understanding these specialized functions is significant in nursing assessments because it enables practitioners to identify the etiology of neurological impairment, thereby enhancing the precision of intervention plans. Outside the cortical regions, subcortical components like the thalamus, hypothalamus, and limbic system have equally important functions. The thalamus is a sensory relay and it filters and routes signals to the appropriate areas of cortex. The hypothalamus, with its important homeostatic functions such as thermoregulation and balance of hormones, suggests its role in autonomic control. The limbic system, which includes structures responsible for emotion and memory, molds survival-related behaviors. An understanding of these neural structures is thus necessary for neurologically evaluating nurses. Without such information, therapists might overlook essential symptomatology that could indicate underlying neurologic disorders, which is vital in providing integrated care. Moreover, the peripheral nervous system (PNS) offers an additional reach of the CNS by connecting it with limbs and organs to facilitate voluntary and involuntary actions. The PNS is again subdivided into the somatic nervous system, responsible for voluntary muscle control, and the autonomic nervous system, responsible for controlling involuntary functions such as heart rate and digestion. The autonomic nervous system branches into the sympathetic and parasympathetic systems, which function in opposition to regulate arousal and relaxation states, respectively. This differentiation highlights the necessity of an integrative approach to neurological assessment in nursing because understanding both CNS and PNS function serves to aid directed therapeutic intervention. Nurses are hence capable of better anticipating complications or complications due to dysfunction of such critical neurological structures, hence maximizing patient care outcomes in neurological rehabilitation settings (Altman et al., 2011; Souza et al., 2007).

Test Your Knowledge

1. What are the major components of the neurological system, including the central and peripheral nervous systems, and what are their primary functions?
2. How does understanding neurological anatomy assist nurses in identifying abnormalities during assessment?

14.2. Common Neurological Assessment Techniques

Learning Outcome

1. Patient History and Symptom Evaluation
2. Physical Examination Methods
3. Use of Diagnostic Tools and Technologies

Neurological evaluation techniques are central to the profession of nursing, allowing neurological disorders to be identified and interventions consequently guided. One of the most frequent techniques is the use of an extended neurological examination consisting of a number of aspects such as cognitive function screenings, cranial nerve examinations, and motor and sensory tests. These tests allow nurses to establish a baseline of neurological function and detect changes that may indicate underlying pathology.

Standardized tools such as the Glasgow Coma Scale and the Mini-Mental State Examination provide systematic methods of evaluating consciousness and cognitive impairment to promote consistency in patient examination and enable early intervention in neurological disorders. By detailed documentation and findings analysis, nurses can communicate findings effectively to interdisciplinary teams, consequently enhancing patient outcomes from care and allowing collaborative management strategies.

Cognitive testing is a critical element of neurological examination since it provides information regarding a patient's mental status and function. Measurement tools such as the Mini-Mental State Examination and the Montreal Cognitive Assessment are designed to assess cognitive impairment and monitor change, and conditions such as traumatic brain injury or dementia are diagnosed based on the ability to identify these changes. In particular, health care clinicians must be able to employ these measures to detect changing patterns of cognitive functioning that would not be otherwise apparent. As emphasized in recent studies, the majority of primary care providers have indicated that they prefer simpler screening tools, like the Mini Mental Status Exam, since they are easy to use and effective in quick assessments.

It can assist nurses in selecting the optimal strategies when screening patients and that the highest priority cognitive impairments are not missed (Bizon et al., 2017). In addition to cognitive assessment, another vital component of neurological exam is the investigation of motor function and reflexes.

These include the assessment of muscle strength, coordination, and sensory response, which are important to ascertain neurological deficits. Tests such as deep tendon reflex testing and proprioception demonstration assist in identifying whether there is any central or peripheral nervous system abnormality. Nurses need to be taught these skills in order to make accurate assessments and implement the appropriate interventions for conditions that are likely to impact mobility or sensory perception. With the prevalence of conditions such as stroke or multiple sclerosis becoming increasingly common within clinical practice, it is important to learn about the impacts of neurological assessment skills. The inclusion of evidence-based practices, as such defined by expert consensus, will further ensure a formal framework for effective patient management, leading ultimately to improved outcomes and supporting the nursing profession in carrying out adequate neurological care (Braun et al., 2018) (Figure 14.6).

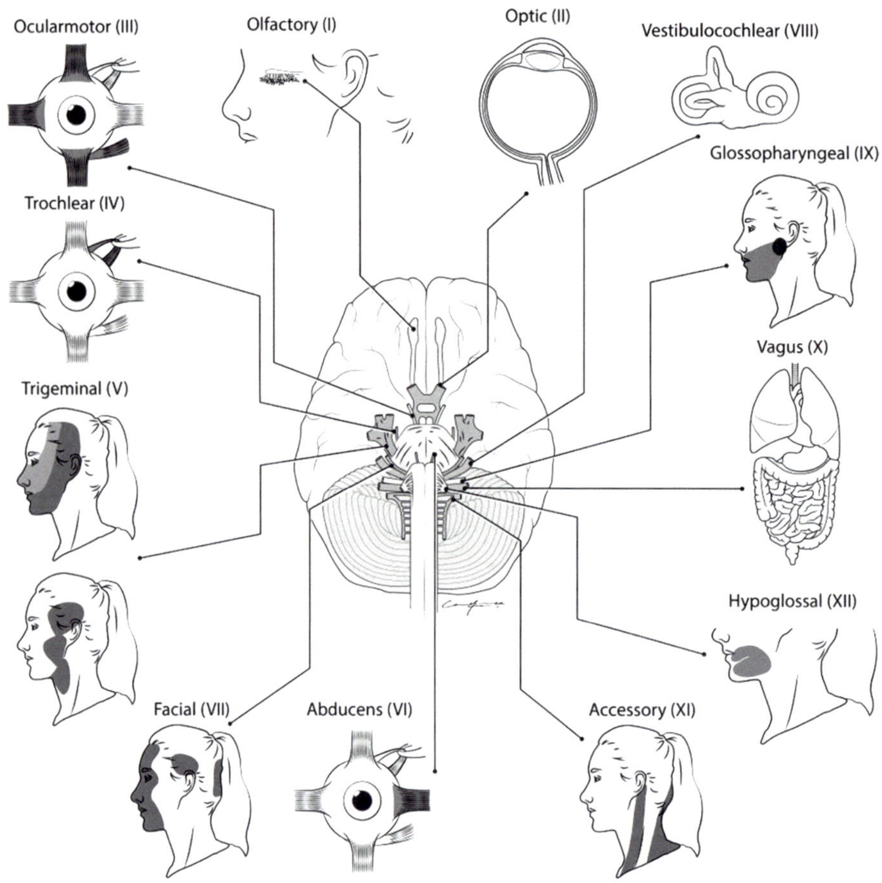

Figure 14.6. Clinical techniques: The neurological assessment.

Source: https://iastate.pressbooks.pub/app/uploads/sites/37/2020/01/Cranial-Nerve-Pathways-Greyscale-Brain-971x1024.jpg.

14.2.1. Patient History and Symptom Evaluation

Patient history collection is important in the assessment of neurological disorders. The collection of complete information assists clinicians to formulate a baseline of the patients neurological function and identify any deviation from standard patterns. Historical details can reveal very useful information, such as previous medical diagnoses, genetic history, and lifestyle factors, which may influence the presenting symptoms of the patient. Careful documentation of such information augments symptom evaluation by correlating the onset and evolution of symptoms with potential underlying disease. Furthermore, awareness of the patient's medical history aids in formulating more individualized treatment plans, which ensures enhanced patient involvement and cooperation with care regimens. The correlation between proper patient history and efficient symptom evaluation cannot be overstressed, as it offers the basis for establishing accurate diagnoses and planned therapeutic intervention. Symptom assessment is a fundamental component of nursing practice, especially when assessing patients with neurological conditions. It not only involves identifying and documenting presenting symptoms but also ranking them based on severity and potential impact on the quality of life of the patients. A more refined understanding of symptom clusters, as emphasized by more recent studies, allows healthcare clinicians to identify patterns related to specific neurological conditions. For instance, patients undergoing hemodialysis can experience a range of symptoms that compromise their general well-being and signal the need for symptom management targeting their particular needs (Zheng et al., 2025). In addition, recognizing the multi-dimensionality of symptoms including physical, emotional, and cognitive forms requires a patient care practice that is likewise inclusive in scope.

This thorough evaluation eventually assists nurses in creating effective interventions aimed at minimizing suffering and overall patient outcomes. For the provision of neurological care, the importance of efficient and prompt communication cannot be overemphasized. The ability of the nurse to effectively interpret and communicate patient symptoms to the broader healthcare team is paramount to continuity of care and effectiveness of treatment interventions. Research has shown that nurses play a core role in end-of-life decision-making, particularly in neurological illness where the difference between progressive symptoms and imminent death is subtle but important (Jonsdottir et al., 2025). Ongoing training in symptom recognition and communication skills is thus essential for nursing staff to achieve their highest level of skill in patient assessment. Interventions to enhance these skills will assist in making more informed decisions in resource plans such that nursing inputs are harmonious with best practices in neurological assessment. By creating a patient-focused mode of practice, the nurses are able to facilitate the dialogue to aid the patient and the family members during periods of adversity (Figure 14.7).

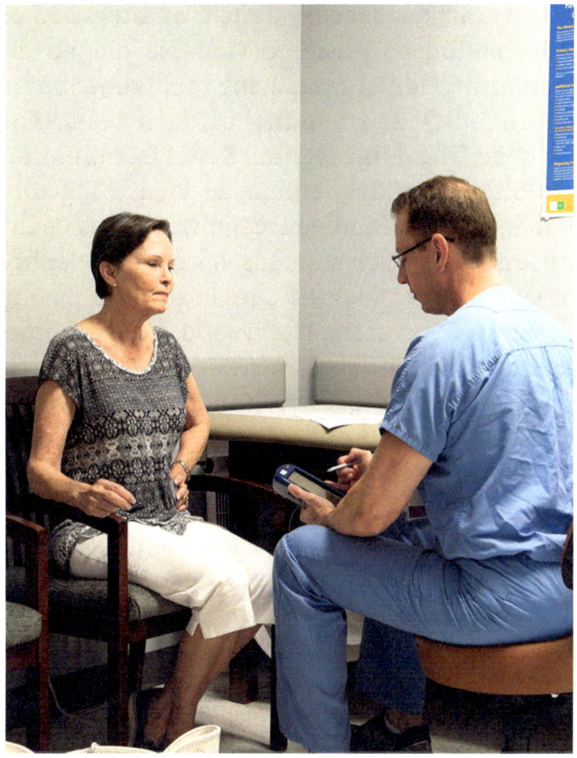

Figure 14.7. Patient history and symptom evaluation of neurological conditions.

Source: https://www.neurologysolutions.com/wp-content/uploads/2018/05/howcanourwellnessclinichelppic-5afdb8b799253.jpg.

14.2.2. Physical Examination Methods

The physical examination methods applied in the evaluation of the neurological system play a significant role in establishing a thorough understanding of a patient's health condition. Comprehensive neurological examination involves a process-based approach that assesses various functions, including motor and sensory function, reflexes, and cognitive function. Practitioners typically apply a combination of observation, palpation, and systematic tests to enable effective evaluation of these aspects. Particularly, targeted testing can reveal abnormality in terms of impairment of motor function, sensory deficit, or alteration of coordination and lead to valuable diagnoses. Standardization of measuring tools contributes to reliability and validity of such tests. For instance, the Mini-Mental State Examination (MMSE) is a widely employed measuring tool that invites streamlined cognitive assessment process. Using such methods, nurses can identify impending neurological issues in advance, paving the way for successful interventions and a better quality of patient care. Further, the integration of advanced diagnostic techniques into physical examination methods plays a crucial role in sharpening neurological assessments. Nurses often collaborate with multidisciplinary teams to facilitate the use of imaging studies, such as magnetic resonance imaging (MRI) and computed tomography (CT), to provide extremely valuable information regarding structural changes. These imaging modalities can confirm impressions obtained at the bedside to ensure that any indicator of pathology is not overlooked. Secondly, electrodiagnostic workup—such as electroencephalograms (EEGs) and electromyograms (EMGs)—provides further information regarding neural function and aids in the diagnosis of specific disorders. By integrating data from both physical examination and advanced diagnostics, doctors can better discern a picture of the patient's neurological health and are better positioned to formulate effective, evidence-based care plans. Finally, continuous education in contemporary physical examination techniques is imperative for nursing practice, particularly neurology. As healthcare practices continue to evolve, remaining up-to-date on the latest methodologies and diagnosis conditions is imperative for nursing practitioners. Noteworthy is emphasis on telehealth examination techniques, which have been vital during the COVID-19 pandemic. The ability to transform physical examinations into virtual modalities accentuates the learning requirement for nurses to be adept at both traditional methods as well as telehealth methods. Additionally, familiarity with new technology enhances the overall effectiveness of neurological examinations. As the field continues to advance, ongoing training programs will maintain nurses adequately capable of utilizing multiple examination modalities, thereby providing optimum quality of care for neurological patients. This approach compliments the broader end of establishing holistic and responsive healthcare environments, ultimately leading to greater rehabilitation and recovery in patients (Figure 14.8).

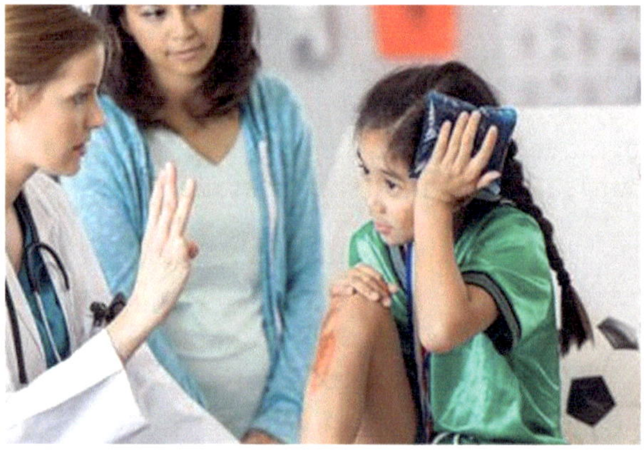

Figure 14.8. Physical examination methods of neurological conditions.

Source: https://images.squarespace-cdn.com/content/v1/5be0663b620b8515f3a9f2b6/1611155154518-6LTU20ZLSUN9VOIBATC6/girlcuncuss.JPG.

14.2.3. Use of Diagnostic Tools and Technologies

Integrating diagnostic technology and equipment into neurological system assessment is significant to nurses since they want to interpret complex patient presentations. Neurological condition assessment occasionally requires a detailed plan that involves advanced imaging techniques, electrodiagnostic examinations, and computer technologies. For example, Magnetic Resonance Imaging (MRI) and Computed Tomography (CT) scans provide nurses with clear and accurate images of the brain structures, which enable them to identify abnormalities such as tumors, hemorrhage, or lesions. Further, technology such as Electroencephalography (EEG) allows measuring the electrical activity in the brain, which is essential for diagnosing epilepsy and other seizure disorders. Use of these diagnostic modalities not only facilitates proper diagnosis but also contributes to early intervention strategies that can impact patient outcomes profoundly. Electronic health records (EHRs) have revolutionized how neurological assessments are documented and shared across the care groups. Not only do EHRs ease documentation, but they also enhance the availability of patient information, thereby improving care coordination across interdisciplinary teams. However, with the implementation of EHRs came issues, such as possible clinician burnout from increased screen time and administrative responsibilities associated with documentation. These issues have to be addressed; as highlighted by recent studies, healthcare professionals' interaction with EHRs could influence their job satisfaction as well as productivity (Downing et al., 2018). Therefore, decreasing the paperwork burden with these technologies is crucial in order to allow nurses to maintain their concentration on patient care so that their focus can be on aptly assessing and treating neurological conditions. The progress of telehealth has also provided variety to the list of devices for neurological assessment in nursing practice. Telehealth technologies enable distant monitoring and consultation to provide patients located in underserved regions with access to specialty treatment in neurology. These facilities are likely to employ video conferencing and remote diagnostics, which allow nurses to conduct tests that were traditionally limited to on-site presentations. The mobile health apps also allow for the constant interaction with patients and offer the capacity to track symptoms as well as compliance with treatment protocols (N/A, 2023). Through the integration of telehealth into practice, nurses can offer patient-centered care through making interventions available to persons with neurological disorders at the appropriate time regardless of location. With continued transformation in healthcare, effective incorporation of these technologies and diagnostic equipment remains a significant aspect of nursing practice in neurology.

Test Your Knowledge

1. What techniques are used to assess neurological function, including mental status, cranial nerves, motor and sensory function, and reflexes?
2. How can a systematic approach to neurological assessment improve the accuracy of findings?

14.3. Neurological Assessment in Different Patient Populations

Learning Outcome

1. Assessing Neurological Function in Pediatric Patients
2. Considerations for Elderly Patients
3. Neurological Assessments in Patients with Chronic Conditions

In the practice of nursing, it is essential to learn to conduct neurological exams in various populations to be able to participate more effectively in optimal care. Neurological function may significantly depend on patient age, history, and some conditions. For instance, those patients with a trauma brain injury history are particularly challenging to examine. Studies indicate that the majority of primary care clinicians are not comfortable with TBI identification and diagnosis due to inadequate training and understanding of available screening tools.

It has been found that many of the available tools like the Mini Mental Status Exam tend to be unsuitable due to the nature of the injuries, and therefore there is a requirement for standardized evaluation instruments tailored for the population. Sealing these disparities by way of education and evidence-based screening tools is required to provide accurate diagnosis and maximal management of TBIs, which are on the rise in primary care (Bizon et al., 2017). Another group of patients requiring advanced neurological assessment is autism spectrum disorder (ASD) patients. The ED nurses play a significant role in caring for autism patients, who typically have typical behavioral and communicative difficulties. Studies have shown that while the majority of ED nurses demonstrate adequate knowledge regarding the condition of autism and its comorbidities, there is a vast amount that is lacking in what is provided to them. Such limited knowledge can impact the quality of care provided to these patients. Additionally, the environment of an ED, with its fast-paced and potentially sensory-overloading atmosphere, presents an obstacle. Therefore, suitable neurological assessment should be in mind the cognitive needs and environmental needs of autistic patients and ways of facilitating effective communication and de-escalation (Miller et al., 2015). Addressing the following issues of neurological assessment in diverse populations not only enhances patient care but also yields a wider understanding among nursing professionals.

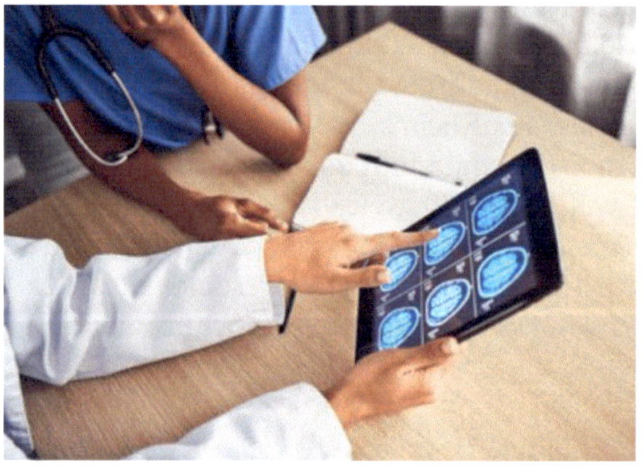

Figure 14.9. Neurological assessment in different patient populations.

Source: https://www.shutterstock.com/image-photo/doctor-tablet-brain-xray-neurology-260nw-2268437167.jpg.

The application of individualized assessment protocols and ongoing education can significantly add to the accuracy and effectiveness of treatment for ASD patients with TBIs. Beyond this, as healthcare evolves and expands, the role of the advanced practice nurse can extend to promoting better training and resources. Through research and development of advanced tools and guidelines, healthcare providers can increase their ability in neurologic assessment. This is particularly crucial because the prevalence of conditions such as TBIs and autism is increasing, necessitating a responsive reaction to patient care interventions and nursing education (Bizon et al., 2017; Miller et al., 2015) (Figure 14.9).

14.3.1. Assessing Neurological Function in Pediatric Patients

Neurological function testing in children is a multi-dimensional approach with integration of clinical observation, standardized testing, and parental report. Assessment begins with thorough medical history and this is followed by a structured neurological examination planned to evaluate various components like consciousness, motor function, and sensory perception. Children, unable to describe their symptoms by words, need the acute observational skills of nurses. By keen observation of physical responses and behaviors, nurses can learn about the neurological status of the patient. Additionally, integration of feedback from family is helpful; parents may provide input on behavioral changes, and developmental milestones that inform the assessment. With an integrated method, there is enhanced capability to monitor and identify neurological disorders effectively and, therefore, intervene in a timely manner tailored to the individualized needs of pediatric patients (Teixeira, 2024). Use of standardized test instruments is vital in the objective evaluation of the neurological function of children. The instruments can range from developmental screening tests to neuropsychological tests that evaluate skills ranging from cognitive and motor skills. For instance, use of the Denver Developmental Screening Test can be used to assist in identifying developmental delay, whereas certain cognitive tests can help evaluate functions such as attention and memory. Repeated advances in evaluation techniques allow nurses to increase their diagnostic accuracy and treatment planning. Furthermore, psychosocial considerations need to be integrated; research indicates that focusing the psychosocial care needs of children can significantly improve health outcomes (Maike et al., 2023). Therefore, merging these devices with clinical inspections provides an overall picture of a child's neurological health, ultimately leading to enhanced care and treatment guidelines unique to pediatric patients.

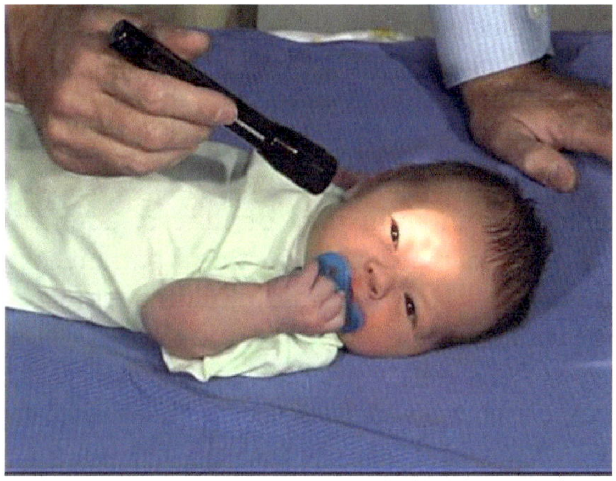

Figure 14.10. Pediatric neurologic examination.

Source: https://cfvod.kaltura.com/p/816122/sp/81612200/thumbnail/entry_id/0_c33kca50/version/100022/width/640/height/512.

Finally, the significance of ongoing neurological observation in pediatric patients cannot be stressed enough, as it tends to lead to enhanced management for identified neurological issues. Regular check-ups can pick up changes that would indicate improvement or deterioration of neurological function, so timely interventions can be instituted. This is particularly valuable in children who have long-term conditions that can affect their nervous system, for example, cerebral palsy or epilepsy. Involvement of a multidisciplinary team of neurologists, nurse practitioners, and psychologists further enriches the process of assessment to allow for complete care that incorporates medical as well as psychosocial elements. Nurses should be well-trained to carry out such assessments because their training directly affects outcomes for the patients as well as the entire health care experience for these patients and their families (Teixeira, 2024) (Figure 14.10).

14.3.2. Considerations for Elderly Patients

When neurological examination is conducted on older patients by healthcare workers, one should recognize the unique physiological and pharmacological changes of aging. Older patients have many comorbid conditions that can disrupt examination and therapy, and thus one should well grasp their history of illness. Cognitive impairment is prevalent in these patients and can be subtle in presentation, influencing how they react to neurological testing. Accordingly, nurses must follow proper communication and obtain a comprehensive history involving any medications and their side effects. The American Geriatrics Society's Beers Criteria® educates the avoidance of some medications for the elderly and demonstrates the necessity of tailored pharmacological interventions to minimize side effects and maximize benefits (N/A, 2019). Having an awareness of the complexities that are a part of neurologic examinations in older patients, it is likewise necessary for nurses to employ a holistic understanding that is not only directed at bodily health but likewise includes psychosocial. Psychological disorders, e.g., depression and anxiety, will have significant effects on cognitive function and overall well-being and thus influence exam results. In addition, environmental factors like social support and the patient's living conditions are also central in care and recovery planning. Nurses may come up with a richer insight into the patients neurological health by evaluating these factors and adjust assessments and interventions accordingly. This holistic assessment agrees with evidence-based practice which advocates for individualized care to enhance older patients' emotional lives (N/A, 2012). Moreover, older nursing evaluations should incorporate pertinent screening tools specifically tailored to meet their needs and exposures. Scales of neurological assessment can effectively enable accurate assessments of motor and cognitive function but must be adapted to accommodate age differences. The complexity of interpretation of results in the elderly necessitates constant education and training for nurses to recognize atypical presentations of neurological disorders. The incorporation of multidisciplinary team feedback will enhance the validity of the assessment and facilitate collaborative care models. With the ongoing research, focused on the development of guidelines considering the unique characteristics of the geriatric population, it will play a vital role in informing nursing practice to improve older adults' health outcomes across different clinical settings (N/A, 2012, 2019) (Figure 14.11).

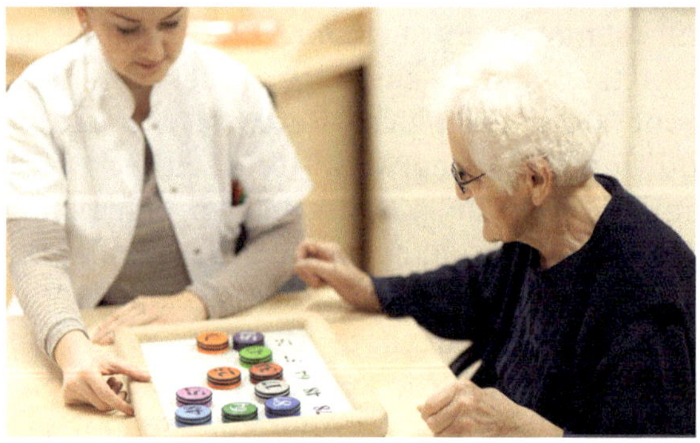

Figure 14.11. Assessing neurological function in elderly patients.

Source: https://i0.wp.com/www.mindworkspsychologists.com/wp-content/uploads/2023/03/psychological-assessment-for-elderly-adults-christian-pass.jpg?resize=800%2C486&ssl=1.

14.3.3. Neurological Assessments in Patients with Chronic Conditions

Assessment of neurological function among patients with chronic conditions is paramount to nursing practice. Nurses are typically the first health care workers to conduct complete assessments of neurological status and to recognize underlying deficits or changes that imply such conditions. Testing usually includes the assessment of cognitive function, reflexes, sensory function, and motor function. Since neurologic changes caused by chronic illnesses like diabetes, multiple sclerosis, or neurodegenerative disorders can have severe effects on neurological health, nurses need to be experienced in identifying the implications of such changes. Such a skill not only helps in creating an efficient care plan but also facilitates patient education and participation. Through early detection of neurologic changes, nurses can justify timely interventions, thereby making a significant contribution to the overall management of the patient's condition. A systematic method of neurological evaluation can better enhance patient outcomes, especially in patients with chronic conditions. The use of standardized measurement instruments, like the Glasgow Coma Scale or neurologic exam protocols, allows nurses to evaluate major neurological functions in a systematic way. Familiarity with the usual impediments in the process of assessment is also crucial. For instance, some patients may have cognitive impairments that are impairing their communication ability and, in the process, making the assessment difficult. A survey of chronic disease transition models demonstrates that good assessments are nested in a comprehensive system of patient-centered care, which is embracing multidisciplinary collaboration (Bagnall et al., 2013). Henceforth, it is necessary for nurses to communicate with other clinicians in order that neurological assessments are thorough and go on to encompass detailed treatment plans on the basis of the individual requirements of each patient. Also, the scenario of chronic illness presents unique challenges when performing neurological checks. As is highlighted in transition process research, chronic illnesses have a tendency to produce complex interactions of neurological and bodily symptoms that can make the clinical presentation complex (Adi et al., 2009). For instance, patients transitioning from child to adult care systems have very demanding manifestations that are neurologically based, such as deteriorating cognitive capabilities in the case of diabetes care. Well-designed evaluations, thus, must consider the state of development of the patient, the specific chronic illness, and the patient's prior medical history. Taking a holistic, as opposed to a fragmented, view in implementing neurological evaluations has the potential not only to enhance the quality of care but also to enable continuity of care at transitional junctures. Such multi-factorial approach ultimately aims towards optimizing patient involvement, engagement, and self-management, thereby empowering individuals to care for their complex disease conditions.

Test Your Knowledge

1. How do neurological assessment techniques differ between adults, children, and older adults?
2. What considerations should be made when assessing neurological function in patients with communication barriers or cognitive impairments?.

14.4. Interpretation of Neurological Assessment Findings

Learning Outcome

1. Identifying Normal versus Abnormal Findings
2. Understanding Neurological Signs and Symptoms
3. Correlating Assessment Findings with Potential Diagnoses

Interpretation of the results of neurological assessments is an important nursing practice, particularly in the management and diagnosis of neurological conditions. There are various assessment tools and techniques used by nurses to evaluate cognitive function, motor function, and sensory responses. Detailed assessment allows healthcare professionals to identify potential neurological impairment and create individualized care plans. For example, the Glasgow Coma Scale is applied to measure levels of consciousness and establish neurological function following traumatic brain injury. These types of tests provide such important information that nurses can use patterns of change in a patient's status over time to identify. This is essential to successful intervention. The finer points of interpretation are based on a deep understanding of healthy as well as diseased neurological function, and therefore highlight the importance of educational origins in nursing education to prepare practitioners for such an integral duty. In addition, neurological examination is not just measuring physical responses; it also significantly includes patients' mental and emotional states. Screening instruments such as mini-mental status tests allow nurses to test for cognitive impairment or psychiatric disorder in the context of a more comprehensive neurological examination. Adopting a broad-based strategy permits practitioners to distinguish between the organic neurological disorders and the possible psychological determinants. Identifying the interface between psychological and neurological findings is essential to effective patient management. For instance, a patient with high stressors might be reported by a nurse as experiencing confusion or changes in behavior, which would be interpreted incorrectly if the emotional underpinning is ignored. Thus, proper training in neurological and psychological assessments enables nurses to deliver holistic care to their patients. Finally, integrating evidence-based practice in the interpretation of neurological assessment findings is essential in nursing. Nurses not only have to rely on traditional assessment tools but also familiarize themselves with emergent research that informs best practice recommendations. The utilization of expert consensus statements, for example, as employed in more current studies of physiotherapy intervention in intubated patients with conditions like community-acquired pneumonia, demonstrates the evolving nature of clinical best practice (Braun et al., 2018). This dynamic approach allows nurses to provide scientifically grounded care as well as tailor the care to meet the individual patient's needs. Additionally, results should be interpreted to include developmental milestones, particularly in pediatric environments, where measurement of skill like sucking non-nutritively is crucial in determining development readiness (Cane et al., 2018). Such contextual and critical knowledge is needed in order to encourage positive patient outcomes and extend nursing practice.

14.4.1. Identifying Normal versus Abnormal Findings

A comprehensive neurological system examination in nursing is an essential element in the identification of normal versus abnormal findings with the potential to influence patient outcomes. Nurses must be proficient in recognizing normal neurological parameters, including consciousness levels, motor strength, and sensory reaction. For instance, a patient who is fully oriented, has suitable stimuli response, and equal strength in all extremities can be termed as normal. Conversely, deviations from these parameters, for instance, decreased consciousness, unilateral weakness, or sensory loss, suggest potential neurological compromise. Having baseline measures in place through systematic evaluations aids early interventions such that the nursing evaluation is not only useful in diagnosis but also essential in monitoring and managing neurological health. Differentiation of normal versus abnormal findings involves an integrative knowledge of several diverse assessment instruments. Nurses typically use the methodical neurovascular examinations that involve assessment of vital signs, pupil reactivity, and movement of the limbs to detect variations that could signal hidden pathologies. Standardized documentation workflows within electronic medical records, which were developed and implemented, have been useful in improving the accuracy and completeness of such examinations. By consolidating key assessment features into a single EHR location, as described in recent research, medical professionals are able to reduce the potential for misplaced or inaccurate documentation, whereby abnormal findings are not just flagged but addressed promptly (Kevin et al., 2024). This streamlined approach not only facilitates better communication among healthcare teams but also to improve patient safety and quality of care. Moreover, neurological examination has come into focus in the case of new medical conditions, i.e., COVID-19, in which abnormal neurological presentations are of utmost significance. The majority of patients hospitalized with COVID-19 have presented with acute neurological presentation, complicating their clinical profile and requiring a judicious assessment strategy (Eligulashvili et al., 2024). Identification of neurological abnormalities in the acute stage is crucial, as such abnormalities have the potential to result in long-term complications, raised mortality, and a requirement for specialized rehabilitation. Neurological examination has to take priority by nursing staff in such patients, with the understanding that early detection of abnormalities from normal observations can pave the way for early intervention and make rehabilitation planning more specific, thereby improving patient prognosis and recovery overall.

14.4.2. Understanding Neurological Signs and Symptoms

In the context of neurological assessment in nursing, it is extremely crucial that early signs and symptoms of neurological disorder are recognized. It has been established that disorders like Alzheimer's disease (AD) can be accompanied by psychological symptoms, i.e., depression and cognitive impairment, often years and even decades before severe neurological deterioration is firmly established. Cognitive impairment might start only approximately 12 years following early signs of memory loss in late-onset Alzheimer's disease, signifying a gradual progression of the disorder that should be detected early by nurses (Bature et al., 2017). Nurses can assist in early interventions that can limit the development of cognitive impairment and improve outcomes by being sensitive to such signs. The nursing role in performing a broader neurological assessment cannot be overstated, particularly in the setting of acute care. It is by current guidelines that nurses are expected to possess a short neurological assessment covering critical evaluation areas such as history taking, level of consciousness, and determination of motor function. These aspects are important in the detection of cerebrovascular conditions such as strokes, which, based on statistics, occur in around 25,000 patients each year in Finland alone (Honkala et al., 2017). Early assessment allows nurses to distinguish between different neurological disorders and act instantaneously, as necessary, so that patients are provided with relevant and required interventions that can help influence their outcome. In addition to the recognition of early warning signs and the making of thorough assessments, evidence-based practice integration within neurological nursing constitutes the foundation.

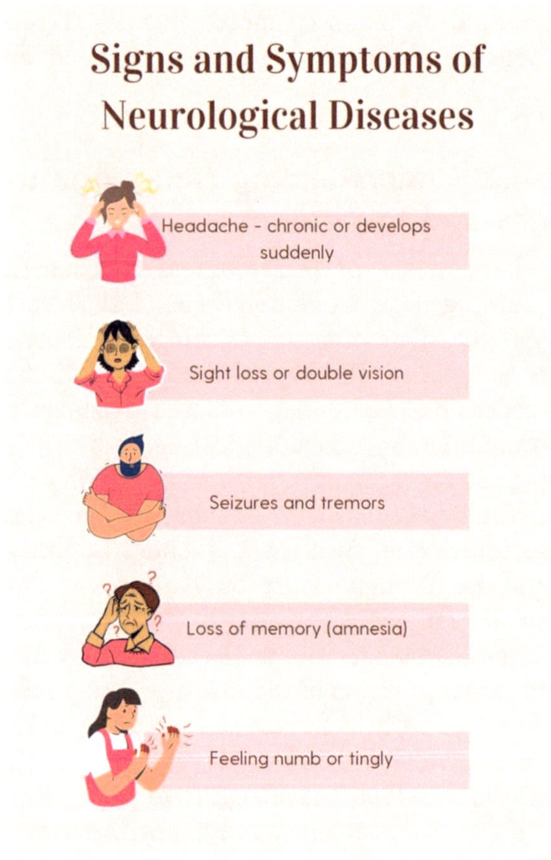

Figure 14.12. Understanding neurological signs and symptoms.

Source: https://external-content.duckduckgo.com/iu/?u=https%3A%2F%2Fwww.grantsformedical.com%2Fwp-content%2Fuploads%2F2022%2F08%2FList-of-Neurological-Symptoms-IG-768x1152.jpg&f=1&nofb=1&ipt=a66e6e217791e765c929d7e3e3e424c896f4735ca1fb50f509184f95ace95cdb.

The value of a systematic system of neurological assessment is expressed in the literature as maximizing uniform assessments to detect abnormalities more effectively. Research informs us that knowledge regarding the subtleties of pupillary response and vital signs is linked with enhanced clinical judgment regarding a patient's neurological status (Honkala et al., 2017). Therefore, ongoing training and education in the latest evidence-based assessment methods are essential for nursing professionals. As they continue to advance their skills, nurses will play increasingly larger roles in the prevention and management of neurological disorder consequences in diverse patient populations, ultimately improving health outcomes (Figure 14.12).

14.4.3. Correlating Assessment Findings with Potential Diagnoses

In nursing, within the context of neurological system assessment, comparing findings from assessment to potential diagnoses is important for the best care of patients. Neurological assessment involves detailed evaluation through observation of patient behavior, testing of cognition, and testing of motor functions. Through systematic gathering of this information, nurses can identify abnormalities that may indicate neurological conditions. For instance, alterations in motor function may suggest anything from stroke to multiple sclerosis. Correlating these findings against a patient's history and symptoms guarantees increased diagnostic accuracy, and therefore interventions can be enacted in a timely manner and have a long-lasting impact on patient outcome. Nurses need to be observant and consider these findings within the broader context of potential neural pathways involved, thereby offering a holistic method of care. That connection is also intensified by the evolution of information about how chronic disease affects neurological health. Kids with neurological or neuromuscular disorders, for example, often present symptoms that can be misattributed or not precisely known. The findings among children in the pediatric patients, as demonstrated in the PELICAN study, emphasize the significance of vigilant observation and interpretation of developmental delays or behavioral changes, which are usually symptoms for serious chronic disease. The symptom burden among children with complex chronic conditions (CCC) highlights the importance of comprehensive assessment taking into account both psychological and physical wellbeing, the study finds. This underlines the role of nurses as lead assessors and coordinators of children's rights to effective palliative care and intervention for their specific needs (Zimmermann et al., 2016). Within this research on stroke childhood survivors, the need for precise neurological assessments is more evident. Research indicates that child cancer survivors who experience strokes have higher risks of mortality and poor health-related quality of life (HRQOL) outcomes. These participants, as discussed in the Childhood Cancer Survivor Study, present distinct issues with memory and cognitive ability that must be identified through targeted screening. The acute incremental risk of death following multiple strokes necessitates nursing assessments to be not only inclusive but also holistic in examining intricate health concerns. By linking assessment information to the diagnoses derived from practice, nurses are in a position to provide valuable back-story context to decisions and interventions that improve general health outcomes for the high-risk populations (Armstrong et al., 2020).

Test Your Knowledge

1. How can abnormal findings in neurological assessments, such as changes in consciousness, motor function, or reflexes, guide clinical decision-making?
2. What patterns in neurological assessment results may indicate acute versus chronic neurological conditions?

14.5. Documentation and Communication of Assessment Results

Learning Outcome

1. Importance of Accurate Documentation
2. Effective Communication with Healthcare Team Members
3. Legal and Ethical Considerations in Documentation

Recording and reporting test results is critical in nursing, particularly in neurological system assessment. Accurate documentation ensures patient information is not lost, and it is easily accessible to health professionals, encouraging continuity of care. This is also the case even when it comes to a multidisciplinary team where occupational and physical therapists all have a crucial role in patient rehabilitation. The International Classification of Functioning, Disability and Health (ICF) is the universal language, enhancing team communication and coordination of rehabilitation services. Applying models such as the ICF allows clinicians to have better communication of assessment outcomes and clinical roles definition, thereby improving the collaborative environment that can augment patient outcomes from stroke rehabilitation and other neurological diseases (McIntyre et al.,

2006). Successful communication of the findings of the assessment is more than just recording; it also entails active exchange of ideas among the members of the team regarding patient care strategies. Through the culture of open communication, practitioners are able to share their perceptions and experience in terms of teamwork in neurological rehabilitation. Sharing is necessary since it uncovers effective and ineffective elements that influence patient care.

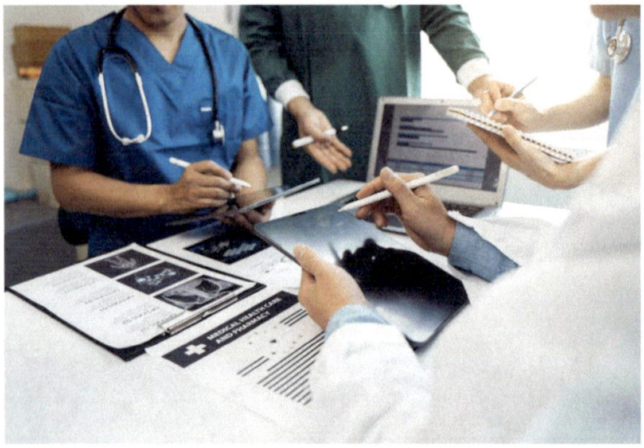

Figure 14.13. Documentation and communication of assessment results in nursing.

Source: https://www.intelycare.com/wp-content/uploads/2023/07/documentation-for-nurses.jpg.

Through qualitative exploration, as highlighted, certain core themes of team dynamics like shared practices, environment, and communication problems emerge as crucial in the evaluation process. Having knowledge of these aspects not only contributes to individual roles but also enhances the overall competence of the team, which eventually leads to enhanced clinical decision making and patient care (Souza et al., 2007). Also, the nature of neurological assessments is that documentation needs to be a comprehensive record of both patient status and care interventions. Well-documented assessments enable nursing practitioners to track change over time, that proper interventions are applied and adjusted as needed. This exchange process not only benefits specific patient cases but also feeds into the larger body of knowledge about neurological rehabilitation practice. By precise and thorough documentation, medical practitioners can look back at their practice and enhance clinical competence. Lastly, good communication and documentation within the ambit of assessment of neurological system is a foundation for quality patient-centered care and hence facilitates interrelatedness of assessment, intervention, and outcome of rehabilitation (Figure 14.13).

14.5.1. Importance of Accurate Documentation

Complete documentation in the case of neurological system assessment in nursing is needed for numerous reasons, particularly patient safety and continuity of care. The neurological system is also highly complicated, as the assessment can have significant implications on treatment plans and outcomes. Erroneous or incomplete neurological assessments may lead to misdiagnosis or delay in treatment, which can damage the patient's health. Through proper documentation in depth and accuracy, nurses provide a valid source of reference to future caregivers to facilitate informed decision-making. Such a degree of clarity is especially crucial as traumatic brain injuries, which form the majority of neurological cases, go undetected or misdetected without proper documentation and appropriate screening instruments as evident in the recent study (Bizon et al., 2017). Consequently, correct documentation is not merely a clerical task but rather an integral part of sound nursing practice that serves as a basis for quality patient care. The consequences of correct documentation extend beyond the patient-to-patient relationship; they also affect interdisciplinary communication among healthcare teams. Such communication and the sharing of correct patient information by team members affect successful team working in neurological rehabilitation. As evident in collaborative dynamics studies among occupational and physiotherapists, the provision of holistic assessments is dependent on each professional's familiarity with up-to-date documentation (Souza et al., 2007). Inadequate documentation leading to miscommunication can lead to piecemeal care and undermine the rehabilitation process. Also, because nurses are often the first to touch patients when assessing the neurological condition of a patient, it is essential that nurses document their findings meticulously so that all healthcare professionals are fully informed. This dependence underscores the necessity for sound documentation practices as a way to facilitate interdependent, integrated patterns of care. Second, accurate documentation is an important part of legal and ethical concerns in nursing practice. Medical professionals are legally bound for what they do, and paperwork errors can have severe legal repercussions. In neurology assessments where specific information could make or break the course of treatment, leaving out precise details could nullify legal immunity for nurses and healthcare institutions. Furthermore, proper documentation assists in upholding the ethical standard of patient care, where patients receive suitable interventions based on accurate historical details. Such an ethical component is underpinned in assessing conditions like traumatic brain injury, as noted in evidence on having reliable screening tools at primary care (Bizon et al., 2017). Lastly, adhering to strict documentation requirements in nursing not only shields individual professionals but also improves the levels of care delivered to patients in the healthcare system.

14.5.2. Effective Communication with Healthcare Team Members

Successful communication between health care teams is of vital importance, particularly in nursing neurological system assessment. Nurses are part of the multi-disciplinary team (MDT) and serve as the intermediary among various specialists working on patients care. A standard language, for example, the International Classification of Functioning, Disability and Health (ICF), is utilized to enhance the effectiveness of communication and the level of understanding regarding members of the team and their responsibilities. This coordination encourages improved coordination among the team members, ultimately translated into improved patient outcomes. The ICF provides a forum where nurses and other health care providers can share information more effectively on the needs of patients so that everyone is at the same level of understanding during the treatment and assessment of neurological disorders, thereby facilitating holistic care strategies (McIntyre et al., 2006). Besides, effective communication improves clinical decision making, especially when multiple members of the team are conducting examination and intervention with neurological conditions. Regular open communication among clinicians can clarify treatment plans, debate potential complications, and review other methods of patient care. For instance, nurses can initiate discussions during patient examinations that highlight observations and results regarding a patient's neurological condition. Such team discussion not only enhances the understanding of the patient's condition but also establishes trust within the team members. Effective communication thus minimizes misunderstandings and facilitates timely adjustment of the care plan to ensure that each team member's skills are being used efficiently in the context of neurological assessments (Bagnall et al., 2013). Also essential to successful healthcare team communication is the role of ongoing education and training. Regular interdisciplinary team meetings provide frequent opportunities for the team members to share information about best practices, updated research, and individualized patient treatment plans. Having everyone educated and on the same page enables the team to better navigate the complexities of neurological exams, with a focus on a patient-centered delivery of care. These education programs ought to accentuate the learning of soft skills such as empathy and active listening, which are critical in fostering a team-oriented collaborative culture. With enhanced communication strategies, healthcare teams are able to optimize neurological assessments and interventions to improve patient outcomes and satisfaction in general (Bagnall et al., 2013; McIntyre et al., 2006) (Figure 14.14).

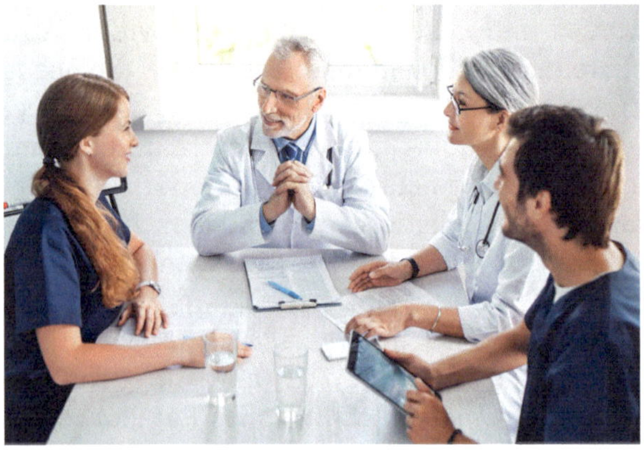

Figure 14.14. Effective communication with healthcare team members.

Source: https://www.welcomeware.live/wp-content/uploads/2023/10/medical-staff-engaging-in-team-building-strategies-in-healthcare.jpg.

14.5.3. Legal and Ethical Considerations in Documentation

The documentation for nursing neurological system examination is one that is under a variety of legal and ethical issues. Primarily, the ethics of informed consent are the basis of practice, wherein patients are provided with the knowledge of the nature of the examination conducted and the data collected. This is particularly the case in neurological patients who have impaired cognitive function and need to have their ability to consent weighed seriously before they participate in testing. Court proceedings mandate this process to be thoroughly documented, the patients' comprehension and consent to proceed continuing to be documented. This degree of detail not only supports patient rights but also safeguards practitioners against potential legal repercussions arising from negligence or ethical misconduct allegations. Ethical documentation that as accurately as possible portrays the consent process is then critical in maintaining trust and adhering to legal standards in nursing practice. In nursing documentation, particularly in neurological examinations, specificity and clarity are crucial. This meticulous attention to detail is not only required to deliver quality patient care, but also to fulfill the ethical imperative for precise record-keeping. Documentation is not merely a device employed in the clinic, but a legal document that could be challenged in the case of litigation or regulatory audit. Because neurological exams typically involve sophisticated tests, including cognition, sensory, and motor function, complete documentation ensures continuity of care and provides accountability for nursing interventions. Moreover, incorrect or illegible documentation can lead to miscommunications among healthcare professionals, and can compromise patient safety. Thus, nurses ought to be taught the ethical standards of documentation and how they can establish a culture where accurate and clear record-keeping is respected as a vital component of their practice. The ethics of documentation go much further than that when documenting with individuals who are vulnerable groups, such as those with disorders of consciousness (DOC). Ethical issues here become more important due to the fine balance between increasing knowledge through research and protecting individuals who cannot articulate themselves. Practitioners and researchers dealing with these patients need to navigate a complex series of legal and ethical guidelines so that their documentation protections are compatible with the best interests of the patients. For instance, even though there is a need for additional neuroimaging in DOC, institutional review boards and funding agencies impose stringent controls on the basis of ethical concerns regarding consent and patient interests. Respect for these ethical and legal documentation requirements is paramount for facilitating responsible research while upholding the dignity and rights of individuals with neurological impairments, as in the literature on this sensitive issue (Chiong et al., 2018; Tovino et al., 2008).

Test Your Knowledge

1. How should neurological assessment findings be documented to ensure clarity and continuity of care?
2. What key information should be communicated to the healthcare team when reporting abnormal neurological findings?

14.6. Challenges in Neurological Assessments

Learning Outcome

1. Variability in Patient Responses
2. Limitations of Assessment Tools
3. Cultural and Language Barriers in Assessment

The intricacies of neurological screening present a critical challenge to nursing professionals, requiring advanced understanding of physiological and cognitive dimensions. The variety of neurological conditions such as strokes, neurodegenerative diseases, and traumatic brain injury compel nurses to possess the ability to recognize an array of symptoms and their interpretations. During neurological rehabilitation, as emphasized in recent literature, effective interdisciplinary cooperation between health professionals like occupational therapists and physiotherapists is essential in the overall management of patients. Interdisciplinary use of various therapeutic disciplines relies on communication and cooperative working attitudes, which are typically inhibited by differences in professional backgrounds and communication styles. Thus, as noted by Souza et al. (2007), such determinants can lead to ineffective interaction, ultimately affecting patient outcomes and further complicating the process of assessment within the nursing environment. Additionally, the assessment process itself can be disrupted by cognitive and communicative barriers presented by patients with neurological disorders. Conditions like autism, characterized by definite social and communicative impairment, further complicate the nurse assessment environment. Research indicates that ED nurses face difficulties in recognizing and treating properly patients with autism due to inadequate training and educational resources concerning the condition. The findings of Miller et al. (2015) indicate that while the majority of ED RNs possess some level of information on autism, there exists a significant gap that must be addressed through targeted education measures. This deficit highlights the importance of guaranteeing that nurses have sufficient resources and training to perform thorough evaluations sensitive to the disparate neurological histories of patients. Environmental factors also contribute to the challenges in performing neurological assessments. Stressed, high-priority settings, such as emergency departments or rehab units, often lead to time constraints that compress patient exams. Nurses may be juggling a list of tasks—ranging from patient treatment to charting—amid the complexities of neurological illness.

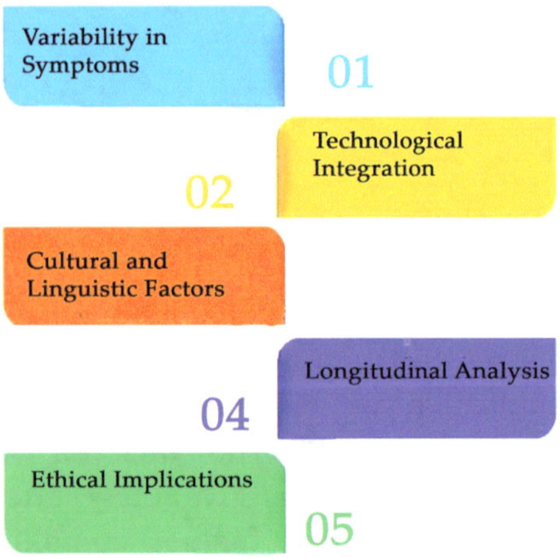

Figure 14.15. Challenges in neurological assessments.

Source: https://fastercapital.co/i/Neurological-Assessment-Tools--Startup-Synapses--Building-Resilience-Through-Neurological-Assessment--Challenges-and-Considerations-in-Neurological-Assessments.webp.

All these stresses can result in omissions or less than thorough assessment, ultimately compromising patient care. The interaction of organizational systems and external determinants, as discussed in Souza et al. (2007), emphasizes the importance of institutions providing nurses with sufficient resources—such as time for evaluation and collaborative systems that enhance interdisciplinary practice. Resolution of these issues is essential for optimizing the effectiveness of neurological examinations and patient outcomes in nursing practice (Figure 14.15).

14.6.1. Variability in Patient Responses

The quantification of patient reactions in neurology is inescapably defined by variability, an element influencing numerous factors like personal physiology, the nature of the neurologic illness, and the therapeutic environment. Variability can take the shape of measurable behaviors, e.g., different in motor function or mental response, or subjective protestations of pain or distress. Knowledge of this variation is important for nurses, as it means they can apply more individualized and effective interventions. For example, things like age, underlying health status, and even psychological status may have a profound effect on how patients integrate neurological stimuli and react to treatment. This underscores the importance of individualized care in nursing assessment, with holistic understanding of the individuals profile permitting informed optimization of care delivery to best practice in patient management, as identified in consensus statements on physiotherapy approaches for particular groups of patients (Braun et al., 2018). The employment of communication is essential to patient response variability management in neurological assessment. Nurses must be adept at determining not only information about the patients' immediate status but also about their emotional response and coping style. Anxiety has the potential to exacerbate neurological symptoms and produce amplified variability in response. In addition, the heterogeneity of stroke recovery rates among survivors is a case in point for the need for more advanced assessment tools that take into account different recovery phases and types of neurological deficits. As scholarship on functional assessment scales points out, the use of such measures as the National Institutes of Health Stroke Scale can help refine knowledge by offering quantifiable parameters. Still, it is crucial to note that it is not remotely possible to use a single measure for all cases because whether to use an assessment scale will have to be determined on the basis of the individual patient's context and nuances of presentation (Harrison et al., 2013). On top of that, professional judgment and expert opinion are required to address the technicalities involved in variability in the response of patients. The most critical challenge is finding appropriate interventions that are responsive to variable reactions experienced during neurological assessment. Evidence-based practice, for instance, from expert consensus of physiotherapy practice in intubated patients, reflects systematic approaches that can enhance nursing practice in diverse clinical settings. With consensus statements being published that address many neurological disorders, they present the opportunity to establish target assessment strategies in recognition of patient heterogeneity. Such an evidence-based approach not only improves optimal care but also provides optimal research into specific neurological interventions, thereby promoting improved patient outcomes within nursing practice (Braun et al., 2018).

14.6.2. Limitations of Assessment Tools

The efficacy of assessment tools in measuring neurological well-being is usually overshadowed by their drawback. Most of the common screening instruments, such as the Mini Mental Status Exam or the Montreal Cognitive Assessment, are beset by considerable degrees of subjective interpretation on the part of the health practitioner, which can lead to some measure of unreliability and inconsistency. Furthermore, tools may not be able to measure the intricacy of neurological disorders, including the co-morbidity of conditions. For instance, a study ascertained that despite the availability of validated screening tools, practitioners were more inclined to use those tools which were simpler to administer due to simplicity, regardless of depth of understanding required in diagnosis (Bizon et al., 2017). Hence, this is a great challenge in the delivery of effective neurological care, particularly in complex cases where sensitivity in assessment is needed in reaching conclusive determinations on a patient's status. Another basic limitation of the use of assessment tools in neurological evaluations is their useability across cultures and contexts. Many standardized tests are developed from specific populations and are not easily transferable across diverse populations. This can potentially lead to imbalances in treatment and diagnosis since these tools may fail to capture unique neurological expressions across different demographic categories, particularly those in low- and middle-income environments (Altman et al., 2011). Furthermore, the use of a single method may overlook cognitive ability or neurological wellness variations by socioeconomic status, education, and culture. While nursing professionals aim to deliver patient-centered care, it is critical to acknowledge the limitations of these assessment measures in order to offer individualized interventions that are representative and inclusive of diverse patient populations. Finally, the dynamic presentation of neurological conditions creates further challenges to the use of assessment measures. Neurological conditions change quickly, and hence symptom presentation and severity may vary over time. Most traditional evaluation instruments are not geared to handle these changes, and thus a snapshot of a patient's status at one point in time might not accurately represent the current changes or developing problems. For instance, even though tools like the CDC Acute Concussion Evaluation may be extremely enlightening, they are at times not sufficient due to the fact that they are unable to address the perpetually shifting and variable symptomatology of traumatic brain injuries (Bizon et al., 2017). It is therefore important that nursing clinicians review and update their use of such instruments constantly, employing an integrated process involving repeat observation, feedback from patients, and new clinical evidence to inform neurological assessment effectively.

14.6.3. Cultural and Language Barriers in Assessment

Effective neurological system assessment in nursing involves a culturally sensitive understanding and recognition of cultural and language barriers that may have a significant impact on patient examination and treatment. These barriers will complicate the communication between healthcare providers and patients, leading to misdiagnosis, inappropriate care, or failure to diagnose specific neurological conditions. The culture of a patient can influence his or her own understanding of illness and symptomatology, which may be different from traditional Western medical assessment. For instance, differences in perceptions of health and wellness can cause patients to underreport and misreport their symptoms, complicating the process of assessment. Therefore, nurses must learn cultural competence that will enable them to modify communication patterns in order to meet the multifaceted needs of the patient population while considering beliefs and values on an individual basis during the assessment process. Differences in language further complicate neurological assessment, particularly among more heterogeneous populations. Non-English-speaking patients may struggle to describe their symptoms or understand clinicians' questions, leading to incomplete or misinterpreted assessments. The use of interpreters and translation services has been proven to enhance communication and prevent misunderstandings within clinical practice. Effective communication channels are required, according to research, to ensure available and appropriate healthcare services for patients belonging to different ethnic groups (Clay et al., 2005). In the absence of such arrangements, the patients are not going to receive proper neurological evaluations, thereby ending up affecting their care and health outcomes. Nursing practitioners therefore have to encourage and establish mechanisms that can facilitate effective communication despite differences in language. Moreover, health systems must also prioritize the inclusion of cultural sensitivity training to address these barriers effectively. This is clearly seen in equitable care discussions where palliative and end-of-life care must be extended to all patients, including those with varied cultural or language backgrounds (N/A, 2009). This philosophy can even be applied to the realm of neurological testing when nurses can miss significant symptoms if they are not able to approach diverse populations respectfully and effectively. Building alliances with community organizations and accessing culturally competent resources creates an environment where patients are respected and appreciated. Thus, nursing educational programs should give significance to strategies for the transcendence of cultural and language barriers in order to promote health equity and improve the quality of neurological assessment of diverse patient populations.

Test Your Knowledge

1. What factors, such as patient cooperation, anxiety, or acute illness, can complicate neurological assessment?
2. How can nurses overcome challenges to ensure accurate and comprehensive neurological evaluation?

SUMMARY

Neurological system assessment in nursing practice is a complete part that plays a major role in affecting patient outcomes. With the growing complexity of the healthcare system, the nurses are most likely to be the first point of contact for those with neurological problems. It is hence crucial that they are proficient in conducting thorough assessments. Inconsistency in instruments used across various practices, as highlighted by studies, has implications for uniformly followed processes to enhance diagnostic accuracy and improve patient care strategies. There is a need to cover topics of traumatic brain injury screening and cognitive testing. Utilization of proven tools like the Mini Mental Status Exam will close gaps in confidence and competence among primary care providers, which are critical for early and efficient intervention in neurological conditions (Bizon et al., 2017). Furthermore, the provided evidence stresses the relevance of continuous education and training of nursing personnel in neurological testing. Comprehending the neurological implications of conditions like autism is also essential, particularly in critical settings where early intervention will probably be life-changing. The connection between educational shortages among nurses and able delivery of best care must be actualized. As indicated by recent studies, increasing educational resources can foster more sophisticated care habits to ultimately enhance the quality of nursing service provided for individuals suffering from complicated neurological disorders (Miller et al., 2015). Thus, it is critical to invest in specialized training programs, which will help nurses make informed observations and interventions, establishing a proactive healthcare setup. Finally, the development of nursing procedures based on neurological system assessments requires consideration from policymakers, schools, and healthcare organizations. Joint efforts must address concerns in creating comprehensive training modules with the highest evidence-based practices. Regular evaluation of screening tools and techniques will ensure that nursing professionals are best suited to handle the complexities of neurological exam. With advancements in healthcare, the creation of an educated nursing workforce will maximize the effectiveness of care given to patients, reducing the consequent morbidity and mortality from unidentified or inadequately treated neurological disorders. Overall, putting education first, standardizing practice, and resource reallocation are measures that are required to enhance the integrity of neurological exams in nursing.

Accurate neurological system assessment is essential in nursing since it provides relevant information regarding patient status and directs clinical practice. Full assessment involves the evaluation of cognitive function, motor skills, sensory perception, and reflexes. This multi-mobility perspective allows nurses to identify potential neurological disorders early and make changes to practice accordingly. Also, knowledge about occupational health history and neurological outcomes becomes increasingly relevant in clinical practice. Apart from the significance of occupational history taking, many healthcare settings do not accord priority to this element as less beneficial to patient care. Such inattention can hide underlying neurological disorders based on occupational exposures, emphasizing the need for uniformly standardized processes for history taking as suggested in relevant initiatives (Paek et al., 2024). Nurses also need to recognize the importance of inpatient falls as significant events affecting neurological health. According to reports, falls represent a major type of avoidable in-patient harm in the hospital setting, with elderly patients at greatest risk of severe injury. A review showed that optimal falls assessment, linked to recommended guidelines, measurably enhanced patient outcomes through organizational reviews. A high increase in the quality of reviews of falls was observed following the use of structured proformas, implying that standardization of assessment methods improves clinical effectiveness. This highlights the importance of thorough neurological assessment in fall prevention, which can result in serious consequences such as head injury or fractures, complicating the neurological status of the patients (Geraghty et al., 2024). Finally, the use of thorough neurological assessment in nursing practice is a key to improving patient safety and outcomes. By using standardized tools and structures, nurses can guarantee that assessments are systematic, total, and consistent across various clinical settings. Merging occupational health data with neurological assessments can help guide a holistic view of the status of patients and ultimately more specific interventions. As the health landscape keeps evolving, the incorporation of contextualized history and evidence-based standards of assessment can improve the quality of neurological care. Continuing education and training of nurses on the same is essential to ensuring high quality care while keeping in mind the multifaceted nature of neurological health in various patient groups (Paek et al., 2024).

KEY TERMS FROM THIS CHAPTER

Central Nervous System (CNS)	Peripheral Nervous System (PNS)
Cranial Nerves	Reflexes
Deep Tendon Reflexes (DTR)	Superficial Reflexes
Motor Function	Sensory Function
Cerebellar Function	Coordination
Balance	Gait
Mental Status	Level of Consciousness (LOC)
Glasgow Coma Scale (GCS)	Pupil Response
Muscle Strength	Sensory Perception
Aphasia	Neuropathy

CRITICAL THINKING QUESTIONS

1. **Which cranial nerve is assessed by asking the patient to smile, frown, and raise their eyebrows?**
   a. Cranial Nerve V (Trigeminal)
   b. Cranial Nerve VII (Facial)
   c. Cranial Nerve IX (Glossopharyngeal)
   d. Cranial Nerve X (Vagus)
2. **During a neurological assessment, the nurse tests the patient's ability to feel light touch and pain on the skin. This assesses:**
   a. Motor function
   b. Sensory function
   c. Reflexes
   d. Coordination
3. **A positive Babinski sign in an adult indicates:**
   a. Normal plantar reflex
   b. Upper motor neuron lesion
   c. Peripheral neuropathy
   d. Cerebellar dysfunction
4. **When assessing coordination, the nurse asks the patient to touch their nose with their finger and then the nurse's finger alternately. This is testing:**
   a. Gait
   b. Fine motor skills
   c. Cerebellar function
   d. Muscle strength
5. **The Glasgow Coma Scale assesses which of the following?**
   a. Sensory and motor function
   b. Level of consciousness
   c. Cranial nerve function
   d. Reflexes

Short Answer Questions

1. What are the major components of the neurological system that should be assessed during a physical examination?
2. Describe the steps for assessing a patient's level of consciousness and orientation.
3. How is cranial nerve function evaluated, and which nerves are most commonly assessed in a routine exam?
4. What techniques are used to assess motor function, including muscle strength and coordination?
5. How can a nurse assess sensory function, including touch, pain, temperature, and vibration?

Answer to Critical Thinking Questions

1. (b) 2. (b) 3. (b) 4. (c) 5. (b)

REFERENCES

1. Adi, Y., Carter, Y., Doug, M., Manjo, K., et al. (2009). Transition to adult services for children and young people with palliative care needs: A systematic review. https://core.ac.uk/download/44454.pdf (accessed on 16th July 2025).
2. Altman, D., Araya, R., Bolton, P., Campbell, C., Chatterjee, S., Chinn, S., Chisholm, D., et al. (2011). Non-specialist health worker interventions for mental health care in low- and middle-income countries. https://core.ac.uk/download/13113977.pdf (accessed on 16th July 2025).
3. Alzheimer's Association. (2023). 2023 Alzheimer's disease facts and figures. *Alzheimer's & Dementia, 19*, 1598–1695. https://doi.org/10.1002/alz.13016 (accessed on 16th July 2025).
4. American Diabetes Association. (2012). Standards of medical care in diabetes—2013. *Diabetes Care, 36*, S11–S66. https://doi.org/10.2337/dc13-s011 (accessed on 16th July 2025).
5. American Geriatrics Society. (2019). American Geriatrics Society 2019 updated AGS Beers Criteria® for potentially inappropriate medication use in older adults. *Journal of the American Geriatrics Society, 67*, 674–694. https://doi.org/10.1111/jgs.15767 (accessed on 16th July 2025).
6. Armstrong, G. T., Buerki, R. A., Chen, Y., Fullerton, H., et al. (2020). Stroke impact on mortality and psychologic morbidity within the Childhood Cancer Survivor Study. https://core.ac.uk/download/286362114.pdf (accessed on 16th July 2025).
7. Bagnall, A., Day, R., & Kime, N. H. (2013). Systematic review of transition models for young people with long-term conditions: A report for NHS Diabetes. https://core.ac.uk/download/29018738.pdf (accessed on 16th July 2025).
8. Baird, K. M., Sheehan, T. O., Johnson, M., & Jacobson, D. (2024). Abstract TP43: Optimizing system-wide nursing assessment documentation in the stroke population. *Stroke*. https://www.semanticscholar.org/paper/717b31a25ccbc77a6aa9a739e956f6ffb2b357a9 (accessed on 16th July 2025).
9. Bature, F., Guinn, B. A., Pang, D., Pappas, Y., et al. (2017). Signs and symptoms preceding the diagnosis of Alzheimer's disease: A systematic scoping review of literature from 1937 to 2016. https://core.ac.uk/download/130975123.pdf (accessed on 16th July 2025).
10. Bizon, L. J. (2017). Traumatic brain injury screening tools in primary care. https://core.ac.uk/download/79664900.pdf (accessed on 16th July 2025).
11. Braun, V., Dennis, D., Hodgson, C., Hsu, C. C., McMillan, S. S., & Portney, L. G. (2018). Expert consensus for respiratory physiotherapy management of mechanically ventilated adults with community-acquired pneumonia: A Delphi study. https://core.ac.uk/download/213607876.pdf (accessed on 16th July 2025).
12. Cane, C., Cockerill, H., Harding, C., Law, J., et al. (2018). Using non-nutritive sucking to support feeding development for premature infants: A commentary on approaches and current practice. https://core.ac.uk/download/323057633.pdf (accessed on 16th July 2025).
13. Chiong, W., & Vaishnav, N. H. (2018). Informed consent for the human research subject with a neurologic disorder. https://core.ac.uk/download/286362450.pdf (accessed on 16th July 2025).

14. Clay, D., Gumber, A., Johnson, M. R. D., et al. (2005). An overview of the research evidence on ethnicity and communication in healthcare. https://core.ac.uk/download/105291.pdf (accessed on 16th July 2025).

15. De Souza, L. H., & Suddick, K. (2007). Therapists' experiences and perceptions of teamwork in neurological rehabilitation: Critical happenings in effective and ineffective teamwork. https://core.ac.uk/download/336329.pdf (accessed on 16th July 2025).

16. Díaz-Pacheco, J., & Cabanillas-Chávez, M. T. (2024). Nursing process applied to a preschooler with spinal muscular atrophy and chronic respiratory failure. *Multidisciplinary (Montevideo)*. https://www.semanticscholar.org/paper/c7ca40f0b8c183ae2f05dbcc22702cd2bdbb2825 (accessed on 16th July 2025).

17. Dougherty, L., Endacott, R., Ibarreta, G. I., Ironside, P. M., & Ricketts, B. (2015). Learning to nurse: Combining simulation with key theory. https://core.ac.uk/download/80693445.pdf (accessed on 16th July 2025).

18. Downing, N. L., Bates, D. W., & Longhurst, C. (2018). Physician burnout in the electronic health record era: Are we ignoring the real cause? *Annals of Internal Medicine, 169*, 50–50. https://doi.org/10.7326/m18-0139 (accessed on 16th July 2025).

19. Eligulashvili, A., Gordon, M., Lee, J. S., Lee, J., Mehrotra-Varma, S., Mehrotra-Varma, J., Hsu, K., et al. (2024). Long-term outcomes of hospitalized patients with SARS-CoV-2/COVID-19 with and without neurological involvement: 3-year follow-up assessment. *PLOS Medicine, 21*. https://www.semanticscholar.org/paper/118077fb1a9dc1c4f2138f5d4b266acf100af05d (accessed on 16th July 2025).

20. Geraghty, T., Boyle, N., McNamee, M., Kelly, J., Lucey, K., & Harkin, E. (2024). Retrospective review of falls in medical inpatients following introduction of a falls proforma at Wexford General Hospital. *Age and Ageing*. https://www.semanticscholar.org/paper/150caef6f5a24488a98545e523d4c78915e73e7f (accessed on 16th July 2025).

21. Harrison, J. K., McArthur, K. S., & Quinn, T. J. (2013). Assessment scales in stroke: Clinimetric and clinical considerations. https://core.ac.uk/download/16457850.pdf (accessed on 16th July 2025).

22. Honkala, E., Karvonen, E., Koistinen, T., Tolonen, H., et al. (2017). Guidelines for a brief neurological nursing assessment in acute care: A literature review. https://core.ac.uk/download/84795764.pdf (accessed on 16th July 2025).

23. Jonsdottir, G., Vilhjálmsson, R., Sigurdardottir, V., Hjaltason, H., Klinke, M., & Jónsdóttir, H. (2025). Nursing contribution to end-of-life care decision-making in patients with neurological diseases on an acute hospital ward: Documentation of signs and symptoms. *BMC Nursing, 24*. https://www.semanticscholar.org/paper/1a462bce6760e11295246ac8a0f835a25e16d4f9 (accessed on 16th July 2025).

24. Kitsiou, A., Caforio, A. L. P., Porta-Sanchez, A., Vahanian, A., Iung, B., Carrera, C., Szymanski, C., et al. (2013). ESC core curriculum for the general cardiologist (2013). https://core.ac.uk/download/55756305.pdf (accessed on 16th July 2025).

25. McIntyre, A., & Tempest, S. (2006). Using the ICF to clarify team roles and demonstrate clinical reasoning in stroke rehabilitation. https://core.ac.uk/download/335601.pdf (accessed on 16th July 2025).

26. Miller, S. M. (2015). Nurses caring for adults with autism in an emergency department: A survey of knowledge. https://core.ac.uk/download/70419788.pdf (accessed on 16th July 2025).

27. Molina-Aroca, A., Bernstein, J., Luque-Moreno, C., Cho, S., Choi, Y., Lucena-Anton, D., De Miguel, A., et al. (2019). Effectiveness of mechanical horse-riding simulators on postural balance in neurological rehabilitation: Systematic review and meta-analysis. https://core.ac.uk/download/288159209.pdf (accessed on 16th July 2025).

28. N/A. (2009). EoL: Towards quality care at the end of life. https://core.ac.uk/download/71365016.pdf (accessed on 16th July 2025).

29. Paek, D., Zoh, K., Kim, Y., Kang, M. Y., Kim, J., Yoon, J. H., Choi, E., et al. (2024). P-094 Taking occupational history into electronic database in public health, the key to the integration of two different systems; occupational versus public health. *Occupational Medicine*. https://www.semanticscholar.org/paper/94bfe566a5675ea3b7b07931931683960cda9d02 (accessed on 16th July 2025).

30. Schwenkreis, P., Kozak, A., Gonschorek, A. S., Schmehl, I., Seddigh, S., Fürst, A., Wohlfahrt, K., et al. (2024). Conception and development of a neurological registry of patients with persistent health impairments following work-related COVID-19 disease in Germany. *GMS Hygiene and Infection Control, 19*. https://www.semanticscholar.org/paper/faafeedc4ca2ff6b98333ffc666d6eb29bf533ea (accessed on 16th July 2025).

31. Teixeira, L. (2024). Nursing assessment and care for a patient with a neurological disorder. *British Journal of Nursing, 33(5)*, 252–255. https://www.semanticscholar.org/paper/34db26716a219ee21838fd8111888641af4ef29f (accessed on 16th July 2025).

32. Tovino, S. A. (2008). Neuroimaging research into disorders of consciousness: Moral imperative or ethical and legal failure? http://scholars.law.unlv.edu/facpub/80 (accessed on 16th July 2025).

33. van Niekerk, M., Richey, A. E., Vorhies, J., Wong, C., & Tileston, K. R. (2023). Effectiveness of psychosocial interventions for pediatric patients with scoliosis: A systematic review. *World Journal of Pediatric Surgery, 6*. https://www.semanticscholar.org/paper/fe94541257e382d8108c44c4de603310e6f2f539 (accessed on 16th July 2025).

34. Widiawati, & Farhan, Z. (2025). Nursing care for neurological system disorders on carotid infarction stroke through the provision of mirror therapy intervention. *Nursing Case Insight Journal*. https://www.semanticscholar.org/paper/aa493b060d1544f26350c1fb9e98ae3f09e1eccf (accessed on 16th July 2025).

35. Zheng, X., Yang, Z., Xu, L., & Wang, A. (2025). Decoding symptom complexity for clinical nursing assessment: A systematic review of simplification strategies in hemodialysis patients. *Worldviews on Evidence-Based Nursing, 22(2)*, e70007. https://www.semanticscholar.org/paper/4cb336020f7d07dc5661fcfd3d795a62c46e971c (accessed on 16th July 2025).

36. Zimmermann, K. (2016). Pediatric end-of-life care needs in Switzerland (PELICAN): Current end-of-life care practices and the perspectives of bereaved parents. https://core.ac.uk/download/84007654.pdf (accessed on 16th July 2025).

BREAST AND AXILLAE ASSESSMENT IN NURSING

15

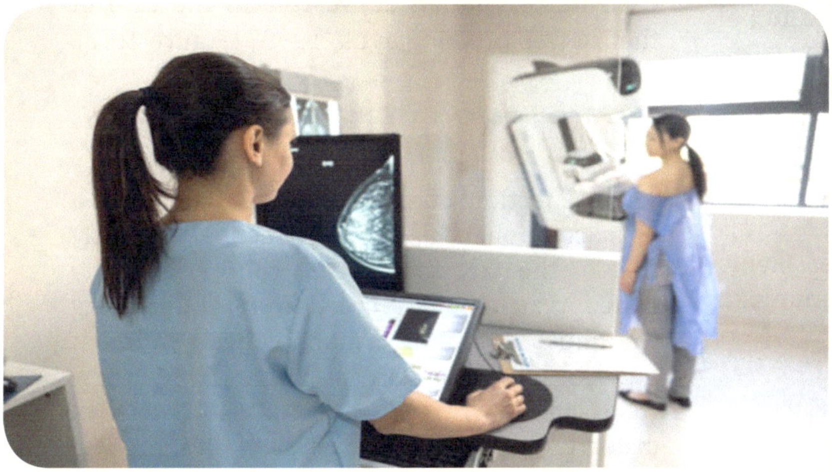

LEARNING OBJECTIVES

After studying this chapter, you will be able to:

1. Understand the anatomy of the breast;
2. Give an importance of axillary assessment;
3. Explain the techniques for breast assessment;
4. Describe the techniques for axillary assessment;
5. List the common findings in breast and axillary assessments;
6. Discuss about the patient education and communication.

Introduction

Assessment of the breast and axillae is a key nursing competency that is part of comprehensive patient care. Apart from the physical assessment, this is also a process that includes consideration of the patients psychological and emotional status. Complete assessment facilitates prompt identification of abnormalities and likely pathologies, such as cancer of the breast, enhancing patient outcomes significantly. Given the vulnerability of breast health, such examinations need to be conducted with cultural competence and emotional sensitivity by nurses in order to provide a safe space where patients will feel free to share their problems. This concise introduction to axillae and breast assessment establishes its role within holistic nursing practice and paves the way for a later detailed examination of approaches, pitfalls, and nursing interventions that guarantee effective patient assessments. Being aware of the anatomy and physiology of the breast and axillae is imperative for nurses undertaking such an assessment.

Knowledge of anatomical sites pertinent to the problem at hand, for example, lymphatic drainage pathways, is essential in order to identify potential problems. The axilla is a specific zone that is of particular importance for lymph node palpation, as it is directly involved in metastatic disease spread from diseases of the breast. Additionally, the interaction of hormonal influences with breast tissue must also be recognized because these will complicate results from evaluations. As explained in existing nursing texts, as well as the educational model of nursing competencies, the focus on thorough evaluations mirrors the greater goals of patient-centered care. Such understanding not only fosters clinical competence but also signifies commitment to professional standards of nursing in the 21st century (Berman et al., 2015). Successful breast and axillae assessments rely as well on establishing communication and rapport between patient and nurse.

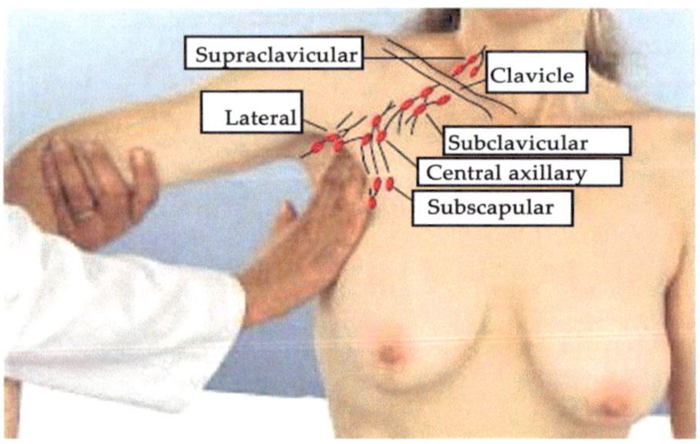

Figure 15.1. Breast and axillae assessment in nursing.

Source: https://img.brainkart.com/imagebk33/CC10ayO.jpg.

Rapport building is necessary because patients can become anxious or embarrassed during intimate examination. Through person-centered care approaches, nurses are able to effectively reassure patients and enhance their comfort levels, promoting effective communication around breast health. Informing patients about their own breast health at the time of assessment also turns out to be a teachable moment, promoting aware action and health. In accordance with nursing texts, e.g., Kozier and Erbs Fundamentals of Nursing, integrating critical thinking and clinical decision-making into assessments underlines this connection. In establishing a respectful and empathetic atmosphere, nurses not only fulfill their professional responsibilities but also allow patients to take an active role in the care of themselves (Cheung et al., 1999) (Figure 15.1).

Importance of Breast and Axillae Assessment in Nursing

The inspection of the breast and axillae is a basic component of nursing practice, primarily due to the fact that breast cancer is highly widespread among women worldwide. Being the most common female cancer in most nations, including Italy, with over 55,900 new cases annually, timely detection is crucial in order to improve patient results and survival (Alfonsi et al., 2024). The World Health Organization guidelines emphasize the Breast Self-Examination (BSE) practice beginning at age 20, encouraging women to become actively involved in checking their own health through routine self-examination (Alfonsi et al., 2024). Being active in such a way is very important in identifying any possible anomalies, thus making it easier for the doctor to intervene in time and foster an environment of health literacy for patients. Thus, nursing practice must incorporate adequate breast and axillary examination to support early detection programs and enhance health care quality. Moreover, identification and education of breast and axillary examination procedures can significantly empower patients and nurses alike. As primary health care workers, nurses play an important role as patient educators, teaching instruction in BSE procedures and general breast health knowledge. However, studies have shown that many healthcare providers are not well educated regarding the use of BSE, which disrupts their capacity to educate patients appropriately and sensitively (Alfonsi et al., 2024). Therefore, investing in specialized training courses for nurses is essential to enhance their knowledge and competency in breast examination, thereby patient engagement with preventive measures. Through the furnishing of information and resources, nurse education can bridge gaps in awareness and prevent disparity of risk perception between individuals, thus promoting a more informed adoption of regular breast health screening. Moreover, the importance of proper breast and axillary examination goes beyond individual patient management and impacts public health interventions at a population level. Because early detection and survival from breast cancer are interconnected complicatedly, nurse activities can make significant contributions to public health programs aimed at increasing the screening and awareness of breast cancer. Using the principles of social ecology in practice has the potential to provide a more comprehensive view of how systemic-level factors affect breast health and screening behavior. Furthermore, through establishing a supportive community environment in which breast health discussion is fostered, nurses are able to engage directly in the changing of attitudes and reduction of stigma around breast self-exam and screening. Lastly, effective breast and axillary assessment not only enhances patient healthcare outcomes but also augments collective community efforts aimed at reducing breast cancer morbidity and mortality in society.

Overview of Assessment Techniques

A proper inspection of the breast and axillae is crucial in the field of nursing practice and is one of the fundamental components of women's health care. There are various assessment techniques that can be employed to properly evaluate these areas. The visible inspection of the breasts, such as examining for any asymmetries, skin changes, or masses, forms the basis of the assessment process. Second, palpation is an important skill, performed with the patient seated and on the supine position, enabling the nurse to detect any abnormal findings such as lumps, alteration in texture, or nipple discharge. With systematic palpation methods such as circular or wedge technique, full coverage is ensured as well as increased chances of the detection of any pathologies. Practitioners' consistent use of these approaches facilitates competency and confidence, ultimately facilitating enhanced patient outcomes through the early detection of potential complications as well as fostering patient and health professional trust. Complemented by traditional assessment approaches, new imaging technology increasingly forms part of breast assessment. Imaging techniques such as mammography, ultrasound, and, where necessary, magnetic resonance imaging (MRI) significantly improve nurses' ability to detect as well as describe breast lesions. Mammography remains the gold standard for screening, particularly in women over 40 years, for helping to identify malignancies early. Ultrasound is now more used as an adjunct tool, particularly in discriminating between solid masses and cystic lesions. Advances in imaging strategies expand the nursing role in identification as well as interpretation of findings that need further workup. The integration of such imaging modalities into the hospital workflow, combined with detailed manual examination, allows nurses to provide holistic care to patients, facilitating early intervention in breast health care. With advances in healthcare, so too does the assessment methodology employed by nursing practitioners in breast and axillary examination have to evolve. Increasing emphasis on patient-centered and personalized care necessitates attention to patient education and shared decision-making as part of the evaluation process. Nurses are uniquely positioned to educate patients about methods of breast self-examination, further spreading the benefits of self-education and proactive health management.

Multidisciplinary coordination within the health team becomes essential, especially in managing complex cases such as those in geriatric patients, who might report unusual symptoms because of comorbidities and frailty. The recognition of these nuances is particularly significant in developing good management plans since presentation of breast cancers can widely vary among populations. Thus, the establishment of sound assessment protocols from the most current evidence and guidelines is important to optimize care and to meet the needs of varied patient populations and attain improved health outcomes in breast and axillae assessment in nursing practice (Melanie et al., 2020; Spyridon et al., 2021) (Figure 15.2).

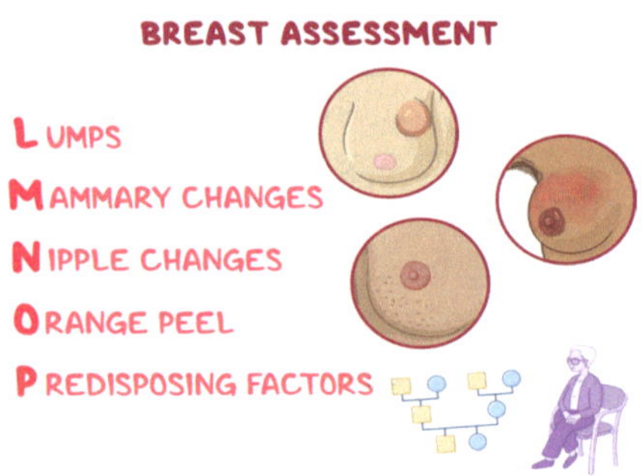

Figure 15.2. Overview of assessment techniques breast and axillae.

Source: https://www.osmosis.org/_next/image?url=https%3A%2F%2Fd16qt3wv6xm098.cloudfront.net%2Fk8d5tiZNS3WVga95EJGx6B4xR2yd-OZ2%2F_.png&w=1920&q=75.

15.1. Anatomy of the Breast

Learning Outcome

1. Structure and Function of Breast Tissue
2. Lymphatic Drainage and Its Significance
3. Variations in Breast Anatomy

Understanding breast anatomy is crucial for nurses who conduct assessments of the breast and axillae. The breast, composed primarily of glandular tissue, fat tissue, and connective tissue, is crucial for lactation and overall breast function. Within each breast, 15 to 20 lobes are present, which further divide into lobules — the functional units that secrete milk. These lobes project out from the nipple and are connected to the nipple by ducts that transfer milk to the exterior during suckling. Furthermore, the presence of various supporting factors, including ligaments and suspended adipose tissue, also contributes to the shaping and positioning of the breasts. A thorough understanding of the anatomy allows nurses to properly identify normal variants and potential pathologies, hence facilitating early intervention on identifying abnormalities, making a skilled anatomical knowledge base in nursing essential. Vascular and lymphatic systems also play a vital role in breast anatomy and need to be evaluated during nursing examinations. The breast is primarily perfused by the internal mammary and lateral thoracic arteries, which reiterate the significance of the cardiac status to breast tissue viability. Moreover, lymphatic drainage of the breast typically proceeds to the axillary lymph nodes, which reiterate a pathway along which malignancies are permitted to disseminate. Nurses need to assess lymph node involvement, that is, for any tenderness or swelling, as such indicators can expose subpathologies such as infections or tumors. The precise knowledge regarding such anatomical and physiological relationships is crucial in ensuring nurses' capacity to conduct evaluations effectively, applying critical thinking during the interpretation of results and responding to patients' unique health needs (Garcia et al., 2018). In addition, comprehensive education in breast anatomy extends beyond physiological facts to include culturally sensitive care as an essential priority. Because nursing assessments involve intimate examination techniques, understanding the diverse cultural environments under which individuals engage with their breast health is pertinent. Texts that inform nursing practice, such as those centered on inclusive conceptual frameworks for assessing health, emphasize integrating cultural responsiveness when conducting breast examinations. As per pertinent educational material, such knowledge facilitates nurses' capacity to recognize not merely the physiological signs but also patients' subjective feelings related to their personal context (Accettola et al., 2023). The employment of the holistic method while assessing the anatomy of the breast is thus in line with optimal nursing practice, enhancing patients' experience and outcomes overall (Figure 15.3).

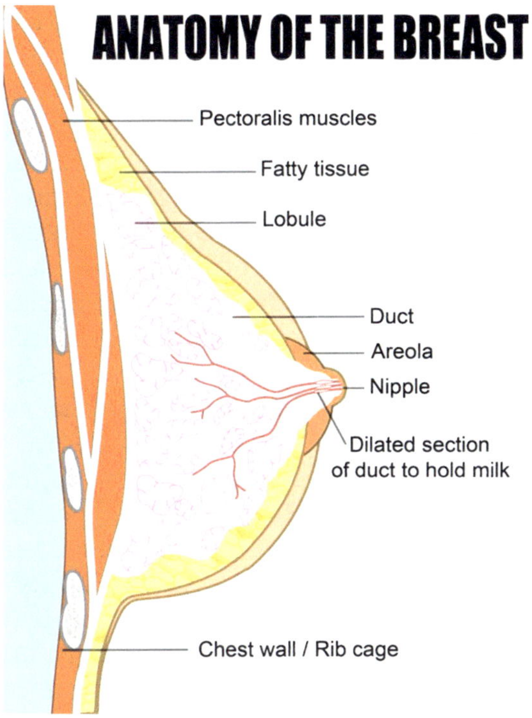

Figure 15.3. Anatomy of the breast.

Source: https://www.southernplasticsurgery.com/wp-content/uploads/2014/09/anatomy-of-female-breast-779x1024.jpg.

15.1.1. Structure and Function of Breast Tissue

The breast tissue architecture is specifically designed to serve its various functions, most of which are related to lactation. Comprising primarily glandular tissue with sparse adipose and connective tissues, the breast is composed of lobes and lobules that contain the acini where milk secretion occurs. The glandular component, consisting of approximately 15 to 20 lobes, is a network that converges into the nipple and allows milk to pass through easily during lactation. This anatomy's complexity is significant in nursing evaluations, as pathology anomalies in the anatomy of breasts or tissue distribution are indicative of diseases. A clear understanding of the breasts' anatomy is core to nursing professionals who are tasked with evaluating breast health and conducting practices. Not only is it useful in determining physiology changes, but it also makes it easier to educate patients regarding breast self-examinations and pathologic symptomatology. In structure, the breast tissue is largely integrated into the endocrine system, functioning in a manner that is based on hormonal control to help in lactation and be involved in reproductive health. Estrogen and progesterone, produced by the ovaries, are responsible for preparing the breast for milk production during pregnancy and lactation. In the postpartum situation, prolactin level rises to trigger milk synthesis and oxytocin is the one that causes the milk ejection reflex. This hormonal interaction is essential to successful lactation but may have implications for the health of the breast tissue as well. Changes in hormone levels may lead to such conditions as fibrocystic changes of the breast, creating difficulties with nursing diagnoses. It is important for nurses to be aware of these functional components so that they may assist and educate the patient about breast care, particularly as they undergo different phases of reproduction and encounter potential complications. Moreover, palpation of the breast and axillary tissue is a fundamental aspect in breast cancer detection and overall health maintenance. Regular follow-ups are required to identify any abnormality, such as lumps or change in breast tissue consistency, which is indicative of a host of conditions, including cancers. A good understanding of breast anatomy enables medical personnel to distinguish benign from malignant disease, hence influencing timely intervention. In survivorship, the understanding of the particular needs of breast cancer survivors like physical changes and risk of recurrence becomes of utmost relevance. Most healthcare providers lack adequate knowledge of the current survivorship guidelines, which can act as a disabler to offering optimal patient care (Scott et al., 2019). An informed nursing practice that is comprised of ongoing monitoring not only encourages early detection but also ensures patients receive well-rounded care according to their individualized needs throughout their recovery process (Figure 15.4).

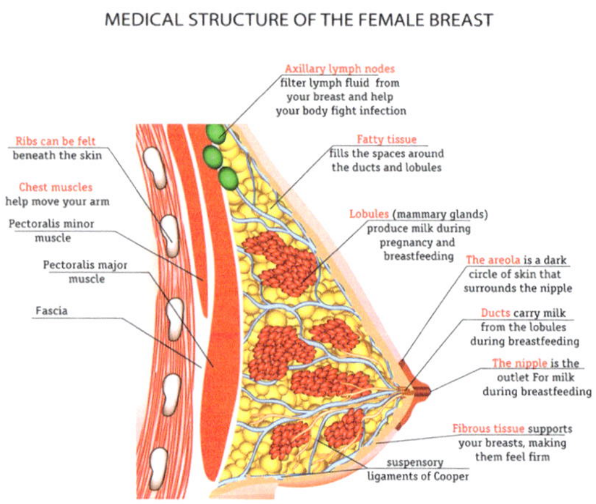

Figure 15.4. Structure and function of breast tissue.

Source: https://www.jackiebellnaturalhealth.com/uploads/3/8/3/1/38313077/5403342_orig.jpg.

15.1.2. Lymphatic Drainage and Its Significance

The lymphatic system plays a role in fluid balance maintenance and supporting the immune response, which has particular significance to breast and axillary assessment in nursing. Patients who have received breast cancer surgery, i.e., mastectomy or lymphadenectomy, are at risk of complications related to lymphatic drainage, the most noted being lymphedema, which is characterized by chronic limb upper swelling. This condition not only affects physical health but also diminishes quality of life (QoL) for those involved. Nurses, in turn, must have great importance assigned to understanding lymph function and its impact while evaluating and providing care for postsurgical patients in order to recognize high-risk patients for lymphedema. Moreover, educating the patients on self-management strategies and potential symptoms of lymphedema can empower them to become active participants in the process of recovery, a concept in holistic care that promotes encouraging patients to take active participation in health management. Breast and axillary assessment nursing practice must also address the necessity of early intervention in the cases of lymphatic drainage complications. Literature indicates that the majority of health providers have the tendency to overlook breast cancer patients' systemic education regarding lymphedema, and it is of larger long-term impacts on patient health. Including focused education on lymphatic system health in nursing programs can potentially improve significantly the quality of care being provided to survivors of breast cancer. These educational advancements would enhance the ability of nurses to practice systematic care and better equip them to teach patients about risks of lymphedema. In the end, this proactive care provides a setting for patients to receive optimal pre- and post-surgical care, a deciding factor in their overall medical results. In addition to clinical assessment and education courses, a complete system for monitoring lymphatic drainage post-op is essential for maximum nursing practice. Continuous assessment of fluid balance and potential swelling is crucial in the early detection of lymphedema, which manifests over time following surgery. This necessitates the integration of individualized care plans that take into account patient-related risks as well as associated medical histories. The significance of lymphatic drainage not only includes initial post-operative needs but also extended follow-up procedures that consider the chronic nature of lymphedema. By treating these practices initially, nurses can improve health-related quality of life (HRQoL) among patients receiving breast cancer care, so they gain from the multidisciplinary care needed to survive the ordeal of their present healthcare path (Haapiainen, 2015; Joanne et al., 2015).

15.1.3. Variations in Breast Anatomy

The anatomically variant human breast is regulated by several factors such as genetics, age, and hormone status. Differences may also occur in different dimensions such as size, shape, and tissue composition. Breast morphology can differ from round to conical or asymmetrical forms, for instance, and these are significant in both aesthetic issues as well as clinical assessment. It is crucial for nursing practitioners who are performing axillary and breast examination to realize these anatomical differences, as they can affect palpation technique, mass identification, and overall assessment of breast health. Unusual anatomical presentations can also complicate imaging studies and lead to potential diagnostic challenges that emphasize the importance of individualized assessment techniques that accommodate differences in breast anatomy. In addition to the environmental variations in breast size and texture, internal anatomic variations also possess the ability to have profound effects on the assessment of the patient. Glandular to fat tissue ratio, which is influenced by the hormone levels, influences mammographic density and associated breast cancer susceptibility. Increased glandular tissue causes imaging difficulty since it has higher density, obscuring lesions. Nursing professionals must be prepared to interpret differences such as these, understanding that increased tissue density will require additional imaging modalities to be applied appropriately for diagnosis. With ongoing education in breast health, nurses must become familiar with variations in breast anatomy and their potential meaning for the detection and treatment of disease and thereby improving outcomes in breast care.

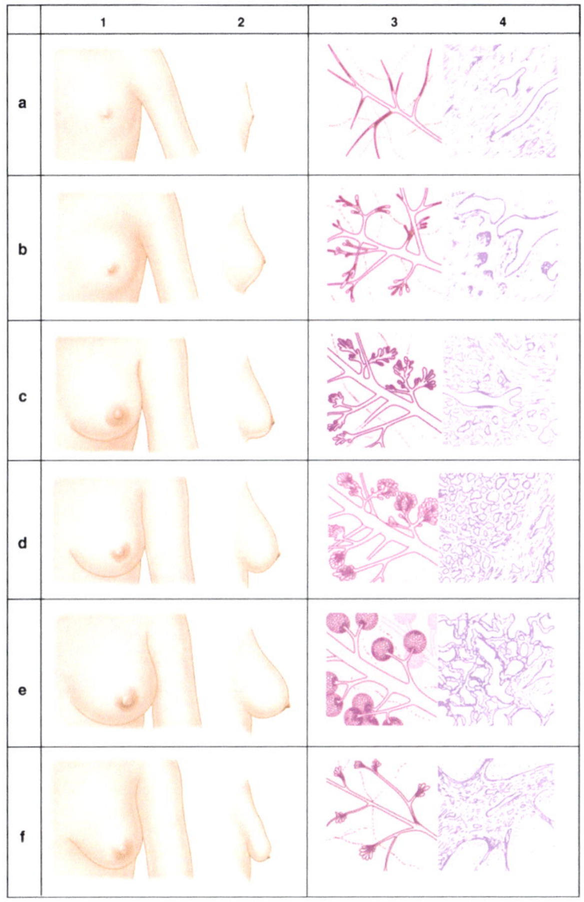

Figure 15.5. Variations in breast anatomy.

Source: https://media.springernature.com/lw685/springer-static/image/chp%3A10.1007%2F978-3-030-45951-2_2/MediaObjects/71577_2_En_2_Fig14_HTML.png.

Furthermore, the identification of anatomical differences extends beyond the breast to the axillary area, where lymphatic drainage patterns can greatly differ. Axillary lymph nodes play a significant role in staging and treatment planning in breast cancer. Compromised drainage or altered lymphatic anatomy as a consequence of surgical intervention, such as lumpectomy or mastectomy, can lead to complications like lymphedema. Understanding these variations is critical to effective nursing assessments as they inform preoperative imaging assessments and postoperative care. With the inclusion in their practice of an understanding of both breast and axillary anatomical variation, nurses can enhance their diagnostic skills and communicate with patients more effectively about their individual anatomical health variations, thus resulting in high quality of care in breast and axillary assessment (Figure 15.5).

Test Your Knowledge

1. What are the primary components of the breast tissue, and how are they arranged?
2. How do the lobes, lobules, and ducts function together in lactation?

15.2. Importance of Axillary Assessment

Learning Outcome

1. Role of Axillary Lymph Nodes in Disease Detection
2. Common Conditions Affecting the Axillae
3. Implications of Axillary Assessment in Patient Care

The significance of axillary examination to nursing surpasses mere physical examination; it is an indispensable diagnostic and therapeutic tool in the care of breast health. The axilla contains lymph nodes that can serve as indicators of systemic disease, particularly when there is breast cancer. Proper examination of such nodes may help stage the cancer, influence treatment, and impact patient results. As breast cancer remains the most common cancer in women, with increasing rates being reported particularly in the elderly, early detection through axillary examination is important to improve cure rates. Through an orderly strategy of palpation and imaging, clinicians can pick up abnormalities that may predispose metastatic spread and thus allow for appropriate early interventions in treatment. Axillary examination is also important to determine patient-specific issues influencing treatment pathways. As breast cancer cases become more complex with advancing age, individualized treatment strategies are imperative. Comprehensive evaluation may guide advice on the need and degree of surgical procedures as well as the indication of adjuvant treatments. As an example, radiological assessments may need to be individualized in order to establish evidence of axillary disease before surgery can be planned. The nursing professionals have an important role to play in this context, especially ensuring that holistic care is provided to the patients addressing both physical and psychosocial needs. The importance of these assessments is underlined by a growing literature on the advantages of collaborative strategies to the care of older patients (Drabi et al., 2021) and the imperatives for evidence-based guidelines. Also, evolving knowledge of volatile organic compounds (VOCs) in relation to breast tissue is an appealing field of axillary examination research.

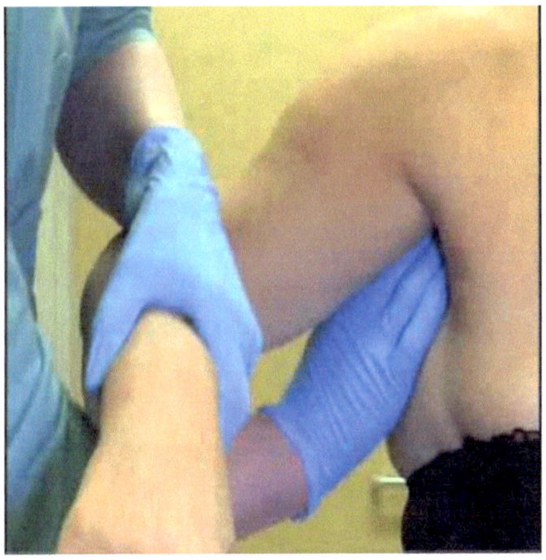

Figure 15.6. Axillary assessment.

Source: https://i.ytimg.com/vi/zfKVu1PlTEQ/hqdefault.jpg?sqp=-oaymwEmCOADEOgC8quKqQMa8AEB-AHeA4AC6AKKAgwIABABGDkgWyhyMA8=&rs=AOn4CLB8b8OlIl9uYmCLUIlLh9u8siqLsA.

New studies have identified a vast range of VOCs from human tissues, which hold diagnostic value for the identification of underlying illness, e.g., cancer (Drabi et al., 2021). With continued practice in nursing using these advances, the integration of information from new sciences like metabolomics into axillary examination can enhance earlier detection and diagnosis. The possibility for VOC analysis as a non-invasive diagnostic tool provides new avenues for enhancing care standards in breast health. By remaining vigilant in assessing both the anatomical and biochemical markers, nursing clinicians are empowered to contribute significantly toward enhancing treatment outcomes as well as quality of life for breast cancer patients (Figure 15.6).

15.2.1. Role of Axillary Lymph Nodes in Disease Detection

The role of the axillary lymph nodes in disease detection is at the forefront in diagnosis and treatment planning, notably in breast cancer. Axillary lymph nodes are vital components of the lymphatic system, serving as a filter for lymph fluid and helping to capture cancer cells that may be spreading away from the primary tumor site. In cases of suspected breast cancer, sentinel lymph node biopsy (SLNB) is often employed to find out the status of these lymph nodes. A positive result can indicate metastasis, followed by further interventions, like surgical removal of the affected lymph nodes or systemic treatment. In doing so, understanding axillary lymph node anatomy and physiology enhances nursing care management and patient care interventions, whereby early intervention is employed to achieve an enhanced prognosis, with emphasis placed on the significance of ongoing education on axillary examination for nurses (Keohane et al., 2020). Furthermore, the prevalence of axillary lymph node involvement is crucial in breast cancer staging, as well as in determining the individual therapeutic strategy. Staging in turn has direct influence on the treatment plans, such as the need for chemotherapy or radiotherapy, and hence it is important that the nursing practitioners are adept at recognizing the signs of axillary examination. Recent studies have shown inconsistent rates of axillary node involvement across different patient populations and tumor sites, indicating the need for advanced approaches in nursing assessments. Additionally, integration with newer imaging technologies, such as high-frequency ultrasound or MRI, can aid in the evaluation of node involvement, offering better clarity for healthcare providers and patient-specific care planning (Torgbenu et al., 2020). By understanding these dynamics, nurses can battle on behalf of proper screenings and create effective working relationships within multidisciplinary teams to advance the best possible patient outcomes. Management of patients with axillary lymph node disease involves more than initial diagnosis and continues through extended surveillance and treatment. Following surgical operations, nursing's role includes instructing patients about potential complications, including lymphedema, which can significantly reduce quality of life when monitored. Research has indicated that the impact of lymphedema can be minimized with early detection and intervention, and therefore it is important for nurses to develop patient education plans on self-examination and symptom management. Furthermore, frequent follow-up management offers a chance to observe changes in lymphatic function, hence shaping long-term health outcomes. With the advancement in understanding the role of axillary lymph nodes in breast cancer staging, nursing practices must also advance through an integrative model that encompasses not only treatment but also patient education and support systems (Keohane et al., 2020) (Figure 15.7).

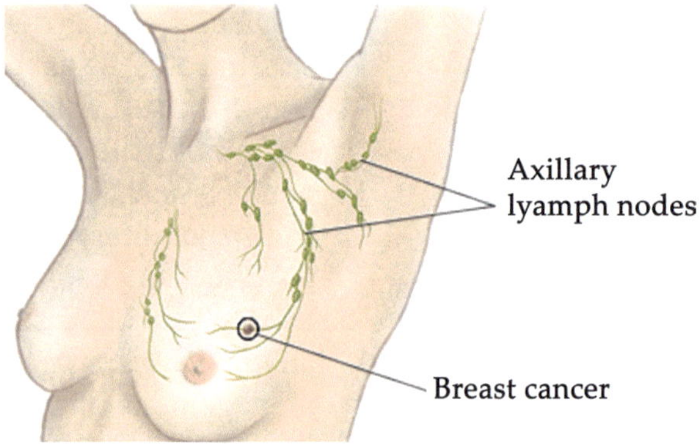

Figure 15.7. Role of axillary lymph nodes in disease detection.

Source: https://www.drnicoleyap.com.au/wp-content/uploads/2021/06/AXILLARY-LYMPH-NODE-ASSESSMENT-1.png.

15.2.2. Common Conditions Affecting the Axillae

The axillae, which are often overlooked in clinical assessment, are prone to various dermatologic conditions that must be appropriately assessed, particularly in nursing. Intertrigo, as manifested by inflammation because of friction and retained moisture in the skin folds, is one of the common conditions present in this area. As pointed out by research, intertrigo in the inguinal area and sub mammary folds is a significant region where it occurs, showing a clear link with secondary factors like diabetes mellitus and urinary incontinence, which can make skin irritation worse (Everink et al., 2021). An awareness of these dynamics is crucial to nursing practitioners, who must not only assess the physical presentations of such conditions, but also uncover latent risk factors and broader implications for patient care. A further condition that is often encountered in the axillae is hyperhidrosis, with potential consequences of skin irritation and secondary infection due to excessive sweating. This condition is not only physically distressing but also carries psychological implications, changing a patient's way of life. Hyperhidrosis is generally managed by modifying one's lifestyle, such as wearing loose clothing and applying topical antiperspirants. More vigorous methods like botulinum toxin injections may be required in severe cases. The nurse's role here is more than the assessment of symptoms; it is educating patients on effective management strategies, hence an equal engagement in care through both physical intervention and emotional support. Folliculitis is also a common axillary condition that is inflammation of the hair follicles. It typically develops due to friction, occlusion, or infections, causing pain and potential complications. Particularly, the axilla's warm, humid environment creates an ideal breeding ground for bacterial and fungal infections, which must be carefully evaluated and managed. In recurrent or severe folliculitis, differential diagnoses can sometimes have to be examined by nurses, such as hidradenitis suppurativa, a chronic skin condition that could indicate an underlying systemic issue. Hence, comprehensive nursing assessments of the axillae must address both overall conditions and how those conditions may be complicated, so that care plans are tailored specifically to the needs of each patient while addressing overall dermatological health (Figure 15.8).

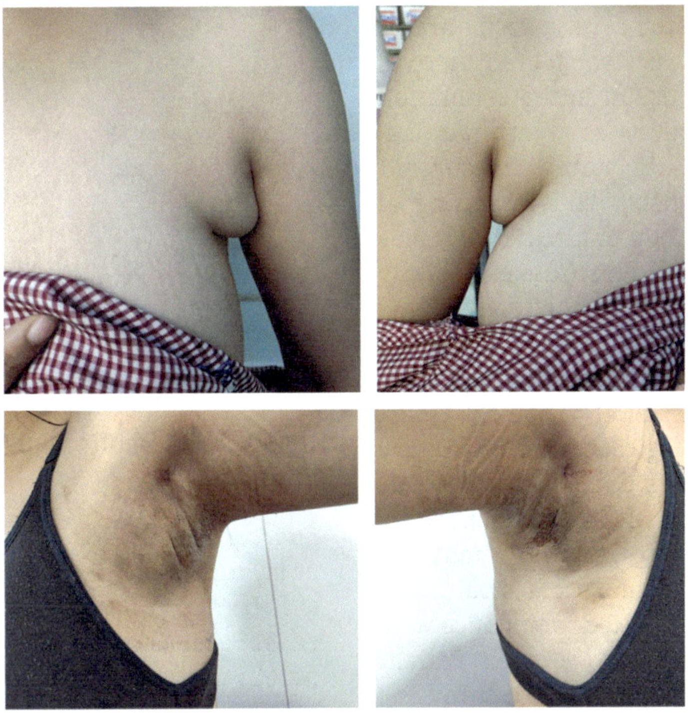

Figure 15.8. Common conditions affecting the axillae.

Source: https://www.drbhupendraplasticsurgeon.com/wp-content/uploads/2023/02/1.jpeg.

15.2.3. Implications of Axillary Assessment in Patient Care

Axillary examination is crucial in the care of the patient, particularly given its relevance in breast and axillary disease diagnosis and management. The axilla is an important anatomical region with lymph nodes clustered in it, and therefore it is crucial that clinicians examine this area for any abnormalities. Axillary abnormalities are a sign that there exists metastasis of breast cancer or any other systemic diseases. Moreover, correct axillary assessment can help define the extent of the disease, which is an important factor for identifying treatment and prognostic factors. Incomplete axillary assessment may result in inappropriate treatment planning, consequently having a bearing on the outcome of patients. Therefore, the inclusion of detailed axillary assessments in the context of daily clinical routines can lead to the early detection and more effective intervention measures, thus enhancing the quality of patient care. The implications of axillary assessment extend beyond simple identification of disease occurrence; they also encompass an influence on surgical management and postoperative care. For instance, data obtained from an axillary exam can inform surgery, such as the requirement for sentinel lymph node biopsies or axillary dissections. Surgical interventions based on axillary assessment have been proven to have a significant impact on the recurrence of breast carcinoma and patient survival. Moreover, total axillary assessment is useful in the estimation of complications, such as lymphedema, arising post-surgery. As noted in current nursing practice, extensive understanding of both axillary and breast examination enables healthcare practitioners to institute exclusively tailored actions that are proportional to the unique needs of patients and regional health guidelines, thus ensuring optimum aggregate clinical outcomes (Michael et al., 2023). Apart from the clinical and surgical concerns, axillary examination also enables patient education as well as patient involvement in treatment to be maximized. By informing patients about the importance of axillary examinations, healthcare providers can guarantee better compliance with follow-up tests and treatment protocols. Patient participation is critical, especially in confronting the complex emotional and psychological climate that accompanies a diagnosis of breast cancer. In addition, an understanding of the function of axillary health can empower patients to assume active responsibility for their own care, including the incorporation of lifestyle changes and regular schedule of screenings. Here, addition of axillary evaluation serves not just as a clinical method but also as an instrument to improve the quality of the care being given as a whole, which fits into broader objectives of patient-focused care and improved health literacy (Chopra et al., 2023) (Figure 15.9).

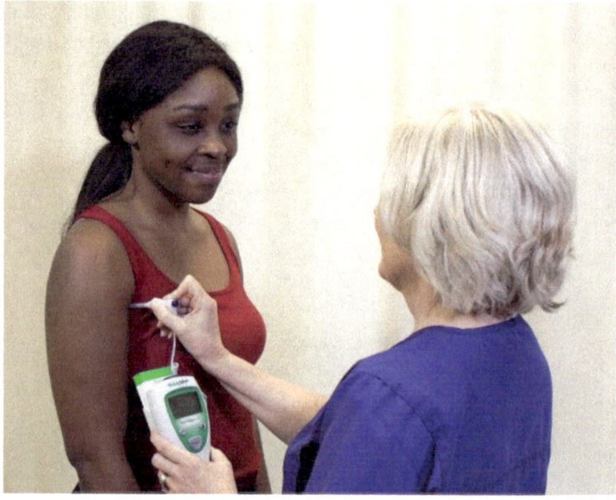

Figure 15.9. Implications of axillary assessment in patient care.

Source: https://external-content.duckduckgo.com/iu/?u=https%3A%2F%2Fpressbooks.library.torontomu.ca%2Fassessmentnursingmain%2Fwp-content%2Fuploads%2Fsites%2F421%2F2017%2F12%2FAxilla-Temperature-1-1024x795-1-768x596.jpg&f=1&nofb=1&ipt=21dbfdb31ddd12c0a7734db155b05762cfe42944b0c69ee2ed6d28239b80f08b.

Test Your Knowledge

1. Why is the axillary assessment crucial in detecting early signs of breast pathology?
2. How can changes in axillary lymph nodes indicate systemic or localized diseases?

15.3. Techniques for Breast Assessment

Learning Outcome

1. Visual Inspection Methods
2. Palpation Techniques for Breast Examination
3. Use of Imaging Technologies in Assessment

Assessment of axillary and breast health is an integral part of nursing practice, and this is why systematic approaches are required to ensure complete assessments. The primary methods are visual inspection, palpation, and interview of the patient's history. With complete visual examination, nurses can identify abnormality such as asymmetry, skin change, or masses that are indicative of underlying disease. Palpation is focused on the systematic examination of breast tissue and axillary lymph nodes to identify any potential lump or swelling. Having good knowledge of the anatomical layout is crucial for the nurse to position his hands accurately during the assessment so he doesn't miss key information that might constitute a diagnosis or carry out further investigative procedures. The integration of patient history during breast examination allows nurses to gather key contextual data on the patients history of illnesses, family risk, and previous breast problems or surgeries. This holistic approach enhances the effectiveness of the physical examination since it equips nurses with knowledge of risk factors related to breast disease. Other aspects such as age, menstrual history, and lifestyle can also play an essential role in determining breast health. A thorough appreciation of these determinants makes it possible to individualize patient education, facilitating active involvement in their own care and resulting in earlier intervention and detection of abnormalities. Methods of integration of this information can dramatically enhance personalized assessment methods, making it more patient-centered. New methods in breast assessment, including the application of sophisticated imaging technologies and biomarkers, complement the age-old techniques of physical examination. Imaging modalities like digital mammography and ultrasonography produce more precise images that are capable of detecting malignancies which do not manifest as palpable. Furthermore, the exploration of volatile organic compounds (VOCs) as biomarkers of breast health is in harmony with the advanced metabolic standards, and research in the future may reclassify assessment protocols. As reviewed in recent literature, such advancements support the need for continued education and practice updating of nursing to encompass enhancing techniques in breast examination, ultimately towards improved patient outcomes (Drabi et al., 2021; Chandler et al., 2018).

15.3.1. Visual Inspection Methods

Visual inspection procedures play a critical role in breast and axillae evaluation, alerting healthcare professionals to significant information about a patient's status. Visual inspection procedures involve methodical visual inspection for the detection of any abnormal signs or changes, such as lumps, skin changes, or asymmetry, which could indicate suspected malignancies, namely breast cancer. The World Health Organization (WHO) highlights the use of frequency of Breast Self-Examination (BSE) as a women's preventive behavior starting at 20 years old, both visual and palpable examination of breast and axillary regions for searching for persistent changes (Alfonsi et al., 2024). Early detection with these visual inspection methods enhances survival and overall prognosis among women with breast cancer, which highlights the need to empower nursing professionals with effective knowledge and skills in these inspections. Incorporating visual inspection methods into nursing education comprehensively can significantly enhance the skill level of nursing students and practitioners in performing breast exams. The latest studies indicate a high percentage of women who are unaware of the BSE recommended practice due to a lack of education that may be solved by nurses. For instance, a study revealed that 95% of female students had inadequate knowledge regarding BSE prior to having a structured educational program, but following the intervention, the majority had sufficient knowledge (Ambika et al., 2014).

This tremendous increase in awareness subsequent to concentrated training highlights the significance of adding visual inspection training to nursing education programs. By equipping future nurses with the skill to conduct effective visual inspections, it becomes possible to enable early detection, facilitate patient education, and eventually enable improved health outcomes in women. Despite the seeming advantages of visual examination techniques, issues persist, particularly in terms of use and frequency of BSE procedures among women.

Differences in levels of knowledge of BSE techniques, as evidenced by research that reported a high percentage of study participants had no knowledge of recommended positions for examination and timing (Alfonsi et al., 2024), illustrate the need for a systematic strategy in nursing education to promote awareness and develop hands-on skills. It fills these gaps both by educating nursing students and through ongoing community outreach to raise the level of awareness about self-examination among women. The efficacy of such educational intervention can also be explored with hands-on workshop or simulation training, to illustrate the correct visual examination techniques and promote regular self-examination among patients as a part of a complete breast health regimen (Figure 15.10).

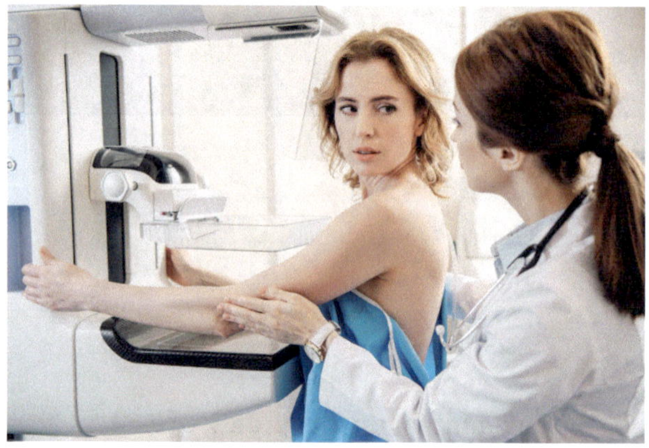

Figure 15.10. Visual inspection methods for breast assessment.

Source: https://external-content.duckduckgo.com/iu/?u=https%3A%2F%2Fwww.statpearls.com%2FCmeImg%2FRetrieveImage%2F18583&f=1&nofb=1&ipt=62b474513a21b81507e25fd09d47335e54752cf17d4c0047225ac72377bf2c40.

15.3.2. Palpation Techniques for Breast Examination

Palpation techniques applied during breast examinations are key to breast and axillae assessment, enabling nurses to identify abnormalities such as masses or areas of pain. The structured procedure is instrumental in helping no area be left out during the examination process. Practitioners mostly employ various palpation techniques, such as the vertical strip, wedge, and circular methods. Both methods allow for effective coverage of the breast tissue, which makes detection of any suspicious mass more likely. For instance, the vertical strip technique's up-and-down motion is most effective at covering the surface of the entire breast. This method is particularly useful in the early breast cancer detection because meticulous palpation can identify conditions like fibrocystic changes or neoplasms that would otherwise go undetected. Furthermore, the role of proper palpation is also extended to the axilla where lymph node examination is relevant. Palpation of the axillae is a key part of breast examinations in an attempt to identify lymphadenopathy, which may represent metastasis or regional spread of breast carcinoma. Size, consistency, tenderness, and mobility should be checked for the lymph nodes because these characteristics are of paramount importance in determining the potential malignancy. Utilization of a standardized technique for both axillary and breast palpation allows for the clinician to provide a more accurate assessment. Such dual focus not only makes the test more effective but also allows clinicians to engage in informed dialogue with patients, leading to mutual decision-making regarding further testing or treatment (Sprakel, 2020).

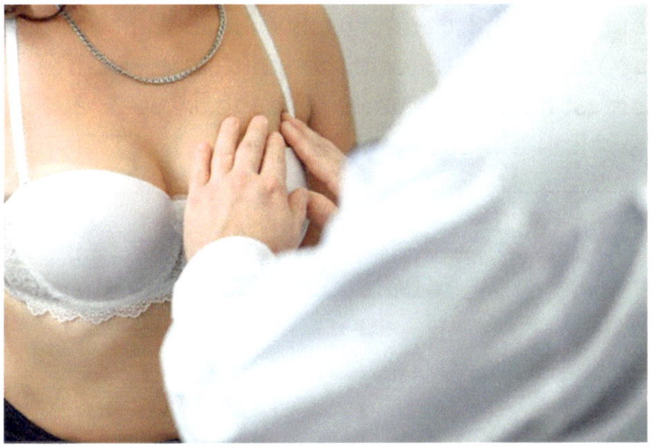

Figure 15.11. Palpation techniques for breast examination.

Source: https://external-content.duckduckgo.com/iu/?u=https%3A%2F%2Fst3.depositphotos.com%2F1546698%2F36245%2Fi%2F450%2Fdepositphotos_362453584-stock-photo-consultation-examination-mammary-gland-mammologist.jpg&f=1&nofb=1&ipt=40fb90535fa5085c239485564752f1b8314cd69bc601d71ae4a50e9824f84f76.

Awareness of psychological factors that accompany breast examination is equally important. Patients may be fearful of the test process and its implications, which may deter a complete evaluation if not properly addressed. Nurses need to employ a gentle touch in palpation, explaining each step of the examination slowly and reassuring the patient. Taking care of the emotional impact of the examination has played an essential role in trust development and positive patient experience. In a vital step, a phenomenon such as breast edema that may develop after cancer treatment also requires not just technical skill but also emotional sensitivity. Sensitively assessing breast edema calls for skilled palpation and highlights the importance of effective communication and empathy as part of practice nursing (Todd, 2017). Identification and the integration of these factors can lead to more holistic care and better patient outcomes (Figure 15.11).

15.3.3. Use of Imaging Technologies in Assessment

Imaging technology applied in the assessment of breast and axillae represents a significant advancement in nursing practice, supporting diagnosis and patient results. Mammography continues to be the gold standard for the identification of breast cancer, and it allows early detection of malignant lesions even before they are palpable. This technique employs low-dose X-rays to visualize internal breast anatomy, providing valuable information regarding breast tissue density and the detection of abnormalities, such as calcifications or masses. Additionally, the introduction of digital mammography has improved image quality and allowed complex imaging analysis, thereby facilitating health workers to assess high-risk populations more effectively. As technology advances in the area of nursing, it also becomes more necessary for clinicians to remain competent in interpreting the results of mammography because it has direct implications on clinical practice and patient education regarding breast health. Use of ultrasound as an adjunct imaging method over the past few years has made breast and axillae exams even more sophisticated. It is particularly useful in distinguishing between solid and cystic masses identified through mammography, thereby providing more reliable diagnoses. Breast ultrasound uses sound waves to form images and offers real-time visualization that is useful in the management of biopsies as well as the evaluation of axillary nodes. Also, since it is non-invasive and no ionizing radiation is used, it is an appealing option for particular patient groups, such as pregnant women or for patients with extremely dense breast tissue in which mammography may be less useful. Training of nursing professionals in the skills of breast ultrasound enhances competency and autonomy, enabling them to efficiently contribute to screening programs and follow-up management plans.

Magnetic Resonance Imaging (MRI) has been an effective modality for complete evaluation of breast and axillae, particularly in high-risk patients or in the case of inconclusive mammographic findings. Breast MRI provides high-resolution images and can detect tumors invisible to other imaging modalities. Such an approach is especially worthwhile in evaluating the degree of registered cancers and identifying potential multifocal disease, which is critical in planning treatment. MRI is also priceless in evaluating patient response to neoadjuvantly administered treatments, thereby allowing for timely adjustment of the treatment regimens. The growing reliance on such imaging technologies goes to further highlight the need for nurses to become familiar with such modalities. This information not only enables nurses to play an active role in early detection and intervention but also inspires interprofessional collaborative approaches with teams committed to enhancing breast health outcomes (Choudhary et al., 2019; Kwok et al., 2015).

Test Your Knowledge

1. What are the key steps involved in a clinical breast examination?
2. How does the positioning of the patient affect the accuracy of breast palpation?.

15.4. Techniques for Axillary Assessment

Learning Outcome

1. Inspection of the Axillary Region
2. Palpation of Axillary Lymph Nodes
3. Identifying Abnormalities in the Axillae

The axillary examination is an important aspect of nursing practice, particularly in breast care. Nurses use a variety of methods to evaluate the axilla for abnormal findings such as lymphadenopathy, which may reflect underlying pathologies such as breast cancer. Cautious examination begins with visual inspection whereby the clinician examines for asymmetry, alteration in skin, or masses. This is followed by palpation to assess lymph nodes size, consistency, mobility, and tenderness. Knowing the anatomical positions and characteristics of the axillary lymph nodes is necessary in order to decide on normal or abnormal findings. Axilla assessment is not only a physical examination clinical skill but also a powerful instrument for patient education, enabling patients to become sensitized to the importance of self-examination in disease detection at an early stage, particularly in breast cancer scenarios, underpinning the necessity of routine assessment in nursing practice. Acquisition of axillary assessment skills requires strong knowledge of anatomical landmarks and potential pathological presentation. The axilla contains several lymph nodes, divided into several levels, all providing critical information regarding systemic states. One example is the central lymph nodes, which are significant because they preferentially take drainage from numerous points, including the breast. Understanding the differences in lymph drainage will assist nurses in understanding the consequences of the enlarged nodes. Additionally, the nurse should be familiar with common conditions that may disguise themselves as axillary pathologies, i.e., infection or cystic change. Developing an informed viewpoint on these approaches improves the nurse's potential to make well-rounded evaluations and emphasizes the necessity of ongoing training and education in clinical practice, because accurate evaluation has a close link to patient outcomes and management strategies. In addition, the combination of imaging procedure development with technology has revolutionized axillary assessment in contemporary nursing practice. Diagnostic modalities such as ultrasound and magnetic resonance imaging (MRI) enable non-invasive assessment of axillary abnormalities to supplement conventional physical assessment methods. The imaging technologies provide enhanced visualization of the lymph nodes and surrounding tissue, and the nurses and healthcare providers are able to utilize the modalities to guide decisions for further diagnostic procedures or interventions. As more becomes known about breast cancer, so do the means for early detection become accessible, underscoring the necessity for nurses to stay up-to-date on best practices and continue to refine axillary assessment skills. The ever-evolving breast health landscape is grounds enough for increased clinical examination, for these are the platform upon which quality screening and attendant treatments are based, ultimately affecting patient care and healthcare outcomes.

15.4.1. Inspection of the Axillary Region

Axillary examination is a component of axillae and breast assessment in nursing. It is a largely underappreciated but clinically significant region, particularly as a site for detecting abnormalities which may indicate underlying disease such as breast cancer. The axilla contains a dense cluster of lymph nodes which serve as an integral component of the immune apparatus. Therefore, any mass, irregularities, or swelling noticed during the examination can point towards the existence of malignancies or infection. A systematic assessment process has to be employed, making use of visual examination and palpation to identify suspicious changes. In addition to physical change, there also has to be an assessment of the emotional and psychological impact of potential findings since patients can become anxious about risk for breast cancer and how it affects their overall health and well-being. With the inspection, the nurse begins with a good visual examination of the axillary region, checking the color, texture of the skin and taking a look for lesions or asymmetry. Observation skill of the nurses is essential since variation in the appearance of the skin might be indicative of as benign to as malign. Aside from that, there is a requirement to assess for any abnormality, such as lymphadenopathy, which is lymph node enlargement and might be indicative of disease processes. This is followed by an adequate patient history, which also encompasses knowledge about risk factors such as family history of breast cancer or prior breast-related issues. This interdisciplinary method optimizes diagnostic accuracy and promotes effective communication between patient and health professional, thereby facilitating an interactive environment for care decision and intervention planning. In conjunction with visual and physical examination, other diagnostic evaluations could be required based on the findings upon examination of the axilla. If abnormalities are present, such as hard, fixed, or irregular palpable lymph nodes, the patient should be referred to further imaging studies or biopsies. Prompt intervention is the key to breast cancer treatment outcomes; the state of the axillary areas normally serves as a general indicator. Further, advances in breast cancer screening and awareness, reflected in literature, highlight the importance of regular assessment in increasing early detection rates and improving outcomes among women globally. Through gaining a profound understanding of the axillary regions inspection, nurses can positively drive patient education and advocacy toward enhancing the continuum of breast health care, as emphasized through the emerging guidelines for evidence-based practice (Akram et al., 2017; Sprakel, 2020) (Figure 15.12).

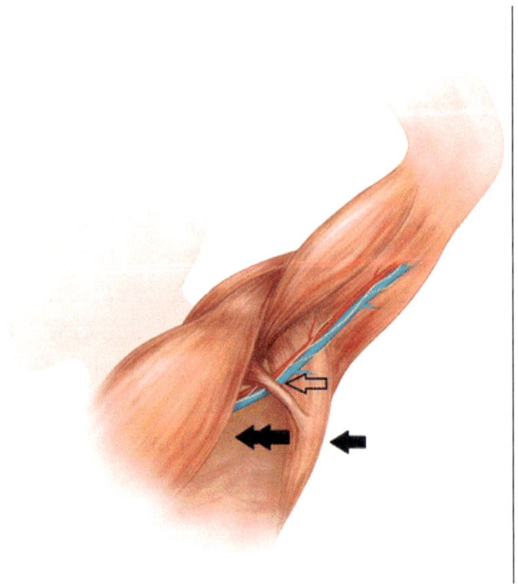

Figure 15.12. Inspection of the axillary region.

Source: https://www.researchgate.net/publication/320334218/figure/fig4/AS:941388770320409@1601455981344/An-artist-rendition-of-Langers-axillary-arch-Open-arrow-points-toward-the-arch-Solid.gif.

15.4.2. Palpation of Axillary Lymph Nodes

In breast and axilla assessment, palpation of the axillary lymph nodes is a significant maneuver that aids clinicians in diagnosing future malignancies and assessing the patient's overall condition. An understanding of the anatomy and physiology of the axilla is essential for effective examination. The axilla has a group of lymph nodes categorized into levels and each level serves a different purpose in lymphatic drainage. On palpation, the clinician closely inspects these nodes, with attention being paid to parameters such as size, mobility, and tenderness. Changes in these parameters could signify underlying pathological processes of infections or malignancy. It is on this basis that proper assessment of axillary lymph nodes is crucial in the early diagnosis and consequent management of breast disorders, stressing the need for competence-based practical training in nursing education in such critical examination procedures. Additionally, palpation is not just a technique issue but also one of patient comfort and cultural sensitivity. Effective communication with the patient during this type of examination can enhance patient compliance and reduce anxiety. On a clinical level, nurses are required to explain the procedure to patients and respond to issues of discomfort or exposure of the area of interest. This discussion is towards cultivating a therapeutic nurse-patient relationship that is core in creating a supportive clinical environment. Sensitivity towards anatomical differences in varied populations also becomes a must for effective assessment. Enforcement of guidelines based on well-studied literature, as suggested in literature provided, will go a long way in ensuring validity in findings with palpation and augmenting best practices in breast and axillae examination, ultimately leading to better patient outcomes (Sprakel, 2020). Finally, the results of palpation of axillary lymph nodes should be carefully documented and communicated among the health team. This information not only informs future clinical care but also impacts care plans for patients. Communication with oncologists and radiologists may be required in cases where abnormal results are obtained, hence the need for interdisciplinary care in managing issues of breast health. With the complexity of breast cancer management, ongoing education on up-to-date evidence-based practice guidelines, such as the ones disseminated through contemporary literature, remains a necessity for nursing professionals. A well-defined process for evaluating axillary lymph nodes, as disseminated through concerted multidisciplinary consensus, provides a common guideline for proper evaluation and collaborative decision-making that ultimately enhances the continuity of patient care across disparate healthcare environments (N/A, 2020) (Figure 15.13).

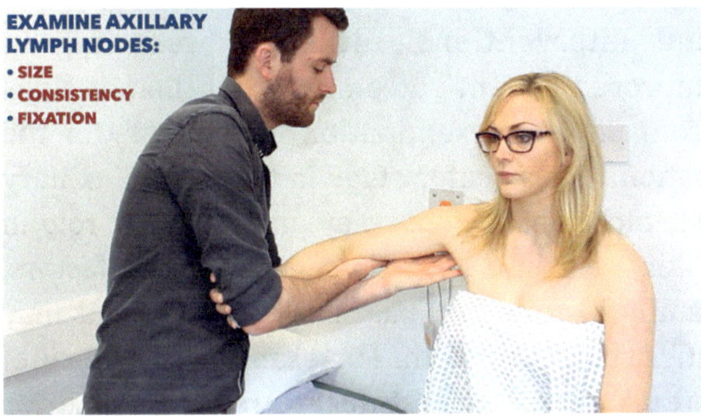

Figure 15.13. Palpation of axillary lymph nodes.

Source: https://geekymedics.com/wp-content/uploads/2013/04/Examine-axillary-nodes.jpg.

15.4.3. Identifying Abnormalities in the Axillae

Finding abnormalities in the axillae forms part of breast and axillae examination in nursing. Axillary region, with its rich lymph tissue, is a very critical area in the evaluation for potential malignancies and systemic disease. Abnormalities may be the presence of enlarged lymph nodes, which may represent infection, inflammation, or neoplastic disease. Besides, abnormalities can be in the form of alteration in the skin such as rashes or the development of abnormal masses, which need comprehensive evaluation. Using systematic palpation techniques, health workers can detect alteration that can be presumptive of underlying disease states. Early detection cannot be overemphasized, particularly with breast cancer, where metastatic spread to the axillary lymph nodes usually features an advanced disease process. Thus, careful and precise observation of the axillae is needed for optimal nursing practice and patient care. Also, anatomical landmark and variation knowledge in the axillary region is significant during observation for abnormalities. The axilla has structures such as the brachial plexus and large vessels, along with numerous lymph nodes. Anatomical configuration knowledge assists nurses in identifying normal versus abnormal results. For instance, the palpable lymph nodes in groups tend to be of a size, consistence, and tenderness that may provide a clinical impression of a patient's health status. The differentiation between malignant lymphadenopathy and reactive hyperplasia relies on careful assessment techniques and palpation ability. Additionally, any conspicuous change in skin contour or texture or underlying tissue, such as retraction or edematous skin, must be further investigated because it may be the sign of more serious pathologies, such as malignancy or infection. Educational procedures in self-examination and clinical examination cannot be eliminated in nursing. Increasing awareness and knowledge of patients towards self-examination of the axillary region can prove helpful for the early detection of potential abnormality. Additionally, nursing professionals need to emphasize the importance of early clinical evaluation, especially among high-risk groups. The increasing incidence of breast cancer necessitates an aggressive approach to community health education, which will eventually lead to successful intervention and improved outcomes. Breast and axillary assessment competency among nursing professionals is vital to improve general patient care. As breast cancer remains a significant public health problem all over the world, involving thorough axillary evaluations in routine examinations is essential for raising awareness and enforcing early detection strategies, especially with the life-threatening hazard posed by untreated conditions as identified by research (Akram et al., 2017).

Test Your Knowledge

1. What is the proper method to palpate axillary lymph nodes during an assessment?
2. How should a nurse differentiate between normal and abnormal axillary findings?.

15.5. Common Findings in Breast and Axillary Assessments

Learning Outcome

1. Normal Findings and Variations
2. Abnormal Findings and Their Implications
3. Documentation of Assessment Results

Breast and axillae examination forms a significant aspect of the nursing profession, facilitating identification of abnormalities and early treatment. Breast tissue tenderness, palpable mass, or cutaneous changes are some of the prevalent findings on such examinations. Visual inspection and palpation are usual methods of systematic examinations utilized by healthcare providers for the identification of these signs. Notably, lymphadenopathy in the axilla may be a sign of underlying disease, including breast cancer, and should undergo additional clinical evaluation. Research reveals that a significant percentage of breast cancer survivors have complications such as lymphedema, highlighting the importance of thorough axillary examination in practice and patient education (Wilson et al., 2012). By recognizing these red flags early on, nurses are able to make effective referrals and interventions, ultimately resulting in improved patient outcomes. Other than findings from physical examination, the history of the patient takes center stage in breast and axillary examinations. Nurses play an important role in taking pertinent details regarding risk factors, family history, and past breast issues that may affect current health. For example, a history of breast cancer in first-degree relatives or prior breast surgery could elevate the chances of developing new conditions in a patient. Having such data included in the assessment facilitates more individualized and comprehensive practice, which renders the care being provided more efficient. Besides, education on self-examination techniques and regular screening is a critical component of prevention. Awareness of normal vs. abnormal results empowers patients and supports individual responsibility toward health. The impact of these assessments doesn't end at immediate outcomes; they lay the foundation for ongoing conversation about health control and prevention measures (Anderson et al., 2016). The impact of patient education coupled with breast and axillary examination cannot be overstated. Nurses educate patients on breast health matters, stressing the value of early detection and patient advocacy for the use of routine examination. Findings such as differences in texture, shape, or the presence of an abnormal discharge should prompt discussions about the value of reporting such results to health care providers. Preventive education on lymphedema is also important, especially in high-risk breast cancer survivors. Evidence supports the utilization of educational programs to increase nursing personnel's knowledge about the risk factors and prevention of lymphedema, eventually leading to better patient outcomes (Wilson et al., 2012). In an interdisciplinary environment, nurses are capable of enhancing the quality of care and enabling patients to feel empowered to take care of their breast health by themselves, therefore highlighting the significance of assessment in nursing practice.

15.5.1. Normal Findings and Variations

Among breast and axillae examination, normal results and variations are significant for health care providers and nurses to appreciate. The breasts ought to normally display a range of anatomical features, like disparity in size, form, and texture, which may vary from individuals and through the phases of life. For instance, the majority of young women appreciate that their breasts exhibit an irregular appearance, and such is typically considered a normal finding. Differences may also encompass differences in skin color and texture based on hormonal changes, age, and previous pregnancies. Professional assessment should seek to advise patients on such normal variations to facilitate self-knowledge and early identification of abnormal changes such as lumps or abnormal discharge necessary for early intervention and treatment in the case of breast cancer, the most prevalent malignancy among women globally according to Alfonsi et al. (2024). In addition to anatomical variation, physiological aspects of breast health also require careful examination. Normal findings on breast examination are soft, mobile tissues with no masses appreciable by palpation and no tenderness other than in association with the menstrual cycle. Underlying such physical examination is the realization that varying density and tenderness of the breast tissue do indeed happen as a result of cyclic hormonal change. Nurses must be able to explain these fluctuating events as normal findings, which alert patients to their presence in normal breast physiology. Moreover, abnormalities in the axillary region, e.g., the number of lymph nodes, may also be assessed as normal if they are not tender and adherent. These observations again emphasize proper education in breast self-examination and recognizing what a normal breast feels like in multi-ethnic populations, closing knowledge gaps reported among healthcare providers, including midwives, as reported by Alfonsi et al. (2024). Through extensive education and assessment procedures, nurses are able to create a setting which normalizes variations so that patients are more interested in keeping track of their breast health. Regular self-examinations, if initiated at 20 years of age as recommended by the World Health Organization, are crucial for the establishment of familiarity with normal anatomical variations, which will make one more aware of reporting significant changes early. Unfortunately, the majority of women lack sufficient knowledge regarding when and how they should perform the breast self-examination, leading to the lacunae in early detection. As suggested by nursing education needs to encompass thorough training on breast assessment skills to bridge this knowledge gap. This integration promotes the adoption of best practices in the management of breast health, ultimately resulting in improved patient outcomes through early detection and education on normal findings and breast anatomical variation (Figure 15.14).

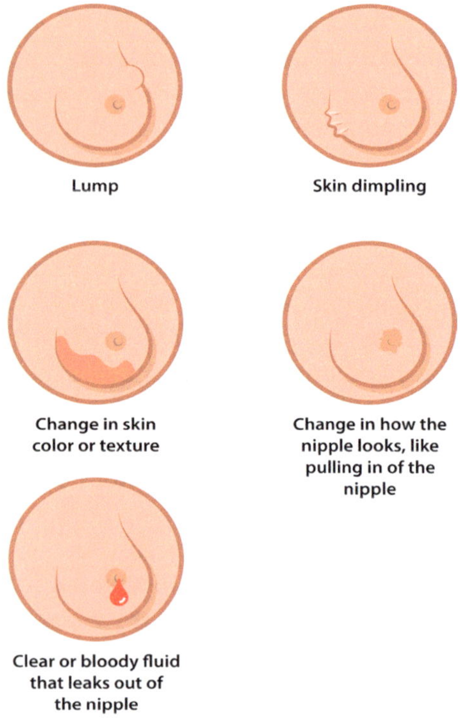

Figure 15.14. Normal findings and variations in breast and axillary assessments.

Source: https://stanfordmedicine25.stanford.edu/the25/BreastExam/_jcr_content/main/panel_builder_0/panel_0/panel_builder_1/panel_0/panel_builder/panel_0/image.img.full.high.png/2.png.

15.5.2. Abnormal Findings and Their Implications

The axillae and breast examination is a critical nursing responsibility that involves the detection of abnormal findings, whose consequences for patient health can be severe. Abnormalities such as lumps, asymmetry, or skin are typically indicative of related pathologies, such as malignancy or benign conditions. A recent study emphasizes the importance of early detection in preventing death due to breast cancer, with breast cancer incidence being also high in Italy at 55,900 new cases per annum and 15,500 related deaths (Alfonsi et al., 2024). The statistic emphasizes that nurses should be competent enough to recognize abnormal findings during routine screenings. Further, effective communication of the implications of such findings to patients is crucial because it encourages compliance with further diagnostic testing and resulting referrals to specialist care, ultimately enhancing patient outcomes. BSE education is central to enabling women to be actively involved in their breast care; however, evidence suggests that most women are poorly informed regarding how to undertake BSE effectively (Alfonsi et al., 2024). This shortfall is of particular concern owing to the consideration that a significant percentage of women do not perform regular self-examinations, and this has the potential to lead to opportunities for early detection being lost. Unusual findings, for example palpable masses or changes in the texture of the breast tissue, need swift reaction and follow-up treatment, which makes nurse education campaigns a necessity. Through the provision of intensive education and information on the signs of breast abnormalities, medical professionals are in a position to increase awareness and encourage patients to seek early medical treatment, thereby contributing to high rates of early detection. Besides physical examination competency, nurses also must be aware of the psycho-social consequences that accompany abnormal breast and axillary findings. Patients become anxious, scared, and bewildered as they discover irregularities on tests, something that can deeply affect their mental and emotional well-being. It is important for nurses to use an empathic, patient-centered approach when imparting abnormal results, reassuring them and appropriate counseling when necessary. By offering a supportive environment, healthcare practitioners are able to help patients solve their dilemmas and decisions regarding follow-up diagnostic workups or treatment. Overall, an integrated appreciation of the physical and emotional impacts of atypical results upholds the critical role of nursing assessment in promoting patient care for the whole person and maximizing overall health outcomes.

15.5.3. Documentation of Assessment Results

Accurate documentation of assessment results in axillae and breast assessment matters in nursing care because it enables continuity of care and clinical decision-making. Documentation of nursing assessments, especially for sensitive areas like the breast and axillae, is extremely crucial to ensure that results are well communicated to other health care practitioners. Documentation should include pertinent information on the history of the patient, physical examination results, laboratory tests, and patient complaints. For instance, documentation of abnormal findings such as masses, tenderness, or changes in skin texture can guide future diagnostic and treatment approaches. More significantly, thorough documentation allows for alterations over time, which is essential for patient care to be timely and effective. In this regard, accurate assessments not only aid in the detection of possible issues but also serve as valuable records for determining treatment protocol effectiveness over time. Moreover, the documentation process should adhere to set guidelines to generate clarity and professionalism. Proper documentation is attained through embracing standardized language and templates that are founded on best practice nursing. In assessing axillae and breast, set instruments and frameworks can help nurses gather the right information in an effective manner. Not only does this promise record consistency, but it also maximizes the ability of every team member to effectively interpret findings. Multidisciplinary treatment necessitates clear communication; hence, each nursing assessment entry must succinctly summarize important findings and propose potential implications for patient management. For instance, where imaging diagnosis is indicated following an abnormal report, it is necessary to record justification for such recommendations before forwarding input towards the collaborative treatment plan, thereby creating a team-oriented system of managing patient health. Furthermore, confidentiality respect and ethical data management are key considerations during recording assessment results. Each entry should be hand-written individually with utmost care for patient confidentiality and respect for legal requirements in reporting health information of a sensitive nature. This is particularly important in recording findings that will necessitate further research or treatment. Nurses should make sure that all conversations of patient health regarding the outcomes of evaluation are carried out confidentially to prevent confidentiality breaches. Additionally, with the progress of clinical practice and guidelines, constant training in documentation guidelines is required. For example, education on ergonomic practices, highlighted in recent addresses, can lead to better documentation practices and reduce the risk of injury that may compromise a nurses ability to conduct thorough assessments (N/A, 2018). Careful recording of findings from assessment is not an automatic task; it is an essential aspect of nursing directly evident in-patient outcomes and overall quality of healthcare service.

Test Your Knowledge

1. What are typical benign breast findings that can be detected during assessment?
2. Which axillary findings should prompt further diagnostic evaluation?.

15.6. Patient Education and Communication

Learning Outcome

1. Importance of Educating Patients About Self-Exams
2. Communicating Findings to Patients
3. Addressing Patient Concerns and Questions

Effective patient education and communication are part of nursing practice, particularly regarding breast and axillae examination. Nurses most often serve as the point of contact for health information concerning the importance of early detection and screening of diseases of the breast. A part of their educational role is to educate patients regarding the purpose and procedure of breast examination and the necessity of self-examination. Effective communication allows for patient understanding and active participation in their health care process. Furthermore, establishing trust through effective communication allows patients to be able to express their concerns, therefore producing a motivating environment that can lead to improved health outcomes. Therefore, the role of patient education is not merely information transmission; it instills a comprehensive consciousness and empowers patients to take care of their own health. Furthermore, the dynamic nature of patient education requires nurses to render their communication plans malleable to accommodate different patient requirements. This is particularly relevant when assessing the health of breasts and axillae, where misconceptions or fear can destroy patients willingness to utilize proper health habits. For instance, cultural beliefs and personal experiences strongly influence patients attitudes towards healthcare and their receptiveness to examinations and treatments. Through these considerations, nurses may utilize culturally responsive communication that is respectful to patients backgrounds yet delivers pertinent health information. Every educational encounter should be tailored to foster understanding through the use of plain language, visual aids, or demonstration as required. Educating patients with empowerment in tailored education not only maximizes compliance but also inspires trust in their capacity for self-care of healthcare, which is pivotal within the prevention and early detection of breast conditions. Moreover, evidence-based practice in patient education has a high likelihood of enhancing breast and axillae examination communication.

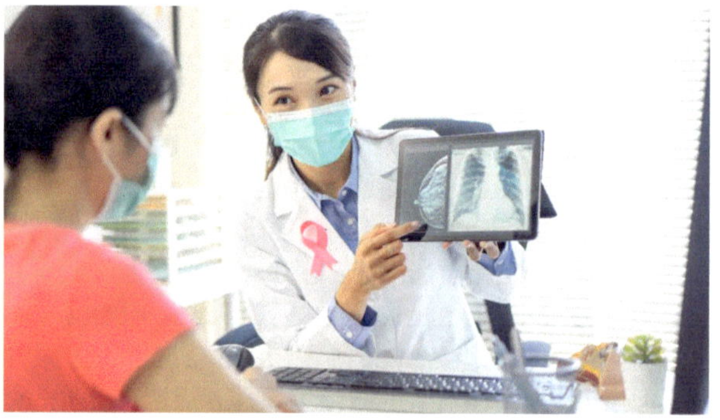

Figure 15.15. Patient education and communication in breast and axillae evaluation.

Source: https://i0.wp.com/oncospark.com/wp-content/uploads/2022/10/Blue-Gradient-Background-6.png?fit=1024%2C576&ssl=1.

Studies recently underscored the importance of feedback and ongoing support in engendering active patient participation and acquisition of skills in health-related activities. For instance, providing the possibility of question and doubt clarification by patients during the examination can lead to the more precise comprehension of procedures and expectations and subsequently reduced anxiety levels and increased satisfaction levels. Active engagement with patients following examination and continued education on breast self-examination are a model way forward in proactive patient care. Lastly, the inclusion of evidence-based practices in patient communication and education not only strengthens the relationship between patient and nurse but also encourages a health literacy culture and improved patient outcomes that are among the goals of successful nursing practice in breast and axillae assessment (N/A, 2020; Ubas-Sumagasyay et al., 2020) (Figure 15.15).

15.6.1. Importance of Educating Patients About Self-Exams

Educating patients on self-examination is a crucial aspect of breast and axillae assessment in nursing. The information apprises the patient of what is abnormal for them, fostering early detection of potential health issues, particularly breast cancer. Empirical findings indicate that self-exams enable patients to establish a criterion for what feels normal for them, which encourages timely consultations with health care providers upon noting abnormalities. In addition, integrating educational initiatives into nursing practice can demystify self-examination and aid in compliance. This is particularly important within populations historically underrepresented within routine screenings, where health disparities are most evident. Through cooperation with patients in the education of self-examination, nurses enhance health literacy, ultimately improving individual health outcomes and supporting active health management behaviors. Furthermore, patient education about self-exams enhances patients' participation in their own health care, making it a partnership between the patient and nurses. Open communication in patient education allows nurses to address misinformation or misconceptions regarding self-exams, mere presence of which discourages people from engaging with breast health information. For instance, most people are unaware of how to correctly conduct a self-exam, and confusion and fear result. Nurses play an important part in providing step-by-step guidance and open conversation that can demolish these barriers. In addition, visual aids and educational materials can also facilitate its comprehension for the patients, thus making them feel more at ease while assessing their breast health. This preventive approach not only empowers the patient but can also lead to greater numbers of early diagnoses and treatment success rates, positively impacting overall community health. Finally, education on self-exam instills a preventive and aware culture, key elements of breast health activism. By encouraging patients to self-monitor, nurses can allow patients to establish lifetime consciousness regarding their axillae and breast health. This proactive role is necessary in order to promote community health, especially because research indicates the importance of early detection in promoting survival. It also prepares one to actively participate in clinical screenings and to bring concerns regarding one's health forward assertively. Focusing on access to routine clinical exams alongside self-exams allows for an integrated approach to breast health management. In doing so, integration of self-exam instruction into nursing curricula not only equips future health professionals with the right skills but also promotes a patient-centered philosophy that positions empowerment and informed decision-making as paramount values in healthcare settings.

15.6.2. Communicating Findings to Patients

Effective communication of outcomes to patients is a vital component in the assessment process of breasts and axillae in nursing. Clarity within information provided can significantly affect a patient's understanding and reaction to their own state of health. When conveying diagnostic procedures, results, or treatment, nurses must make certain that patients comprehend the meaning of their outcomes. This involves application in layman's language, avoiding clinical terminology, and placing information in relation to individual patients' circumstances. Additionally, it's also important to establish an environment in which patients can ask questions without hesitation because participation and informed choice are enhanced. The process is not so much about conveying facts as it is about sensitiveness to the emotional weight a finding such as a lump in the breast or an abnormal imaging may carry. Development of rapport with patients has the ability to improve communication of results and is thus a fundamental aspect of nursing practice. Trust can improve the communication of critical information better, with patients who feel respected more likely to receive and value the information concerning their health assessment. An empathetic response in consultation can include active listening to patients' concerns and provision of reassurance as well as the provision of required medical information. Studies demonstrate that a positive communication style will decrease patient anxiety, particularly useful in reporting potentially disturbing results of breast examinations. Moreover, the use of visual aids or model representations can enhance patients' comprehension, particularly in explaining complex diagnoses or treatment regimens, as consistent with best practices for patient education. Lastly, timing and style of reporting results can play an important role in patient outcome. For instance, talking about outcomes after an assessment may be daunting and need early consideration in order to enable patients to adequately make sense of such information. Second opinion consultations or talks can also increase understanding and dispel any lingering questions. In cases where patients require additional investigations or referral, nurses need to outline the subsequent steps and expectations of the patient clearly. Such proactive communication aids in generating a sense of control among the patients, ensuring they are being actively involved in their own healthcare journey. In general, a strategic approach to sharing findings, incorporating emotional intelligence and patient-centric practice, is imperative in optimizing patient comprehension and satisfaction with breast and axillae assessments in nursing.

15.6.3. Addressing Patient Concerns and Questions

In the nursing practice, answering questions and alleviating patient concerns during axillae evaluation and breast is essential to patient involvement and trust. Patients generally come in with a laundry list of concerns that are at the very least fear, but may also include ignorance of process. Active listening is central; nurses must be understanding and empathetic, easing worries. Besides, education of patients regarding the intention and procedure of breast examination can empower them to feel involved in their own care. Because of the serious implication of this conversation, nurses should try their best to create an open conversation environment. This not only serves to treat short-term problems but also equips patients with knowledge so they can make the right choices about their healthcare, thereby enhancing their general satisfaction and experience with healthcare services. Moreover, the heterogeneity of breast cancer survivorship also imposes additional aspects on patient problems, for example, follow-up and long-term care of their health. As noted, most survivors of breast cancer face long-term physical and emotional challenges even after the cessation of treatment. Nurses also play a key role in conveying these concerns and providing appropriate information in terms of survivorship guidelines. Answering inquiries about lifestyle changes, signs and symptoms to monitor, and what to expect in regular follow-up visits can make a significant difference in patient outcomes. Improved understanding by nurses of current survivorship guidelines will better equip them to provide personalized care, as the majority are not aware of the most recent advancements. Thus, by creating a sound communication framework, not only does it help manage patients' main issues but also fosters confidence among survivors as they navigate their post-treatment existence (Scott et al., 2019). Lastly, nurses have to recognize the patient's diverse backgrounds and experiences, which can influence concerns and issues regarding breast and axillae assessments. Individual variation—anything from cultural beliefs to personal histories—may influence the nurse's patient to view his or her health and treatment. To offer wholeness care, nurses can engage with each patient with a culturally responsive attitude, being open to learning about their individual understandings. In this way, nurses can better respond to specific concerns and adapt their communication strategies appropriately. Combining knowledge from multidisciplinary sources, such as midwives' knowledge of patient communication and health education, can render the strategy for addressing these issues stronger (N/A, 1994). Lastly, a personalized and respectful form of communication not just relaxes anxiety but also empowers the patient, enabling a helpful setting that is essential to successful nursing practice.

Test Your Knowledge

1. How should nurses educate patients about performing regular breast self-examinations?
2. What strategies can be used to communicate sensitive findings without causing undue anxiety?.

SUMMARY

The important role of axillae and breast examination in the domain of nursing practice must not be overemphasized. While breast cancer remains a top health issue for women globally, the nuances of breast self-examination (BSE) are paramount for midwives as well as nurses. It is evidence that demonstrates early detection to be directly linked with better survival rates and treatment response. Hence, instilling the skills of medical experts to adequately counsel patients in regard to the BSE is key since most women are ill-informed and poorly practicing the process. An improvement in curriculum designs in nursing schools incorporating adequate prevention and screening of breast cancer could lead to improved outcomes and survival rates among women suffering from this illness, as noted by existing literature (Alfonsi et al., 2024). It is important that nursing programs address these needs in order to better prepare subsequent generations of health care professionals. Moreover, the outcomes of several research studies indicate the importance of more rigorous training programs that emphasize the significance of BSE for nurses. The knowledge gaps that presently exist revealed while midwives demonstrate a greater understanding than nursing students, there remains a considerable percentage that is unaware of available guidelines for conducting BSE optimally (Alfonsi et al., 2024). As the pillars of preventive health care among women, midwives and nurses ought not just to be well-versed but be experts at relaying this critical information to patients. Comprehensive training may demystify self-examination techniques and encourage regular practice, essential in fostering an active mindset towards breast health among women. Institutionalizing a culture of education and awareness has the capacity to redefine the context of breast cancer prevention. Finally, the application of this study's findings into nursing practice and education is an important challenge for enhanced health outcomes. Not only can we ensure that healthcare professionals are properly equipped with skills and knowledge to deliver effective BSE, but we are also able to promote a proactive healthcare model centered on early detection and patient education. By improving interprofessional working between nursing stakeholders and employers, it is possible to develop programs that address existing areas of noted knowledge gaps in the nursing workforce. Lastly, investing in the education and training of nursing personnel with regards to breast and axillae examination will create an educated base that empowers women to be responsible for their bodies and health. The move is crucial in mandating involvement in screening programs and ultimately improving overall public health results.

Assessment of the breast and axillae is a key aspect of nursing practice, heavily emphasizing early detection of deviation and patient education. Nursing professionals are trained to perform systematic assessments, emphasizing the key aspects of inspection and palpation. These assessments allow detection of the many conditions such as lumps, tenderness, or skin alterations, which are suspect of underlying conditions, such as malignancy. An intimate knowledge of the breast anatomy and normal and abnormal findings is required in patient management. Patient education on self-examination is also important and can help the patient become a part of his or her own care, facilitating early detection and treatment outcomes as outlined in modern nursing policies (Cheung et al., 1999). The significance of the axillary examination cannot be overstressed, particularly regarding the examination of lymph nodes, a significant determining factor in the direction of disease. Nurses must be skilled at palpating axillary lymph nodes to note any sign of enlargement or tenderness that can represent systemic involvement of disease processes such as breast cancer. Also, understanding the anatomic landmarks of the axilla guarantees a comprehensive examination that lessens the chances of overlooking relevant abnormalities. Continuing education and training are essential to guarantee nursing staff are updated on best practices so they can perform comprehensive examinations that comply with National Guidelines or local standards in breast health screening (Durand et al., 2020). In the long term, the inclusion of breast and axillary examinations in wide-ranging nursing practice allows for comprehensive patient care. The assessments are not only technical procedures but also avenues for rapport and trust development between patients and healthcare professionals. Through a setting where patients feel free to discuss delicate matters, nurses are able to significantly enhance the quality of care delivered. Moreover, the combination of clinical skill with empathetic communication fosters follow-up compliance and aids in patients developing lifelong health awareness. These interventions are critical because they result in enhanced health outcomes and are consistent with the radical goals of contemporary nursing practice for tackling women's health issues (Cheung et al., 1999).

KEY TERMS FROM THIS CHAPTER

- Breasts
- Axillae
- Lobes
- Lobules
- Milk Ducts
- Nipple
- Areola
- Montgomery Glands
- Cooper's Ligaments
- Lymph Nodes
- Tail of Spence
- Breast Symmetry
- Skin Changes
- Retraction
- Dimpling
- Nipple Discharge
- Palpation
- Mammary Tissue
- Self-Breast Examination (SBE)
- Clinical Breast Examination (CBE)

CRITICAL THINKING QUESTIONS

1. **During a breast assessment, the nurse notes a fixed, hard lump in the upper outer quadrant of the breast. Which action is most appropriate?**
   a. Document as a normal finding
   b. Teach the patient breast self-examination techniques
   c. Refer the patient for further diagnostic evaluation
   d. Apply a warm compress and reassess in one week
2. **Which position is BEST for a nurse to assess the upper outer quadrant of the breast and axilla?**
   a. Patient lying supine with arm at side
   b. Patient sitting with hands on hips
   c. Patient supine with arm raised above head
   d. Patient standing with arms relaxed
3. **Which finding during axillary palpation is considered abnormal?**
   a. Small, soft, mobile lymph nodes
   b. No palpable lymph nodes
   c. Firm, fixed, non-tender lymph nodes
   d. Tender, mobile lymph nodes after recent infection
4. **When teaching a patient about breast self-examination, which statement is correct?**
   a. "Check your breasts only if you notice pain."
   b. "Perform the exam once a year during your annual checkup."
   c. "The best time is a few days after your menstrual period ends."
   d. "Use only the tips of your fingers to examine the breast."
5. **Dimpling of the breast skin may indicate:**
   a. Fibrocystic changes
   b. Normal aging process
   c. Underlying malignancy
   d. Hormonal fluctuations

Short Answer Questions

1. Describe the structure of the breast, including the location of the lobes, ducts, and lymphatic drainage. Why is knowledge of lymphatic drainage important in breast assessment?
2. What are the differences between the vertical strip, circular, and wedge methods of breast palpation, and which is considered the most effective for detecting lumps?
3. What signs should a nurse look for during the visual inspection of the breasts and axillae that may indicate underlying pathology?
4. How can nipple discharge be assessed, and what are the clinical implications of unilateral, bloody, or spontaneous discharge?
5. What is the proper technique for axillary lymph node assessment, and which nodes are commonly palpated?

Answer to Critical Thinking Questions

1. (c) 2. (c) 3. (c) 4. (c) 5. (c)

REFERENCES

1. Accettola, E., Bogdan, A., Callahan, S., Chawda, H., et al. (2023). Introduction to health assessment for the nursing professional: Part II. https://core.ac.uk/download/622362029.pdf (accessed on 16th July 2025).
2. Akram, M., Iqbal, M., Daniyal, M., & Khan, A. U. (2017). Awareness and current knowledge of breast cancer. *Biological Research, 50*. https://doi.org/10.1186/s40659-017-0140-9 (accessed on 16th July 2025).
3. Alfonsi, C. (2024). Breast self-examination (BSE) among midwives and midwifery students: A national survey. https://core.ac.uk/download/636341424.pdf (accessed on 16th July 2025).
4. Ambika, L. (2014). A study to evaluate the effectiveness of video assisted teaching programmed on knowledge regarding breast self-examination among III year female students studying at Nandha Arts and Science College, Erode. https://core.ac.uk/download/235655204.pdf (accessed on 16th July 2025).
5. American Medical Association. (1998). Fiction. *JAMA, 279*, 962. https://doi.org/10.1001/jama.279.12.962-jbk0325-3-1 (accessed on 16th July 2025).
6. Anderson, G. C., Bergman, N., Medley, N., Moore, E., et al. (2016). Early skin-to-skin contact for mothers and their healthy newborn infants. https://core.ac.uk/download/80780222.pdf (accessed on 16th July 2025).
7. Araújo Vilar, D., Castro Pais, A., Cobelo Gómez, S., Fernández Pombo, A., et al. (2021). Variable expressivity and allelic heterogeneity in type 2 familial partial lipodystrophy: The p.(Thr528Met) LMNA variant. https://core.ac.uk/download/395735347.pdf (accessed on 16th July 2025).
8. Australasian Sonographers Association. (2018). ORAL PRESENTATIONS. *Sonography, 5*, 3–31. https://doi.org/10.1002/sono.12141 (accessed on 16th July 2025).
9. Berman, A., Dwyer, T., Erb, G. L., Hales, D., et al. (2015). *Kozier and Erb's Fundamentals of Nursing* [3rd Australian edition]. https://core.ac.uk/download/303778222.pdf (accessed on 16th July 2025).
10. Chandler, D., & Fuller, L. C. (2018). A review of scabies: An infestation more than skin deep. *Dermatology, 235*, 79–90. https://doi.org/10.1159/000495290 (accessed on 16th July 2025).
11. Cheung, K. L. (1999). Clinical examination of the breast. https://core.ac.uk/download/37967700.pdf (accessed on 16th July 2025).
12. Chopra, A., Tillu, G., Chuadhary, K., Reddy, G., Srivastava, A., Lakdawala, M., Gode, D., et al. (2023). Co-administration of AYUSH 64 as an adjunct to standard of care in mild and moderate COVID-19: A randomized, controlled, multicentric clinical trial. *PLOS ONE, 18*, e0282688. https://doi.org/10.1371/journal.pone.0282688 (accessed on 16th July 2025).
13. Choudhary, K., Singh, R. K., Garg, A. S., Verma, N., Purohit, A., & Deora, D. (2019). An updated overview of polycystic ovary syndrome. *Innovare Journal of Medical Sciences*. https://doi.org/10.22159/ijms.2019.v7i3.34248 (accessed on 16th July 2025).
14. de Buys, M., Moodley, K., Cakic, J. N., & Pietrzak, J. R. T. (2023). Staphylococcus aureus colonization and periprosthetic joint infection in patients undergoing elective total joint arthroplasty: A narrative review. *EFORT Open Reviews, 8*, 680–689. https://doi.org/10.1530/eor-23-0031 (accessed on 16th July 2025).

15. Drabińska, N., Flynn, C., Ratcliffe, N., Belluomo, I., Myridakis, A., Gould, O., Fois, M., et al. (2021). A literature survey of all volatiles from healthy human breath and bodily fluids: The human volatilome. *Journal of Breath Research, 15*, 034001. https://doi.org/10.1088/1752-7163/abf1d0 (accessed on 16th July 2025).

16. Durand, K., Loos, H., Saxton, T., Schaal, B., et al. (2020). Olfaction scaffolds the developing human from neonate to adolescent and beyond. https://core.ac.uk/download/288435873.pdf (accessed on 16th July 2025).

17. Everink, I. H. J., Halfens, R., Kottner, J., Schols, J., et al. (2021). Skin areas, clinical severity, duration and risk factors of intertrigo: A secondary data analysis. https://core.ac.uk/download/395601318.pdf (accessed on 16th July 2025).

18. Garcia, W., & Lapum, J. L. (2018). *Vital Sign Measurement Across the Lifespan* (1st Canadian edition). https://core.ac.uk/download/622362086.pdf (accessed on 16th July 2025).

19. Haapiainen, T. (2015). Taking the lymphatic system into consideration in nursing: How lymphedema affects breast cancer patients' quality of life. https://core.ac.uk/download/pdf/38121708.pdf (accessed on 16th July 2025).

20. Keohane, S., Botting, J., Budny, P. G., Dolan, O. M., Fife, K., Harwood, C. A., Mallipeddi, R., et al. (2020). British Association of Dermatologists guidelines for the management of people with cutaneous squamous cell carcinoma 2020. *British Journal of Dermatology, 184*, 401–414. https://doi.org/10.1111/bjd.19621 (accessed on 16th July 2025).

21. Kwok, C., Ong, A. J., Babakinejad, P., Arunjuna, N., Derrick, E., Storan, E. R., Aalto, L., et al. (2015). Bristol Cup posters. *British Journal of Dermatology, 173*, 21–76. https://doi.org/10.1111/bjd.13761 (accessed on 16th July 2025).

22. Lester, J. L. (2015). Surgical treatment of breast cancer. *OR Nurse*. www.ORNurseJournal.com (accessed on 16th July 2025).

23. Marinopoulos, S. S., Dimitrakakis, C., Kalampalikis, A., Zagouri, F., Andrikopoulou, A., & Rodolakis, A. (2021). Adjuvant treatment of elderly breast cancer patients: Offer the best chances of cure. *Breast Care, 17*, 71–80. https://doi.org/10.1159/000513708 (accessed on 16th July 2025).

24. Morscher, M. A., Thomas, M., Sahgal, S., & Adamczyk, M. J. (2020). Onabotulinum toxin type A injection into the triceps unmasks elbow flexion in infant brachial plexus birth palsy. *Medicine, 99*, e21830. https://doi.org/10.1097/md.0000000000021830 (accessed on 16th July 2025).

25. N/A. (1994). Newsletter, 1994–07, no. 12. https://core.ac.uk/download/154211309.pdf (accessed on 16th July 2025).

26. Neal-Boylan, L. (2020). Resolutions. https://doi.org/10.1002/9781119603238.part11 (accessed on 16th July 2025).

27. Saaty, H. P. (2007). A feasibility study for establishing a dedicated breast magnetic resonance imaging center in the city of Redlands. https://core.ac.uk/download/227028256.pdf (accessed on 16th July 2025).

28. Scott, L. E. (2019). Development of a breast cancer survivorship care toolkit. https://digitalscholarship.unlv.edu/cgi/viewcontent.cgi?article=4675&context=thesesdissertations (accessed on 16th July 2025).

29. Sprakel, J. (2020). A systematic review of the research gaps in breast cancer in the Gulf region. https://doi.org/10.11606/t.17.2020.tde-09042021-092805 (accessed on 16th July 2025).

30. Todd, M. (2017). Identification, assessment and management of breast oedema after treatment for cancer. *International Journal of Palliative Nursing, 23*, 440–444. https://doi.org/10.12968/ijpn.2017.23.9.440 (accessed on 16th July 2025).

31. Torgbenu, E. L., Luckett, T., Buhagiar, M. A., Chang, S., & Phillips, J. (2020). Prevalence and incidence of cancer related lymphedema in low and middle-income countries: A systematic review and meta-analysis. *BMC Cancer, 20*. https://doi.org/10.1186/s12885-020-07079-7 (accessed on 16th July 2025).

32. Ubas-Sumagasyay, N. A., & Oducado, R. M. (2020). Perceived competence and transition experience of new graduate Filipino nurses. *Deleted Journal, 23*, 48–63. https://doi.org/10.7454/jki.v23i1.1071 (accessed on 16th July 2025).

33. Wilson, D. (2012). The effect of education on healthcare personnel's knowledge of lymphedema detection and prevention. https://core.ac.uk/download/53025763.pdf (accessed on 16th July 2025).

34. WoCoVA Organizing Committee. (2020). Abstracts from the postponed 6th World Congress on Vascular Access (WoCoVA 2020–June 17–19th). *The Journal of Vascular Access, 21*, NP1–NP68. https://doi.org/10.1177/1129729820953245 (accessed on 16th July 2025).

INDEX

A

Abdomen Contour 409
Abdominal assessments 117, 383, 386, 387, 396, 397, 402, 404, 405
Absent Sounds 409
Active assessment 2
Active listening 37, 48, 51, 60, 64, 84, 85, 512
Acute illness 18, 320
Adventitious Sounds 342
Adverse childhood experiences (ACEs) 86
Age-related macular degeneration (AMD) 256
Alopecia 185, 205
Anatomical landmarks 16, 117, 386, 387, 418, 503
Ancient nursing practices 8
Androgenetic alopecia 185
Anterior cruciate ligament (ACL) 126
Aphasia 482
Apical Pulse 376
Assessment method 16, 117, 407
Assessment skills 3, 10, 14, 26, 119, 120, 200, 219, 236, 239, 247, 251, 290, 315, 316, 327, 349, 359, 368, 381, 384, 387, 390, 453, 456, 461, 503, 507
Asthma 328, 329, 330
Asthma Control Test (ACT) 329
Atrophy 409, 445
Auditory assessments 122
Auricle 306
Auscultation 2, 14, 17, 18, 30, 107, 108, 109, 110, 119, 121, 122, 123, 124, 125, 132, 134, 135, 151, 157, 165, 219, 221, 280, 313, 315, 316, 318, 320, 321, 325, 327, 328, 331, 338, 339, 349, 364, 365, 376, 381, 382, 383, 387, 388, 389, 391, 404, 407, 408, 409

B

Barrel Chest 306, 342
Baseline Data 147
Biographical Data 100
Biomechanics 128
Biopsychosocial integration 80
Blood Circulation Process 355
Blood pressure 18, 141, 142, 143, 145, 148, 151, 152, 153, 154, 155, 156, 157, 158, 160, 162, 164, 165, 166, 168, 272, 351, 355, 357, 358, 360, 361, 364, 365, 367, 368, 373, 375, 378, 449
Body Build 169
Body-focused repetitive behavior disorders (BFRBDs) 186, 188
Body language 49, 113
Body Mass Index (BMI) 169
Body position 49, 123, 321
Body posture 50, 77, 111, 112
Bowel Sounds 409
Brain natriuretic peptide (BNP) 365
Breast Symmetry 515
Breath Sounds 342
Bronchial asthma 82, 105

Bronchial constriction 124
Bronchial Sounds 342
Bronchovesicular Sounds 342

C

Capillary Refill 376
Cardiac Cycle 355
Cardiovascular diseases (CVD) 360
Cardiovascular system 347, 348, 349, 350, 351, 352, 353, 355, 356, 357, 358, 359, 361, 363, 364, 365, 366, 375, 379, 380
Carotid Artery 376
Central Nervous System (CNS) 482
Cerebellar Function 482
Cervical Nodes 240
Chest Expansion 342
Chief Complaint 30, 100
Chronic conditions 2, 24, 142, 144, 151, 163, 224, 263, 324, 468, 469, 473
Chronic obstructive pulmonary disease 124, 314, 319, 324, 333, 334, 340, 346
Chronic otitis media (COM) 287
Chronic suppurative otitis media (CSOM) 287
Clinical Breast Examination (CBE) 515
Clinical decision 1, 7, 12, 14, 16, 17, 73, 80, 93, 94, 99, 117, 122, 131, 135, 141, 143, 144, 145, 150, 160, 162, 163, 165, 176, 192, 193, 201, 218, 220, 221, 238, 251, 264, 280, 292, 299, 301, 304, 325, 326, 336, 348, 365, 400, 422, 433, 474, 475, 488, 509
Clinical decision-making 1, 7, 16, 73, 80, 93, 94, 99, 117, 122, 135, 141, 143, 144, 145, 150, 160, 162, 163, 176, 192, 193, 218, 220, 221, 238, 251, 264, 292, 299, 301, 304, 325, 326, 348, 365, 400, 422, 433, 488, 509
Clinical evaluation 18, 50, 313, 314, 505, 506
Clinical history 4
Clinical Judgment 30
Clinical management decisions 132
Clinical standards 17, 176, 233, 379
Clinician-patient therapeutic relationship 47
Closed-Ended Questions 65
Cognitive function screenings 461
Cognitive impairments 50, 461, 469
Communication failures 37
Comorbid patients 81
Competency assessment 7
Complex care management systems 7
Comprehensive assessment 1, 6, 145, 150, 175, 211, 213, 247, 349, 391, 393, 406, 473
Computer-aided history-taking systems (CAHTS) 92
Computer-assisted history-taking systems (CAHTS) 84
Computer decision-support software (CDSS) 92, 108
Computerized provider order entry (CPOE) 23
Concealed dysfunctions 116
Concealed Information Test (CIT) 127
Confidentiality 56, 57, 58, 95, 96
Congestive heart failure (CHF) 371
Conjunctiva 273
Consensual Response 273
Coopers Ligaments 515
Cornea 273
Coronary Artery Disease 367
Cranial nerve examinations 461
Cranial Nerves 482
Crepitus 445
Cultural competence 14, 19, 38, 52, 53, 60, 62, 193, 198, 297
Cultural Competence 30, 52
Culturally sensitive nursing 21
Cultural Sensitivity 65
Cyanosis 205, 342

D

Data privacy 78, 272
Deep Tendon Reflexes (DTR) 482
Deformity 445
Dementia patients 15
Demographic information 81, 142, 149
Dermis 205
Diagnostic abilities 110, 291
Diagnostic accuracy 93, 121, 299, 300, 301, 305, 326, 389, 467, 472, 481, 503
Diagnostic imaging 109

Diagnostic precision 79, 125, 128, 262, 406
Dietary supplements 182
Disease diagnosis 119, 326, 497
Disease prevention 2, 105, 147, 212, 272, 349
Doctor-patient dynamics 78
Documentation 10, 13, 130, 131, 132, 164, 166, 200, 231, 232, 264, 265, 333, 336, 400, 403, 436, 473, 474, 476, 485, 506, 509
Dysphagia 289, 309
Dyspnea 342

E

Ear anatomy 282
Ear disorders 286, 287, 288
Ear, Nose, Mouth, and Throat (ENT) region 279
Eczema 182
Edema 205, 376
Effective communication 37, 39, 40, 59, 89, 166, 201, 230, 259, 266, 398, 457, 475, 476, 480, 504, 510, 511
Effective interviewing 14, 37, 38
Electrocardiograms (ECGs) 349, 363
Electronic documentation 131
Electronic health records (EHRs) 2, 14, 22, 74, 130, 143, 159, 200, 233, 246, 251, 264, 265, 267, 465
Emotional care 87
Emotional state 14, 15, 48, 49, 112, 295
Empathetic questioning 41
Empathy 65, 86
Epidermis 205
Erythema 205
Ethical responsibility 28, 37, 96
European Stroke Organization (ESO) 158
Eustachian Tube 306
Evidence-Based Practice
External Auditory Canal 306
Extraocular Muscles 273
Eye assessment technology 267, 270
Eye testing technology 270

F

Facial Symmetry 240
Factual information 41
Fall risk–augmenting medications (FRIDs) 78
Family Adoption Program (FAP) 55
Family health histories 78
Family History 100
Fear of Falling Avoidance Behavior Questionnaire (FFABQ) 263
Fetal Alcohol Spectrum Disorders (FASD) 43
Fever of unknown origin (FUO) 109
Fluid accumulation 16, 217, 327, 355
Focused Assessment 135
Fontanelle 240
Fractional exhaled nitric oxide (FeNO) 330
Functional Assessment 100

G

Gag Reflex 306
Gas Exchange Process 320
General Appearance 169
General Health Survey 141, 142, 144, 148
General Survey 135
Genetic disorders 43, 82
Genetic tendencies 82, 251
Glasgow Coma Scale (GCS) 454, 482
Glaucoma 247, 256, 258, 259, 276
Good communication skills 11, 64, 84, 382
Good interviewing skills 41
Gynecology 115

H

Hair disorders 183, 185, 186
Hair health 183, 184, 185, 186, 187
Hard Palate 306
Head-to-Toe Assessment 135
Health Assessment 1, 5, 10, 14, 18, 22, 26, 30, 37, 41, 48, 60, 242, 254, 275, 378
Health assessment history 5, 7
Health assessment interviews 37, 60
Health assessment process 3, 29, 39, 44, 49, 52, 54, 62
Health assessment techniques 2, 14
Health Buddy Patient Telemonitoring Program 147
Healthcare continuum 16

Health care delivery 13, 38, 302
Healthcare delivery 3, 19, 52, 74, 75, 94, 108, 119, 149, 150, 159, 220, 271, 303, 398, 449
Healthcare environment 2, 7, 19, 23, 82, 95, 96, 131, 142, 146, 247, 304, 313, 430
Health care environments 14
Health care systems 2
Health challenges 10, 48
Health data 37, 58, 94, 97, 147, 153, 482
Health hazards 62, 78, 195
Health History 30, 73, 76, 80, 84, 88, 92, 95
Health history interview 43
Health history taking 73, 74, 75, 76, 77, 78, 79, 82, 83, 84, 85, 86, 87, 88, 89, 90, 91, 92, 93, 94, 95, 96, 97, 98, 99, 100
Health information 2, 24, 39, 42, 46, 49, 53, 58, 60, 74, 75, 85, 86, 89, 90, 94, 95, 96, 130, 150, 158, 167, 214, 232, 233, 261, 264, 279, 280, 375, 396, 509, 510, 511
Health Insurance Portability and Accountability Act (HIPAA) 133
Health interviewing 56
Health management 20, 42, 65, 83, 142, 143, 151, 154, 161, 236, 303, 305, 375, 489, 492, 511
Health miscommunication 40
Health needs 10, 19, 29, 38, 143, 221, 317, 380, 383, 427, 490
Health outcomes 2, 3, 5, 11, 13, 16, 19, 20, 21, 26, 28, 29, 30, 38, 40, 43, 47, 52, 53, 60, 64, 75, 76, 77, 82, 85, 87, 89, 90, 98, 107, 108, 145, 149, 150, 153, 154, 157, 162, 164, 165, 166, 176, 178, 180, 183, 185, 193, 195, 197, 198, 203, 204, 218, 225, 229, 230, 232, 235, 255, 282, 283, 289, 292, 296, 303, 310, 314, 321, 332, 336, 337, 341, 348, 349, 357, 359, 360, 361, 369, 371, 373, 390, 393, 408, 417, 422, 426, 432, 434, 440, 444, 445, 456, 467, 468, 472, 473, 480, 490, 496, 500, 502, 508, 510, 511, 514, 515
Health-related quality of life (HRQoL) 177, 178, 493
Health screening 38
Healthy behavior 41, 356, 372
Hearing Acuity 306
Heart Failure 367, 372
Heart rate 18, 142, 145, 151, 152, 154, 155, 157, 160, 161, 162, 163, 164, 165, 168, 357, 358, 361, 364, 365, 375, 460
Heart Sounds 376
High-quality patient care 3, 129
High-resolution computed tomography (HRCT) 287
Hip replacement 132
Hirsutism 205
History of present illness (HPI) 80
Holistic Assessment 30
Hygiene 169, 486
Hyperactive Sounds 409
Hyperresonance 342
Hypertension 367, 368, 376
Hypoactive Sounds 409
Hypotension 376

I

Immunization History 100
Informed consent 12, 56, 57, 73, 85, 96, 97, 98, 260, 476
Initial assessments 4
Inspection 14, 15, 16, 30, 110, 111, 121, 134, 135, 219, 220, 222, 252, 254, 290, 291, 325, 326, 388, 389, 418, 422, 423, 424, 499, 502, 503, 504
Integrative care 80, 114, 121, 183, 185, 226, 371, 443
Integumentary system abnormality 191
Intercostal Spaces 342
Interpersonal communications 1
Interprofessional educational (IPE) 285
Interprofessional team-based practice 2
Intervention planning 2, 42, 112, 341, 504
Interviewing skills 40, 45
Iris 273

J

Jaundice 205
Joint effusion 117

K

Kyphosis 445

L

Legal and ethical documentation 132
Lesion 205
Level of Consciousness 169, 482
Long short-term memory (LSTM) 160
Lordosis 445
Lymphadenopathy 223, 226
Lymphatic system 213, 214, 217, 218
Lymph Nodes 240, 494, 502, 515

M

Magnetic Resonance Imaging 97, 464, 502
Magnetic resonance imaging (MRI) 110, 464, 489, 503
Mammary Tissue 515
Medical care 81, 134, 141, 242, 269, 316, 484
Medical examination 16, 111
Medical history 8, 10, 12, 14, 41, 43, 73, 74, 77, 80, 82, 93, 95, 99, 104, 111, 118, 145, 147, 148, 149, 176, 177, 194, 239, 261, 289, 295, 302, 363, 394, 404, 422, 462, 467, 469
Medical treatment 3, 20, 96, 118, 183, 249, 401, 508
Medication administration 13
Medication History 100
Melanin 205
Mental Status 454, 461, 466, 479, 481, 482
Milk Ducts 515
Mindfulness interventions 61
Mini-Mental State Examination (MMSE) 464
Mobile health 92, 94
Modern nursing 5, 8, 9, 514
Modern ophthalmoscopes 114
Montgomery Glands 515
Motivational interviewing 41, 42, 46, 51, 54, 55, 60, 64, 67, 68, 69, 107, 372
Motivational interviewing techniques 41
Motor Function 482
Multi-communication online training (MOT) 40
Multidisciplinary healthcare team 13
Muscle Strength 445, 482
Muscle Tone 445
Musculoskeletal tissues 115
Myofascial pelvic pain (MFPP) 117, 121, 384, 392, 424, 433

N

Nail abnormalities 188, 189, 190, 191
Nail analysis 190
Nail assessment 175, 177, 188, 190, 191, 202, 203, 205
Nail Clubbing 205
Nail evaluation 188
Nail structure 188, 189
Nasal disorders 286, 288, 289
Nasal Mucosa 306
nasal passages 280, 282, 284, 291, 292, 299
Nasal Septum 306
Neck pain 223, 225
Neonatal intensive care units (NICUs) 125
Neurological disease 127, 220, 245, 455, 457
Neurological examination 454, 456, 458, 461, 463, 467, 468, 470, 471
Neurological function 127, 214, 215, 455, 456, 458, 461, 462, 467, 468, 470
Neurological health assessment 454
Neurologic function 454
Neuromuscular physiology 117
Neuropathy 482
Nipple Discharge 515
Nonverbal communication 48, 49
Nursing documentation practice 13
Nursing education 2, 4, 5, 7, 8, 13, 18, 20, 21, 25, 26, 32, 34, 35, 119, 161, 175, 176, 193, 197, 221, 229, 232, 236, 254, 266, 271, 272, 285, 291, 299, 309, 317, 327, 344, 349, 357, 368, 373, 374, 375, 382, 390, 391, 397, 398, 417, 427, 436, 444, 456, 467, 470, 499, 500, 504, 507
Nursing evaluations 7, 150, 161, 226, 284, 317, 444, 468, 491
Nursing health assessment 1, 4, 29
Nursing practice 3, 209, 453
Nursing practitioners 11, 17, 22, 191, 201, 204, 212, 239, 247, 249, 251, 255, 256, 257, 258, 259, 265, 272, 291, 342, 347, 349, 350, 351, 360, 369, 381, 383, 397, 406, 408, 417, 418, 427, 437, 464,

474, 489, 493, 495, 496
Nursing Process 30
Nutritional History 100

O

Objective Data 30
Observational information 7
Ocular structural assessment 113
Open-ended questioning 11, 39, 61, 86, 150
Open-Ended Questions 65
Ophthalmoscope 111, 113, 248, 254, 260, 273
Optic Disc 273
Oral/oropharyngeal squamous cell carcinoma (OSCC) 212, 231
Otoscope 111, 113, 290, 291, 293, 306
Oxygen Saturation 169

P

Pain Assessment 169
Painstaking observation 454
Palmar Surface 135
Palpation 14, 16, 30, 110, 115, 117, 118, 135, 151, 177, 191, 192, 193, 194, 219, 220, 221, 254, 290, 292, 293, 325, 326, 388, 390, 409, 422, 424, 499, 500, 501, 502, 504, 505, 515
Palpation examination 115, 192
Parotid Gland 240
Past Medical History 100
Patient assessment 13, 18, 25, 27, 74, 120, 144, 146, 152, 154, 157, 158, 160, 164, 165, 166, 175, 201, 202, 212, 213, 214, 217, 218, 219, 221, 233, 237, 246, 247, 255, 262, 350, 356, 357, 364, 381, 387, 391, 392, 409, 422, 429, 436, 438, 454, 455, 463
Patient autonomy 11, 12, 27, 57, 97, 258, 260
Patient care experience 48, 98
Patient-centered care 2, 5, 8, 11, 25, 28, 29, 43, 47, 57, 64, 74, 85, 86, 93, 97, 98, 132, 148, 150, 178, 184, 198, 213, 215, 221, 239, 258, 280, 289, 293, 295, 296, 301, 302, 305, 306, 320, 339, 341, 382, 393, 406, 432, 436, 444, 457, 465, 469, 474, 479, 488
Patient confidentiality 95, 96, 97
Patient data 1, 2, 14, 22, 26, 39, 58, 60, 84, 149, 158, 159, 264, 267
Patient dissatisfaction 38, 75
Patient engagement 45, 54, 61, 88, 93, 95, 98, 100, 107, 145, 154, 228, 229, 395, 489
Patient health 4, 5, 7, 10, 15, 18, 23, 25, 29, 45, 60, 82, 144, 145, 146, 148, 151, 164, 165, 168, 176, 183, 184, 220, 233, 239, 246, 255, 286, 315, 318, 330, 352, 357, 361, 362, 383, 385, 395, 408, 417, 460, 492, 508, 509
Patient hesitation 88
Patient history 1, 8, 74, 90, 93, 94, 126, 127, 131, 149, 150, 166, 177, 190, 194, 219, 224, 260, 261, 279, 294, 295, 296, 305, 329, 330, 339, 360, 363, 364, 365, 381, 382, 392, 397, 408, 415, 428, 430, 432, 433, 453, 462, 499, 503
Patient information 7, 10, 22, 23, 28, 39, 58, 64, 88, 90, 92, 93, 96, 130, 132, 165, 200, 232, 246, 266, 401, 402, 465, 473, 474
Patient perception 8
Patient-physician trust 39
Patient-provider relationship 19, 76, 77
Patient safety 13, 18, 23, 24, 26, 32, 55, 78, 80, 93, 126, 130, 131, 133, 142, 143, 144, 146, 147, 153, 155, 157, 159, 161, 163, 165, 168, 169, 171, 180, 200, 202, 204, 221, 226, 229, 232, 233, 234, 235, 262, 265, 266, 268, 282, 300, 305, 317, 327, 333, 363, 366, 383, 390, 401, 402, 403, 404, 436, 438, 448, 471, 474, 476, 482
Patient satisfaction 3, 11, 12, 14, 19, 20, 22, 38, 39, 40, 45, 49, 50, 51, 54, 64, 77, 85, 86, 88, 95, 108, 109, 155, 166, 183, 197, 198, 230, 246, 297, 302, 304, 330, 338, 396, 398, 430
Patients feeling 42
Patient's health condition 40, 122, 463
Patient spontaneity 74
Patient status 16, 22, 75, 200, 279, 315, 325, 474, 481
Patient wellness 8
Peak expiratory flow (PEF) 330
Percussion 30, 110, 119, 120, 121, 135, 292, 325, 327, 342, 409
Percussion sounds 119, 121, 122

Perioperative complication 123
Peripheral Nervous System (PNS) 482
Peripheral Pulse 376
Peripheral Vision 273
Personal health-related information 86
Personal history 40, 149, 329
Personalized patient care 7
Person-centered treatment plans 43
Pharyngitis 289, 290
Pharynx 306
Phonocardiography 124
Physical assessment 12, 42, 117, 119, 120, 121, 122, 151, 193, 229, 252, 316, 327, 329, 344, 348, 360, 363, 388, 416, 432, 439, 440, 487, 503
Physical examination 1, 38, 107, 108, 109, 110, 111, 112, 113, 114, 115, 117, 118, 119, 120, 121, 122, 123, 124, 125, 126, 128, 130, 131, 132, 133, 134, 135, 137, 139, 140, 150, 151, 177, 194, 197, 201, 223, 226, 235, 290, 294, 299, 305, 326, 330, 359, 363, 364, 381, 382, 383, 386, 409, 415, 428, 430, 463, 464, 494, 499, 502, 504, 506, 507, 508, 509
Physical symptoms 10, 26, 83, 185, 213
Physician Assistants (PAs) 51
Pleural Friction Rub 342
Pneumonia 325, 328, 331, 332
Postauricular Nodes 240
Practice-based learning 51
Preauricular Nodes 240
Precordium 376
Primary care delivery 89
Probing questions 45, 47, 48
Psychosocial assessment 1
Psychosocial History 100
Psychosocial setting 79
Public health 5, 29, 30, 40, 70, 75, 76, 77, 82, 90, 97, 142, 144, 147, 153, 161, 166, 185, 240, 247, 273, 315, 334, 360, 406, 429, 436, 438, 444, 450, 486, 489, 506, 514
Public health promotion 40
Pulmonary diseases 119, 340
Pulmonary health 124
Pulse Rate 376
Pulse Rhythm 376
Pupil 273, 482
Pupillary Light Reflex 273

Q

Qualitative data 11, 45
Quantitative data 11, 40, 425
Quantitative evidence 11

R

Range of Motion (ROM) 445
Rapport development 87, 398
Real-time imaging 110
Real-time information 3, 158, 163, 165
Rebound Tenderness 409
Recurrent neural networks (RNN) 160
Reflection 65, 344
Refractive errors 256, 257
Remote assessments 22, 24, 25
Remote monitoring technology 144
Renin-angiotensin-aldosterone system (RAAS) 353, 358
Respiration 154, 169, 346
Respiratory rate 18, 121, 141, 142, 148, 151, 152, 153, 154, 156, 157, 160, 162, 166, 168, 314, 316, 321, 322, 325, 333, 339, 346
Respiratory Rate 342
Retina 273
Review of Systems 30, 100, 150
Rhonchi 342
Rinne Test 306
Routine assessment 176
Routine examination protocols 117

S

SBAR (Situation, Background, Assessment, Recommendation) 234, 264, 438
Sclera 273
Scoliosis 445
Sebaceous Glands 205
Self-Breast Examination (SBE) 515
Self-management skills 77, 434
Sensitive health information 24, 38, 382

Sensory Function 482
Sensory perception 454, 456, 457, 458, 460, 461, 467, 481
Sensory Perception 482
Sentinel node biopsy (SNB) 212, 219, 231
Sexual health 62, 74, 75
Sexual History 100
Skin disinfection practices 176
Skin pathology 192
Skull 240
Snellen Chart 273
Social determinants of health (SDOH) 86
Social History 100
Socioeconomic status 26, 53, 78, 81, 340, 404, 479
Soft Palate 306
Sound communication 38, 202, 512
Special tests 126, 128, 425
Speculative evidence 12
Spinal Alignment 445
Standard documentation protocols 130
Stethoscope 17, 25, 122, 123, 124, 135, 325, 327, 328, 391
Subcutaneous Tissue 205
Subjective Data 30
Subjective data collection 10, 11
Submandibular Gland 240
Submandibular Nodes 240
Submental Nodes 240
Subtle pathology 118
Summarization 65
Superficial Reflexes 482
Supraclavicular Nodes 240
Surgical intervention 258
Sweat Glands 205
Systemic disease 111, 178, 180, 192, 204, 211, 212, 215, 217, 219, 224, 237, 245, 254, 261, 296, 408, 494, 505
Systemic lupus erythematosus (SLE) 177, 178

T

Tactile Fremitus 342
Technical and Vocational Education Training (TVET) 110
Telehealth 22, 24, 25, 27, 92, 93, 94, 140, 150, 167, 172, 174, 267, 269, 270, 302, 334, 465
Telehealth systems 39, 165, 269
Telehealth technologies 22, 24
Temporal Artery 240
Temporomandibular joint (TMJ) dysfunction 223
Therapeutic Communication 65
Therapeutic nurse-patient relationship 1, 14, 504
Therapeutic Relationship 65
Thoracic Cage 342
Thoracic Cavity 316
Thoracic examination 326
Throat disorders 286, 289
Thyroid Gland 240
Tonsils 306
Training programs 49, 76
Traumatic brain injuries (TBIs) 453
Treatment regimes 38, 424
Trichotillomania 185
Turbinates 306
Turgor 205
Tympanic Membrane 306

U

Ultrasound 110, 346, 489
Urology 115
Uvula 306

V

Valvular heart disease 124
Vascular anatomy 113, 214
Ventilator-Associated Pneumonia (VAP) 325
Verbal Communication 65
Vesicular Sounds 342
Vestibular evoked myogenic potentials (VEMP) 283
Visual Acuity 273
Visual acuity testing 252, 253, 260
Visual assessment 111, 112, 134, 191, 192, 220, 280, 423
Visual examination 191, 193, 220
Visual inspection methods 191, 192, 499, 500
Visual observation 112
Vital sign assessment 18

Vital sign measurement 156
Vital Signs 30, 135, 141, 143, 152, 154, 156, 160, 161, 162, 164, 169

W

Weber Test 306
Wheezes 342
World Dental Federation 55